Practitioner's Guide to Psychoactive Drugs for Children and Adolescents

SECOND EDITION

Practitioner's Guide to Psychoactive Drugs for Children and Adolescents

SECOND EDITION

Edited by

John Scott Werry, M.D.

Emeritus Professor of Psychiatry
University of Auckland
Auckland, New Zealand

and

Michael G. Aman, Ph.D.

Professor of Psychology and Psychiatry
The Ohio State University
Columbus, Ohio

PLENUM MEDICAL BOOK COMPANY
New York and London

Library of Congress Cataloging-in-Publication Data

Practitioner's guide to psychoactive drugs for children and
  adolescents / edited by John Scott Werry and Michael G. Aman. -- 2nd
  ed.
      p.   cm.
  Includes bibliographical references and index.
  ISBN 0-306-45885-3
  1. Pediatric psychopharmacology--Handbooks, manuals, etc.
I. Werry, John S. II. Aman, Michael G.
  [DNLM: 1. Psychotropic Drugs--pharmacology handbooks.
2. Psychotropic Drugs--therapeutic use handbooks. 3. Mental
Disorders--in infancy & childhood handbooks. 4. Mental Disorders-
-in adolescence handbooks. 5. Monitoring, Physiologic handbooks.
QV 39P895 1998]
RJ504.7.P7 1998
618.92'8918--dc21
DNLM/DLC
for Library of Congress   98-29332
                                                               CIP

The information in this book is based on the experiences and research of the editors and authors. This material is for informational purposes only and should not be construed as prescribing information for individual patients. The editors, authors, and publisher assume no responsibility for any treatment undertaken by the practitioner with individual patients. Companies, interventions, and products are mentioned without bias to increase your knowledge only.

ISBN 0-306-45885-3

© 1999, 1993 Plenum Publishing Corporation
233 Spring Street, New York, N.Y. 10013

http://www.plenum.com

Plenum Medical Book Company is an imprint of Plenum Publishing Corporation

10 9 8 7 6 5 4 3 2 1

Printed in the United States of America

For Dianne and Marsha

Contributors

Michael G. Aman, Ph.D. Director of Research, The Nisonger Center for Mental Retardation and Developmental Disabilities, Ohio State University, Columbus, Ohio 43210-1296; Professor of Psychology and Psychiatry, Ohio State University, Columbus, Ohio 43210

L. Eugene Arnold, M.Ed., M.D. Professor Emeritus of Psychiatry, Ohio State University, Columbus, Ohio 43210; *mailing address*: 479 S. Galena Road, Sunbury, Ohio 43074

Russell A. Barkley, Ph.D. Professor of Psychiatry and Neurology, Department of Psychiatry, University of Massachusetts Medical School, Worcester, Massachusetts 01655

Kelly Botteron, M.D. Assistant Professor of Psychiatry (Child) and Radiology, Mallinckrodt Institute of Radiology, Washington University School of Medicine, St. Louis, Missouri 63110

Richard O. Carpenter, M.D. Private practice; *mailing address*: 5450 Errol Place, Atlanta, Georgia 30327

Daniel F. Connor, M.D. Associate Professor of Psychiatry, Department of Psychiatry, University of Massachusetts Medical School, Worcester, Massachusetts 01655

C. Keith Conners, Ph.D. Professor of Medical Psychology, Department of Psychiatry, Division of Medical Psychology, Duke University Medical Center, Durham, North Carolina 27710

Michael Dragunow, Ph.D. Department of Pharmacology and Clinical Pharmacology, School of Medicine, University of Auckland, Auckland, New Zealand

Kenneth S. Duckworth, M.D. Clinical Director, Massachusetts Mental Health Center, Boston, Massachusetts 02115; Instructor in Psychiatry, Harvard Medical School, Boston, Massachusetts 02115

George J. DuPaul, Ph.D. Professor of School Psychology, Department of School Psychology, Lehigh University, Bethlehem, Pennsylvania 18015

Andrea Eisner, M.D. Clinical Assistant Professor, Department of Psychiatry and Behavioral Sciences, University of Washington, Seattle, Washington 98195

Monique Ernst, M.D., Ph.D. Associate Director of the Brain Imaging Center, National Institute on Drug Abuse, National Institutes of Health, Baltimore, Maryland 21224

Kenneth D. Gadow, Ph.D. Professor of Psychiatry, Department of Psychiatry and Behavioral Science, State University of New York at Stony Brook, Stony Brook, New York 11794

Barbara Geller, M.D. Professor of Psychiatry, Department of Psychiatry, Washington University School of Medicine, St. Louis, Missouri 63110

Regina George, M.D. Brain Imaging Center, National Institute on Drug Abuse, National Institutes of Health, Baltimore, Maryland 21224

Nilda M. Gonzalez, M.D. Department of Psychiatry, Henry Ittleson Center, Bronx, New York 10471

Igor Janke, M.D. Assistant Professor of Psychiatry, Director of Research, Training, Chief Child Psychiatry Consultation Service, Department of Psychiatry, Ohio State University, Columbus, Ohio 43210

Richard P. Malone, M.D. Assistant Professor of Psychiatric and Director of Child and Adolescent Psychiatry Research, Department of Mental Health Sciences, Philadelphia, Pennsylvania 19102

Jon McClellan, M.D. Assistant Professor, Department of Psychiatry and Behavioral Sciences, University of Washington, Seattle, Washington 98195

Antony Milch, M.B.B.S., F.R.A.N.Z.C.P. Queenscliff Health Centre, Manly Hospital and Community Health Services, North Manly, New South Wales 2100, Australia

James William Paxton, Ph.D. Senior Lecturer, Department of Pharmacology and Clinical Pharmacology, School of Medicine, University of Auckland, Auckland, New Zealand

Deborah A. Pearson, Ph.D. Assistant Professor, Department of Psychiatry and Behavioral Sciences, University of Texas Medical School at Houston, Houston, Texas 77030

Amy B. Rowan, M.D. Director, Child and Adolescent Psychiatry, The Children's Hospital of Philadelphia, Philadelphia, Pennsylvania 19104

Raul R. Silva, M.D. Director, Child and Adolescent Psychiatry Department, St Lukes/ Roosevelt Hospital, New York, New York 10025

Ronald Shouten, M.D., J.D. Director, Law and Psychiatry Service, Massachusetts General Hospital, Boston, Massachusetts 02114; Assistant Professor of Psychiatry, Harvard Medical School, Boston, Massachusetts 02115

Elizabeth P. Sparrow, M.A. Ph.D. candidate in Clinical Neuropsychology, Department of Psychiatry, Washington University, St. Louis, Missouri 63130

John O. Viesselman, M.D. Children's Services, Ventura County Behavioral Health, and private practice, Ventura, California 93003; Consulting Child Psychiatrist, Casa Pacifica Residential Facility and Shelter Care, Camarillo, California 93012

Eileen P. G. Vining, M.D. Associate Professor, Departments of Neurology and Pediatrics, Johns Hopkins University School of Medicine, Baltimore, Maryland 21287

Brent Waters, M.D., F.R.C.P., F.R.A.N.Z.C.P. Consultant Child Psychiatrist, Edgecliff Centre, Edgecliff, New South Wales 2027, Australia

John Scott Werry, M.D.   Emeritus Professor of Psychiatry, University of Auckland, Auckland, New Zealand; *mailing address*: 19 Edenvale Crescent, Mount Eden, Auckland 3, New Zealand

Emily M. Yamada, M.S.   Department of Psychology, University of Washington, Seattle, Washington 98195

Alan J. Zametkin, M.D.   Office of the Clinical Director, National Institute of Mental Health, Bethesda, Maryland 20892

Preface to the First Edition

Psychoactive drugs are those used to modify emotions and behavior and to treat psychiatric illnesses. Technical information about these drugs is contained in the field of psychopharmacology, which began in the 1930s with the introduction of the modern barbiturates, the psychostimulants, and the antihistamines. However, it was not until 1950 and the introduction of chlorpromazine (Largactil®, Thorazine®), the first of the many antipsychotic (neuroleptic or "major tranquilizer") drugs, that it developed as a major part of the medical specialty of psychiatry. With the introduction of antidepressants, lithium, and the benzodiazepines or "minor tranquilizers"—all before 1965—the use of psychoactive drugs soon spread to embrace the treatment of less severe illnesses. Interestingly, while psychopharmacological knowledge has advanced considerably, there have been no major new psychoactive drug groups discovered since. Together with psychosocial programs, the antipsychotics helped revolutionize the care of the severely mentally ill and shifted the emphasis from custodial institutional care to community habilitation. Today, the use of such drugs is widespread and, as always in the history of medicine, there has been overuse and abuse of these very valuable treatments that has led to both legitimate and misinformed public concern.

Though pediatric psychopharmacology actually began in Providence, Rhode Island, in 1937 with the introduction of psychostimulants, the use of drugs in children and adolescents has been much slower to get started, partly because the severe psychiatric illnesses are infrequent until later adolescence, partly because of a reluctance to resort to such treatment in the immature, and partly because of the laudable, but false belief that all emotional and behavioral problems in children should be resolvable by psychological and social means. Nevertheless, there has been a substantial amount of systematic study of psychoactive drugs in children and adolescents, though clinical usage has lagged far behind. However, fifty or more years on from the birth of psychopharmacology, the use of these drugs in children is now widespread, as witnessed in 1990 by the launching of a scientific journal (*Journal of Child and Adolescent Psychopharmacology*) devoted to that topic. As in adults, there has been intermittent reasonable and prejudicial public concern about the use of these drugs in young persons.

There is now a need for a ready reference text that summarizes our knowledge about psychoactive drugs for children and adolescents for all those who seek information. This book aims to do this for practitioners, professionals in health, welfare, and education, and interested laypersons, including parents. This is no easy task, since the levels of technical knowledge vary from that of the special education teacher seeking information about the drugs that many such pupils will be receiving, to that of the modern young child and adolescent psychiatrist whose grasp of the difficult fields of pharmacokinetics (how drugs are absorbed, distributed, and eliminated) and neurotransmitter physiology (via which most psychoactive drugs work) is daunting to the editors, who grew up in the bucolic clinical–empirical era. Inevitably there are sections of the book that will prove too technical for any except the medically qualified, but considerable effort has been applied to make much of the text, especially that discussing the clinical uses and side effects of the drugs, comprehensible to anyone used to getting information by reading. We also take comfort in the fact that many of the major contributions in pediatric psychopharmacology have been made by nonmedical professionals, notably psychologists, suggesting that an audience beyond the medically qualified is practicable.

One other problem confronted us—whether to organize the book by psychopathological symptoms (e.g., hyperactivity) and disorders (e.g., autism) or by drugs. Since the limited number of psychoactive drugs available are used across a wide variety of disorders and symptoms in children and adolescents, and since there are a number of good texts available operating from the basis of psychiatric disorders, it was decided that this book should be about the psychoactive drugs, that is, **essentially a pediatric psychopharmacology text, not a textbook of child and adolescent psychiatry**. Further, none of the latter provides the detailed information about psychoactive drugs that most practitioners now need. However, when the starting point is a disorder rather than a drug, Chapter 7 ("Disorders, Symptoms, and Their Pharmacotherapy") will identify what drugs are indicated. Then it will be necessary to go to the chapter(s) detailing those drugs.

One last point: Chapter 12, on antiepileptic (anticonvulsant) drugs, may seem out of place in a psychopharmacological text. The reason for its inclusion is not to teach nonspecialists how to treat the epilepsies; rather, when these disorders are associated with psychopathological problems, mental health professionals often are consulted and (along with special educators) need to be knowledgeable about these drugs, which have important incidental influences on behavior and learning. Many also have important emerging direct psychoactive uses in addition to those in epilepsy.

As with most things in life, this book evidences compromises—in this case eschewing detailed scholarly discussion of the evidence in print, in favor of the author's statement of critical appraisal of that evidence. We hope that this volume will serve the practical needs of professionals and consumers who require ready information about psychoactive drugs, at the same time signposting the important scholarly work in this area.

John S. Werry
Michael G. Aman

Auckland, New Zealand and Columbus, Ohio

Preface to the Second Edition

The *Practitioner's Guide to Psychoactive Drugs for Children and Adolescents* is intended for an array of professionals and advanced students in health and education, including practitioners, academics, and students in child psychiatry, pediatrics, neurology, psychology, nursing, social work, and special education. However, the book is also for consumers, especially parents and caregivers. As in the first edition, we have striven to make the *Practitioner's Guide* intelligible to as large an audience as possible without sacrificing accuracy and precision. Most sections (e.g., clinical indications, side effects) will be readily understood by a wide audience, whereas some sections that are intrinsically technical (e.g., neurochemistry, mechanisms of action) will inevitably be comprehensible only to a smaller group, such as those with knowledge of chemistry and physiology. As in the first edition, this book is primarily organized around drug groups rather than psychiatric disorders. This arrangement is much more efficient for readers wanting information about *drugs*. For those seeking basic information on the clinical or diagnostic indications for psychoactive agents in children, there is Chapter 7, "Disorders, Symptoms, and Their Pharmacotherapy."   In keeping with the practical orientation of this book, we have avoided exhaustive discussions of the research literature. Authors were asked to make *conclusions* for clinical usage based on their extensive knowledge of the relevant research. The hard evidence for these conclusions is supported by extensive referencing to what has become a vast literature.

A major reason for the second edition is that several new drugs with novel features have been added to the choices open to practitioners. First, the availability of the specific serotonin reuptake inhibitors (SSRIs) (fluoxetine, sertraline, paroxetine, and fluvoxamine), barely mentioned in the first edition, has had a profound impact on all of psychiatry, including child psychiatry. Other innovations include naturally occurring substances like melatonin and hypericum (the active ingredient in St. John's wort). Second, there have been major strides in developing antipsychotics with promising new neurochemical profiles, such as clozapine, risperidone, olanzapine, remoxipride, and so forth. Third, recently there has been a proliferation of new antiepileptic drugs, including gabapentin, lamotrigine, tiagabine, topiramate, and vigabatrin. Some of the antiepileptic drugs (valproic acid, carbamazepine) have established psychiatric applications, and others (e.g., lamotrigine) may eventually be found to do so as well. In addition to these high-profile developments, there have been other new medications more closely related to their ancestors, such as Adderal® (an amphetamine preparation), and the empirical literature on some of the older drugs continues to grow.

Other major events have also prompted this newer edition. The transition from the third revised edition (DSM-III-R) to the fourth edition of the *Diagnostic and Statistical*

Manual of Mental Disorders (DSM-IV) has resulted in changes in diagnostic terminology and in the composition of some disorders. There have been major changes in the many instruments available for assessing medication effects. For example, the Conners scales—widely used in assessing attention-deficit hyperactivity disorder (ADHD)—have been revamped, and an empirically derived instrument (the New York Teacher Rating Scale) is available for assessing hostile and disruptive behaviors associated with conduct disorder. Newly developed and/or refined instruments are now available for assessing a wide range of other disorders as well. Finally, some readers of the first edition suggested that information on drug combinations and on the management of overdoses would be helpful. Therefore, all of the drug chapters have been expanded to include this information also.

These days, many parents and professionals get much of their information by searching the Internet. Much of this information is impressionistic and unresearched. We believe that, in keeping with rapid progress in the field of pediatric psychopharmacology, the second edition is a significant advance over the first edition of *Practitioner's Guide to Psychoactive Drugs for Children and Adolescents*. In blending optimism with caution to offer a truly informed summary, we hope that readers will find the *Practitioner's Guide* to be user-friendly, authoritative, practical, and safe.

ACKNOWLEDGEMENTS. The editors thank Marsha Aman for extensive logistical help in preparing manuscripts for this volume.

John Scott Werry

Auckland, New Zealand

Michael G. Aman

Columbus, Ohio

Contents

4. Monitoring and Measuring Drug Effects. I. Physical Effects **69**

Alan J. Zametkin, M.D., and Emily M. Yamada, M.S.

II Specific Drugs

Russell A. Barkley, Ph.D., George J. DuPaul, Ph.D.,
and Daniel F. Connor, M.D.

12. Antiepileptics (Anticonvulsants) 355

Eileen P. G. Vining, M.D., Richard O. Carpenter, M.D.,
and Michael G. Aman, Ph.D.

13. Psychoactive Effects of Medical Drugs   387

*L. Eugene Arnold, M.Ed., M.D., Igor Janke, M.D.,
Brent Waters, M.D., F.R.C.P., F.R.A.N.Z.C.P.,
and Antony Milch, M.B.B.S., F.R.A.N.Z.C.P.*

14. Nootropics and Foods   413

C. Keith Conners, Ph.D., and Elizabeth P. Sparrow, M.A.

I

General Principles

1

Introduction: A Guide for Practitioners, Professionals, and Public

JOHN SCOTT WERRY, M.D.

I. INTRODUCTION

A. Preamble

This chapter, more than any other, is written for nonmedical professionals and parents to introduce them to what may at first seem a dauntingly arcane field and to empower them to seek good information. It sets the scene for all the other chapters by introducing some basic terminology and concepts, most of which are familiar to prescribers. However, hopefully even they will benefit from a quick overview and reminder of things they know.

B. Definitions

This book is about the use of chemical substances for the modification of emotional, intellectual, or behavioral function of children and adolescents, that is, the medical discipline called pediatric psychopharmacology. The substances used for this purpose are known as psychoactive, psychotropic, or psychiatric drugs.

Unfortunately, drug has different meanings; strictly, it means any substance produced primarily for medical reasons, but it is now popularly used for any mind-affecting substance and subdivided into legal or illegal. To get away from this confusion, psychiatry is promoting the use of the term substance to designate drugs that are used illegally, coverage of which can be found in Chapter 11.

Child and the medical equivalent *pediatric* will be used in this book to include adolescents or teenagers whom society considers still dependent on and responsible to parents or guardians. While there are separate subspecialties of medicine concerned with adolescence, these have not yet become widespread. Instead, there is increasing acceptance

JOHN SCOTT WERRY, M.D. • 19 Edenvale Crescent, Mt. Eden, Auckland 3, New Zealand.

Practitioner's Guide to Psychoactive Drugs for Children and Adolescents (Second Edition), Werry and Aman, eds. Plenum Publishing Corporation, New York, 1999.

that the traditional child-oriented medical specialties should also be responsible for the care of adolescents. The most concrete example of this can be seen in the American Academy of Child Psychiatry's changing its name (and that of its prestigious journal) to include "Adolescent."

C. The Multidisciplinary Team

The medical specialty that deals with emotional or behavior disorders is called psychiatry; but child and adolescent psychiatry is typically carried out by a multidisciplinary team containing psychiatrists, psychologists, social workers, occupational therapists, nurses, speech and language therapists, special educators, and so on. Only the psychiatrists in this team are medically qualified (physicians) and can prescribe drugs. Unlike others in the team, psychologists, social workers, and speech and language therapists are usually trained in universities away from medical and health science campuses. Further, most such professionals do not work in the medical area, but those who do, usually have some extra training in medical settings. The presence of these basically nonmedical professions in the team is a recognition of the large psychosocial component of child and adolescent mental health. But, in addition to their own health professionals, child psychiatric teams usually also have strong working relationships with other child health professionals in pediatrics and neurology, a recognition of the other firm base of the team. The multidisciplinary team is likewise increasingly becoming a feature of all pediatric medical subspecialities, not just psychiatry. Sorting out who each member of the team is, and who does what, can be very confusing for parents, teachers, and others, and they should have no hesitation in seeking clarification.

D. Child Psychiatry, Behavioral Pediatrics, and Pediatric Neurology

In recent years, with the increase in the number of pediatricians and the decline in the prevalence of many childhood diseases, there has developed a medical subspecialty of behavioral pediatrics, which may cause confusion with child psychiatry. No hard-and-fast lines can be drawn between the domains of child psychiatry, behavioral pediatrics, and pediatric neurology since all three medical subspecialties have certain elements of training and practice in common. However, pediatricians spend most of their residency training with children, while child psychiatrists must first train in adult psychiatry. Thus, it would be expected that pediatricians would be better trained in childhood physical diseases, in pediatric pharmacology, and in normal childhood, while child psychiatrists would be more knowledgeable about the full range of disorders of emotion and behavior and about psychopharmacology and have more training in extended listening to people. Pediatric neurologists are more familiar with brain diseases like epilepsy or cerebral palsy but generally do not have much experience in psychiatry. With one or two exceptions (notably attention-deficit and tic disorders; see Chapter 7), adult-type psychiatric disorders occurring in childhood now constitute the main indications for the use of psychotropic drugs in children, and this trend toward a disorder-focused approach is increasing markedly. Further, most of the psychoactive drugs used in children were developed originally for use in adults; so that, at the moment, through their training in adult psychiatry, (modern) child psychiatrists are somewhat better positioned for considering the full range of possible psychiatric disorders (differential diagnosis) and for administering psychotropic drugs in children, especially in serious or complicated cases. However, credentials alone do not make a good physician (see below).

II. HISTORICAL OVERVIEW

A. Foundations

The use of drugs to control children's behavior is not new. In the past, English nannies used brandy to soothe fretful infants, and proprietary "teething powders" were administered by parents, sometimes with disastrous results like "pink disease" due to mercury poisoning. There was also a range of sedating drugs like the barbiturates, paraldehyde, and opiates, which were undoubtedly used widely. However, modern pediatric psychopharmacology probably is best dated as beginning with the publication of "The behavior of children receiving Benzedrine" in 1937 by Charles Bradley[1] at the Emma Pendleton Bradley Hospital in Rhode Island. At that time, Benzedrine® (amphetamine) had only just been synthesized and was a drug of great popularity and interest in medicine. Until very recently, Bradley's observation that stimulants settled overactive and behaviorally disturbed children was (with the possible exception of the use of antihistamines by Lauretta Bender at Bellevue Hospital; see Conners[2]) the only major contribution to pediatric psychopharmacology from child psychiatry, as opposed to hand-me-downs from adult psychiatry.

Bradley's work was soon lost owing to a shift during and after World War II away from medical aspects of child psychiatry because of the growing influence of psychoanalysis, which seemed to offer greater hope than the medical science of that time for understanding and treating emotional and psychiatric problems.

In the early 1950s, in the search for better anesthetic drugs, the first of the modern psychiatric drugs, chlorpromazine, was discovered quite serendipitously to be effective against schizophrenia. This heralded a whole new era that has given us most of the modern psychoactive drugs and most of our understanding of their action and use as well as pointers as to what might be the causes of psychiatric disorders.

Child psychiatry had independent beginnings in two main streams, community and pediatric. The community stream began in the Chicago and Boston juvenile courts with William Healy and led in the 1920s to the development of child guidance/mental hygiene clinics. The medical stream started in pediatric hospitals in Berlin with Professor Tramer and in Baltimore with his enormously influential pupil, Dr. Leo Kanner (who discovered infantile autism). After World War II, the influence of community child guidance clinics declined somewhat, certainly as intellectual and political driving forces, as did the influence of pediatrics when child psychiatry became a subspecialty of psychiatry.

From then on, the main influences on pediatric psychopharmacology derived from adult developments—with a lag phase of several years. Most of the adult drugs were tried in children in what were mostly very crude studies but which seemed good enough to show that most children did not respond. The rise of psychopharmacology seems to have set the scene and the search for better drugs led to the reemergence of Bradley's work with amphetamine in the late 1960s. (For a good historical review, see Conners.[2])

Until the late 1970s, child psychiatry was still preoccupied with psychoanalytic theory though its star was already beginning to wane in adult psychiatry. As a result, pediatric applications of psychopharmacology were slow getting started. Pediatric psychopharmacology was greatly influenced by some psychologists [such as C. K. Conners, Virginia Douglas, Rachel (Gittleman) Klein, and R. L. Sprague] with understandably better training in research methods than some child psychiatrists who, realizing this lack, had turned to them for help. This prominence of psychologists not only persists today but has had some important consequences that have differentiated pediatric and adult psychopharmacology. The first is earlier use of better experimental designs for clinical trials and complex statistical analyses, notably multivariate methods like factor analysis, which have both clinical and research applicability (see Sprague and Werry[3]). The second is greater emphasis on formal, structured (including laboratory) measures of drug effects and, most important and unique, the early and general acceptance of the need to look at effects on learning and academic performance. The third is that, in the reverse of the situation in the adult area, there has been strength in psychosocial and some weakness in biological measures.

The history of pediatric psychopharmacology is not without its ups and downs. When hyperactivity [also known as minimal brain dysfunction, and now, attention-deficit hyperactivity disorder (ADHD)] finally caught on in the mid-1960s, it almost completely overrode interest in any other disorder (or any drugs other than the stimulants) until the 1980s. Only a very few like Bender, Fish, and Campbell at New York's Bellevue Hospital focused on other disorders and other drugs. The advent of the American Psychiatric Association's classification system for psychiatric disorders, DSM-III[4] *(Diagnostic and Statistical Manual of Mental Disorders, 3rd ed.)*, now updated in 1994 as DSM-IV,[5] has helped refocus research in child and adolescent psychopharmacology on the whole range of psychiatric disorders rather than just ADHD, which almost totally preoccupied it in from the sixties to the mid-eighties. It has also remedicalized psychiatry in general, though the creation of DSM-III was itself a sign of this change. This remedicalization has helped increase interest in pediatric psychopharmacology, which has mushroomed in the last decade.

Nevertheless, the former near-exclusive preoccupation in child psychiatry with ADHD and with one drug, methylphenidate, had one beneficial effect—it produced most of the methodology for evaluating drugs in children, providing a ready-made matrix (or at least a model) for subsequent study of any disorder and any drug.

One other important influence on pediatric psychopharmacology is also worth noting and that is the field of mental retardation, now called developmental disabilities. Apart from those whose disability is so severe that they are bedridden and require constant nursing care, most of those in developmental centers, special hospitals, and other institutions for the mentally retarded are there because of associated behavior problems that made their maintenance in the community difficult. This led to the widespread use of major tranquilizers (neuroleptics) for their behavioral control as detailed in Chapter 3. Thus, until the 1980s, though biological child psychiatry interested itself primarily in ADHD, those working in mental retardation (mostly psychologists again) contributed much of the work on the pharmacotherapy of aggressive, self-injurious, and stereotyped behavior (see Ref. 6 and Chapter 10).

In concluding, it is worth noting one other historical phenomenon. Most of the types of major psychotropic drugs in current use were discovered before 1965, and, with few exceptions, the discoveries were serendipitous.[7] We might thus call the first epoch "pharmacological fiddling."

B. Current Trends and Future Directions

Since the mid-1980s, pediatric psychopharmacology has become increasingly popular, respectable, and scientific, highlighted by the launching in 1990 of a specialist publication, the *Journal of Child and Adolescent Psychopharmacology*. At the same time, there has been an increase in the number and, to a lesser degree, in the quality of articles in other child psychiatric journals (though mostly confined to North American publications).

Medical science, especially neuroscience, is overtaking the psychosocial sciences, which dominated psychiatry for so long. This is partly due to scientific developments such as the increasing knowledge of genetics and molecular biology, of brain function, and of methods of studying the brain such as magnetic resonance and positron-emission organ imaging (see Chapter 4) and the availability of biochemical analyses using receptor physiology. But also, though all the initial major psychotropic agents were discovered by accident, 30 years' study of their action has led to shifts from empiricism to theory. We now have good ideas of how drugs work and thus of what the underlying pathological mechanisms might be. Not only does this make psychopharmacology more focused and exact, but it portends an era in which drugs are being developed with specific cellular actions on the brain in mind. While there has yet to be any real innovation as a result of this shift, there is good reason to hope that in the 21st century psychopharmacology will be as revolutionized as was medicine by the rise of bacteriology and cellular pathology in the 19th. With one or two exceptions like ADHD, much of the drug use in children had been symptomatic. DSM-III has caused a burgeoning interest in psychiatric disorders (or diseases), as any perusal of a leading journal in child psychiatry (*Journal of the American Academy of Child and Adolescent Psychiatry*) makes clear. A shift toward disorder- or diagnosis-dictated pharmacotherapy is both inevitable and well under way as current interest in childhood depression, manic, panic, tic, obsessive–compulsive, and psychotic disorders illustrates (see Chapter 7). It will be unfortunate if behavioral pediatrics does not show similar shifts, which will require much more training in psychiatry and less in pediatrics.

In normal clinical practice, medication is only one part of a multimodal treatment program. Child psychopharmacology has shown more interest than adult psychiatry in interaction between psychosocial treatments like behavioral and educational therapies and medication, but the volume of research has still been far too low. There is also a need for more emphasis on what is one of the main features of child and adolescent psychiatry, the multimodal, multifocus, multidisciplinary approach that starts from the premise of a psychobiosocial organism called a child set in a social matrix called family, school, and peer group. Any approach that looks only at one aspect is bound to be limited. Another important and very neglected area is that of development, which implies the concepts of change and of differentiation of functions. One may criticize psychoanalysis for many things but not for its emphasis on this dimension. Apart from interest in learning, and then only mostly short-term learning, there has been little study of the impact of pharmacotherapy on biological, psychological, or social development. Yet there are some important indicators of the need to look at drugs and development. Schizophrenia, antidepressant-responsive major depression, mania, and suicide are not common until adolescence, but their effect on development can be devastating, and schizophrenia particularly is thought in some cases to be a developmental disorder beginning at birth.[8] And their treatment is primarily psychopharmacological. Family and peer relationships are critical in socialization, yet there have been few studies of psychopharmacological effects on these processes (see Chapter 8). But the biggest shortfall has been in longitudinal studies where children have been kept on drugs for good reason for some years. Understandably, these studies are difficult to prosecute because of the time span and of subject (and investigator) attrition, but they can[9] and should be done.

III. CLASSIFICATION OF PSYCHOACTIVE DRUGS

There are various ways of classifying psychoactive drugs: (1) by the chemical grouping of the drug (e.g., barbiturates), (2) by the action of the drug (e.g., stimulants, dopamine blockers), or (3) by the therapeutic use (e.g., antidepressant, antipsychotic, antianxiety, anticonvulsant).

On the whole, medicine is increasingly favoring the third method for main classifications and the second and then the first for subclassifications, as can be seen in Table 1 and elsewhere in this book. [The persistence of "neuroleptic" (i.e., classified by action) for "antipsychotic" in North America is an exception.] Nevertheless, designation by therapeutic indication can create problems, since drugs may have more than one therapeutic use, and this has been particularly true of pediatric psychopharmacology, where the drugs have come through adult psychiatry but are often put to rather different uses in children. A good example is the use of antidepressant drugs for ADHD or the use of antipsychotic drugs for aggressive behavior in children who are developmentally disabled.

Understandably, drugs also acquire popular classifications such as "tranquilizer," "speed," and "crack," especially when they are used illegally. The term tranquilizer has been an albatross around the neck of psychopharmacology that persists despite efforts for 30 years to get rid of it.[10] It was introduced originally to describe the new form of sedation (calming without sleep) produced by the antipsychotics. In a most unfortunate manner, the term was used by the drug companies to introduce benzodiazepines like diazepam (Valium®) in the mid-1960s to emphasize that these drugs were different from the older central nervous system depressants used as sedatives or sleeping pills. In fact, this difference has proven to be more apparent than real. In the majority of cases, the antipsychotics are not used to tranquilize but for the treatment of psychosis, and the continued use of the term tranquilizer is both stigmatizing to persons who take them for this purpose and grossly deceptive when applied to modern antianxiety drugs like the benzodiazepines. The attempt to distinguish the latter from the former by introducing qualifying adjectives (i.e., minor versus major tranquilizers) is not helpful, and the terms are better avoided altogether.

A. Names of Drugs

By now, most will know that drugs have a trade, proprietary, or brand name that is carefully chosen to be euphonious and catchy and often to emphasize the drug's main function, e.g., Serenace® for a major "tranquilizer" or Oblivon® for a sleeping pill. Trade names like Tegretol® that come from foreign languages may lose this therapeutic suggestiveness. Trade names are always written with an initial uppercase letter and often carry the superscript ® for registered trade name.

There is also a generic name, which is always lowercase and derived from the chemical structure of the drug. As a result, generic names are often difficult to pronounce—e.g., carbamazepine (Tegretol®)—and this is exploited to commercial advantage in the careful development of trade names. Thus, on the whole, physicians tend to use trade names

TABLE 1. Types of Psychoactive Drugs[a,b]

Antidepressants
- Heterocyclics
    Tricyclics (imipramine, amitriptyline, clomipramine, desipramine, protriptyline, doxepin, trimipramine)
    Dibenzoxazepines (amoxapine)
    Quadricyclics (maprotiline)
    Phenylpiperazines (trazodone, nefazadone)
  Selective serotonin reuptake inhibitors (SSRIs) (fluoxetine, fluvoxamine, paroxetine, sertraline)
    Other (non-MAOI) (buproprion, nomifensine, venlafaxine)
- Monoamine oxidase inhibitors (MAOIs)
    General MAO inhibitors (isocarboxazid, phenelzine, tranylcypromine)
    Selective (MAO-A) inhibitors (moclobemide)
Antipsychotics (neuroleptics, major tranquilizers)
- Phenothiazines (all end in -azine, e.g., chlorpromazine, thioridazine, trifluoperazine, fluphenazine, perphenazine, prochlorperazine)
- Benzamides (remoxipride)
- Butyrophenones and diphenylbutylpiperidines (haloperidol, droperidol, pimozide)
- Dibenzoxazepines (loxapine)
- Dihydroindolones (molindone)
- Thioxanthenes (chlorprothixene, flupenthixol, thiothixene)
    Atypical (clozapine, olanzapine, quetiapine, risperidone, sertindole, ziprasidone)
Antimanics
- Lithium carbonate
- Carbamazepine
- Valproate
Anxiolytics (antianxiety) and sedatives
- General brain depressants (alcohol, barbiturates, meprobamate, chloral, paraldehyde, solvents, older anticonvulsants)
- Selective brain depressants Benzodiazepines and related compounds (chlordiazepoxide, diazepam, lorazepam, oxazepam, nitrazepam, flunitrazepam, temazepam, triazolam, clonazepam, zopiclone)
- Antihistamines and anticholinergics (diphenhydramine, promethazine)
- Serotonin antagonists (buspirone)
- Opiates and narcotics (these have additional, analgesic properties) *— retalin*
Stimulants
    Sympathomimetic and allied drugs (dextroamphetamine, methylphenidate, pemoline, cocaine)
Cannabis and hallucinogens
    Cannabis
    Hallucinogens (LSD, mescaline, PCP)
Miscellaneous drugs (psychoactive use)
    Adrenergic blockers (clonidine, guanfacine, propanolol) *— antihypertension*
    Anticonvulsants (phenytoin, carbamazepine, valproate)
    Calcium-channel blockers (verapamil, nifedipine)
    Fenfluramine
    Opiate antagonists (naloxone, naltrexone)
    Dietary substances (choline, glutamic acid, piracetam, vitamins, minerals, tyrosine, tryptophan)

[a]Note: Inclusion of a drug on this list does not mean that its efficacy and safety have been established (see individual chapters for this information).
[b]This list is not complete, and new drugs are being introduced each year. Not all these drugs are available in all countries.

despite the fact that only generic names appear in good journals or books that discuss, review, or research the properties of drugs. While such an impression is not entirely accurate, the use of trade names does suggest that information is coming to that physician by way of drug company publicity rather than from the more objective medical journals and should be a cause for concern.

B. Look-Alike Drugs

Once a successful new drug has been introduced, not surprisingly, other companies seek to find a competitive product. Apart from some borrowings from other areas of medicine (e.g., the antihypertensive clonidine discussed in Chapter 15), there have been no major new classes of psychiatric drugs over the original four groups (antipsychotics, antidepressants, antimanics, and selective anxiolytics) introduced by the mid-1960s.[7] While these major classes have produced enormous benefit, none of them can be described as truly curative (like penicillin or antibacterials), with the power to dispose of the underlying disorder swiftly and effectively. Even the most successful, such as the antidepressants, the stimulants, lithium, and the newer antipsychotics, require to be continued over the natural course of the disorder, and the disorder usually continues to be detectable to the patient or relatives through minor symptomatology or dysfunction.

Over 100 different psychotropic drugs have appeared since the introduction of the prototypic drugs of these four classes. Some are new subtypes that offer real advances over the prototypic drugs in their main class [e.g., newer antipsychotics and the selective serotonin reuptake ingibitors (SSRIs) antidepressants]. Some also offer prospects for enhancing research because of their somewhat different pharmacological profile. However, many of these new drugs are merely look-alike variations within a major therapeutic class or newer subclass as pharmaceutical companies seek to keep up with their competitors. Improvement in drug licensing regulations in most countries now requires that a new drug have distinctive, valuable differences from already licensed ones. Sometimes these differences stem from pharmacokinetics (longer or shorter duration) and side-effect spectrum rather than therapeutic efficacy. While such differences may be valuable, they are of limited value therapeutically, especially in treating those who have failed to respond to prototypic drugs.

What psychopharmacology needs to move ahead in a substantial way is the development of therapeutically novel major classes of drugs similar to the introduction of the four classes of drugs 30–40 years ago. Particularly needed are psychoactive drugs which are truly curative and have highly specific actions (i.e., relatively free from side effects).

IV. DRUG EVALUATION

Before the advent of modern, scientific medicine, the worth of drugs and other therapeutic procedures was spread by word of mouth and by armchair treatises such as those by Aristotle or Galen. The most important factor was the reputation and influence of the promulgator. Beginning largely in the mid-19th century, paralleling previous developments in the physical sciences, there was a shift away from assertion to observation, hypothesis induction, and then hypothesis testing. This gradually gave us the modern way in which drugs are evaluated. Chapter 2 describes this process in detail, as do reviews.[3,6] The basis of the testing in human patients is called a clinical trial, and there are well-developed rules by which the safety and efficacy of a drug are established. Drug licensing agencies like the Food and Drug Administration (FDA) in the United States now require that new products be tested by these strict methods.

It might be believed that the old methods of assertion and charisma have disappeared, but this is wrong. The supremacy of the human species over others is based on adaptability, and this in turn is based on observation, hypothesis induction, and crude personal confirmation of the hypothesis. In the clinical situation, this means that the physician unwittingly or gradually begins to try out the drug in slightly different ways than originally indicated or notices effects on other symptoms, etc. This leads to informal "experimentation" and the drawing of conclusions. This phenomenon is called clinical experience. This is excellent for generating hypotheses; an example of this is the discovery of AIDS by a skillful clinician noting an unusual but consistent pattern of symptoms/disease in several patients. However, the confirmation of AIDS required the full panoply of modern laboratory immunology, quite beyond the scope of clinical observation. The scientific method was developed primarily as a device to prevent the fallacies that arise from human observation and conclusion. The clinician rarely goes about testing the hypothesis in the systematic way that is needed to eliminate error, and so the conclusions reached are likely to be in serious error. Obviously, sometimes the clinician is correct—in fact, the introduction of antipsychotics and antidepressants was based on shrewd clinical observation—but most of the easy, obvious hypotheses have now been made and tested by the legions of ambitious and skillful researchers so that for the clinician the possibility of error is far greater than that of success.

It is useful in thinking about clinical experience as a way of evaluating treatment in medicine to remember the use of bleeding and purging or the galenicals (or herbal medicines) that dominated medicine for centuries. Their use may now seem incomprehensible, but not if one recognizes that it was driven by the desire to help based on "clinical experience."

From a practical point of view, then, it is important that practitioners and consumers learn to distrust uses of psychotropic drugs that are based on clinical experience and that differ from those set out in competent reviews of the scientific literature. On the whole, the scientific findings tend to be more limited and conservative in scope and size. Enthusiasm for a drug and positivity about its value should immediately cause suspicion and invoke a request for the basis (preferably with references) upon which such judgments were made. There is an unfortunate misconception in the public and the media that qualified answers are a sign of weakness in physicians—quite the opposite is true. In nature, things are rarely so clear or scientific knowledge so advanced that we can put aside all doubt.

V. DETERMINANTS OF PRESCRIBING

The act of prescribing a drug is a complex human transaction set in a social field at a particular historical time and subject to a variety of unseen influences. If one believes that Homo sapiens is at least in part a rational being, knowledge of these factors may lead to better prescribing by practitioners and more informed participation by consumers in the process.

A. Medical Knowledge

It should be clear that the use of drugs is dictated by knowledge about the disorder/symptom or behavior involved and the available treatments. Unfortunately, medical knowledge about children's behavioral and emotional disorders is quite limited, and what is known is largely atheoretical or empirical, though this is changing with the growth of the neurosciences. Thus, most of what we know in pediatric psychopharmacology is rather like twiddling the knobs on a television set in the absence of any real understanding of radio-physics. What this means in practice is that within broad diagnostic guidelines such as ADHD or tic disorder suggesting that some such children may respond to medication, there is only one way to find out whether or not pharmacotherapy has a useful role for any particular child and that is to try it. This may seem rather crude, but it is a truthful reflection of the state of medical knowledge. However, it does require that the prescriber set up proper ways of evaluating the effect of medication, which ordinarily should include both parent and school observations.

It is worth noting one other important medical knowledge factor—it dictates the way that physicians view phenomena. Before the advent of DSM-III,[4] psychiatrists tended to view abnormal behavior within a psychodynamic or psychological process framework. DSM-III produced a marked shift toward disorder or disease focus. This in itself is likely to increase a set toward a drug-based treatment program. One would like to think that such shifts in medical thinking were dictated by accumulating knowledge, but DSM-III had large ideological as well as knowledge-based reasons for its development. In a sense, it was a statement of prospect for psychiatry based firmly within medical science which was only partly justifiable by actual developments in knowledge in areas such as neurobiochemistry and psychopharmacology. As a result, DSM-III and its successors, in a manner reminiscent of French psychiatry in the 19th century, overreached itself in an attempt to classify most aberrant human behavior and contains a number of categories which are almost certainly invalid. Fortunately, there is some developing resistance, seen by the failure to include in DSM-IV some popular (with media and lawyers) so-called "mental diseases" like Munchausen by proxy, battered wife, and false memory syndromes which are better subsumed either under existing broader categories or as social or psychological phenomena.

B. Patient and Parent Factors

Among patient and parent factors, the most obvious factor is the disorder or symptom or behavior that the child has, but there are a number of other factors in this category. Consumers come to the physician with a set of expectations and attitudes. Mostly, these are that the doctor will diagnose the problem, identify its cause, indicate the likely outcome, and institute treatment. While there is much wild assertion but little firm data on this, there seems little doubt that parents may both expect and, more often now in this "green" and bucolic era, resist physicians' suggestions for drug treatment. Parent knowledge and attitudes are shaped by a multiplicity of factors, not too many of which are based on accurate medical knowledge.

One important parent factor may be to see the cause of the child's problem as within the child. Medication may then be seen as confirming that the child is "sick" rather than "sinful." Society and parents themselves generally believe that children's problems stem from the family so that the prescription of medication may be an eagerly sought talisman of innocence before an accusing world.

C. Physician Factors

Factors such as the physician's competence and familiarity with the most recent developments are fairly apparent. What is not, though, are subtle, powerful, and often unconscious processes that the prescriber brings, namely, human fallibility, and personal needs such as to be helpful, to project an image of confidence, to dominate, or to make a living in a field that is becoming increasingly competitive. The main implication for both prescribers and consumers is to recognize that the motivation for prescribing is only partly influenced by objective medical knowledge and to look for and discuss the less obvious factors frankly before a decision is made. When in doubt, consumers should always ask for a second opinion, which is their right, well recognized in medicine though sometimes resisted.

D. Social Factors

Both physician and consumer operate in a complex social environment. The parents may be under pressure from the school to do something about their child's disruptive behavior. Relatives and friends may see medication as doping or defining the child as mentally ill. Certain nonmedical professional groups involved with disturbed children may have attitudes toward prescribing of psychoactive drugs that are based on prejudice or even competition. There are also certain lay groups who totally oppose medication or even the whole profession of psychiatry. All these factors impinge on both physician and patient. There is also the movement of consumerism and, in the United States, the national sport of suing for damages.

Some of these social factors are set out in Chapters 3 and 6, and some of the very little systematic study of such factors (especially peer and school influences) is considered in Chapter 8.

E. Economic Factors

Pharmaceuticals are big business, and drug companies invest millions of dollars in promoting their products. There are almost no medical journals that would survive without drug company advertising. Drug companies use every legitimate marketing technique to sell their products, with an increasing emphasis on projecting an image of being interested in helping physicians to help their patients. It is always surprising to see the extent to which a well-paid profession will respond to a free dinner or breakfast at a convention. There is nothing wrong with this, as long as physicians understand that drug companies are there to make money and physicians to help patients, and the two objectives are not necessarily convergent. It is the responsibility of the profession to resist corruption and seduction, not that of the drug company. It is now well known that generic brands are often cheaper than brandname drugs, yet prescribing and physician communication are typically through brand names. This is why the use of brand names by physicians must raise suspicion that one is dealing with less than optimal competence.

Studies[11] suggest that many drugs prescribed for children are wasted in that physicians tend to overprescribe and for too long. This is expensive and dangerous, as other children in the family may have access to the drugs, and amounts to poor practice.

But economic factors can operate in the opposite direction. Among the poor, access to good medical care and to drugs may be restricted by economic factors, and children may be deprived of drugs that could make things a lot better for them. Much is said about the corruption of physicians by pharmaceutical houses but not enough about society's failure to make it economically possible for all its children to have equality before medicine.

F. The Powerful Placebo

Placebo is Latin for "I will please" and is used to describe beneficial effects that arise from the act of giving medication rather than the medication itself. It is usually demonstrated by giving a substance known to be inert but presented as if it were genuine medication. The caption "powerful placebo" is taken from a classical monograph by Beecher of Harvard describing studies done in the late 1940s showing that even in something as clearly physical and "real" as postoperative pain, placebos had a strong effect.

Though even among the lay public the placebo effect is well known, it is mostly ignored, and this allows useless, mostly harmless, but occasionally potentially dangerous substances to litter the shelves of drugstores, health shops, and supermarkets. But the medical profession is equally at fault. An analysis of all the studies of psychotropic drugs in children to that date allowed Sulzbacher[12] to show that those that did not employ a placebo control reported far higher success rates than those that did. Unfortunately, many of the published reports in pediatric psychopharmacology still lack proper placebo controls, and there is a need for editors to tighten up on paper selection.

The placebo effect is now often referred to as an "expectancy" effect because it stems primarily from the patient's and the physician's expectancy that the physician can help. It illustrates in a graphic way that prescribing is a complex interpersonal transaction between patient and physician.

VI. PRINCIPLES OF DRUG USE*

A. First Do No Harm (Primum non nocere)

This dog Latin phrase is well known to physicians as one of the fundamental principles of medicine; history shows that it has often been ignored. In the worst scenario, physicians have used painful and harmful treatments without benefit to the patient of which bleeding and purging are the best known examples. Many will recall from school history books the miserable time that Charles II of England (apologizing for being so long in dying) was put through by his physicians. At the turn of the century, removing colons, teeth, and tonsils was carried out because of a quite mistaken belief in "focal infection." In our era, there is hardly any treatment that is not used to excess in conditions in which it may be properly

*After Ref. 13.

indicated and in a range of conditions in which it is not. Antibiotics, antihypertensive agents, and, of course, "minor tranquilizers" like diazepam (Valium®) are all used far beyond their proper indications by physicians in most countries. In pediatric psychopharmacology, the use of excessive dosages of neuroleptic drugs in patients with developmental disabilities described in Chapter 3 provides but one example.

While drugs have important benefits, there is no effective drug that does not have side effects. Fortunately, these side effects are usually not life-threatening, but they can cause quite significant discomfort, nevertheless. For example, the stimulants may cause stomachache or the "miseries" (see Chapter 8), and the neuroleptics, a most unpleasant inability to sit still called akathisia (see Chapter 10).

A good but seldom-followed principle in medicine, and in prescribing in particular, is "when in doubt, don't."

B. Know the Disorder and Use Drugs When Indicated

There is an understandable reluctance by some physicians to prescribe medication for children, and for parents to allow their children to have medication. However, when the disorder/symptom/behavior has been properly diagnosed, and where it is seriously interfering with the child's adjustment or happiness, and where the state of medical knowledge shows that treatment is likely to be both effective and safe, it is wrong for both parent and physician to withhold treatment. Among examples of this would be manic–depressive or schizophrenic disorder (these are more common in adolescents than children), severe ADHD, and disabling Tourette (multiple tic) disorder (see Chapter 7). However, in most instances of pediatric psychopharmacology, the situation is not so clear-cut, and a cautious, limited trial with careful evaluation of effects and side effects involving independent observers such as teachers is to be preferred to pressuring parents or overenthusiasm by physicians, which elides the equivocal nature of much pediatric psychopharmacotherapy.

One more point: most illnesses, including children's behavioral and emotional disorders, wax and wane on their own and/or are self-limiting. Rushing in with drug or any treatment may make physician and parent happy but may be unnecessary. The conditions and symptoms for which use of psychotropic drugs with children and adolescents is indicated are now well established (see Chapter 7), and there is little defensible in giving medication outside these indications. In general, pediatric psychopharmacotherapy is a job only for those with specialist knowledge and training in child emotional and behavioral disorders.

C. Choose the Best Drug

Usually, there are a number of options of classes of drugs and also of subtypes. Then it becomes important to choose the drug that has the best risk/benefit ratio. For example, studies have shown that stimulants, antidepressants, and neuroleptics all can improve ADHD (see Chapter 7). However, the stimulants have both the best result qualitatively and the least side effects, so that there is little reason to use the others except when stimulants fail or produce unacceptable side effects (such as weight loss and growth retardation). Subclasses of medication sometimes also differ in their effectiveness but more often in their duration of action and side-effect profile. For example, in the initial treatment of psychotic disorders like mania or schizophrenia (see Chapter 7) where neuroleptics (antipsychotics) are indicated, there is little to choose between about 20 different drugs in terms of efficacy,[14] but some cause predominantly atropinic side effects (dry mouth, constipation) whereas others cause extrapyramidal effects (tremor, muscle rigidity, restless legs). When there is a range of lookalike drugs, as with the neuroleptics or antidepressants, then it is best that the physician become thoroughly familiar with one or two with different side-effect profiles and eschew all others in that class.

D. Understand the Drug and Its Properties

One might have thought this admonition unnecessary. However, there are far too many instances in which it is clear that the prescriber seems unaware of some properties of the drug. For example, it is common for preferences for antipsychotics to be expressed in terms of ability to influence particular symptoms in schizophrenia, despite the fact that this is without foundation.[14] Or antipsychotics may be given three or four times a day when, because their action is actually very long (several days), once a day would suffice and be a lot more convenient. Antidepressants are frequently prescribed for enuresis as a cure (see Chapter 9) though they can merely suppress the symptom only as long as they are given. Further, escape from the effect is common, and this may result in higher and higher dosage with greater risk of side effects.

E. Minimize Drug Use and Dosage

Most disturbed children are dealt with (or ought to be) by multidisciplinary teams, and for very good reason–drugs are only one small part of the therapeutic armamentarium available. Except in certain disorders like ADHD, psychoses, and Tourette syndrome (see Chapter 7), drugs have weak or limited effects whereas psychosocial interventions can be very powerful. Most distressed children are best soothed with tender loving care, not sedatives. To this point, drugs have not been effective against learning problems, where educational interventions seem more logical (though they too are less effective than is often believed[15]).

However, it is less a matter of "either/or" than of using drugs in combination with psychosocial procedures. While synergist effects acting to reduce the frequency and dosage of medication seem logical and should be presumed, studies have not been as supportive as might have been hoped, though they are few in number and mostly only in ADHD (see Chapter 8).

Dosage should also be the minimum possible, though not so low that the drug is nothing more than a placebo. Most drugs probably have what has been picturesquely called "a therapeutic window"—too low or too high a dosage and one cannot see the view. There is an insidious tendency in medicine to operate on the principle that more is likely to be better. The clearest example of this is in the treatment of schizophrenia and of aggression in the developmentally disabled, where the doses given are often several times that which has been shown to be effective. Though still a matter of controversy (Chapter 8), Sprague and Sleator[16] suggested that commonly used doses of stimulants may be too high and could affect learning adversely in some children. One factor that operates to increase dosages is that there is often a lag phase of even 2 to 6 weeks before psychoactive drugs begin to act or are pharmacodynamically stable (see Chapter 2). The apparent lack of effect in this phase may lead to unwarranted increases in dosage.

F. Keep Things Simple

Physicians often forget that parents and children lead busy lives and have other things to do than take medication. Also, communication between physician and patient still has some way to go, especially when the two are from different cultural or educational backgrounds. Patients are polite and often in awe of the physician and say yes when they do not fully understand. One way to illustrate this graphically is to ask the parent to repeat back your instructions before they leave the office. The simpler things can be kept, the greater are the chances of compliance. Many psychoactive drugs can be given once a day in the evening or on rising. If one drug can do the job, it is simpler than juggling two or three. Each prescribing situation needs to be examined in the light of the chances of accurate execution, and some compromises often have to be made between ideal and practicable.

G. Avoid Polypharmacy

The trend in medicine—and in pediatric psychopharmacotherapy[17]—increasingly is to give several drugs. Sometimes this is to counteract the side effects of the primary drug [e.g., anticholinergics to treat extrapyramidal symptoms caused by antipsychotic drugs in the treatment of schizophrenia (Chapter 10)]. Another situation is where a partial effect has been obtained and an attempt is made to amplify the effect (e.g., fluoxetine added to methylphenidate in the management of ADHD). In some instances, several drugs may be given to reduce the dosage of each individual medication needed to achieve a therapeutic effect [e.g., use of antipsychotics and benzodiazepines in acute mania (Chapter 15)]. There are, as yet, only a few established instances in pediatric psychopharmacology where more than one drug should be given at a time, and none of these is obligatory—a wait-and-see and carefully staged response is preferable.

It is basically a matter of a cost/benefit trade-off. There is no such thing as either a "cost-free" or 100% effective pharmacotherapy in psychiatry. Even our most effective drugs such as stimulants in ADHD or antidepressants in major depression cannot achieve a 100% successful response in any individual child. Nor do most useful drugs fail to produce side effects of small but significant annoyance to the patient. Doctors who cannot accept this level of imperfection put their patients at risk in a futile search for the holy grail through tactics like adding more drugs. Polypharmacy usually increases the cost of treatment; but it also can reduce the prospect of compliance through making things more complicated for the patient. The second drug usually has side effects of its own (such as dry mouth, constipation, or urinary retention from anticholinergics) which can then lead to the administration of yet another drug (such as pilocarpine) to treat these second-level side effects and which then produces its own side effects. Polypharmacy increases the chances of drug interactions that reduce or increase the effect of the main drug, for example, fluoxetine and other useful newer antidepressants can interfere with the metabolism of the antipsychotic clozapine, leading to very high and potentially toxic drug levels. In combination with monoamine oxidase inhibitor (MAOI) antidepressants, clozapine can produce a life threatening disorder called hyperserotonergic syndrome (see Chapter 9). The possibilities of drug interactions can be checked before prescribing through reference to the package inserts of the drugs, pharmacological texts, and, increasingly, specialized software and data bases. There is also a useful monograph on drug interactions in psychiatry available in paperback.[18]

In contrast to the above situations (managing side effects and amplifying therapeutic effect), which, carefully weighed, can be indications for combined drug use, a quite indefensible yet common form of polypharmacy is giving different drugs from the same class. There is little evidence that this is indicated even with antipsychotics,[14] where in theory it might cancel out side effects (such as to reduce both sedation and extrapyramidal side effects).

Current snowballing enthusiasm for combinations of medication in pediatric psychopharmacology outruns by some distance the research to support their safety and efficacy. When the U.S. media picked up a rumor that the combination of methylphenidate and clonidine (see Chapters 8 and 15) might be implicated in sudden death in children with ADHD, an FDA official[19] caustically pointed out that though "thousands" of children were receiving this drug combination, there were no clinical trials attesting to either its efficacy or its safety. Clinical use of medication should always reflect what research suggests is correct, not what clinicians feel may help.

On the whole, combinations of medication in pediatric psychopharmacology should raise suspicion in the minds of parents and invoke requests for a well-argued rationale for such a practice from the prescriber. A second opinion should be sought if any doubts remain.

H. Don't Be a Fiddler

Understanding the time frame of drugs and the disorder is essential to therapeutic simplicity, compliance, and success. With the possible exception of stimulants in ADHD, therapeutic response in pediatric psychopharmacology, compared with the rest of medicine, tends to occur in slow motion. For example, treatment of schizophrenia rarely shows a good response before 6 weeks. Chopping and changing drugs and dosages before that interval of time has elapsed makes no sense unless it is specifically to target emergent side effects. It takes sure knowledge of psychopharmacology and of psychiatric disorders to resist fiddling, while drugs and/or disorder operate to a different drummer.

I. Don't Follow Fads

The history of medicine illustrates that just as with clothes, there are fashions with drugs—what is new is often modish. One medical cynic described the history of the typical new drug as progressing from panacea to placebo to poison. Drug companies have a limited time of patent protection during which to recoup very expensive investments in the development of new products. They thus use every market ploy to improve sales. The media too have a habit of picking up initial promising research results, often inflating and sensationalizing the results. Unfortunately, these are much more likely to be published than negative results and are often found not to hold up subsequently. Publication is a legitimate signal to researchers to assist in firmly establishing these initial findings; to sensation-hungry media, it is simply news. A good example of this is to be seen with the first reports of use of fenfluramine in autism, which led to media reports that raised false hope in parents of children with this very distressing disorder (see Chapter 15). It does not appear that the media subsequently were very interested in correcting initial enthusiasm when more extensive work showed this drug to be of limited value (see Chapter 15).

The best policy to follow is to wait until several independent centers have reported on both safety and efficacy of new drugs before prescribing.

J. Take Particular Care with Children

Children are vulnerable in that they cannot make informed decisions for themselves. The complex ethics of this are discussed in detail in Chapter 6. Also, their minds and bodies are developing at a very rapid pace and are therefore, in theory at least, much more liable to major and serious disruptions that may not just delay but misdirect development. They may be physically more susceptible to the actions of the drug though the opposite is generally true in that they typically require relatively higher doses (see Chapter 2). Since most of the breakthroughs in psychopharmacology occur first in adult psychiatry, it is better to allow proper trials to be carried out there before applying them to children. There have been innumerable instances in which apparently safe drugs have subsequently been shown to have serious long-term effects. Tobacco is a good example. A number of psychoactive drugs have had to be withdrawn because of effects not shown in initial trials. It took about 20 years of use of neuroleptics to discover that they may produce neurological disability after several years of use (tardive dyskinesia).

But it is not just serious risks that must be borne in mind. Minor side effects can be quite discomforting, and children hate to be seen to be different by their peers—taking psychotropic medication is one such clear difference with particularly adverse social connotations (see Chapter 8). It is the overall picture that must be in balance and clearly reflect the child's best interests.

K. Establish a Therapeutic Alliance

One of the more persistent requests that the public makes is for more personalized medicine. Parents are now much better informed, more aware of their rights, and less subservient to authority figures like physicians. Taking the parent on as a partner and involving the child as much as possible not only meets ethical considerations (see Chapter 6) but also will pay dividends in terms of compliance and enhancement of the effect of medication through expectancy (placebo) effects. The drug is invested with the personality of the physician. Time taken to establish an alliance with the patient is merely part of holistic medicine, which is not new but part of the tradition of medicine and one of the reasons that, warts and all, it is still a respected profession.

L. Compliance (Adherence) with Treatment

Getting patients to take medication as directed or to continue with medication is a serious problem in medicine. Eighty-five percent of pediatric patients stop acute medical treatment before the end of the full course, and among those who need long-term medication, less than 50% continue.[20] This problem area is usually referred to as "compliance" though this word has found disfavor because it suggests a servile relationship between the precriber and the patient. "Adherence" is now preferred.[20] In a useful overview, Stine[20] reviews this topic with respect to pediatric psychopharmacology, noting that there are only a few good studies, which, as elsewhere in medicine, suggest that adherence is a significant problem. There are two theoretical formulations of adherence[20]—the health belief model (the consumer's perceived seriousness of the illness, benefits of treatment, costs, etc.) and the locus-of-control model (how much power consumers perceive themselves to have).

The most proximate sections of this chapter have outlined, if indirectly, some of the factors that may enhance or reduce adherence. Stine[20] summarizes factors associated with psychostimulants in ADHD—oppositional symptoms and passivity in the child, parental concerns about safety of medication, parent and child reaction to the diagnosis of "illness," media misinformation, and stigma. Despite the growth of interest in pediatric psychopharmacology, there continue to be few formal studies of adherence—apparently only one in 1995.[21] One of the most important findings of the limited recent research is to confirm the importance of parental and child beliefs about medication. A study[22] showed that even though the professional literature shows that medication in ADHD is by far the most regularly and dramatically useful treatment, parents still, on the whole, prefer psychosocial treatments. Under such circumstances, many parents who are persuaded or politely agree to try medication are at high risk of not following through. Unfortunately, it is no easy task to change attitudes to medication. A study[21] not only confirmed the importance of attitudes to medication but showed that efforts to improve knowledge about the particular medication prescribed seemed to have little effect on attitudes and failed to improve adherence. There is a need for far more systematic research of this type on how to improve adherence.

It is tempting to conclude that a well thought-out and continuing campaign of education to overcome deep-rooted prejudice against medication among the public and in the media is needed. However, it should be noted that the medical profession is not entirely blameless and needs to cleave more to research findings and show less tearaway, unbridled enthusiasm for medication. The scare over the unresearched methylphenidate–clonidine combination in ADHD discussed above[19] shakes public confidence and imperils adherence.

VII. CONCLUSION

This chapter has attempted to show a number of things: (1) that drugs are an integral part of modern child psychiatry and behavioral pediatrics; (2) that there is a rich technology of diagnosis and of pharmacology with which physicians must be thoroughly familiar before prescribing; (3) that there is a code of proper ways to evaluate whether drugs are helpful and safe; (4) that prescribing drugs is a complex human transaction involving not only the main actors, the physician and the patient, but also a host of unseen forces ranging from relatives to school to economics; (5) that there is a set of canons for the prescriber to follow, only a few of which will be found in books on the pharmacology of the drugs concerned; and (6) that the use of psychoactive drugs in children should be but one part of a multidisciplinary multimodal treatment program, in which all parts work harmoniously together to enhance the end result.

Parents should take great care in choosing their doctor and share the suspicion of doctors that those within the profession have of some of their colleagues. Public popularity, or the size of the practice, is the most fallible of all ways to choose a doctor. Physicians are seldom so evaluated by their peers, not because of envy but because of professional assessment. Credentials are some guide. On the whole, the best care is likely to come from those who are trained and specialize in the treatment of children and adolescents. Because of their more relevant training, child psychiatrists should ordinarily be regarded as the most expert in the proper assessment and diagnosis of child emotional and behavior problems and in pediatric psychopharmacology, and difficult cases or requests for second opinions should be referred to them. However, this alone is insufficient since it is possible to divide even child psychiatrists into "wets" who embrace medication with enthusiasm, using high doses and combinations of drugs in almost every patient they see, and "drys" (often psychotherapists) who are prejudiced against any use of medication. Neither posture is defensible. The position and number of enthusiasts is being strengthened by a somewhat irresponsible willingness of major journals to publish, at length, uncontrolled studies, which now dominate reports in pediatric psychopharmacology. These do have value in stimulating proper research or theory but should be confined to a maximum of one full page, set in small type, relegated to the back pages of journals and carry an editorial disclaimer to the effect that these are unsubstantiated findings, reported to stimulate proper study and not to be cited as having established clinical efficacy.

Guides to recognizing a doctor about whom further inquiries may be needed are:

1. Not board certified in a child medical specialty
2. Working alone
3. Not credentialed to a good hospital
4. Making a diagnosis after a few minutes
5. Overpositivity and "coming on strong"
6. Not seeking information from schools or other caretakers in addition to parents
7. Not using some standard published assessment techniques, (see Chapters 4 & 5)
8. Overuse of expensive medical tests or hi-tech equipment (see Chapter 4)
9. Use of higher doses than those recommended throughout this monograph
10. Use of combinations of drugs at the start
11. Failure to explain carefully effects, symptoms not affected, and potential side effects (usually including written information), to monitor the effects of medication at frequent intervals, assess impact in school, talk with the child about what he or she feels after taking medication, and to provide means of phone or emergency advice after hours.

At the moment there are no miracles or indeed any real cures from psychoactive drugs, but life for some disturbed or distressed children and their caretakers can in many instances be enhanced through the knowledgeable, humane, and careful use of psychoactive drugs. There are a number of organized and individual opponents of pharmacotherapy; but most of these are ill informed or have vested interests in other treatment methods. Unlike most other treatments for child emotional and behavior problems, medication, when properly indicated and carefully prescribed and monitored, is usually cheap and simple to administer, does not disrupt routines like school with frequent visits to the therapist, and is highly cost-efficient. This important and beneficial role for pharmacotherapy should increase rapidly over the next decade. Even so, a responsible prescriber should rarely, if ever, offer pharmacotherapy as sufficient treatment on its own.

REFERENCES

1. Bradley C: The behavior of children receiving Benzedrine. *Am J Orthopsychiatry* 9:577–585, 1937.
2. Conners CK: Pharmacotherapy, in Quay HC, Werry JS (eds): *Psychopathological Disorders of Childhood.* New York, John Wiley & Sons, 1972, pp 316–347.

22 1. Introduction

3. Sprague RL, Werry JS: Methodology of psychopharmacological studies in the retarded, in Ellis N (ed): *International Review of Mental Retardation*. New York, Academic Press, 1971, vol 5, pp 147–219.
4. American Psychiatric Association:*Diagnostic and Statistical Manual of Mental Disorders*, ed 3. Washington, DC, American Psychiatric Association, 1980.
5. American Psychiatric Association: *Diagnostic and Statistical Manual of Mental Disorders*, ed 4. Washington, DC, American Psychiatric Association, 1994.
6. Aman MG, Singh NN: *Psychopharmacology of the Developmental Disabilities*. Berlin, Springer, 1988.
7. Lehmann HE: Strategies in clinical psychopharmacology, in Lipton MA, Di Mascio A, Killam KF (eds): *Psychopharmacology: A Generation of Progress*. New York, Raven Press, 1978, p 13.
8. Werry JS: Child and adolescent schizophrenia: A review in the light of DSM-III-R. *J Autism Dev Disord* 22:601–624, 1992.
9. Weiss G, Hechtman LT: *Hyperactive Children Grown Up*. New York, Guilford Press, 1986, pp 240–256.
10. Efron DH: *Psychopharmacology: A Review of Progress 1957–1967*. New York, Raven Press, 1968.
11. Werry JS, Carlielle J: The nuclear family, suburban neurosis and iatrogencsis in mothers of preschool children. *J Am Acad Child Psychiatry* 22:172–179, 1983
12. Sulzbacher S: Psychotropic medication with children: An evaluation of procedural biases in results of reported studies. *Pediatrics* 51:513–517, 1973.
13. Schoonover SC: Introduction: The practice of pharmacotherapy, in Bassuk EL, Schoonover SC, Gelenberg AJ (eds): *The Practitioner's Guide to Psychoactive Drugs*, ed 2. New York, Plenum Press, 1988, pp 1–18.
14. Kane JM: Treatment of schizophrenia. *Schizophr Bull* 13:147–170, 1987.
15. Feagens L: A current view of learning disabilities. *J Pediatr* 102:487–493, 1983.
16. Sprague RL, Sleator E: Methylphenidate in hyperactive children: Differences in dose effects on learning and social behavior. *Science* 198:1274–1276, 1977.
17. Wilens TE, Spencer T, Biederman J, Wosniak J, Connor D: Combined pharmacotherapy: An emerging trend in pediatric psychopharmacology. *J Am Acad Child Adolesc Psychiatry* 34:110–112, 1995.
18. Ciraulo DA, Shader RI, Greenblatt DJ, Creelman W: *Drug Interactions in Psychiatry*, ed 2. Baltimore, Williams and Wilkins, 1995.
19. Fenichel RR: Combining methylphenidate and clonidine: The role of post-marketing surveillance. *J Child Adolesc Psychopharmacol* 5:155–156, 1995.
20. Stine JJ: Psychosocial and psychodynamic issues affecting noncompliance with psychostimulant treatment. *J Child Adolesc Psychopharmacol* 4:75–86, 1994
21. Bastiaens L: Knowledge, attitudes and compliance with pharmacotherapy in adolescent patients and their parents. *J Child Adolesc Psychopharmacol* 5:39–48, 1995.
22. Wilson LJ, Jennings JN: Parents' acceptability of alternative treatments for Attention-Deficit Hyperactivity Disorder. *J Attention Disord*, 1:114–121, 1996.

2

Pharmacology

JAMES WILLIAM PAXTON, Ph.D., and MICHAEL DRAGUNOW, Ph.D.

I. INTRODUCTION

In this chapter we shall consider how drugs get into the body; their fate within the body; how they are eliminated; their time course within the body (their pharmacokinetics); and also the general mechanisms by which they produce a response (their pharmacodynamics). In addition, we shall cover some of the reported differences between adults and children with regard to the fate and effects of drugs in the body. To date, these have been confined mainly to pharmacokinetic differences. This topic is naturally one of the more technical and does require some knowledge of high school biology and chemistry. We shall cover the general principles, but also some of the more technical aspects (mostly for prescribing physicians) will be addressed. These may be skipped by those seeking only some basic understanding of how drugs work.

II. FATE OF DRUGS IN THE BODY

Drugs are mainly small organic molecules, typically with molecular weights in the range of 200–1000 daltons, which are foreign to the body. A drug can only produce the desired response when it is in the immediate vicinity of its site of action. However, most drugs do not enter the body at or even near their site of action and must move from the site of administration to the tissue or cells where they act. To do this, the drug must pass through various cells and tissues, which tend to act as barriers to this movement. These barriers show a certain degree of selectivity in the ease with which they permit drugs and chemicals to pass through, depending on the physicochemical properties and structural configuration of the barrier, as well as the chemical nature of the migrating drug molecule. Once the drug has gained entry into the body, it (1) is diluted in the bloodstream; (2) may be bound by plasma proteins; (3) is carried to the kidney, where it may be excreted unchanged in the urine; and (4) is also carried to the liver, where it may be transformed into a more water-soluble (and usually inactive) metabolite, which may be excreted in the urine or the bile and

JAMES WILLIAM PAXTON, Ph.D., and MICHAEL DRAGUNOW, Ph.D. • Department of Pharmacology & Clinical Pharmacology, School of Medicine, University of Auckland, Auckland, New Zealand.

Practitioner's Guide to Psychoactive Drugs for Children and Adolescents (Second Edition), Werry and Aman, eds. Plenum Publishing Corporation, New York, 1999.

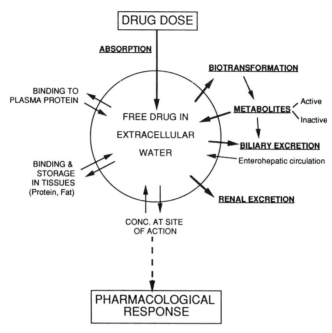

FIGURE 1.   Summary of the fate of a drug within the body.

thence, via the feces, out of the body (Fig. 1). All these processes are working toward reducing the effect of this foreign molecule and removing it from the body. However, if a sufficiently large dose of drug is administered, a small fraction of the drug molecules will survive the journey to the site of action to produce a response.

A. Passage of Drugs across Biological Membranes

Reduced to its most simplistic description, the body consists of billions of cells mostly bound to each other in some way, floating in a sea of water (interstitial fluid or blood) containing electrolytes, nutrients, and breakdown products. Passage of drugs through tissues such as the intestinal wall or the skin usually occurs via the cell. Exceptions to this include the glomerular capillaries of the kidney, which contain unusually large pores that permit passage by simple filtration of all the plasma constituents (except macromolecules such as proteins of >30 kDa). Indeed, in keeping with their role of bringing essential supplies like oxygen and glucose and taking away breakdown products, most blood capillaries are generally relatively porous, allowing rapid interchange of drug molecules between the blood and (interstitial) fluid surrounding cells.

In order for a drug to pass through a cell, it must first penetrate the cell membrane, which thus becomes the ultimate barrier to the migration of drugs through any biological structure. Membranes from all types of cells are remarkably similar, consisting chiefly of two layers of phospholipids (fats) in which cholesterol and proteins are embedded, but the details of membrane structure are still widely debated. Some of the protein molecules act as specific *transporters* of nutrients (or waste products) or may form *channels* with their charged groups through which small water-soluble molecules and ions may pass. Cholesterol is thought to fit closely within the phospholipid bilayer, giving the structure some rigidity but not solidifying it. The ability of membranes to restrict and sometimes prevent the passage of many molecules is believed to arise from this compact phospholipid bilayer.

There are several mechanisms by which molecules can cross cell membranes. Of these, *passive diffusion* is by far the most important for drugs. It applies to drugs that are fat-soluble and thus can easily dissolve in the lipid bilayer and move down the concentration gradient into the cell (or out again). However, many drugs are weak electrolytes and, in an aqueous environment like blood or interstitial fluid, partially ionize; e.g., a weak acidic drug (HA) may lose a proton (H$^+$) to become negatively charged:

$$HA \leftrightharpoons H^+ + A^-$$

where A$^-$ represents drug anion. If the concentration of protons in the system increases for any reason, the reaction will tend to be driven to the left to maintain the equilibrium, in accordance with the law of mass action. Thus, as the H$^+$ concentration rises (i.e., the pH falls or the fluid becomes more acidic), the ionization of the acidic drug decreases and more will be in the uncharged fat-soluble form, favoring transfer across any biological membrane. In contrast, bases are proton acceptors, and in aqueous solutions a weakly basic drug will gain a proton to become positively charged. As the pH falls, more of the weak base will become charged, reducing its potential to pass across a biological membrane. Thus, the pH of the aqueous environment greatly influences the degree of ionization of weak electrolytes and hence their passage across membranes, since it is the nonionized form of the molecule that is more fat-soluble. This is important since blood, gastrointestinal, and kidney systems have a variable pH depending on the state of digestion, exercise, and respiration.

Dissociation of weakly acidic and basic drugs is characterized by a "pK_a" value, which is the negative log of the association constant (K_a) and is a measure of strength as an acid; thus, the stronger the acid, the lower is its pK_a, since the ionization of a strong acid is less suppressed by a high H$^+$ concentration (i.e., a low pH) than is the ionization of a weak acid. For example, the pK_a of sulfuric acid is 2.0, while the pK_a of phenytoin, a weak acidic drug, is 8.4. The pK_a is identical to the pH at which the weak electrolyte is 50% dissociated. Thus, in an aqueous solution with a pH of 8.4, phenytoin would exist in equal concentrations of charged and uncharged forms. A knowledge of the pK_a value along with the chemical nature of the drug (i.e., whether it is a weak base or acid) is useful, as it enables the prediction of the effect of pH changes on ionization and the possible passive diffusion through biological membranes.

Other methods of drug transfer across biological membranes include the *passage of small water-soluble molecules (<100 Da) through water-filled pores* and *carrier-mediated (active) transport*. The latter requires energy, which is supplied by the cell, and has the ability to move molecules against their concentration gradient. Active transport of a wide variety of molecules such as ions, sugars, amino acids, nucleotides, some water-soluble vitamins, and various other compounds vital to the cell has been shown to occur in specialized membranes such as those of the nervous system, gut, kidney, and liver. The physiological need for active-transport systems that will allow a cell to accumulate substances essential for growth and maintenance, and to eliminate waste products against a concentration gradient, is obvious. However, active transport of drugs appears to be limited to agents that are structurally similar to endogenous (existing within the body) molecules, such as the dopamine precursor dihydroxyphenylalanine (DOPA), which is transported into the brain by an amino acid active-transport system.

B. Routes of Drug Administration

In order to produce the desired pharmacological response, an appropriate concentration of drug must be achieved at its target site of action. The chemical nature of the drug molecule will influence the speed at which this is achieved, by affecting the drug's absorption and distribution. Absorption into the body will vary according to (1) the route of administration and (2) the ease with which the drug crosses cell membranes. Most drugs, other than those applied locally, such as skin lotions, must enter the bloodstream to be carried to their receptor sites.

The most efficient route for drug administration is *intravenous (IV) injection*. This ensures that the entire dose is available for distribution by the bloodstream to its site of action, since it does not have to undergo the vagaries of absorption in the gastrointestinal tract (see later) or through the skin (transdermal preparations). Thus, the amount of drug entering the bloodstream can be controlled with an accuracy not possible by other routes. Electronically controlled infusion pumps may also be used to guarantee a constant supply of drug over a long period of time, as is required for some kinds of pain relief. In addition, IV administration is rapid, with no lag time associated with absorption. It takes 10–15 sec for drug injected into an arm vein to proceed through the heart to the brain, and approximately 1 min for a complete circulation of the body.

Oral administration is the most common method of drug administration. Although the most convenient, it is the most unpredictable with regard to both extent and rate of absorption into the bloodstream. With oral administration, in contrast to IV administration, it takes approximately 30 to 90 min to achieve the maximum concentration of drug in the bloodstream. Apart from the physicochemical properties of the drug molecule, additional factors determining the extent and rate of absorption are the dosage form (i.e., tablet or capsule) and formulation factors, such as degree of tablet compaction, size of drug particles, crystal and salt form of the drug, and the presence of excipients, such as inert binding agents, various fillers (starch, lactose, sucrose, calcium sulfate), and wetting agents. Also, after ingestion, the dosage form must disintegrate in the stomach and/or intestines and release the active drug. Drug release may be very rapid but can also be very slow in the case of special pharmaceutical formulations, such as sustained-release preparations. Before absorption into the body, the drug particles must dissolve in the gastrointestinal (GI) fluids and must be capable of withstanding degradation by gastric enzymes (e.g., peptidases) and gastric acids. The absorption process may be slowed down or even prevented by numerous factors such as changes in stomach acidity, the presence of food or other drugs, and changes in the rate of stomach emptying or intestinal motility due to other drugs (e.g., opiates or anticholinergics) or due to diarrhea and/or gastroenteritis or general debility.

After absorption from the stomach or the intestines, drugs are carried by the portal (gut) blood supply to the liver and, after passage through the liver, enter the systemic circulation for distribution to the main body and their sites of action. During this first circuit through the liver, some drugs undergo substantial extraction and deactivation.[1] This is known as *first-pass elimination* and is observed for a number of drugs [e.g., the antidepressant imipramine (Chapter 9)]. *Bioavailability* is the term used to indicate the relative amount of an administered dose that reaches the main cardiovascular circulation. The bioavailability of drugs may be greatly increased during hepatic disease, resulting in unexpected overdosage. Many other drugs, such as morphine, have such extensive first-pass elimination that they are rarely given orally. The absolute bioavailability of an oral dose (or a dose administered by any other route) can only be determined by comparison of the amounts of drug in the bloodstream (as measured by the area under the blood/plasma concentration–time curve) after the oral dose and after the same dose is given IV in the same subject. Variation in the absorption process and extraction and deactivation by the liver after oral administration are major contributing factors to the wide range of response to a standard dose observed in the patient population.

Other routes for drug administration are used less frequently, but each has advantages and disadvantages depending on the situation and the drug. For example, the *intramuscular route* is usually very slow and incomplete and often results in some precipitation of the drug at the injection site, which may irritate the tissue. Some formulations, such as fluphenazine decanoate used in schizophrenia (Chapter 10), are specially formulated to provide a slow release from intramuscular sites, thus providing a greatly prolonged effect over 2–4 weeks. The *rectal route* for the administration of drugs (e.g., prochlorperazine suppositories for severe nausea) has obvious advantages in patients where vomiting is a problem with oral administration. In addition, much of the blood supply to the rectum bypasses the liver, avoiding a possible reduction in bioavailability with first-pass elimination. Other routes, such as *sublingual,* are only suitable for a small amount of drug with rapid dissolution; e.g., sublingual glyceryl trinitrate affords rapid entry into the bloodstream and rapid relief of angina. Recently, interest has been shown in the skin as a route of drug administration using stick-on skin patches.[2] These transdermal preparations are only suitable when small doses are involved, and usually employ a rate-controlling membrane that allows a small amount of drug onto the skin to diffuse through. They are useful for drugs that have a short elimination half-life or that are destroyed in the gut and liver and have been successfully applied to glyceryl trinitrate, scopolamine (for the prevention of motion sickness), and clonidine (used psychotropically; Chapter 15).

The *respiratory tract* may also be used to gain entry of a drug into the body. The most obvious examples are the gaseous anesthetics or volatile solvents used in adolescent drug abuse (Chapter 11). These compounds are relatively nonpolar, highly lipid-soluble molecules so that they diffuse across the lung (alveolar membranes) and rapidly enter the bloodstream. Absorption will continue as long as the partial pressure of the gas in the alveolar air exceeds the partial pressure of the gas in the pulmonary capillary. Once anesthetic administration (or sniffing) ceases, the partial pressure of the alveolar air falls and backdiffusion of the gas from pulmonary to alveolar air occurs. The respiratory route is also used most effectively with inhalers in asthma, the most common chronic disorder of children (Chapter 13).

C. Distribution

After introduction into the bloodstream, a drug is subjected to the multiple processes of distribution, governed by its lipid solubility, its pK_a, the pH of body fluids, the extent of protein and tissue binding, and differences in regional blood flow. Organs such as the heart, liver, kidney, brain, and endocrine glands are richly perfused with blood, and rapid equilibration of the drug between plasma and tissue takes place. In contrast, in tissues such as muscle and adipose that have a lesser blood supply, equilibration takes much longer. Entry of drugs into the brain may also be less readily achieved as the brain capillaries are surrounded with a protective cellular sheath of glial cells (the so-called *blood–brain barrier*), resulting in permeability characteristics more closely resembling those of tightly bound tissue cell walls than those of the more porous capillary endothelia.[3] To gain access to the brain, a drug must be (1) highly lipid-soluble or (2) subject to active-transport mechanisms.

Another important source of variation in drug distribution is the pronounced interindividual differences in the binding of many drugs to proteins in the tissue and in blood. This varies with age and also environmental and pathological factors. For example, most drugs exist in blood in a dynamic equilibrium between a form that is *free* in the plasma (blood minus cells) and one that is *bound* to plasma proteins. This binding is reversible, with very fast rates of association and dissociation in the range of milliseconds. It is therefore not a limiting factor in the uptake of drug from the bloodstream by major organs (e.g., the liver), where perfusion time (i.e., complete passage) may be several seconds or more. The role of plasma proteins in drug distribution and elimination is variable, depending on the relative affinity of the plasma protein for the drug and the affinity of the various uptake mechanisms that the drug might encounter. If the affinity between the plasma protein and drug is greater than the uptake mechanism of the eliminating organ, the plasma protein binding would be expected to give some protection from elimination, and vice versa. In addition, for drugs that might otherwise have solubility problems in plasma, these proteins act as very efficient carriers, aiding drug absorption and transport around the body. As large protein molecules (with bound drug) are unable to leave the bloodstream, it is the unbound drug that diffuses out of the circulation to interact with metabolic and transport sites or reach effector sites to produce a response. There is increasing evidence indicating a better correlation between drug response and *unbound rather than total drug concentration in plasma at steady state*.[4] However, most laboratory methods for drug measurement provide a total drug concentration in plasma. Consequently, all commonly used therapeutic ranges are based on total drug concentrations in plasma. Fortunately, the unbound drug concentration is a relatively constant fraction of the total concentration over the range achieved after administration of therapeutic doses for most drugs. Thus, total concentration is a reasonable index of activity for many drugs. However, situations are increasingly being recognized in which the plasma protein binding of the drug is significantly altered. This can assume major importance in evaluating plasma drug concentrations. With a change in the ratio of unbound to total drug concentration, the commonly accepted therapeutic range will not be applicable.[5]

The major plasma protein involved in drug binding is albumin, which binds both acidic and basic drugs, and which occurs at a concentration of approximately 0.7 mmole/liter (42 g/liter) in normal plasma. Few drugs are used at such high concentrations to achieve a therapeutic effect, and thus only a small fraction of the available binding sites will be occupied in most situations. Consequently, the unbound fraction remains relatively constant and independent of drug concentration. Exceptions to this include salicylate and valproate (Chapters 9 and 12), which are used at millimolar concentrations and which can saturate the binding sites of albumin. For these drugs, the unbound fraction is dependent on drug concentration and can change significantly within the therapeutic range, affecting the interpretation of total plasma concentration.

Another plasma protein that may play a major role in the plasma binding of a number of basic drugs is α_1-acid glycoprotein (AAG) (also known as orosomucoid).[6] Extremely low AAG concentrations (3–5 μmole/liter) are observed in neonates, rising to adult levels (10–20 μmole/liter) by about 10 months. Because AAG is an acute-phase reactant protein, AAG concentrations are elevated in a large number of conditions characterized by *physiological stress* such as inflammatory disease, cancer, myocardial infarction, and trauma from surgery, burns, and severe injury. Elevated AAG levels are associated with increased binding of basic drugs, such as chlorpromazine and imipramine (Chapters 9 and 10) and may cause a significantly reduced unbound fraction of drug in plasma.

D. Elimination

Elimination may be defined as the process that contributes to the drug as such ceasing to exist in the body. There are two processes of elimination: (1) excretion of unchanged drug (e.g., in the urine or feces) and (2) chemical conversion (biotransformation/metabolism), giving rise to one or more metabolites, which are subsequently excreted or further metabolized. For most drugs, the processes of absorption and distribution determine the *speed of onset* of drug effect, while the processes of excretion and biotransformation terminate the action of drugs by removing the active form of the drug from the body (i.e., these processes determine the *duration of drug activity*).

1. Excretion

Excretion is the process whereby compounds are removed from the body to the external environment. The kidney is the most important excretory organ, but other potential excretory pathways are the biliary tract, respiratory tract, sweat, tears, saliva, vaginal secretion, and breast milk. Of these, only the biliary tract is of major quantitative importance with regard to drugs; and also the respiratory tract in the special case of anesthetic gases and volatile solvents (Chapter 11). *Water solubility* is the decisive factor that determines whether a drug is excreted unchanged in the urine. All plasma constituents, except macromolecules such as proteins, are filtered to urine in the glomerulus by the simple action of blood pressure. However reabsorption into the blood of all drugs that easily cross membranes (i.e., fat-soluble) takes place in the proximal tubule, loop of Henle, and distal tubule of the kidney. In this regard, the *pH of the urine* is important for some drugs [(e.g., dextroamphetamine (Chapter 8)], as it determines whether they are present in the ionized (water-soluble) or in the nonionized (fat-soluble) form. As tubular reabsorption is by passive diffusion and is dependent on a concentration gradient, it will also be affected by *urinary flow rate*. Low rates of urine flow, as in dehydration, kidney disease, or shock, will enhance concentration gradients, with consequently increased passive reabsorption of fat-soluble drug molecules from urine into plasma. Conversely, increased urinary flow decreases tubular absorption and thus enhances excretion.

The glomerular filtration rate (GFR) is the total volume of glomerular filtrate produced per unit time by all functioning nephrons. In healthy subjects, the GFR is approximately 120–130 ml/min, equivalent to 10% of renal blood flow, producing approximately 180 liters of filtrate per day. Of this original filtrate, 99% is reabsorbed in the proximal tubule and to a lesser extent in the distal tubule, giving a daily total urinary output of 1–2 liters. The GFR is decreased when the number of functioning glomeruli is decreased (as ultimately occurs in all disease affecting the nephron) or with severe reduction in renal blood flow. Reduced GFR will result in a reduced elimination of those drugs [e.g., lithium (Chapter 9)] that are largely excreted in the urine unchanged. In these circumstances, such drugs should be given at the reduced dose and/or less frequently; otherwise, there is a risk of substantial accumulation and toxicity. The most commonly used clinical method for determining GFR is the measurement of the *renal clearance of creatinine*, an endogenous breakdown product of the body (Chapter 4).

Apart from filtration and passive reabsorption, the third mechanism controlling the composition of the filtrate is *active transport*. After passing through the capillaries around Bowman's capsule, the unfiltered fraction of plasma and blood cells pass into the vessels surrounding the proximal convoluted tubules, which possess two highly active but non-specific active-transport systems, one for acidic and one for basic drugs. Transport may occur in either direction; for example, penicillin is almost exclusively secreted, while bile acids are almost exclusively reabsorbed. Drugs and metabolites must be in their ionized form for secretion by these mechanisms. Many drugs are biotransformed in the liver by conjugation with a glucuronide or sulfate molecule, both of which are ideal substrates for these transport systems. Both free and protein-bound drug can be removed from plasma and secreted into urine by these high-affinity transport mechanisms; as free drug is removed from plasma by the tubular cells, there is a rapid dissociation of the bound drug from the transporting plasma protein to maintain the equilibrium in plasma. These active-transport processes are saturable and specific only for a particular ionic species; thus, competition for secretion may occur between like-charged compounds. This is sometimes used to prevent too rapid excretion of some drugs.

Less is known about the mechanisms involved in biliary drug excretion. Bile is formed by active secretory processes in the liver bile canaliculi. The primary event is the active secretion of bile salts, with secretion of water and electrolytes osmotically controlled. Most drugs excreted in the bile are highly polar, have ionizable groups, have a size of >300–400 Da, and are thought to be transported by an active carrier-mediated process. After secretion in the bile, drugs and metabolites are concentrated in the gallbladder, which, upon contraction, releases its content into the lumen of the gut. Thereafter, drugs and/or metabolites may be excreted with the feces, metabolized by the bacterial flora normally resident in the gut, and/or reabsorbed back into the portal bloodstream and carried to the kidney for excretion in urine. Drugs excreted in the bile as conjugates (particularly glucuronides) may also be hydrolyzed by bacterial enzymes in the gut to form the original, less polar parent drug, which is more readily absorbed. This is known as the enterohepatic circulation and is thought to be partially responsible for the long elimination half-life of digitoxin,[7] but its importance in the case of psychotropic drugs remains to be demonstrated.

2. Biotransformation

The majority of drugs are fat-soluble and thus cannot be excreted unchanged in the (aqueous) urine. However, their fat solubility allows a wider distribution of the drug in the body and also gives the drug access to enzymes that generally lie beyond several lipid membranes within the liver cell. The enzymatic biotransformation of drugs in the liver generally results in *more water-soluble products*, which facilitates their excretion in the urine or bile. These enzymatic reactions can be divided into two phases. In a phase I reaction, the drug's structure is modified by either adding or unmasking a functional group, such as a hydroxyl or amine group, so that the drug is in the appropriate chemical form to be acted upon by the phase II or conjugating enzymes. In a phase II reaction, the drug is joined to a polar endogenous molecule such as glucuronide, sulfate, or glutathione, rendering it more water-soluble and an ideal substrate for the excretory processes of the liver and kidney. If an appropriate functional group is already present in the drug, the phase II biotransformations need not necessarily be preceded by a phase I reaction; for example, morphine is converted to morphine 3-glucuronide by direct conjugation with glucuronic acid before excretion. The conjugated metabolite products of phase II reactions are generally devoid of pharmacological activity, whereas the metabolites generated after phase I may or may not retain the pharmacological activity of the parent drug; for example, imipramine is biotransformed to desipramine, which has equivalent or greater antidepressant activity. Indeed, some molecules need to be chemically converted to produce their pharmacological effect and are known as prodrugs; for example, DOPA is the precursor "prodrug" of dopamine, the active metabolite responsible for the therapeutic effect in Parkinson's disease, but dopamine cannot cross the blood–brain barrier while DOPA does. Once in cerebral tissue, DOPA is decarboxylated to dopamine by an enzyme involved in the normal production of catecholamines such as noradrenaline in the brain.

The phase I biotransformations consist of oxidation, reduction, hydrolysis, and hydration reactions. Of these, oxidation is by far the most common and is carried out by a superfamily of more than 30 closely related enzymes, the *cytochrome P450* isoenzymes (CYP450), which are located largely in the endoplasmic reticulum of the hepatocytes (liver cells) but are also found in other tissues such as the kidney, lungs, brain, and gastrointestinal tract. At present, some ten or so different human isoenzymes in the CYP450 family are known to be involved in the oxidative metabolism of drugs. However, the actions of these enzymes are not confined to drugs but also include compounds that occur naturally in the body, such as steroids, fatty acids, leukotrienes, prostaglandins, bile acids, biogenic amines, and also dietary compounds and toxicants.[8] Indeed, it may have been for protection from naturally occurring toxicants that the CYP450 superfamily evolved. The liver's location and the portal venous blood supply make it well suited to modify chemical compounds, especially those absorbed from the gut, the major route by which chemicals enter the body. The wide variety of chemicals to which organisms may be exposed requires that the biotransformation enzymes in the liver have broad substrate specificity and can adapt to increased exposure to certain chemicals. Both characteristics are exhibited by the CYP450 system. This system is also important in drug interactions such as the augmentation of clozapine concentrations by selective serotonin reuptake inhibitors (SSRI antidepressants) (see later in this chapter).

3. Variability in Human Drug Biotransformation

Individuals may show a wide variation in their responses to the same dose of a drug. Much of this interindividual variability in drug response can be explained by differences in absorption, distribution, excretion, and in particular biotransformation; for example, a 36-fold difference has been observed in steady-state levels of desipramine in patients on a standard dose, which was attributed to different rates of oxidation of imipramine (Chapter 9).[9] The basal rate of drug biotransformation of an individual is determined by genetic factors but, in addition, varies with age, sex, and environmental factors, such as diet, smoking, exposure to chemicals, disease states, and concurrent use of other drugs.

The importance of *genetic regulation* of drug biotransformation was revealed in studies of commonly used clinical drugs in dizygotic and monozygotic twins.[10] Little variation in the elimination half-lives was observed in monozygotic twins, but marked variation was observed between dizygotic twins (6- to 22-fold). Thus, hereditary differences in the amount or structure of key metabolizing enzymes may result in significant variations in the rate of drug biotransformation. This variability can be of two distinct types, continuous or discontinuous. The former is more common and arises when inherited characteristics are controlled by several genes of small effect (i.e., multifactorial inheritance). The distribution of the given characteristic in the population will show a continuous variation and will yield a unimodal or Gaussian distribution curve. On the other hand, where a characteristic depends on a single gene of major effect, a bi- or trimodal distribution in the population may be observed. This monofactorial inheritance is much less common and so far has been restricted to a few specific examples, the best known of which is the hepatic enzyme *N*-acetyltransferase. For example, 60% of Europeans are "slow acetylators," and the remaining 40% "rapid acetylators," in contrast to 80–90% rapid acetylators in most Asian populations.[11] So far, this polymorphism has not been shown to affect psychotropic drugs.

A more important polymorphism with regard to psychopharmacology is that of the CYP2D6 isoenzyme involved in the oxidative metabolism of a considerable number of drugs, including psychoactive drugs such as amitriptyline, nortriptyline, imipramine, desipramine, fluoxetine, paroxetine, perphenazine, thioridazine, remoxipride, risperidone, trazodone, and venlafaxine (Table 1). Approximately 5–10% of Caucasians and 1% of Asians are deficient in this enzyme and are known as "poor metabolizers" or PM phenotypes, as compared with the normal "extensive metabolizers" or EM phenotypes. Individuals who are PMs will exhibit greater bioavailability, greater plasma concentrations, prolonged elimination half-lives, and possibly exaggerated pharmacological responses from standard dose regimens. In addition, a small proportion of the population have been identified as "ultra-rapid metabolizers" (URM) with extremely high CYP2D6 activity. These subjects fail to respond to treatment due to excessively low plasma concentrations[12] and in some circumstances could mistakenly be suspected of noncompliance. Another polymorphism involved in the metabolism of a smaller number of psychoactive drugs such as citalopram, diazepam, imipramine, and possibly moclobemide is the mephenytoin hydroxylation polymorphism (Table 1). The proportion of PMs for this polymorphic enzyme (CYP2C19) is reported to be 18% of Japanese, 19% of African-Americans, 8% of Africans, and 3–5% of Caucasian subjects.[13] Further exploration of drug biotransformation in ethnic groups has indicated other subtle differences; for example, in the case of CYP2D6, Chinese EMs have slightly slower metabolism rates than Caucasian EMs; lower activity of CYP1A2 has been reported in black compared to white subjects; and lower activity of CYP3A4 has been reported in Indian/Bangladeshi subjects compared to Europeans.[14] The latter isoenzyme may account for up to 60% of all CYP450s in human liver and has the widest substrate specificity, metabolizing many drugs. With regard to psychoactive drugs, overall the data suggest that drug doses should be lower in Asians compared to Caucasians to achieve similar steady-state concentrations. However, there are marked interindividual variabilities in all ethnic groups.

Drug biotransformation also *varies with age*, especially at the two extremes, the very young and the very old. Variation of drug biotransformation in the neonate and in children is discussed in Section V. In the elderly there may be a diminished dose requirement for many drugs[15]; for example, significantly higher concentrations of paroxetine and citalopram have been reported in the elderly compared to the young receiving the same dose rate.[16] Population studies failed to show any effect of age on CYP2D6 and CYP2C19 metabolism, but an increased incidence of PMs was observed in elderly unmedicated African-Americans.[12] Age and changes in the environment may alter the activity of CYP1A2, which is inducible by polycyclic aromatic hydrocarbons such as are present in

TABLE 1. Some Substrates, Inhibitors, and Inducers of Human CYP450 Isoenzymes[a]

Enzyme	Substrates	Inhibitors	Inducers	Genetic polymorphism
CYP1A2	Amitryptiline, caffeine, clomipramine, clozapine, fluvoxamine, haloperidol, imipramine, phenacetin, tacrine, theophylline, verapamil, *R*-warfarin	Cimetidine, fluvoxamine, grapefruit juice, viloxazine, fluoroquinolones, furafylline	Cigarette smoke, cabbage (etc.), barbecued meat, polycyclic aromatic hydrocarbons	Possible
CYP2C9	Diclofenac, phenytoin, piroxicam, tenoxicam, tetrahydrocannabinol, ticrynafen, tienilic acid, tolbutamide, torsemide, *S*-warfarin	Sulfaphenazole, phenytoin, sulfinpyrazone, ketoconazole, fluconazole	Rifampin, barbiturates	Possible
CYP2C19	Citalopram, clomipramine, cycloguanil, diazepam, hexobarbital, imipramine, lansoprazole, *S*-mephenytoin, mephobarbital, moclobemide, omeprazole, pentamidine, propranolol	Tranylcypromine, sertraline, ketoconazole, moclobemide	Rifampin	Yes
CYP2D6	Amitriptyline, brofaromine, clomipramine, codeine, debrisoquin, desipramine, dextromethorphan, encainide, flecainide, fluoxetine, haloperidol, imipramine, maprotiline, metoprolol, mianserin, nefazodone, nortriptyline, paroxetine, perphenazine, propafenone, propranolol, remoxipride, risperidone, sparteine, thioridazine, trazodone, venlafaxine	Amitriptyline, chloroquine, chlorpromazine, cimetidine, clomipramine, desipramine, desmethylcitalopram, dextropropoxyphene, diphenhydramine, flecainide, fluoxetine, fluphenazine, haloperidol, imipramine, meclobemide, methotrimeprazine, metoclopramide, metoprolol, mexiletine, nicardipine, norfluoxetine, nortriptyline, paroxetine, phenylcyclopropylamine, pindolol, primaquine, propafenone, propranolol, quinidine, quinine, sertraline, thioridazine, timolol, trifluperidol	Unknown	Yes
CYP2E1	Ethanol, dapsone, halothane, chlorzoxazone, isoflurane, enflurane	Disulfiram	Ethanol, isoniazid	Probable
CYP3A4	Alfentanil, alprazolam, amiodarone, amitriptyline, astemizole, carbamazepine, clomipramine, cyclophosphamide, cyclosporin, dexamethasone, dextromethorphan, erythromycin, felodipine, imipramine, lidocaine, lovastatin, midazolam, nefazodone, omeprazole, quinidine, retinoic acid, sertraline, terfenadine, triazolam, verapamil, vinblastine	Cimetidine, erythromycin, ethinylestradiol, fluconazole, fluoxetine, fluvoxamine, grapefruit juice, ketoconazole, nefazodone, paroxetine, progestins, sertraline, troleandromycin	Carbamazepine, dexamethasone, phenobarbital, phenytoin, rifampin, sulfamethazine, sulfinpyrazone	No

[a]Data from Refs. 8, 12, 13, and 14.

cigarette smoke. The influence of *smoking* (Chapter 11) on drug biotransformation has been extensively studied.[17,18] Most human studies have indicated that heavy smoking caused increased metabolism of imipramine, haloperidol, chlorpromazine, fluphenazine, thiothixene, nicotine, pentazocine, caffeine, and theophylline but not of diazepam, nortriptyline, pethidine, and phenytoin. Diet is also an important source of inter- and intraindividual variability in human drug biotransformation.[17] Cruciferous vegetables such as cabbage and brussels sprouts, barbecued food, and high-protein, low-carbohydrate diets induced CYP1A2 and stimulated the metabolism of model drugs, such as theophylline and phenacetin. Grapefruit juice has also been demonstrated to be a potent inhibitor of CYP3A4 and possibly CYP1A2, causing clinically significant increases in the bioavailability of felodipine due to inhibition of first-pass metabolism.[19] This interaction is probably not limited to felodipine and other dihydropyridine calcium antagonists, but similar effects on psychotropics remain to be demonstrated. Inhibition of drug biotransformation may result in exaggerated and prolonged responses, with an increased risk of toxicity. Cimetidine, widely used in the treatment of peptic ulcers [but with important psychotropic side effects (Chapter 13)], is a potent inhibitor of a number of the CYP450 isoenzymes (Table 1) involved in the oxidation of drugs such as theophylline, nifedipine, phenytoin, carbamazepine, valproate, and many benzodiazepines (Chapters 11 and 12).[18] The mechanism of action of this apparent competitive inhibition involves the binding of cimetidine's imidazole group to the heme moiety of the P450 enzyme, thereby reducing the interaction with other substrates. Similarly, ketoconazole, which also contains an imidazole group, is also a potent inhibitor of a number of CYP450s, including CYP2C9, CYP2C19, and CYP3A4. However, the presence of an imidazole group is not a necessity for inhibition; for example, a number of psychoactive drugs such as the SSRIs (fluoxetine, paroxetine, and sertraline), thioridazine, and meclobemide are potent inhibitors of CYP2D6, increasing the plasma concentrations of coadministered tricyclic antidepressants, neuroleptics, and presumably other CYP2D6 substrates. Fluoxetine and sertraline (plus fluvoxamine) are also reported to inhibit CYP3A4, causing increased concentrations of benzodiazepines and carbamazepine, whereas fluvoxamine has also been associated with inhibition of CYP1A2, and thus the potential for important reactions with theophylline, amitriptyline, clozapine, clomipramine, and imipramine. In addition, noncompetitive inhibition of drug biotransformation may occur after exposure to toxic metals such as cadmium, mercury, lead, and arsenic.

The rate of drug biotransformation can also be increased by a number of drugs and chemicals, including *alcohol* (chronic alcoholism is a major cause of liver disease, leading to abnormal and deficient drug biotransformation). However, more importantly in adolescents, alcohol itself (independently of liver disease) also influences the biotransformation of drugs.[20] Acute exposure generally depresses the rate of biotransformation; thus, higher plasma concentrations of many benzodiazepines, including diazepam and chlordiazepoxide, occur with acute ethanol intake. In contrast, chronic alcohol intake has been associated with increased biotransformation (CYP2E1) and a lesser response for some drugs (Chapter 11). Similarly, chronic use of anticonvulsant drugs including phenobarbital, phenytoin, and carbamazepine and some antibiotics such as rifampin, sulfamethazine, and sulfinpyrazone leads to induction of CYP450s and low plasma concentrations of concurrent drugs metabolized by these isoenzymes. This may lead to insufficient efficacy.

Much of the data on the potential for drug–drug biotransformation *interactions* has been obtained through the use of in vitro models, such as human microsomal liver preparations. Caution must be exercised in the extrapolation of these data to the clinical situation. In vivo, the severity of any drug–drug interaction will depend on many factors, such as the route of drug administration (e.g., whether oral or intravenous); whether the clearance is dependent on hepatic blood flow or the capacity of the metabolizing enzymes; and the presence of metabolites. The clinical significance of potential interactions between drugs may only be determined by the concomitant use of these drugs in vivo in patients. To date, most information on drug–drug interactions and ethnic differences in the biotransformation of psychotropics has been confined to the CYP450 family, in particular, CYP2D6 (for reviews, see Refs. 12, 13, 14, and 21), but this is a rapidly expanding area of research and similar advances will occur with other biotransformation reactions such as those of the phase II systems.

III. PHARMACOKINETICS

The goal in drug therapy is to get the appropriate drug into the tissue (where the receptor is present) at the appropriate concentration for the appropriate length of time, in order to achieve the desired therapeutic response. If concentrations in the desired tissues are too low, therapy will be ineffective; if concentrations are too high, toxicity may result. Thus, the key determinants in effective therapy are appropriate tissue concentrations as a function of time. The tissue profile of a drug is determined by (1) the dosage regimen (i.e., the rate of drug input into the body), (2) the subsequent absorption, (3) the distribution, and (4) the elimination of the drug. The study of the relationship between drug input rate and the time course of drug concentration in the body is termed pharmacokinetics and encompasses drug absorption, distribution, and elimination.

From the previous section it is apparent that these pharmacokinetic processes are very variable between patients and within a patient, depending on disease state, diet, and concurrent drugs. *Thus, for many drugs (especially psychoactives) the relationship between dose and resulting therapeutic effect is quite unpredictable.* However, measurement of drug concentration in the body can help to overcome some of this variation and allow a more appropriate and rational adjustment of drug dose rate for an individual patient. Obviously, the most appropriate site to measure the drug concentration would be in the vicinity of its receptor, but this is not usually possible, and most often drug concentrations are measured in the blood (i.e., plasma). For many drugs (especially under steady-state conditions), the plasma concentration is a reasonable index of the concentration at the site of action.

The plasma therapeutic range (i.e., the concentration range that has the highest probability of giving the desired response with a minimum amount of side effects) has been defined for a number of psychoactive drugs, including anticonvulsants [phenytoin, phenobarbital, carbamazepine, and ethosuximide (Chapter 12)], antidepressants [amitriptyline plus nortriptyline, and desipramine (Chapter 9)], and antimanics [lithium and carbamazepine (Chapter 9)]. However, it must be emphasized that the *therapeutic range is only a statistical concept and is not rigidly applicable to all patients.* Some patients may have quite adequate clinical responses at drug concentrations below those considered therapeutic; likewise, some patients may require plasma concentrations that would be toxic for most. It must always be remembered that the ultimate determinant of drug efficacy is not achievement of a plasma concentration within the therapeutic range but the achievement of the desired therapeutic effect. Obviously, if the optimal drug dose regimen can be established directly by accurate quantitation of its pharmacological actions (such as the reduction in blood pressure during antihypertensive therapy), that is the preferred method of individualization of dose rate, and drug concentration measurements are not necessary. However, for a drug like lithium, which exhibits a small difference between the concentration that has therapeutic benefit and that which is toxic (i.e., a low therapeutic index) and where the therapeutic endpoint is difficult to determine or is arrived at over several days, a knowledge of its pharmacokinetics and therapeutic drug monitoring is essential for its safe clinical use. For most psychotropics, which, in general, have high therapeutic ratios and highly variable blood levels, the therapeutic range is most useful only in cases of non-response or unexpected toxicity.

The most important pharmacokinetic parameters are (1) the apparent volume of distribution, (2) the plasma clearance, and (3) the elimination half-life. Some knowledge of these parameters is useful for the most effective use of many drugs.

A. Apparent Volume of Distribution

The concept of distribution volume is used to relate the plasma drug concentration to the dose administered (if no elimination has occurred) or to the amount of drug in the body. The apparent volume of distribution (V) of a drug can be defined as a volume into which all the drug in the body would appear to be distributed to achieve a concentration the same as that in the plasma. For most drugs, this does not represent a true anatomical volume, as drugs are taken up to different extents by various organs and tissues, depending on the nature of the tissue and the physicochemical properties of the drug. For example, fat-soluble drugs such as nortriptyline, which are avidly taken up by tissues, have a large volume of distribution of 1500 liters, which is many times the actual anatomical volume of the body; on the other hand, lipophobic drugs such as the antibiotic gentamicin, which are ionized and are more or less confined to the interstitial fluid, have a small volume of distribution of 17 liters, considerably less than the total body volume.

The volume of distribution can be used to estimate the loading dose required initially to produce a target concentration (C_t):

$$\text{Loading dose} = VC_t \tag{1}$$

B. Clearance

Elimination of drugs depends mainly on two processes: biotransformation by the liver and excretion by the kidney. The efficiency of elimination by these organs or any other organ is measured by clearance (CL). It is commonly observed that the elimination rate of a drug is proportional to its concentration (C); i.e., it is a first-order process (provided the process of elimination is not saturated).

The constant of proportionality is the clearance and thus:

$$\text{Rate of elimination} = \text{CL} \cdot C$$

Hence,

$$\text{CL} = \frac{\text{elimination rate}}{C} \tag{2}$$

The units of clearance are volume per time (e.g., ml/min or liters/hr). An alternative definition of clearance is the volume of plasma from which a drug is irreversibly removed per unit time. For any particular organ, the physiological determinants of drug clearance are (1) organ blood flow and (2) the inherent ability of the organ to extract the drug from the blood. As applied to the liver, the clearance of a drug could be determined either by hepatic blood flow or by the capacity of the drug-metabolizing enzymes of the liver.

1. Dosage, Clearance, and Half-life

The clearance of drugs by various organs (liver, kidney) and tissue is also additive. If known, the systemic clearance of a drug may be used to determine the dosage rate required to maintain a desired steady-state plasma concentration (C_{ss}) by the following equation:

$$\text{Maintenance dose rate} = \text{CL} \cdot C_{ss} \tag{4}$$

In the past, the elimination half-life ($t_{1/2}$), which is the time for the blood concentration to fall by 50%, has been used as an index of elimination. However, in many situations, $t_{1/2}$ is a poor index of drug elimination as it is a hybrid parameter depending not only on the elimination processes (clearance) but also on the volume through which the drug is distributed. Thus, it can be shown that $t_{1/2}$ is directly proportional to the volume of distribution and inversely related to clearance, as described by the following equation:

$$t_{1/2} = (\ln 2)V/\text{CL} \tag{5}$$

However, $t_{1/2}$ is a useful parameter for the determination of a suitable dosage interval (see following section) and also, on cessation of dosing, of the time required to totally eliminate the drug. In theory, owing to the first-order kinetics, an infinite time would be required to eliminate drug totally from the body, but in practice it is useful to note that 50% of drug is removed in $t_{1/2}$, 75% in two $t_{1/2}$, 87.5% in three $t_{1/2}$, and 93.75% in four $t_{1/2}$. Thus, after an interval of time corresponding to four $t_{1/2}$, less than 10% remains in the body, and this is conveniently regarded as the total elimination time. Similarly, *the time required to attain the steady-state situation during repeated dosing is taken as four $t_{1/2}$.*

C. Multiple Dosing and Steady-State Drug Concentrations

Most drugs are not given in a single isolated dose but are administered in a repetitive or chronic fashion over a prolonged period when the aim is to have a sustained therapeutic level over several days or weeks without rising to toxic levels. If doses are administered at widely spaced intervals or if elimination of the drug is very rapid, most of the drug will be eliminated before the next dose is given. Therefore, the more common situation is that in which the dosage interval is sufficiently short to allow a buildup of the drug in the body to therapeutic levels and also achieve a "steady state." The latter occurs when the rate of drug administration equals the rate of elimination, such that there is no net change in the plasma concentration with time. As drug enters the body, some is removed, but the concentration continues to rise, as does the elimination rate (CL·C). After four $t_{1/2}$, >90% of the steady-state concentration has been achieved, irrespective of the input rate. Thereafter, if drug input is kept constant and there is no change in elimination rate (e.g., by enzyme induction), input is continuously balanced by elimination and the steady state is maintained. The magnitude of the steady-state concentration (C_{ss}) achieved is a function of the dose rate, the systemic CL, and the bioavailability (F), as shown by the following equation (where D is the repeated dose and T is the interval between doses):

$$C_{ss} = \frac{F \cdot D}{T \cdot CL} \tag{6}$$

During continued oral administration, a true steady-state concentration is not achieved, but rather there is a series of peaks and troughs within a dosing interval. The magnitude of the difference between peak and trough concentration is determined by (1) frequency of dosing, (2) absorption rate, and (3) the elimination $t_{1/2}$. Thus, a drug that is slowly absorbed will not have as exaggerated a peak-and-trough difference as would the identical dose given in a formulation that was rapidly absorbed in the bloodstream. The acceptable magnitude of the peak-and-trough differences is primarily defined by a drug's therapeutic index (i.e., the ratio between the therapeutic and toxic levels). If a drug has a very large therapeutic index [e.g., most neuroleptics (Chapter 10)], it may be administered infrequently in large doses, where high and low concentrations are acceptable for therapeutic effect without producing serious toxic side effects. In contrast, if a drug has a narrow therapeutic index, or where high concentrations are associated with serious toxicity [e.g., lithium and antidepressants (Chapter 9)], it must be given in smaller doses on a more frequent basis in order to maintain therapeutic levels without producing concentrations that cause toxic side effects. In clinical practice, the choice of dosage interval usually represents a compromise between the desire to minimize between-dose variations and the inconvenience of frequent dosing. With many drugs, the extent of fluctuation in concentration is clinically acceptable when the interval between doses does not exceed the $t_{1/2}$, which means that the ratio of peak to trough concentration will be less than 2. Some of the problems of frequent dosing and taking medication during the night may be overcome by the use of sustained-release dose forms, which are available for some drugs that have short $t_{1/2}$. The purpose of such preparations is to reduce the dosing frequency to make therapy more convenient and thus promote better patient compliance. In addition, by maintaining a relatively constant concentration of the drug in plasma, excessive peaks of concentration are avoided and side effects that may be associated with peak concentrations might be lessened. Most psychotropic drugs, however, are long-acting (i.e., $t_{1/2} > 20$ hr); exceptions are lithium and stimulants, for which attempts to develop sustained-release forms had mixed results (Chapter 8).

D. Saturation Kinetics

In the foregoing discussion it has been assumed that all the systems operating on the drug are first-order. This means that the pharmacokinetic parameters (i.e., CL, V, $t_{1/2}$, and F) are independent of drug concentration. Most drugs are administered therapeutically in amounts that lead to concentrations well below saturation levels of the eliminating systems, and drug elimination is always proportional to the concentration present (rate out = $C_{ss} \cdot CL$). Under these conditions, drug accumulation is a linear function of dose, and any change in dose rate will produce proportional changes in C_{ss}. Some drugs do not have such linear characteristics, the most common cause of which is the limited capacity of their metabolizing enzyme systems. In some situations, drug concentrations can rise sufficiently high to cause saturation of the enzyme system, causing the elimination to occur at a maximum constant rate (i.e., zero-order kinetics), independent of any increases in drug concentration. Thus, for some drugs, upon increasing the dose, the elimination rate increases only until saturation occurs; then a constant elimination rate will be achieved (i.e., Michaelis–Menten kinetics, which is a mixture of first- and zero-order kinetics), and drug accumulation will not be readily predictable. Once saturation has been reached, the plasma concentration

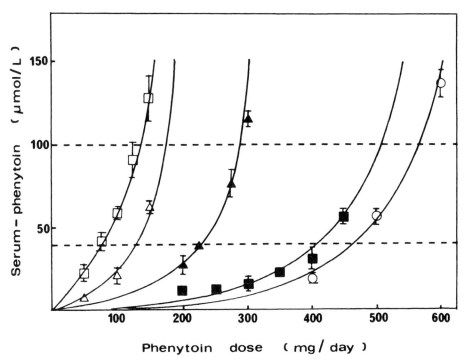

FIGURE 2. Relationship between phenytoin dose and steady-state concentration in five epileptic patients. The dashed lines represent the therapeutic range. (Reproduced with permission from Richens and Dunlop, *Lancet* 1975.)

will increase disproportionately with subsequent dosing. In addition, the time required to reach the steady state will increase with the increasing $t_{1/2}$. Well-known examples of compounds whose metabolism becomes saturated at clinically achievable concentrations include alcohol and phenytoin.

Figure 2 illustrates the relationship observed between dose and C_{ss} for phenytoin, which exhibits Michaelis–Menten kinetics within the therapeutic range.[22] Once the maximum capacity of the metabolizing enzyme system has been surpassed, small increases in the dose lead to disproportionately large increases in C_{ss}, and may bring a subtherapeutic level into the toxic range for some patients. Since the individual capacity for metabolizing phenytoin varies, prediction of the dose required to achieve a desired plasma steady-state concentration is difficult, and therapeutic drug monitoring is necessary to individualize the dose rate for each patient. The zero-order kinetics of alcohol also result in a number of deaths each year in adolescents (Chapter 11).

IV. TIME COURSE OF PHARMACOLOGICAL EFFECT

A complete description of the way in which the plasma concentration of a drug changes with time does not, by itself, predict how the pharmacological effect will change with time. In fact, the pharmacological effect may often follow a very different time course from the plasma concentration. Possible reasons for this divergence are considered in the following sections.

A. Nonlinear Concentration–Response Curve

The intensity of the pharmacological effect increases in a nonlinear fashion until a maximum is reached. In the range of 20–80% of maximum response, there is usually an approximately linear relationship between the intensity of the pharmacological effect and the logarithm of the drug concentration. Appreciable changes in response only occur during the period when the drug concentrations are within this range. Changes of drug concentration above or below this range will result in very little alteration in the intensity of drug effect (always providing, of course, that the concentration is well below the toxic level).

B. Slow Equilibration with Site of Drug Action

After a single dose, the concentration–time profile of the drug in the tissue where the receptor resides may be very different from the plasma concentration–time profile. For example, if the drug experiences a slow uptake and equilibration into the tissue where it elicits its response, the concentration in the plasma may be falling but that within the tissue still rising to reach a maximum. For example, the maximum effect of lysergic acid diethylamide (LSD) on mental performance occurs 30 min after the peak concentration in plasma but coincides with the peak tissue concentration and declines in parallel with tissue concentrations. Thus, although a significant relationship may exist between tissue concentration and response, this is not apparent from the plasma drug concentration.

C. Presence of Active Metabolites

The presence of active metabolites can often distort the concentration–response relationship for unchanged drug, and hence the expected time course of drug action. Where active metabolites are more slowly eliminated from the body than parent drug, it may be difficult to relate the changes in plasma concentration of parent drug to changes in response. After repeated doses, the active metabolite may accumulate to a greater extent than unchanged parent and be responsible for most of the effect. For many of the benzodiazepines [diazepam, chlordiazepoxide (Chapter 11)], the tricyclic antidepressants [amitriptyline, imipramine (Chapter 9)], and the selective serotonin uptake inhibitor fluoxetine, which are metabolized to active metabolites, the $t_{1/2}$ of the parent drug may have little relationship to the time course of pharmacological response; for example, fluoxetine has a $t_{1/2}$ of 1–4 days, whereas for the active metabolite norfluoxetine, $t_{1/2}$ is 7–15 days. Thus, on repeated dosing, the plateau concentration of norfluoxetine (and maximum response) might be expected to occur at 4–8 weeks. Similarly, on halting therapy, therapeutic effects may outlast significant concentrations of parent drug by days or weeks, depending on the $t_{1/2}$ of the active metabolite.[23]

D. Indirect or Slow Biochemical Response

For some drugs, the elicited biochemical or physiological response may take time to develop, compared with the alterations in plasma drug concentrations. Such drugs may have time courses of drug action that have a complex relationship with the changes in drug plasma concentration. Similarly, where the drug effect is mediated by transcription factors that regulate gene expression, the response may lag far behind the initial drug presence (see Section VI).

V. PEDIATRIC VARIATIONS IN PHARMACOKINETICS

Generally, childhood has been classified into four discrete periods: the neonatal period (premature and full-term neonates up to 1 month postnatal age), infancy (1–12 months), childhood (1–10 years), and adolescence (11–15 years). Although these age groupings are convenient for comparative purposes, their physiological validity must be treated with caution. The fundamental characteristic that sets the fetus, infant, and child apart from the mature adult is the process of differentiation, growth, and development, which can have a significant influence on a drug's pharmacokinetic profile and pharmacodynamic response. Owing to the development and availability of sophisticated instrumental methods for the measurement of drugs in biological fluids, most attention has focused on the differences in pharmacokinetics and metabolite profiles in the different stages of childhood.[24,25]

A. Absorption

The extent and rate of drug absorption after oral administration is determined by the state of the GI system, including gastric acidity, emptying time, and motility. Postnatally, gastric acid secretion appears to display a biphasic pattern, with the highest acid concentration occurring within the first 10 days and the lowest between 10 and 30 days of extrauterine life. The lower limits of adult values are approached by 3 months of age. Motility of the GI tract is also irregular and unpredictable, making extrapolation of adult absorption data to neonates very difficult. Accordingly, neonates absorb some drugs such as diazepam to the same extent as adults, whereas phenobarbital and phenytoin are absorbed to a lesser extent, and others such as ampicillin to a greater extent. In general, the rate of drug absorption in children and adolescents seems to resemble that in adults.

B. Distribution

Drug distribution in the body is influenced by a number of age-dependent factors such as the size of body water and fat compartments and the quantity and binding capacity of plasma and tissue proteins. The changes in body fat and water with aging have been well characterized.[26,27] Fat is an important repository for highly lipid-soluble compounds, and so the total bulk of body fat will affect distribution of drugs such as diazepam. For practical clinical purposes, it may be assumed that *children have less fat proportionately* than adults and thus will have smaller volumes of distribution for fat-soluble drugs.

Altered binding to plasma and tissue proteins is another possible source of variation in drug distribution and kinetics in the pediatric population. Many factors, such as the amount and type of protein present, the number of binding sites, the presence and amounts of endogenous compounds (e.g., free fatty acids, bilirubin), and the blood and tissue pH, may affect the binding of drugs to plasma and tissue proteins and do change during the various stages of childhood (e.g., low AAG concentration in the neonate). However, there is little information on the clinical significance of these binding changes.

C. Biotransformation and Excretion

The liver has a remarkable capacity for biotransforming foreign chemicals introduced into the body. Neonates, however, are not born with full metabolic capacity.[25,28] This gradually develops over the first year of life, with different enzyme systems developing at different rates. For example, CYP3A4 has been reported to be lowest in neonates and increases to maximum levels in adulthood.[14] Thus, during the perinatal period, the baby may be sensitive to the deleterious effects of drugs and compounds (e.g., bilirubin) that are eliminated by metabolism. In general, during infancy, the metabolic rates are markedly elevated, then gradually decline with age until puberty, when another important reduction in metabolic rate takes place. This decrease in metabolism rates to adult levels at puberty may parallel increases in steroid hormone production as the child matures.

The various renal functions also develop at different rates until adult function is achieved at about 1 year.[25] The GFR appears to increase dramatically after the first week of postnatal life, approaching adult values by 3–5 months of age, whereas tubular secretion and reabsorption capacity appear to mature at a much slower rate, approaching adult values at approximately 7 months. Blood flow, the driving force in renal elimination, approaches adult values by 5–12 months of life.

For clinical purposes, it can be assumed that, outside the first year of life, children will inactivate and eliminate drugs somewhat faster than adults and adolescents and in general require a greater mg/kg dose than adults to achieve the same response.

D. Response

Studies on pharmacological or clinical responses to drugs in children have not kept pace with pharmacokinetic studies, perhaps because of the difficulties experienced in quantitation of pharmacological response, especially in psychiatry. For this reason, the development of rational dosage regimens in much of pediatrics has been mostly based on drug concentrations rather than on pharmacological response. Evidence suggests that children may display altered *drug receptor sensitivity* relative to adults. Thus, the effective serum concentration ranges in children may be somewhat different from those in adults[29]; for example, there is evidence that children require a slightly lower therapeutic range for chlorpromazine, haloperidol, and phenytoin.[30] However, this lower therapeutic range in some instances may be due to *reduced plasma protein binding* and increased free fraction of drug rather than an increased receptor sensitivity. Further studies are necessary in this area.

VI. MECHANISMS OF DRUG ACTION (PHARMACODYNAMICS)

Pharmacodynamics is that part of pharmacology concerned with the mechanism(s) of drug action. The pharmacological response of a small number of drugs is due to their physicochemical properties; for example, anesthetic gases and solvents (Chapter 11) are lipid-soluble and therefore can dissolve in the nerve-cell membranes and may cause general anesthesia by altering the physical state of the membrane lipids and hence the excitability of the neuron/synapse. More commonly, drugs act by binding to a distinct site on a specific biological molecule.[31] These biological molecules must have molecular locales that are both spatially and energetically favorable for binding of specific drug molecules. So far, these drug binding sites have been situated on proteins, glycoproteins, or proteolipids. This is not surprising because of the strong tendency of proteins to undergo folding to form unique three-dimensional structures and thus form special binding sites of the correct three-dimensional shape to accommodate drug molecules. Common targets of drug action include the following.

A. Enzymes

Drugs that work by interacting with enzymes include the monoamine oxidase (MAO) inhibitors [e.g., the antidepressant phenelzine (Chapter 9)]. Inhibition of MAO, which normally breaks down noradrenaline, leads to increased brain concentrations of mono-amines and therapeutically to an elevation of mood.

B. Voltage-Gated Ion Channels

Voltage-gated ion channels are proteins that contain a water-filled pore that allows the passage of specific ions (e.g., K^+, Na^+, Ca^{2+}) across a membrane. The ion selectivity results from the charged groups on the channel's surface. Greater than a million ions per second can pass through an ion channel down an electrochemical gradient. They are voltage-dependent (i.e., changes in the electrical field across a membrane produce changes in the channel's molecular structure, resulting in the opening or closing of the channel) and are responsible for the electrical excitability of nerve cells and their processes.

Drugs that interact directly with voltage-dependent ion channels include the local anesthetics (e.g., lidocaine and chlorpromazine), which are reversible Na^+-channel blockers. They have a higher affinity for Na^+ channels in the open (rather than closed) state; therefore, they block action potentials and nerve impulse conduction and lead to a local anesthetic action. Other drugs, such as nimodipine, are Ca^{2+}-channel blockers and may be useful in treating epilepsy; their psychiatric use is still experimental. Most psychotropic drugs affecting ion channels [e.g., benzodiazepines (Chapters 11 and 15)] do so indirectly through receptors (see below).

C. Reuptake Mechanisms

Many endogenous molecules (e.g., neurotransmitters) are inactivated and removed from their site of action by reuptake mechanisms (mediated by an energy-dependent active-transport system) back into the presynapse, or cell, where they are inactivated. Many cyclic antidepressant drugs [e.g., imipramine (Chapter 9)] work by blocking reuptake of the neurotransmitters serotonin and noradrenaline.

D. Receptors

Many drugs work by binding to specific receptors for endogenous ligands (i.e., body chemicals such as hormones, neurotransmitters, growth factors, and cytokines) and either mimic the action of the natural ligand or prevent (block) the ligand from acting.[31,32]

Receptors have the dual ability of recognizing (binding) a drug with both sensitivity and specificity (selectivity) and then converting the process of recognition into a signal to produce a drug effect. Receptors have the properties of (1) saturability (since there is a finite number of receptors), (2) specificity toward a particular chemical structure (i.e., only certain ligands bind strongly), and (3) reversibility.

The interaction between drug and receptor can be described by (1) affinity, which is a measure of the attraction of the drug to a receptor—if a drug has a high affinity for a receptor, low concentrations of drug can bind, whereas with low affinity, high concentrations of drug are required—and (2) efficacy (intrinsic activity), which is the ability of a drug–receptor combination to produce an effect. Maximum efficacy is given an arbitrary value of 1, and no efficacy is given a value of 0.

When a drug binds to a receptor, it can act as (1) an agonist, (2) a partial agonist, or (3) an antagonist. An agonist binds to a receptor to produce an effect that mimics that of the natural ligand. A full agonist produces maximum effect (efficacy = 1). An agonist usually has both high affinity for the receptor and high efficacy. A partial agonist fails to produce a maximum effect even when all receptors are occupied (0 < efficacy < 1). A partial agonist can have high affinity for a receptor but less than maximal efficacy. An antagonist binds to a receptor (usually with high affinity) but produces no biological effect (efficacy = 0). Antagonists are further subdivided into the following categories: (a) competitive, where the drug competes with the agonist for the same receptor site; (b) noncompetitive, where the drug does not bind to the same site as the agonist and therefore the antagonism is not surmountable or reversible (e.g., botulism); (c) chemical, where one drug binds to another and inactivates it; and (d) physiological, which involves the activation of opposing regulatory pathways [e.g., the use of antiparkinsonian agents such as benztropine for extrapyramidal effects of neuroleptics (Chapter 10)].

1. Dose–Response Curve

The most common way of portraying the effect of a drug on a tissue is the dose–response or concentration–response curve. Responses to low drug concentrations producing an effect on a tissue (or on behavior for that matter) by binding to a finite population of receptors usually increase in direct proportion to the concentration. However, as concentrations continue to increase, the incremental response diminishes; finally, at higher concentrations, the response reaches an asymptote (flattens out) because all available receptors producing the response are saturated. This results in the typical hyperbolic concentration–response curve.

Such a curve is difficult to fit to experimental data, particularly when appreciable scatter is present. Thus, more typically the concentration–response curve is plotted with concentrations on a log scale, which results in essentially a straight line between about 20 and 80% of the maximal response. Such concentration–response curves can also be used to determine the EC_{50} (concentration of drug producing half the maximal effect) and to analyze the interactions of agonists and antagonists and discern if a drug is an antagonist or a partial agonist (Fig. 3A). The addition of a competitive antagonist (X) causes a parallel shift to the right in the agonist (W) concentration–response curve without altering the maximal response. The addition of a noncompetitive antagonist (Y) reduces the maximal response and causes a flattening of the agonist concentration–response curve. The addition of a partial agonist (Z) causes a potentiation at low and an inhibition at higher agonist concentrations (see Fig. 3A).

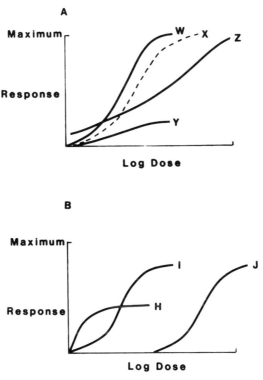

FIGURE 3. (A) Effects of a competitive antagonist (X), a noncompetitive antagonist (Y), and a partial agonist (Z) on the concentration–response curve of an agonist (W). Note that the competitive antagonist produces a parallel shift in the agonist dose–response curve without altering the maximal response. The partial agonist works as an agonist at low concentrations and as a competitive antagonist at higher concentrations. The noncompetitive antagonist greatly reduces the maximal effect of the agonist. (B) Dose–response curves for three drugs H, I, and J. The most potent is H, but I and J have greater efficiency.

Another important concept in drug–receptor interactions is potency, which is a measure of the dose or concentration of drug required to produce a given response. For example, in Fig. 3B, the most potent drug is H, as it produces 50% of the maximal response at the lowest concentration. Note that *potency differs from efficacy*, which is a measure of the size of the drug effect (e.g., clinically, a potent drug may have only a small effect). In Fig. 3B, drugs I and J have greater efficacy than drug H.

2. Receptor Number and Distribution

In many cases, a full agonist does not have to occupy all receptors to produce a maximal effect, because there are "spare" receptors (*receptor reserve*). The number and distribution of receptors are also important in determining the magnitude of the drug's effect; for example, if a drug needs to occupy 30 receptors to produce a maximal effect and tissue M has 40 receptors, the drug will act like a full agonist on this tissue (i.e., it produces a maximal effect). However, if tissue N has 20 receptors, the drug will act like a partial agonist on this tissue (i.e., it produces a submaximal effect). This is why changes in receptor number (up- or downregulation) have important implications for drug action. Chronic administration of drugs can influence receptor number: (1) in general, chronic antagonist treatment produces an increase in receptors (*upregulation*); for example, chronic neuroleptic administration is thought sometimes to cause an increase in dopamine receptors, leading to tardive dyskinesia (Chapter 10); (2) conversely, in general, chronic agonist exposure produces a decrease in receptor number (*downregulation*); for example, chronic diazepam produces a decrease in GABA receptors. Changes in receptor number and/or affinity can be brought about by a number of mechanisms such as receptor internalization, desensitization producing changes in affinity, and changes in the synthesis of receptors (brought about by changes in gene expression). Thus, receptor number or affinity is not static but dynamic, changing in response to environmental signals (e.g., drugs).

3. Receptor Subtypes

Many neurotransmitters, which convey information from one nerve cell to another, bind to several receptor sites to provide varied biological effects[33]; for example, serotonin binds to receptor subtypes 5-HT$_{1A}$, 5-HT$_{1B}$, 5-HT$_{1C}$, 5-HT$_2$, and 5-HT$_3$, each encoded by a different gene. This allows for a diversity in response to a single chemical and is one cause of unwanted (side) effects of drugs such as the extrapyramidal effects from neuroleptics.

4. Modeling of Drug–Receptor Interactions

Over the years a number of mathematical models have been proposed for drug–receptor interactions which are not exclusive.[32] Simple occupancy theory states that the magnitude of the biological response is directly proportional to the amount of drug–receptor complex formed (i.e., affinity of drug for receptor alone predicts biological response). Modifications to simple occupancy theory have suggested that the drug effect is proportional to both affinity and efficacy, whereas rate theory proposes that the drug effect is proportional to the rate of receptor occupation (i.e., the process of receptor occupation, rather than the occupation itself, determines effect). More recent "two-state" models suggest that receptors exist in equilibrium in active and inactive states. Agonists have a higher affinity for the active state, whereas antagonists have a higher affinity for the inactive state, and partial agonists have equal affinities for both states. Mobile or floating receptor models suggest that the drug–receptor complex may interact with a number of effectors in the membrane and that coupling to these effectors is required for drug action.

E. Mechanisms of Receptor Action

When an agonist drug binds to a receptor, it causes some effect in the cell, which is related to drug affinity and efficacy and receptor number, type, and distribution. However, the question remains: how does an agonist drug, by binding to a receptor, cause a biological effect? The mechanism differs depending on the type of receptor.[34–39]

1. Ligand-Gated Ion Channels

Ligand-gated ion channels mediate fast responses inside nerve cells. These are transmembrane proteins with 50% of their length outside the membrane. They are generally constructed of a number of subunits packed together to form an aqueous pore in the center. When a drug (ligand) binds to this type of receptor, it produces a structural change in the subunits comprising the receptor, which opens or closes the ion channel to produce an ion flux, and hence the drug effect.

2. G-Protein-Linked Receptors

G-protein-linked receptors mediate slower responses.[40] G-proteins are guanine nucleotide-binding regulatory proteins, which couple receptors to biochemical second messengers and/or ion channels. G-proteins are composed of three subunits (α, β, and γ). In the absence of a drug, GDP binds to the α-subunit of the complex and the G-protein is inactive. When an agonist drug binds, it produces a replacement of GDP with GTP, and the α subunit dissociates from the $\beta\gamma$ complex, leading to the drug effect. This might involve direct activation of an ion channel (e.g., $GABA_B$ receptor) or generation of another molecule, a second messenger (e.g., D_1 receptor). To terminate the signal, intrinsic GTPase activity replaces the GTP with GDP, and the G-protein returns to its inactive state. There are a number of different types of G-proteins (e.g., G_o, G_i, G_s), which produce different effects; for example, G_i-proteins inhibit adenylate cyclase, whereas G_s-proteins activate adenylate cyclase and elevate levels of the second messenger cyclic AMP. G-protein-coupled receptors tend to be single-unit proteins with seven transmembrane domains. Receptor diversity can be generated by alternative splicing. Activation of some types of receptors can generate third messengers that regulate gene expression.

3. Second and Third Messengers

A number of G-protein-linked receptors produce their effects by inducing the production within cells of second messengers (e.g., cyclic AMP, cyclic GMP, Ca^{2+}/calmodulin, diacylglycerol, arachidonic acid). Second messengers work by activating protein kinases (e.g., protein kinase A, protein kinase C, calmodulin kinase II), which are molecules that phosphorylate proteins, leading to altered structure and function. Protein kinases can phosphorylate constitutively expressed transcription factors (these are proteins that bind to DNA and regulate gene transcription; e.g., cyclic AMP response element binding protein), which activate them and allow them to alter gene transcription. These constitutively expressed transcription factors can directly alter the transcription of structural proteins, enzymes, or receptors and/or can activate a second wave of transcription factor expression by binding to cis-acting elements on DNA (e.g., the cyclic AMP response element, TGACGTCA).[41] These transcription factors (trans-acting elements) themselves bind to certain cis-acting elements on DNA (e.g., the AP-1 site, TGACTCA, the target binding site for the Fos/Jun and Jun/Jun hetero- and homodimer transcription factors) and regulate the expression of target genes. Thus, drug activation of certain types of receptors that activate second messengers, protein kinases, and transcription factors can influence cellular gene expression and produce long-lasting cellular effects. Furthermore, many drugs can interact with different components of these receptor coupling mechanisms to produce their effects at the postreceptor level.

F. Speed of Response of Receptors

In the nervous system, the type of receptor activated influences the onset latency and the duration of the signal (drug action).

Therefore, different receptors mediate different responses in neurons. (1) Ligand-gated ion channel receptors (e.g., $GABA_A$) produce fast-onset responses lasting at most tens of milliseconds. (2) G-protein-linked receptors linked directly to ion channels (e.g., $GABA_B$) produce responses lasting hundreds of milliseconds. (3) G-protein-coupled receptors that generate second messengers (e.g., D_2 dopamine) produce responses lasting tens of seconds. (4) Receptors that produce increases in second messengers and third messengers produce responses lasting hours, days, or months, because these third messengers are transcription factors that regulate gene expression.

G. Summary of Mechanisms of Receptor Activation

Figure 4 summarizes the main routes whereby drug binding to membrane-bound receptors induces biological effects. Some receptors are themselves ligand-gated ion channels (e.g., $GABA_A$ receptor) so that drug binding opens or closes the channel, changing ion flux and causing the drug effect on the cell (1 in Fig. 4). An influx of ions can also generate second messengers. Drugs acting on this type of receptor generally produce quick-onset, short-lasting effects (e.g., neuronal hyperpolarization). Other receptors are linked to G-proteins that can be coupled to ion channels (2), again leading to changes in ion flux (e.g., A_1 adenosine receptors, $GABA_B$ receptors; these can be linked to the same G-protein along with $5-HT_{1A}$ receptors). Other G-protein-linked receptors generate second messengers (3) that activate protein kinases, which in turn phosphorylate specific target proteins. These target proteins can be ion channels, other enzymes, structural proteins, or receptors. Drugs working via these receptor signal transduction mechanisms produce slower-onset, longer-lasting effects. Protein kinases can also phosphorylate constitutively expressed transcription factors (4), which can either directly modify gene expression or activate immediate-early gene proteins (5), which then regulate the expression of late-effector genes (6) and lead to a long-lasting drug effect. Activation of these gene regulatory proteins by drugs may account for such effects as drug tolerance and dependence and for some drug side effects (e.g., tardive dyskinesia produced by neuroleptics).

Many types of molecules (e.g., neurotransmitters, peptide hormones) work on the types of receptors depicted in Fig. 4. However, many growth factors (e.g., epidermal growth factor) bind to cell membrane-bound receptors that have a drug recognition site as well as an intracellular catalytic domain, which provides an enzymatic function. Many of these are tyrosine kinases. Other receptors (e.g., the nerve growth factor receptor) bind their ligand and internalize it, and the receptor–ligand complex is transported retrogradely to the cell nucleus. Nerve growth factor is transported retrogradely by its receptor, down cholinergic axons in the brain to the nucleus, where the complex has its biological effects. Finally, steroid hormone receptors are intracellular. Steroid hormones, derived from cholesterol, are lipid-soluble and penetrate the cell membrane, bind to their receptors (which are transcription factors), and change gene expression inside cells.

Thus, drug action is greatly determined by the type of receptor activated (or blocked) by the drug. As our understanding of receptor signal transduction processes increases, the potential for novel drug action on these transducer molecules increases. Furthermore, with the recent developments in receptor cloning and reconstitution, our increased understanding of the regulation, structure, and function of drug receptors will have enormous potential for the development of new therapeutic agents.

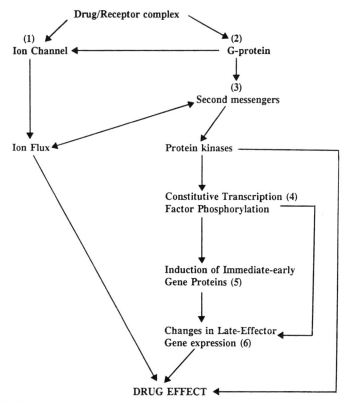

FIGURE 4. Summary of receptor/effector coupling to membrane-bound receptors.

REFERENCES

1. Pond SM, Tozer TN: First-pass elimination. Basic concepts and clinical consequences. *Clin Pharmacokinet* 9:1–25, 1984.
2. Merkle HP: Transdermal delivery systems. *Methods Find Exp Clin Pharmacol* 11:135–153, 1989.
3. Bates IP: Permeability of the blood brain barrier. *Trends Pharmacol Sci* 4:447–450, 1985.
4. Huang J, Oie S: Effect of intra-individual change in serum protein binding on the pharmacological response of *R*- and *S*-disopyramide in the rabbit. *Res Commun Chem Pathol Pharmacol* 41:243–253, 1983.
5. Rowland M: Plasma protein binding and therapeutic drug monitoring. *Ther Drug Monitor* 2:29–37, 1980.
6. Paxton JW: Alpha$_1$-acid glycoprotein and binding of basic drugs. *Methods Find Exp Clin Pharmacol* 5: 635–648, 1983.
7. Rollins DE: Pharmacokinetics and drug excretion in bile, in Benet LZ, Massoud N, Gambertoglio JG (eds): *Pharmacokinetic Basis for Drug Treatment.* New York, Raven Press, 1985, p 77.
8. Klassen CD (ed): *Casarett and Doull's Toxicology; The Basic Science of Poisons.* McGraw-Hill, New York, 1996.
9. Sjöqvist F, Bertilsson L: Clinical pharmacology of antidepressant drugs: Pharmacogenetics, in Usdin E, et al (eds): *Frontiers in Biochemical and Pharmacological Research in Depression.* New York, Raven Press, 1984, p 359.
10. Vesell ES: Pharmacogenetics. Introduction: Genetic and environmental factors affecting drug response in man. *Fed Proc* 31:1253–1258, 1972.
11. Clark DWJ: Genetically determined variability in acetylation and oxidation status; clinical implications. *Drugs* 29:342–345, 1985.

12. Meyer UA, Amrein R, Balant LP, et al.: Antidepressants and drug-metabolizing enzymes–expert group report. *Acta Psychiatr Scand* 93:71–79, 1996.
13. Nemeroff CB, DeVane CL, Pollock BG: Newer antidepressants and the Cytochrome P450 System. *Am J Psychiatry* 153:311–320, 1996.
14. Glue P, Banfield C: Psychiatry, psychopharmacology and P450s. *Human Psychopharmacol* 11:97–114, 1996.
15. Montamat SC, Cusack BJ, Vestal RE: Management of drug therapy in the elderly. *N Engl J Med* 321:303–309, 1989.
16. Catterson ML, Preskorn SH: Pharmacokinetics of selective serotonin reuptake inhibitors: Clinical relevance. *Pharmacol Toxicol* 78:203–208, 1996.
17. Sitar DS: Human drug metabolism in vivo. *Pharmacol Ther* 433:363–375, 1989.
18. Barry M, Feely J: Enzyme induction and inhibition. *Pharmacol Ther* 48:71–94, 1990.
19. Bailey DG, Arnold JMO, Spence JD: Grapefruit juice and drugs: How significant is the reaction? *Clin Pharmacokinet* 26:91–98, 1994.
20. Lane EA, Guthrie S, Linnoila M: Effects of ethanol on drug and metabolite pharmacokinetics. *Clin Pharmacokinet* 10:228–247, 1985.
21. Ereshefsky L: Drug–drug interactions involving antidepressants: Focus on venlafaxine. *J Clin Psychopharmacol* 16(suppl 2):37S-50S, 1996.
22. Richens A, Dunlop A: Serum phenytoin levels in the management of epilepsy. *Lancet* 2:247–248, 1975.
23. Garattini S: Active drug metabolites. An overview of their relevance in clinical pharmacokinetics. *Clin Pharmcokinet* 10:216–227, 1985.
24. Kearns GL, Reed MD: Clinical pharmacokinetics in infants and children: A reappraisal. *Clin Pharmacokinet* 17(suppl 1):29–67, 1989.
25. Morselli PL: Clinical pharmacology of the perinatal period at early infancy. *Clin Pharmacokinet* 17(suppl 1):13–28, 1989.
26. Friis-Hansen B: Body composition during growth: In vivo measurements and biochemical data correlated to differential anatomical growth. *Pediatrics* 47(suppl):264–274, 1971.
27. Friis-Hansen B: Water distribution in the foetus and new-born infant. *Acta Paediatr Scand* 305(suppl):7–11, 1983.
28. Burchell B, Coughtrie M, Jackson M, et al: Development of human liver UDP-glucuronosyltransferase. *Dev Pharmacol Ther* 13:70–77, 1989.
29. Boreus LO: Pharmacokinetics in children, in Boreus LO (ed): *Principles of Pediatric Pharmacology*. London, Churchill Livingstone, 1982, p 135.
30. Gilman JT: Therapeutic drug monitoring in the neonate and paediatric age group: Problems and clinical pharmacokinetic implications. *Clin Pharmacokinet* 19:1–10, 1990.
31. Lamble JW, Abbott AC (eds): *Receptors, Again*. Amsterdam, Elsevier Science Publishers, 1984.
32. Yamamura HI, Enna SJ, Kuhar MJ: *Neurotransmitter Receptor Binding*. New York, Raven Press, 1987.
33. Schofield PR, Shivers BD, Seeburg PH: The role of receptor subtype diversity in the CNS. *Trends Neurosci* 13:8–11, 1990.
34. Alberts B, Bray D, Lewis J, et al: *Molecular Biology of the Cell*, ed. 2. New York, Garland, 1989.
35. Neubig RR, Thomsen WJ: How does a key fit a flexible lock? Structure and dynamics in receptor function. *BioEssays* 11:136–141, 1989.
36. Webster RA, Jordan CC (eds): *Neurotransmitters, Drugs and Disease*. Oxford, Blackwell Scientific Publications, 1989.
37. Birdsall NJM: Receptor structure: The accelerating impact of molecular biology. *Trends Pharmacol Sci* 10:50–52, 1989.
38. Watson SP, James W: PCR and the cloning of receptor subtype genes. *Trends Pharmacol Sci* 10:346–347, 1989.
39. Turner AJ, Bachelard HS (eds): *Neurochemistry—A Practical Approach*. Oxford, IRL Press, 1987.
40. Neer EJ, Clapham DE: Roles of G protein subunits in transmembrane signalling. *Nature* 333:129–134.
41. Dragunow M, Currie RW, Faull RLM, et al: Immediate-early genes, kindling and long-term potentiation. *Neurosci Biobehav Rev* 13:301–313, 1989.

3

Prevalence of Drug Therapy

KENNETH D. GADOW, Ph.D.

I. INTRODUCTION

This book is a guide to psychotropic drug therapy for children and adolescents. But just how common is the medical prescription of such drugs at the moment? Is it too little or too much? Does clinical application precede scientific verification of safety and efficacy? Are recommendations for patient management generally followed in everyday clinical settings? This chapter examines these and related issues to the extent that available data will allow.

The initial impetus for determining the prevalence of pharmacotherapy for child and adolescent psychiatric disorders, particularly the disruptive behavior disorders, was to confirm or disprove allegations of overdiagnosis, and resultant overtreatment. It was thought that by knowing the number of children who were receiving medication, it would be possible to generate a rough estimate of the percentage of all cases receiving treatment. As it turned out, however, this was much more difficult than initially believed because of the inherent ambiguity of psychiatric diagnoses, the nonspecificity of drug effects, and the extraordinary difficulty in obtaining such information from individuals in community settings. Equally troublesome is the absence of a recognized standard for determining overuse. Two likely candidates are establishing that a patient is asymptomatic prior to, or unresponsive after or during treatment. Even if it were possible to conduct such assessments on a representative sample of patients, this would still not resolve all the conceptual problems associated with the notion of overprescribing. For example, if a child does not meet a specific set of diagnostic criteria for hyperactivity (or is not above cutoff on a particular diagnostic device) but nevertheless benefits from stimulant drug therapy, is this an example of overuse? If a child can be effectively withdrawn from medication and managed with a behavioral intervention, is this proof of unnecessary treatment? If medication is withdrawn and there is no change in symptom status, is this a case of overmedication or a failure to evaluate change in clinical progress? As these examples illustrate, the issue of

KENNETH D. GADOW, Ph.D. • Department of Psychiatry & Behavioral Science, State University of New York at Stony Brook, Stony Brook, New York 11794-8790

Practitioner's Guide to Psychoactive Drugs for Children and Adolescents (Second Edition), Werry and Aman, eds. Plenum Publishing Corporation, New York, 1999.

overmedication can only be meaningfully addressed by establishing fairly rigid criteria for diagnosis, the need for intervention, and inappropriate drug prescribing.

Data on the number of children receiving a specific agent are also of interest in determining the significance of specific clinical issues. A recent example is the report of desipramine-related fatalities in prepubertal children.[1-3] In this case, it would be useful (for many reasons) to know the number of children who are and have received this drug. Unfortunately, with the exception of data collected by private companies that monitor certain aspects of prescribing practices for commercial purposes,[4] there really is no national data base on the number of children receiving specific drug products for specific disorders and the duration of treatment.

A. Research Objectives

It should be emphasized that, from the outset, treatment prevalence surveys were much more than a simple exercise in head counting. Investigators were equally, if not more interested in a number of important issues pertaining to the way psychotherapeutic agents were prescribed, evaluated, and monitored in everyday clinical situations. Among the topics that have been addressed in treatment prevalence surveys are the pattern of treatment; physician, patient, and environmental characteristics and other psychosocial variables associated with drug use; and specific procedures for evaluating response to medication. Some investigators have also reported on the perceived efficacy and safety of specific drugs.

The term "pattern of treatment" has been used to refer to the relative frequency with which specific drugs are prescribed, dosage and schedule, polypharmacy, age at onset and duration of treatment, and the use of nondrug therapies prior to, concurrent with, or subsequent to drug treatment. These data have been used to determine whether drugs are being prescribed and used according to generally accepted standards and to identify aspects of treatment that sorely need additional study. The latter is particularly important given the fact that drugs are often prescribed for patients and disorders for which they are not specifically approved and the enormous gaps in the clinical literature with regard to empirically-based assessment procedures.

Some of the psychosocial variables that have been examined in treatment prevalence surveys have been socioeconomic status (SES), race, gender, and birth order. A recent study found that *parental* use of psychotropic medication and whether there are one or two parents in the household also may have significant effects on medication use by the children in these families.[5] Much attention has also been given to environmental variables (particularly in the case of individuals with developmental disabilities) associated with high rates of drug use. These data are generally used to identify specific patient populations that may be at unusual risk for inappropriate drug applications (e.g., children from low-income families) and patient characteristics that are associated with referral and treatment.

Another general topic that has been addressed by treatment prevalence surveys pertains to clinical practices in natural settings. Researchers have examined the sequence of events that lead to referral and diagnosis; interactions among the school, family, and physician during diagnosis, dosage adjustment, follow-up (monitoring), and the termination of medication; and specific procedures for evaluating and monitoring response to medication. The primary applications of these data have been the identification of inadequate treatment practices and the substantive base for arguments for the need for better professional training. These survey findings have also stimulated the formulation of empirically-based drug assessment programs, which are available in some specialty clinics.

B. Scope of the Review

This chapter presents a brief overview of treatment prevalence surveys of various disorders for which psychoactive drugs are prescribed. Because this area of study does not appeal to most scientists and is perceived to have low scientific status (especially when compared with the documentation of the safety and efficacy of drug products), there is generally little research on the prevalence and pattern of drug treatment for most behavior and seizure disorders or patient populations, with the notable exceptions of hyperactivity and individuals with mental retardation. The studies reviewed here vary considerably with regard to methodology, the time interval for which drug use data were collected, and geographic area, which makes meaningful comparisons between studies all but impossible. In deciding the general organization of this chapter, it seemed most logical to begin the discussion with those disabilities that account for the largest number of children receiving chronic drug therapy and to conclude with low-frequency disorders. No attempt has been made to address the numerous methodological issues associated with the collection and interpretation of treatment prevalence data. Readers interested in this topic are referred to another chapter by this author.[6]

As this book was going to press, the *Journal of Child and Adolescent Psychopharmacology* published a special feature that addresses drug prevalence and prescribing patterns in children and adolescents. Unfortunately, owing to publication deadlines, some of this material could not be included in the present chapter. Therefore, readers wanting more up-to-date information or a more comprehensive perspective of this topic are encouraged to consult Vol. 7 (issue no. 4) of this journal, published in 1997.

II. HYPERACTIVITY (ATTENTION-DEFICIT HYPERACTIVITY DISORDER)

The initial interest in the extent of psychotropic drug treatment for hyperactivity stemmed from both allegations and concerns about the unnecessary use of medication. The most celebrated example is a June 1970 newspaper story claiming that 5–10% of the 62,000 students in Omaha public schools were receiving stimulant drugs for hyperactivity.[7] It was later revealed that these figures referred to the number of children in programs for the learning disabled. Regardless, this newspaper account was the catalyst for a number of articles alleging that drugs were being prescribed in a capricious manner to large numbers of schoolchildren as a substitute for much-needed academic reform.[8–10] More recent publications show that this issue is still quite volatile.[11–13]

A. Early Studies

One of the earliest estimates of drug use for hyperactivity was reported by Stephen, Sprague, and Werry.[14,15] Questionnaires were mailed to 700 physicians in the Chicago area, and 255 were returned. On the basis of these physician reports, Stephen et al. estimated that between 2 and 4% of the public and private school enrollment were receiving medication for hyperactivity during the 1970–71 school year. Stimulants were the preferred therapeutic agents. The mean daily dose of methylphenidate was 16.5 mg for children between 6 and 10 years of age.

One early review of treatment prevalence studies of elementary-school-aged children examined the findings from five different geographic locations in the United States:[6] three on the East Coast (midstate New York; Queens, New York; Baltimore County, Maryland), one in the Midwest (Grand Rapids, Michigan), and one on the West Coast (East Bay area of San Francisco). In all studies, school personnel were asked to report the number of treated children, and in two surveys, parents of schoolchildren were also contacted and served as an additional source of information. The findings from these studies showed that prevalence of drug treatment varied from one geographic area to the next, with most studies reporting a prevalence between 1 and 2%. There was also considerable variability in the percentage of students receiving medication for schools within the same geographic locale.

Several variables were shown to account for some of the variability in reported prevalence of drug treatment within school systems and presumably for samples drawn from different geographic areas. Among these were the funding status of the school (public or private); the SES, race, and age of the students; whether the sample included special-education students; and both the year and time of year the data were collected. In general, the rates were lower for private schools, less affluent areas, older students, and schools without self-contained special-education classrooms.

B. Recent Surveys

The most extensive community surveys of drug treatment for hyperactivity (or any disorder for that matter) have been conducted by Safer and Krager in Baltimore County, Maryland, which has a total school enrollment ranging from 85,000 to 100,000 children and adolescents. School nurses were the source of the data base. The surveys began in 1971 and have been conducted biannually since that time.[16] The prevalence of treatment doubled every 4 to 7 years, and by 1987 6% of all public elementary school students were receiving medication for ADHD. The highest rates of drug use have repeatedly been found in third-graders (8- to 9-year-olds). The prevalence of treatment in middle schools and secondary schools was 3.7 and 0.4%, respectively. The rates for private parochial schools were much lower. For the entire school population, Safer and Krager reported that 3.6% had received medication for ADHD at some time during the 1987 school year. The gender ratio was 5:1, male:female. Stimulants accounted for 99% of all drug prescriptions. In rank order, the frequency distribution of stimulants was as follows: methylphenidate (93%), pemoline (4%), and dextroamphetamine (3%).

In addition to calculating rates of treatment, Safer and Krager gathered much additional information about different aspects of treatment. For example, they reported that 79% of the elementary school children received at least one dose of medication in school. Three-fourths of the children were treated by private practitioners, typically a pediatrician. Among the changes in treatment prevalence that occurred over time, Safer and Krager reported increased rates of use in females and older students and in children with attention deficits who did not present with significant concomitant behavioral disturbances.[17] The average duration of treatment (*M*, in years) for each school level was as follows: elementary, $M = 2$; middle school, $M = 4$; senior high school, $M = 7$. A review of the medical folders of a subsample of favorable responders to methylphenidate indicated that the mean daily dose was 18.7 mg during the first year of treatment, and had increased to 24.4 mg three years later.[18] However, when corrected for body growth, the dose at the older age was comparable to the initial dose.

A considerable amount of media attention has focused on production quotas for methylphenidate in the United States. Because the primary clinical indication for this drug is the treatment of ADHD, it has been concluded that these figures indicate a dramatic increase in the number of children receiving medication for ADHD during the 1990s. However, a highly meticulous review of numerous data sources conducted by Daniel Safer and his colleagues[19] indicates a more modest increase in methylphenidate prescribing that is consistent with historical trends. Between 1990 and 1995, there has been a 2.5-fold increase in the number of youths receiving methylphenidate prescriptions, much of which can be explained as follows: (a) children are being treated for longer periods of time, often into middle school/junior high school and senior high school; (b) more students with learning disabilities who have ADHD, predominantly inattentive type, are taking medication; (c) disproportionately larger numbers of females and children between 3 and 6 years old are receiving pharmacotherapy for ADHD; and (d) medication is more likely to be prescribed during the summer months. Furthermore, the increasing popularity of stimulant drug therapy for ADHD in adults also accounts, in part, for the increased use of methylphenidate in general. Using treatment prevalence figures from multiple sources, Safer et al.[19] estimated that between 2.5% and 3% of children and adolescents in the United States between 5 and 18 years old were receiving methylphenidate treatment in mid-1995.

C. Special Education

Drug therapy prevalence rates are much higher for certain special-education programs (compared with regular classrooms) for a number of reasons, most notably the co-occurrence of hyperactivity with other disabilities (academic underachievement, mental retardation, cerebral palsy). The Baltimore County surveys[16] found that 25% of all the children with ADHD in public schools were in special-education classes or schools. Reported treatment rates for different categories of special education are as follows: 19–26% for learning-disabled students in self-contained classes,[16] 6.7% for trainable mentally retarded students (IQs ranging from approximately 55 to 35) in self-contained classes,[20] 7.9% for those in early-childhood special-education programs serving children aged 3 to 5 years,[6] and 13–17% for those in public special-education schools for severely and profoundly mentally retarded, physically handicapped, and seriously disturbed children.[16]

D. Socioeconomic Status

There is little support for the notion that children from either low-SES or minority-group families are more apt to receive drugs for hyperactivity than children from more affluent homes. Even though hyperactivity is no less common among poor children (and quite possibly more common for many well-documented environmental reasons), a few studies have shown that drug treatment is used significantly less often with children from low-SES homes compared with children from more well-to-do backgrounds.[6] It has been demonstrated that this situation can be reversed by the development of public health clinics specializing in the treatment of hyperactivity that make their services available to less affluent families.[16]

E. Treatment Practices

In the early 1970s, the use of methylphenidate for the treatment of hyperactivity received considerable media attention, much of it negative.[8,21] One of the issues that was raised repeatedly in the popular press was the allegation that procedures for evaluating and monitoring treatment regimens were less than adequate. Investigations into the management of drug therapy confirmed, in large part, what many care providers had experienced firsthand.[22–28] Diagnostic practices were idiosyncratic and rarely based on operational definitions of symptoms or normative data. Dosage adjustment was at best haphazard. Direct contact between the treating physician and the classroom teacher was uncommon. Structured instruments for evaluating drug response (e.g., behavior rating scales) at home or in school were rarely used.[22–28] The standard method for obtaining such information was through anecdotal reports from the parents. Many parents adjusted dosage on their own, sometimes with the physician's approval.[24–27] Teachers frequently questioned the appropriateness of the dose of medication[23] and noted that important treatment decisions were often made unilaterally by the patients' parents. Unfortunately, the findings from more recent treatment management studies show that many of the problems identified previously are still with us.[29–33]

F. National Estimates of Treatment Prevalence

The findings from the Baltimore County studies as well as treatment prevalence rates from other geographic locales have been used to estimate the total number of children receiving medication. In mid-1995, Safer et al.[19] estimated that between 1.3 and 1.5 million children and adolescents in the United States were taking methylphenidate for ADHD.

III. MENTAL RETARDATION

People with mental retardation constitute one of the most heavily medicated segments of our population. Given the vulnerability of these individuals to clinical mismanagement, it is not surprising that they have become the focus of considerable study concerning psychoactive drug use. The treatment-related issues associated with mental retardation are much the same as those for ADHD. Are too many people being treated? Is medication being monitored appropriately? The answer to the first question is "yes" if one accepts as proof the success of drug therapy reduction programs.[34,35] The answer to the second question is an unqualified "no" as evidenced by the extensive litigation in this area.[36–38] Results of a recent survey assessing drug prescription in a predominately adult sample suggested that this may be improving in some settings.[39] In the main, psychotropic drug prescription was consistent with established or presumptive indications, but there were significant anomalies as well.

A. Institutional Settings

Largely as a result of lawsuits concerning the mistreatment of people with mental retardation in institutions, a fairly substantial amount of information about how pharmacotherapy is managed in real-world situations is now available. Surveys of psychotropic drug use in institutions have generally shown relatively high treatment rates, ranging from 30 to 60%.[34,35] Interestingly, very little has been done with these data with regard to the age of the residents. Most surveys have failed to report age, which is an important oversight because treatment rates vary with age;[16,20] and some drugs, such as the stimulants, are used primarily for child and adolescent behavior disorders. The most extensive studies of institutions have been conducted by Hill and his colleagues at the University of Minnesota.[40,41] In 1977, they identified 55,438 individuals with mental retardation under the age of 22 in public residential facilities (institutions) in the United States.[40] Staff interviews concerning a randomly selected sample ($N = 281$) of children and adolescents, over three-fourths of whom were severely and profoundly retarded, revealed that 31% were receiving psychotropic medication (stimulants, 0.7%; neuroleptics, 20%).

The biggest challenge to the legitimacy of such extensive pharmacotherapy for people in residential facilities has come from treatment withdrawal programs designed to reduce drug use. In facilities around the world, clinicians have demonstrated that many individuals receiving psychotropic drug therapy can be successfully withdrawn from medication and unnecessary polypharmacy.[34–35]

B. Community-Based Facilities

The most extensive studies of specially licensed community residential facilities (e.g., foster homes, group homes) have also been conducted by Hill and his associates.[40,41] In 1977, they identified 35,751 children and adolescents with mental retardation in community residential placements; approximately half of these youngsters were moderately to severely mentally retarded. Staff interviews concerning a randomly selected sample ($N = 391$) indicated that 19% were receiving psychotropic medication (stimulants, 2.3%; neuroleptics, 13%).

C. Public Schools

Surprisingly little is known about the prevalence of psychopharmacotherapy in children with mental retardation who attend public schools. One statewide study conducted in Illinois[20] and one citywide survey conducted in Auckland, New Zealand,[42] have examined the use of medication in this population. Results of the Illinois study showed that 4.9% of trainable mentally retarded children were receiving medication for behavior disorders and that an additional 1.8% were taking drugs for both behavior problems and seizures (stimulants, 3.4%; neuroleptics, 2.3%). The New Zealand figure was slightly lower: 3.4% of the "special school" children and adolescents were receiving psychotropic medication (neuroleptics, 2.0%).

Information about drug use in educable mentally retarded (IQs ranging from approximately 55 to 75) students is limited to one pilot study by Cullinan et al.[43] They collected drug treatment data for 238 children enrolled in special-education programs for educable mentally retarded children in northern Illinois and found that 15% were receiving medication for behavior disorders. Stimulants accounted for over half of all prescribed drugs. Approximately a third were being treated with a neuroleptic. Given the small sample size and its restricted geographic range, generalizations about and estimates derived from these data obviously must be qualified.

The findings from detailed investigations into the clinical management of children with mental retardation receiving psychotropic medication raise many questions about the adequacy of procedures for assessing response to medication and monitoring efficacy.[23,24] There is little evidence of interdisciplinary collaboration or the use of standardized instruments to assess therapeutic or untoward drug effects.

D. National Estimates of Treatment Prevalence

Gadow and Poling[35] generated estimates of the number of children and adolescents with mental retardation receiving psychotropic medication in the United States. Based on the available data, they calculated that approximately 57,000 and 40,000 were receiving neuroleptics and stimulants, respectively. These estimates exclude children in early-childhood special-education programs (not counting the children labeled mentally retarded) and students labeled learning disabled or emotionally disturbed (behavior disordered) but who would score below 70 on an individually administered IQ test. Such estimates must be interpreted with caution because (1) when one multiplies the estimated drug prevalence from a small sample by the total school enrollment, a very small error of estimate (e.g., 0.01%) makes a very big difference in the absolute number of children estimated to be receiving medication and (2) the well-documented regional variability in the extent of drug use makes the selection of a specific rate arbitrary.

IV. SEIZURE DISORDERS

For a number of reasons, there is considerable variability in the prevalence of seizure disorders (epilepsy) as reported in epidemiological studies. However, when similar methodologies and definitions of epilepsy are used, the rates are fairly consistent. Between 0.4 and 1.0% of children in the United States have active epilepsy,[44] which is defined as receiving antiepileptic medication or having a seizure within a certain period of time prior to interview (usually within 2–5 years). The primary contributor to the variablility in reported prevalence of active epilepsy is whether or not children in institutional settings are included in the study sample. Rates with and without children in residential facilities range from 0.6 to 0.9% and 0.4 to 0.5%, respectively. On the basis of 1980 census figures for the number of children between 5 and 14 years old, this would mean that there are 150,251 to 324,961 cases of active epilepsy in the United States. The highest prevalence of seizure disorders is in children under 2 years old. Seizure disorders are slightly more prevalent in males. In an epidemiological study in Ohio, Aman and colleagues found a rate of 0.56% in 2-year-old children.[45] The findings from treatment withdrawal studies suggest that some children may be receiving antiepileptic medication for longer periods than necessary.[46–48]

In spite of a long history and widespread application, with few exceptions little effort has been made to learn how antiepileptic drug therapy is used in everyday clinical situations.[20,49,50] The available data indicate that interdisciplinary collaboration is minimal and that standardized procedures for obtaining drug response information from care providers are all but nonexistent.

Seizure disorders occur with much greater frequency in people who have experienced some type of injury to the brain. Therefore, it is not surprising that surveys of educational and habilitative programs that serve people with severe or profound mental retardation, cerebral palsy, or multiple handicaps report relatively high rates of antiepileptic drug therapy. It also follows that the care providers who staff these programs and facilities encounter epilepsy on a regular basis, a fact that has important implications for professional training. As for the people who are the recipients of these services, the needs and problems created by their seizure disorders, their underlying handicapping conditions, and their medication often interact in ways that create a special set of treatment-related concerns. For these and other reasons, treatment prevalence data pertaining to people with developmental disabilities are presented here as a separate topic.

A. Autism

Several investigators have reported on the prevalence of seizure disorders in children, adolescents, and adults with autism.[51-53] The findings from these studies suggest that as many as 20–30% of individuals who have this disorder may receive antiepileptic medication for seizures at some time in their lives. The incidence of seizure disorders is higher during early childhood and adolescence compared with other age groups.[51-53]

B. Mental Retardation

The international picture of antiepileptic drug prescribing for people with mental retardation living in residential facilities is fairly consistent. Although there is obviously some variability, approximately 30% of the residents in institutions in Australia, Canada, New Zealand, the United Kingdom, and the United States receive medication for seizure disorders.[34,35] The literature generally supports the conclusion that the treatment regimens of many patients are poorly monitored and that multiple drug therapy is commonplace. Programs to improve the quality of clinical care have shown that a substantial minority of treated individuals can be withdrawn from antiepileptic medication, polypharmacy can be greatly reduced, and the degree of seizure control in patients who require treatment can be increased.[54-57]

Several surveys of community placements (e.g., group homes, foster care) have been conducted, and an accurate description of drug use is emerging for these settings. The incidence of antiepileptic drug use in these facilities ranges from 15 to 20%.[34,35]

As previously noted, much of what is known about the pattern and prevalence of antiepileptic drug use among trainable mentally retarded children in special-education programs comes from one statewide study conducted in Illinois[20] and one citywide survey conducted in New Zealand.[42] The results of the Illinois study showed that 11.9% received medication for a seizure disorder at some time during the school year. This figure includes children who were receiving medication for both a behavior and a seizure disorder (1.8% of the sample were administered drugs for both conditions). Multiple drug therapy was commonplace. Parents reported that the onset of treatment was usually quite early, often between birth and 2 years of age. Interestingly, the New Zealand prevalence data are similar. There, it was found that 17.4% of the "special school" children and adolescents were receiving antiepileptic medication.

C. Preschool-Aged Children

Information about the prevalence of antiepileptic drug therapy for young children (between 3 and 5 years old) comes from one survey of preschoolers diagnosed as trainable mentally retarded[20] and from two studies of youngsters enrolled in early-childhood special-education programs.[6] The study of trainable mentally retarded preschoolers found that 16.1% were receiving antiepileptic medication, which included the 2.1% who were being treated concurrently for both a seizure and a behavior disorder. Of all the age groups participating in this investigation (3 to 21 years), the highest rate of pharmacotherapy was for the 3- to 5-year-olds. The early-childhood special-education surveys found that 6.6% were receiving antiepileptic medication. This figure includes youngsters who were being treated for both a behavior and a seizure disorder (1.1%).

V. AUTISM

One data archive on drug-prescribing practices for children with autism is the Institute for Child Behavior Research (ICBR) in San Diego, California. The ICBR maintains a detailed data bank on thousands of autistic individuals in over 40 countries. On the basis of approximately 4000 questionnaires, completed by the parents of children with autism, Rimland[58] ranked the drugs prescribed on the basis of the respondent's perception of efficacy. The most commonly reported drugs were thioridazine ($n = 724$), phenytoin ($n = 471$), chlorpromazine ($n = 460$), methylphenidate ($n = 426$), and diphenhydramine ($n = 425$). By far the most highly rated treatment with regard to efficacy was a combination of vitamin B_6 and magnesium ($n = 318$), a treatment that has been promoted in ICBR publications. Next was deanol ($n = 121$), which is no longer available in the United States as a prescription drug but is available as a nutritional supplement under the trade name DMAE-H3. Fenfluramine ($n = 104$) ranked with the neuroleptics. The stimulants were rated as being highly ineffective. The Rimland study was not a treatment prevalence survey *per se* and relied on responses to a newsletter, which makes it difficult to know how representative the sample was.

More recently, Aman et al.[59] surveyed the members of the Autism Society of North Carolina. Drug-use information was generated for 838 individuals who ranged in age from infancy to adulthood (median age = 13 years). More than 30% of the study sample was receiving psychotropic medication. The most commonly prescribed drugs (i.e., percentage of individuals treated) were neuroleptics (12%), stimulants (7% of the total sample, 12% of 7- to 13-year-olds), sedatives/hypnotics (6%), and antidepressants (6%). Five percent were taking vitamins specifically for treating autism (vitamin B_6 alone, vitamin B_6 plus magnesium, dimethylglycine). With regard to specific drugs, the most often prescribed (in rank order) were thioridazine, methylphenidate, haloperidol, clonidine, clomipramine, and lithium.

VI. DEPRESSION

There is relatively little research on the treatment of depression in children or adolescents. Kovacs et al.[60] conducted a 5-year naturalistic follow-up study of 65 carefully selected depressed children and reported extremely low rates of pharmacotherapy. Only two cases were prescribed antidepressants, and one individual received an antianxiety agent. Approximately two-thirds of the subjects received some form of psychological intervention. Keller et al.[61] also reported low rates of drug therapy in a sample of 38 adolescents diagnosed as having an episode of major depression. Only one of the youths received medication (an antianxiety agent), and only six received psychotherapy for their depressive symptoms. It is noteworthy that treatment incidence is low for adults as well. For example, Keller et al.[62] found that only 34% of adults with depression who volunteered to participate in a naturalistic follow-up study had received antidepressants prior to their involvement in the study.

VII. ENURESIS

Although enuresis is a fairly common childhood disorder, medical intervention is limited to a minority of patients. For example, one follow-up study of enuretic children to the age of 11 years found that only one-third had been referred for medical evaluation for bed-wetting.[63] A more recent study by Foxman et al.[64] examined bed-wetting in a large sample (1724) of children aged 5 to 13 years from various geographic areas who were enrolled in the Rand Health Insurance Experiment. Participants were administered a bed-wetting questionnaire in which they were asked if their child had wet the bed in the past 3 months. The study was conducted in 1975 and 1976. The results of this survey showed that 14% of the children had wet the bed at least once during the previous 3 months. The percentage who wet the bed at least once a week was much lower (boys, 7%; girls, 6%). Approximately 2% wet the bed "almost every night." According to parental report, 92 children had been seen by a doctor about their problem. A higher rate of physician evaluation was associated with gender (female), parental education (high), and age (older children). Sixty percent of the physician-evaluated group of bed wetters received one or more treatments of enuresis. The most common was medication (usually imipramine), which was prescribed to 31 (34%) of the 92 children who saw a physician. The bed alarm was prescribed for only 3 children.

In the entire sample of 1724 children, at least 2% had received medication for enuresis. The number of children who had ever been treated would be higher than this figure, because the questionnaires were completed only if the child had wet the bed recently (within the past 3 months). If this study[64] sample is representative of the pediatric population, then enuresis is one of the most common disorders for which psychotropic drugs are prescribed. However, until more research in this area is conducted, this conclusion must be considered tentative.

VIII. TOURETTE SYNDROME

Most of what is currently known about drug therapy for children and adolescents with Tourette syndrome is limited to surveys of the membership of the Tourette Syndrome Association of Ohio, the most recent of which was conducted in the spring of 1987.[65] Questionnaires were mailed to the entire membership ($N = 1034$), of which 75% were returned. Questionnaires for individuals under 18 years of age were mailed to their parents or legal guardians. Although medication use for children was not analyzed separately from that for adults, three-fourths of the respondents were under 20 years old: 0–9 years, 10%; 10–14, 37%; and 15–19, 25%. The male-to-female ratio was 4.2:1, which is comparable to gender ratios generally reported in the literature. Onset of Tourette symptoms (most commonly a facial tic) began before the age of 10 years in 83% of the cases. Of all the medical specialties, neurologists were the most likely (45%) to have made the initial diagnosis of Tourette syndrome. Over 20% were self-diagnosed.

A relatively large (71%) portion of the sample reported taking medication for Tourette syndrome at some time, but only 43% were receiving medication (active treatment) at the time of the survey. The active-treatment group was much more likely to report severe symptoms without medication than those who were no longer receiving treatment. The most commonly reported drugs by the active-treatment group (in rank order) were halo-peridol (51%), clonidine (26%), pimozide (15%), and methylphenidate (4%). Treatment history data indicated that over a dozen different drugs were reported as the first medica-tion, the most common being haloperidol (69%), methylphenidate (10%), and clonidine (8%). Twenty percent said that their symptoms worsened on medication, and 60% reported trying an alternate medication (usually clonidine), primarily because the initial medication produced unacceptable side effects.

With regard to the safety and efficacy of specific drugs, 74% of the respondents who were treated with haloperidol reported symptomatic improvement; 14% said their tics got worse. Less than one-third of the respondents who were initially treated with haloperidol were still taking the drug at the time of the survey. Treatment was terminated in 47% of the cases owing to adverse drug reactions.

A diagnosis of ADD/hyperactivity had been made in over 40% of the cases, and the majority (58%) of these respondents had taken stimulant medication at some point in time for this disorder. It is noteworthy that 49% reported that stimulants had made their tic symptoms worse.

In general, there was a fairly high degree of dissatisfaction with drug therapy in this patient sample because of the relatively high rate of unacceptable side effects. Many had tried alternative interventions (e.g., behavioral interventions, dietary restrictions) with some success.

IX. OTHER DISORDERS

As documented in this book, there are a number of other child and adolescent dis-orders for which psychotropic drugs are prescribed (e.g., anxiety, eating, and sleep dis-orders, schizophrenia as it is defined in DSM-IV, conduct disorder as a separate clinical entity from ADHD, substance abuse). It is not possible to comment on these other treatment applications because the research literature is limited to highly restricted samples or is simply nonexistent. The findings from two surveys of child and adolescent psychiatric hospitals do indicate, however, fairly high rates of drug use for more severely impaired patients. One survey of 100 consecutive patients admitted to an acute-care child psychiatry facility in Canada during 1976 and 1977 found that 66% received psychotropic medication during their stay in the hospital.[66] The most common diagnosis was behavior disorder. All of the children with diagnosed psychosis received medication. The most commonly pre-scribed drugs were thioridazine and chlorpromazine. Twenty percent of the entire sample of children received a phenothiazine in combination with an anticholinergic drug.

Another survey of 14 state-operated child and adolescent facilities in New York State during 1 month in 1989 also revealed fairly high rates of drug prescribing.[67] The study sample consisted of 679 primarily long-term chronic patients. The percentages of individuals receiving various classes of drugs were as follows: neuroleptics, 49%; antiparkinson agents, 15%; antidepressants, 14%; lithium, 11%; and antianxiety agents, 7%. None of the patients received more than one drug from the same drug class.

One study of prescribing practices in two university-affiliated child psychiatry outpatient facilities in the United States in 1990 reported relatively low rates of medication use.[68] Of 800 outpatients seen in a one-month interval in one facility, 15% were prescribed medication. In the second facility, 19% were prescribed medication in a 1-year interval. From 11% to 22% of those prescribed medication received more than one psychotropic medication at the same time. The most frequently prescribed medications were antipsychotics, stimulants, and antidepressants. Of the 146 children treated with medication, most were diagnosed as having a disruptive behavior disorder (ADHD, conduct or oppositional disorder). Much less common diagnoses were psychosis ($n = 15$), depressive disorder ($n = 18$), and bipolar disorder ($n = 5$). In 90% of the cases, medication was judged to have been used appropriately.

X. INTERNATIONAL VARIATIONS IN PRESCRIBING

One group surveyed child and adolescent psychiatrists worldwide to examine prescription preferences in different regions.[69] Questionnaires were sent to 135 child psychiatrists, and 38 respondents from 24 countries replied. In addition, 67 of 186 Canadian child psychiatrists responded to the same questionnaire. Whereas 82% of Canadian psychiatrists indicated that they would prescribe methylphenidate for patients with ADHD, only 58% of psychiatrists elsewhere responded similarly. One respondent from Switzerland reported that hyperkinesis is usually considered in that country to represent a "manic-like" symptom within a general psychiatric disorganization. Use of methylphenidate and dextroamphetamine were reported not to be permitted in Argentina and Bulgaria,[69] and the diagnosis of ADHD was said to be rarely made in Italy.[69] Hence the diagnosis and treatment of ADHD still appears to be controversial in many countries other than the United States and Canada.

In contrast, both Canadian and overseas psychiatrists prescribed tricyclic antidepressants for depression but usually not for dysthymia. The majority of psychiatrists, regardless of sample, indicated that they did not prescribe psychotropic drugs for separation anxiety and overanxious disorder, whereas they did for panic and obsessive-compulsive disorders.[69]

XI. SUMMARY

Researchers have used a variety of procedures to obtain information about the prevalence and pattern of drug treatment for childhood behavior and seizure disorders. With the exception of ADHD and behavior disorders in people with mental retardation, not much is known about treatment practices in everyday clinical settings. Most of the studies have been conducted in the United States, although there have been a number of treatment surveys of residential facilities for people with mental retardation in various locales around the world.

Surveys of children with ADHD clearly show that stimulants are the drugs of first choice, with methylphenidate being the most popular. They are most likely to be prescribed by pediatricians, and dosage tends to be conservative (10–20 mg daily), a practice that appears to have remained fairly consistent over a number of years. This finding is note-worthy considering the salience of dosage issues in the stimulant drug therapy literature. The average duration of treatment is 2–4 years. Anecdotal reports from care providers often serve as the basis for assessing response to medication. Approximately 2–5% of elementary school children receive medication for ADHD in the United States. Rates are much higher for children in special-education programs. Over the past 20 years, the number of children receiving medication has increased. The patient population has expanded to include more females, older children and adolescents, and children with attention deficits who do not have significant concomitant behavioral disturbance (disruptive, oppositional, aggressive behaviors).

Surveys of individuals with mental retardation show very high rates of psychoactive drug use in residential facilities, with much lower levels for individuals in community placements and public school special-education classes. Neuroleptics are the primary psychotropic drugs in residential and community facilities, but they are prescribed much less often for children in special-education programs and share preference with the stimulants.

Approximately 1% of children in the United States have active epilepsy, most of whom receive antiepileptic medication. Treatment rates for developmentally delayed individuals are much higher (30% for residential facilities). Most surveys show that multiple antiepileptic drug therapy is a common practice and that there is little evidence of active collaboration among care providers concerning assessment of drug response. Combination psychotropic and antiepileptic treatment regimens are particularly common for children with developmental disabilities.

Studies of psychotropic drug therapy for other childhood disorders are extremely limited. The treatment rate for enuresis reported in one study (2%) makes this disorder a relatively common reason for prescribing psychotropic medication. In contrast, depression in children and adolescents is unlikely to be treated with medication, and many cases go undetected. Drug therapy appears to be the treatment of choice for Tourette syndrome, but few patients take medication for any extended period of time. The clinical utility of haloperidol is greatly limited by annoying side effects.

It is somewhat difficult to deduce general trends in the treatment prevalence literature given such disparate disorders, but several conclusions can be made. First, there is clear evidence that psychotropic drugs are overprescribed if one considers as evidence children who can be successfully switched to nondrug therapies and the findings from studies that show no return of symptoms when medication is withdrawn. Lest this statement be misunderstood, it is important to add that evidence showing a higher rate of use than what would be predicted on the basis of the known prevalence of the disorder (target behaviors) is not compelling. Second, whereas the prevalence of drug use may be decreasing in individuals with severe developmental disabilities (mental retardation), it is increasing in nonintellectually impaired children in public school programs, in part as a result of the introduction of ADD without hyperactivity into the clinical nomenclature. Third, the administration of drugs not specifically approved for certain disorders or age groups or not empirically demonstrated to be effective is not uncommon. Fourth, most physicians show a clear preference for pharmacotherapy over other interventions. Lastly, the existing technology for evaluating and monitoring drug therapy[70–74] is not routinely used in everyday clinical settings. One of the explicit objectives of this book is to present and encourage the adoption of state-of-the art procedures for this purpose.

REFERENCES

1. Abramowicz M (ed): Sudden death in children treated with a tricyclic antidepressant. *Med Lett Drugs Ther* 32:53, 1990.
2. Biederman J: Sudden death in children with a tricyclic antidepressant. *J Am Acad Child Adolesc Psychiatry* 30:495–498, 1991.
3. Riddle MA, Nelson JC, Kleinman CS, et al: Sudden death in children receiving Norpramin: A review of three reported cases and commentary. *J Am Acad Child Adolesc Psychiatry* 30:104–108, 1991.
4. Sprague RL, Gadow KD: The role of the teacher in drug treatment. *School Rev* 85:109–140, 1976.
5. Hong SH, Shepherd MD: Psychosocial and demographic predictors of pediatric psychotropic medication use. *Am J Health-Syst Pharm* 53:1934–1939, 1996.
6. Gadow KD: Prevalence of drug treatment for hyperactivity and other childhood behavior disorders, in Gadow KD, Loney J (eds): *Psychosocial Aspects of Drug Treatment for Hyperactivity*. Boulder, Colo, Westview Press, 1981, pp 13–76.
7. Maynard R: Omaha pupils given "behavior" drugs. *Washington Post*, June 29, 1970.
8. Hentoff N: The drugged classroom. *Evergreen Review*, December, 1970, pp 31–33.
9. Ladd ET: Pills for classroom peace. *Saturday Review*, November 21, 1970, pp 66–68, 81–83.
10. Rogers JM: Drug abuse—Just what the doctor ordered. *Psychology Today*, September, 1971, pp 16–24.
11. Gates D: Just saying no to Ritalin. *Newsweek*, November 23, 1987, p 6.
12. Johnson P: Family: Remedy led to "hell." *USA Today*, April 27, 1988.
13. Schmidt WE: Sales of drugs are soaring for treatment of hyperactivity. *New York Times*, May 5, 1987.
14. Stephen K, Sprague RL, Werry J: Drug treatment of hyperactive children in Chicago (Progress Report of NIMH Grant No. MH 18909, 1970–1973, RL Sprague, Principal Investigator). Urbana, Ill, Children's Research Center, 1973.
15. Sprague RL, Sleator E: Effects of psychopharmacological agents on learning disorders. *Pediatr Clin North Am* 20:719–735, 1973.
16. Safer DJ, Krager JM: A survey of medication treatment for hyperactive/inattentive students. *JAMA* 260:2256–2258, 1988.
17. Safer DJ, Krager JM: Hyperactivity and inattentiveness: School assessment of stimulant treatment. *Clin Pediatr* 28:216–221, 1989.
18. Safer DJ, Allen RP: Absence of tolerance to the behavioral effects of methylphenidate in hyperactive and inattentive children. *J Pediatr* 115:1003–1008, 1989.
19. Safer DJ, Zito JM, Fine EM: Increased methylphenidate usage for attention deficit disorder in the 1990s. *Pediatrics* 98:1–5, 1996.
20. Gadow KD, Kalachnik J: Prevalance and pattern of drug treatment for behavior disorders of TMR students. *Am J Ment Defic* 85:588–595, 1981.
21. Divoky D: Toward a nation of sedated children. *Learning* 1:7–13, 1973.
22. Bosco JJ, Robin SS: Ritalin usage: A challenge to teacher education. *Peabody J Educ* 53:187–193, 1976.
23. Gadow KD: School involvement in pharmacotherapy for behavior disorders. *J Spec Educ* 16:385–399, 1982.
24. Gadow KD: Pharmacotherapy for behavior disorders: Typical treatment practices. *Clin Pediatr* 22:48–53, 1983.
25. Loney J, Ordona TT: Using cerebral stimulants to treat minimal brain dysfunction. *Am J Orthopsychiatry* 45:564–572, 1975.
26. Sandoval J, Lambert N, Yandell W: Current medical practice and hyperactivity. *Am J Orthopsychiatry* 46:323–334, 1976.
27. Solomons G: Drug therapy: Initiation and follow-up. *Ann NY Acad Sci* 205:335–344, 1973.
28. Weithorn CJ, Ross R: "Who monitors medication?" *J Learn Disabil* 8:458–461, 1975.
29. Bennett FC, Sherman R: Management of childhood "hyperactivity" by primary care physicians. *J Dev Behav Pediatr* 4:88–93, 1983.
30. Brulle AR, Barton LE, Foskett JJ: Educator/physician interchanges: A survey and suggestions. *Educ Training Ment Retard* 18:313–317, 1983.
31. Copeland L, Wolraich M, Lindgren S, et al: Pediatricians' reported practices in the assessment and treatment of attention deficit disorders. *J Dev Behav Pediatr* 8:191–197, 1987.
32. Jensen PS, Xenakis SN, Shervette RE, et al: Diagnosis and treatment of attention deficit disorder in two general hospital clinics. *Hosp Community Psychiatry* 40:708–712, 1989.
33. Sindelar PT, Meisel CJ: Teacher–physician interaction in the treatment of children with behavioral disorders. *Int J Partial Hosp* 1:271–277, 1982.

34. Aman MG, Singh NN (eds): *Psychopharmacotherapy of the Developmental Disabilities*. Berlin, Springer-Verlag, 1988.
35. Gadow KD, Poling AD: *Pharmacotherapy and Mental Retardation*. Austin, Tex, PRO-ED, 1988.
36. Gualtieri CT, Sprague RL, Cole JO: Tardive dyskinesia litigation and the dilemmas of neuroleptic treatment. *J Psychiatry Law* 14:187–216, 1986.
37. Sprague RL: Litigation, legislation, and regulations, in Breuning SE, Poling AD (eds): *Drugs and Mental Retardation*. Springfield, Ill, Charles C Thomas, 1982, pp 377–414.
38. Sprague RL, Galliher L: Litigation about psychotropic medication, in Gadow KD, Poling AD: *Pharmacotherapy and Mental Retardation*. Austin, Tex, PRO-ED, 1988, pp 297–312.
39. Aman MG, Sarphare G, Burrow WH: Psychotropic drugs in group homes: Prevalence and relation to demographic/psychiatric variables. *Am J Ment Retard* 99:500–509, 1995.
40. Hill BK, Balow EA, Bruininks RH: A national study of prescribed drugs in institutions and community residential facilities for mentally retarded people. *Psychopharmacol Bull* 21:279–284, 1985.
41. Hill BK, Lakin KC, Bruininks RH: Trends in residential services for mentally retarded people: 1977–1982. *J Assoc Persons Severe Handicaps* 9:243–250, 1984.
42. Aman MG, Field CJ, Bridgman GD: City-wide survey of drug patterns among noninstitutionalized retarded persons. *Appl Res Ment Retard* 6:159–171, 1985.
43. Cullinan D, Gadow KD, Epstein MH: Psychotropic drug treatment among learning disabled, mentally retarded, and seriously emotionally disturbed students. *J Abnorm Child Psychol* 15:469–477, 1987.
44. Hauser WA, Hesdorffer DC: *Epilepsy: Frequency, Causes, and Consequences*. New York, Demos, 1990.
45. Aman MG, Rojahn J, King EH, Logsdon DA, Marshburn EC: Prevalence and pattern of prescribed medication in 2-year old children. *J Dev Phys Dis* 6:87–99, 1994.
46. Emerson R, D'Souza BJ, Vining EP, et al: Stopping medication in children with epilepsy. *N Engl J Med* 304:1125–1129, 1981.
47. Holowach J, Thurstone DL, O'Leary J: Prognosis in childhood epilepsy: Followup study of 148 cases, in which therapy had been suspended after prolonged anticonvulsant control. *N Engl J Med* 286:169–174, 1972.
48. Todt H: The late prognosis of epilepsy in childhood: Results of a prospective followup study. *Epilepsia* 25:137–144, 1984.
49. Gadow KD: School involvement in the treatment of seizure disorders. *Epilepsia* 23:215–224, 1982.
50. Pietsch S (ed): *The Person with Epilepsy: Life Style, Needs, Expectations*. Chicago, National Epilepsy League, 1977.
51. Deykin EY, MacMahon B: The incidence of seizures among children with autistic symptoms. *Am J Psychiatry* 126:1310–1312, 1979.
52. Gillberg C: The treatment of epilepsy in autism. *J Autism Dev Disord* 21:61–77, 1991.
53. Volkmar FR, Nelson DS: Seizure disorders in autism. *J Am Acad Child Adolesc Psychiatry* 29:127–129, 1990.
54. Alvarez N: Discontinuance of antiepileptic medications in patients with developmental disability and diagnosis of epilepsy. *Am J Ment Retard* 93:593–599, 1989.
55. Beghi E, Bollini P, DiMascio R, et al: Effects of rationalizing drug treatment of patients with epilepsy and mental retardation. *Dev Med Child Neurol* 29:363–369, 1987.
56. Collacott RA, Dignon A, Hauck A, et al: Clinical and therapeutic monitoring of epilepsy in a mental handicap unit. *Br J Psychiatry* 155:522–525, 1989.
57. Sivenius J, Savolaninen S, Kaski M, et al: Therapeutic intervention in mentally retarded adult epileptics. *Acta Neurol Scand* 81:165–167, 1990.
58. Rimland B: Controversies in the treatment of autistic children: Vitamin and drug therapy. *J Child Neurol* 3(suppl):S68–S72, 1988.
59. Aman MG, Van Bourgodien ME, Wolford PL, Sarphare G: Psychotropic and anticonvulsant drugs in subjects with autism: Prevalence and patterns of use. *J Am Acad Child Adolesc Psychiatry* 34:1672–1681, 1995.
60. Kovacs M, Feinberg TL, Crouse-Novak MA, et al: Depressive disorders in childhood: I. A longitudinal prospective study of characteristics and recovery. *Arch Gen Psychiatry* 41:229–237, 1984.
61. Keller MB, Lavori PW, Beardslee WR, et al: Depression in children and adolescents: New data on 'undertreatment' and a literature review on the efficacy of available treatments. *J Affect Disord* 21:163–171, 1991.
62. Keller MB, Klerman GL, Lavori PW, et al: Treatment received by depressed patients. *JAMA* 248:1848–1855, 1982.
63. Miller FJW: Children who wet the bed, in Kolvin I, MacKeith RC, Meadow SR (eds): *Clinics in Developmental Medicine: Bladder Control and Enuresis*. New York, JB Lippincott, 1973, pp 47–57.
64. Foxman B, Valdez RB, Brook RH: Childhood enuresis: Prevalence, perceived impact, and prescribed treatments. *Pediatrics* 77:482–487, 1986.
65. Stefl ME, Bornstein RA, Hammond L: The 1987 Ohio Tourette Survey. Milford, Ohio, Tourette Syndrome Association of Ohio, 1988.

66. Ahsanuddin KM, Ivey JA, Schlotzhauer D, et al: Psychotropic medication prescription patterns in 100 hospi-talized children and adolescents. *J Am Acad Child Adolesc Psychiatry* 22:361–364, 1983.
67. Patton K, Personal communication, March 8, 1989.
68. Kaplan SL, Simms RM, Busner J: Prescribing practices of outpatient child psychiatrists. *J Am Acad Child Adolesc Psychiatry* 33:35–44, 1994.
69. Simeon JG, Wiggin DM, Williams E: World wide use of psychotropic drugs in child and adolescent psychiatric disorders. *Prog Neuro-Psychopharmacol Biol Psychiatry* 19:455–465, 1995.
70. Barkley RA, Fischer M, Newby RF, et al: Development of a multimethod clinical protocol for assessing stimulant drug response in children with attention deficit disorder. *J Clin Child Psychol* 17:14–24, 1988.
71. Fine S, Jewesson B: Active drug placebo trial of methylphenidate: A clinical service for children with an attention deficit disorder. *Can J Psychiatry* 34:447–449, 1989.
72. Gadow KD, Nolan EE, Paolicelli LM, et al: A procedure for assessing the effects of methylphenidate on hyperactive children in public school settings. *J Clin Child Psychol* 20:268–276, 1991.
73. Pelham WE, Hoza J: Behavioral assessment of psychostimulant effects on ADD children in a summer day treatment program, in Prinz R (ed): *Advances in Behavioral Assessment of Children and Families.* Greenwich, Conn, JAI Press, 1987, vol 3, pp 3–34.
74. Sleator EK, von Neumann A: Methylphenidate in the treatment of hyperkinetic children. *Clin Pediatr* 13:19–24, 1974.

4

Monitoring and Measuring Drug Effects. I. Physical Effects

ALAN J. ZAMETKIN, M.D., and EMILY M. YAMADA, M.S.

I. INTRODUCTION

The decision to use psychoactive medications in children and adolescents is not taken lightly by parents or clinicians. Many factors are weighed in this decision, including the diagnosis and severity of symptoms, age, preferences of the child and parents, medical and family history, risk of serious adverse effects, and success and failure of previous treatment. Medications are often utilized only after periods of behavioral therapy or psychotherapeutic approaches have failed to ameliorate adequately the presenting symptoms.

This chapter will highlight the importance of conducting a careful baseline physical examination and collecting medical history data of children and adolescents prior to psychoactive drug initiation. Once a child is started on a course of medication, additional physical assessment will be required for maintenance while on drug therapy. Although specific recommendations about particular medications and their follow-up physical studies are reviewed in subsequent chapters, the general approach to the physical assessment (as opposed to behavioral monitoring) of psychoactive medications will be discussed here.

II. BASELINE PHYSICAL ASSESSMENT

Medication produces its effects by altering body function. While the prescriber may target one symptom such as hyperactivity, drugs have a far wider spectrum of activity and so these nonfocused systems must be assessed so that unexpected surprises do not result.

ALAN J. ZAMETKIN, M.D. • Office of the Clinical Director, National Institute of Mental Health, Bethesda, Maryland 20892   EMILY M. YAMADA, M.S. • Department of Psychology, University of Washington, Seattle, Washington 98195-1525

Practitioner's Guide to Psychoactive Drugs for Children and Adolescents (Second Edition), Werry and Aman, eds. Plenum Publishing Corporation, New York, 1999.

The two major reasons for a careful and complete medical history and physical examination are (1) *to exclude medical conditions* as the cause of psychiatric symptoms and (2) *to establish the baseline physical status* prior to initiation of medication therapy against which to monitor any changes.

An integral part of the decision to use psychoactive medication in children and adolescents is the physical status of the patient. The course of the presenting problems always dictates the nature of the initial medical evaluation. For example, a teenager with exemplary grades and excellent interpersonal skills should be examined immediately by either a family physician, a pediatrician, or even a neurologist if he or she presents with a sudden personality change accompanied by gross social disinhibition and headaches. On the other hand, evaluating chronic problems such as long-standing anxiety, affective, or conduct symptoms may only require thorough medical history taking and a recent physical exam by the family physician to permit the judicious use of psychoactive medications. Clearly, the acuteness of the presenting symptoms alone cannot determine a medical cause for psychiatric symptomatology. Tables 1 and 2 highlight the multitude of medical illnesses that can present themselves with psychiatric symptoms.

The minimum prerequisites for all patients prior to medication therapy are a careful and complete documentation of the present illness, past medical history, medical review of systems, history of allergies and drug sensitivities, other prescribed or illicit drug or alcohol use, and a family psychiatric history. In addition, a physical and neurological exam (including a mental status exam) should be conducted to identify any organic factors contributing to the psychiatric symptomatology and any coexisting medical abnormalities. Table 3 presents a standard outline for the medical history and medical review of systems. Reliable documentation of another clinician's physical exam may also be utilized by the treating clinician as long as the exam has been performed within a reasonable time frame.

A complete psychiatric assessment would also include appropriate psychological tests if indicated, resulting in a working diagnosis and comprehensive treatment plan, and baseline behavioral measurements. The treatment plan should be developed in conjunction with both the parents or the primary caretaker and include participation of the child or adolescent as appropriate to his or her understanding. The use of medication, including expected benefits and possible short- and long-term adverse effects, should be reviewed with the parents and child in understandable terminology and documented in the medical record. Treatment with psychoactive drugs should always be part of a more comprehensive treatment program if at all possible.

Particularly for the nonmedical reader, the important components of a complete history taking will be reviewed below.

TABLE 1. More Frequent Organic Causes of Anxiety States[a]

Endocrine disorders	Metabolic disorders	Drugs and medications
Cushing's disease	Hypoglycemia	Caffeine
Hyperthyroidism	Hypocalcemia	Amphetamines
		Withdrawal states from addictive drugs
		Steroids

[a]Reprinted with permission from Schoonover.[54]

TABLE 2. Organic Causes of Psychosis[a]

Space-occupying lesions of CNS	Metabolic and endocrine disorders
Brain abscess (bacterial, fungal, TB, cysticercus)	Adrenal disease (Addison's and Cushing's
Metastatic carcinoma	diseases)
Primary cerebral tumors	Calcium
Subdural hematoma	Diabetes mellitus
Cerebral hypoxia	Electrolyte imbalance
Anemia	Hepatic failure
Lowered cardiac output	Homocystinuria
Pulmonary insufficiency	Hypoglycemia and hyperglycemia
Toxic (e.g., carbon monoxide)	Pituitary insufficiency
Neurological disorders	Porphyria
Alzheimer's disease	Thyroid disease (thryotoxicosis and myxedema)
Distant effects of carcinoma	Uremia
Huntington's chorea	Nutritional deficiencies
Normal-pressure hydrocephalus	B_{12}
Temporal lobe epilepsy	Niacin (pellagra)
Wilson's disease	Thiamine (Wernicke–Korsakoff syndrome)
Vascular disorders	Drugs, medications, and toxic substances
Aneurysms	Alcohol (intoxication and withdrawal)
Collagen vascular diseases	Amphetamines
Hypertensive encephalopathy	Anticholinergic agents
Intracranial hemorrhage	Barbiturates and other sedative–hypnotic agents
Lacunar state	(intoxication and withdrawal)
Infections	Bromides and heavy metals
Brain abscess	Carbon disulfide
Encephalitis and postencephalitic states	Cocaine
Malaria	Corticosteroids
Meningitis (bacterial, fungal, TB)	Cycloserine (Seromycin®)
Subacute bacterial endocarditis	Digitalis (Crystodigin®)
Syphilis	Disulfiram (Antabuse®)
Toxoplasmosis	Hallucinogens
Typhoid	Isoniazid (INH® and others)
	L-DOPA (Larodopa® and others)
	Marijuana
	Reserpine (Serpasil® and others)

[a]Reprinted with permission from Schoonover.[54]

A. Past Medical History

A review of all previous medical illnesses is important, including those listed in the standard medical history outline (Table 3). For example, a practitioner might be interested in any chronic ear infections, which may affect speech and language development. A history of rheumatic fever has been noted in adolescents developing what may seem to be obsessive–compulsive disorder. A history of illnesses such as tuberculosis exposure, diabetes, heart disease (in the form of a heart murmur), and chronic or multiple hospitalizations must be obtained. Often, families will neglect to furnish the most obvious medical history to a "therapist" in a nonmedical setting and are not necessarily any more forthcoming with a physician.

TABLE 3. Standard Medical History Outline

Date: _____
CHIEF COMPLAINTS:
PRESENT ILLNESSES (Active Problems):
Instructions: Circle positive responses and comment appropriately. Underline negative responses. Leave unaltered if information not available.
PAST MEDICAL HISTORY
(a) Pediatric and Adult Illnesses: mumps, measles, chicken pox, rheumatic fever, arthritis, rheumatism, chorea, scarlet fever, pneumonia, tuberculosis, diabetes mellitus, heart disease, renal disease, hypertension, jaundice.
(b) Immunizations:
(c) Hospitalizations:
(d) Trauma:
(e) Transfusions:
(f) Current Medications:
(g) Allergies:
(h) Habits (drug, alcohol, tobacco):
SYSTEMS REVIEW
(a) General: weakness, fatigue, change in weight, appetite, sleep.
(b) Integument: color changes, hair changes, nail changes.
(c) Hematopoietic: anemia, excessive bruising.
(d) Central Nervous System:
    1. General: syncope, loss of consciousness, convulsions, meningitis, encephalitis, stroke.
    2. Mentative: speech disorders, emotional status, orientation, memory disorders, change in sleep pattern, history of nervous breakdown.
    3. Motor: tremor, weakness, paralysis, clumsiness of movement.
    4. Sensory: radicular or neuralgic pain (head, neck, trunk, extremities), paresthesias, anesthesias.
(e) Eyes: vision, glasses/contact lens, date of last eye exam, scotomata.
(f) Ears: tinnitus, deafness, other.
(g) Nose, Throat, and Sinuses: discharge, sinusitis, hoarseness.
(h) Dentition: caries.
(i) Breasts: masses, pain.
(j) Respiratory: cough, tobacco usage, wheezing.
(k) Cardiovascular: chest pain, murmur, syncope, near-syncope.
(l) Gastrointestinal: nausea, vomiting, diarrhea, constipation, food intolerances, abdominal pain, jaundice, use of laxatives.
(m) Urinary tract: renal colic, frequency of urination, nocturia, dysuria, incontinence.
(n) Genito-reproductive System
    Male: history of veneral disease, libido.
    Female:
    A. Gynecologic history: age of menarche, history of venereal disease, last Pap smear.
    B. Methods of contraception:
(o) Musculoskeletal
    Joints: pain, edema, heat rubor.
(p) Endocrine: goiter, heat intolerance, cold intolerance, change in voice, polyuria, polydipsia, polyphagia.
(q) Psychiatric: hyperventilation, nervousness, depression, insomnia, nightmares, memory loss.

B. Immunizations

Are immunizations up-to-date? If not, this may give warning that compliance with the health care system may be an issue in pharmacotherapy.

C. Hospitalizations

Basic questions should be asked concerning any past medical or psychiatric hospitalizations—number of hospitalizations, nature and severity of condition, and length of stay—in order to evaluate factors such as multiple illnesses, adequate supervision of medications, frequency of hospitalizations, accident proneness, and, unfortunately, drug overdose.

D. Trauma

It is essential to obtain a history of traumatic events, including accidents and brain injury. A history of head injury and unexplained or multiple accidents may raise suspicions of abuse or neglect, which may be etiologically related to presenting psychiatric symptoms. Trauma may also be the result of physical or sexual abuse. Head injury may affect action of a drug.

E. Transfusions

Given the current epidemic of HIV (AIDS) infections, a history of transfusions is especially important in children who received blood products prior to the more recent careful screening of blood products for HIV. This is particularly relevant in children with hemophilia.

F. Current Medications

As part of the medical history, inquiries should be made about all medications, including those prescribed by other clinicians and over-the-counter drugs used even occasionally by the patient, and, as appropriate, alcohol and illicit or recreational drug use. Many psychoactive drugs have significant interactions with other medications, and the addition of a psychoactive medication to other specific medications can cause dangerous side effects. For instance, the administration of monoamine oxidase (MAO) inhibitors (Chapter 9) to patients who commonly take sympathomimetics for allergies can be dangerous (i.e., precipitate a hypertensive crisis). One medication may also alter the blood level of another, thereby increasing or decreasing the effectiveness of either of the two medications (e.g., subadrenergic blockers may substantially raise blood levels of common neuroleptic drugs) (see Chapter 2). Medications for asthma, allergies, or seizures can cause side effects indistinguishable from psychiatric disorders (see Chapter 13). For example, the use of phenobarbital for seizures can make children hyperactive, and the use of xanthines (such as theophylline) in the treatment of asthma can produce anxiety as a side effect.

Drug interactions are discussed in Chapter 1 and for each of the classes of psycho-active drugs in subsequent chapters and are beyond the scope of this chapter. It is the prescribing clinician's responsibility to be aware of any medication, prescription or otherwise, that the patient may be taking concurrently and to evaluate the potential interaction before prescribing a new medication. Parents or caretakers and patients, as appropriate to their age and cognitive abilities, should be instructed to inform any treating clinicians of psychoactive medication(s) currently being taken.

G. Allergies

A careful history of previous allergic reactions to medications is essential since these presage such problems with psychoactive drugs.

H. Substance Use History

Particularly for teenage patients, a history of alcohol, tobacco, or illicit drug use (common in psychiatric patients) tempers the decision to use psychoactive medications (see Chapter 11). For example, when tricyclic antidepressants are taken in combination with marijuana, sinus tachycardia may become prominent. Nicotine may decrease the effects of the tricyclic antidepressants by increasing their metabolism, thereby lowering plasma levels. The tricyclics can also increase the central nervous system effects of alcohol. Young patients and families should be warned about the potential danger of taking psychoactive drugs in combination with drugs and alcohol.

I. Social History

A social history can be vital when the use of stimulants in teenagers is contemplated. Have there been problems with the law? Has antisocial behavior occurred? To what kind of peer group does the teenager belong? How involved is the teen with his or her family? Will the parents provide careful supervision and feedback for the prescribing clinician? (This is covered in more detail in Chapters 1 and 5.)

J. Pregnancy and Birth History

Pregnancy and birth history is important to obtain, especially information on drug and alcohol use and smoking during pregnancy. Other vital information includes birth weight, complications during delivery, and time in neonatal intensive care.

K. Family Medical History

Although frequently neglected, family medical history is often critical in decision making. Inherited medical problems such as thyroid disease, Huntington's disease, and

Tourette syndrome may present with psychiatric symptoms. A family history of sudden cardiac death is particularly relevant to treating minors with tricyclic antidepressants. Given recent reports of cardiac deaths in minors treated with tricyclics[1-5] (see also Chapter 9), a complete family medical history should not be omitted. There is also a suggestion that side effects of drugs such as extrapyramidal symptoms may be familial in some cases.

L. Family Psychiatric History

A family psychiatric history can be especially helpful in diagnostically difficult cases and is an integral part of all evaluations. Additionally, a positive response to a particular tricyclic antidepressant in a parent might assist the clinician in choosing a medication for a depressed offspring since genetic factors influence pharmacokinetic and probably therapeutic response. Of particular importance is the search for a family history of Tourette syndrome or a motor movement tic disorder in children being considered for stimulant treatment (see Chapter 8).

III. MEDICAL REVIEW OF ORGAN SYSTEMS

Once the above history has been clarified, a medical review of systems should be conducted to help rule out other medical illnesses and to establish the baseline rate of complaint for all organ systems. The review of systems can be of critical importance in children who are "somatizers," particularly anxious children who may have a high baseline rate of physical complaints. These premedication complaints may involve multiple organ systems and be manifested as headaches or gastrointestinal symptoms. Without a careful multisystem review, medical illnesses may be missed, and preexisting physical complaints will be attributable to any medication that is prescribed, as has been noted with the use of stimulants in attention-deficit hyperactivity disorder (ADHD) (Chapter 8).

The following review of systems is a brief synopsis of how information gained can directly alter decision making in choosing an appropriate pharmacological intervention for a child or adolescent. It is not meant to be a complete review of systems but rather highlights certain critical questions for each organ system.

A. General Health and Appearance

In querying the general health of a psychiatric patient, useful information about fatigue, eating habits, growth rate, sleeping pattern, and general state of physical health is obtained. Clearly, a history of poor eating habits and slow growth might moderate the decision to use stimulants or be useful in evaluating appetite disturbance during treatment. Although being a "picky" eater should not be a contraindication to stimulant use, extra surveillance would be recommended for a child who has a less than optimal appetite as well as a weight-conscious teen who resists medication such as neuroleptics or antidepressants that may add more pounds. Similarly, the presence or absence of sleep difficulties in depressed adolescents may be used to decide between sedating or activating forms of antidepressant medications and what time of day the medication should be administered.

In these days of high-tech medicine, it should also be remembered that much can be learned from observing the appearance of the child. For instance, Down's syndrome, fragile X syndrome, fetal alcohol syndrome, and a number of genetic and chromosomal disorders (Klinefelter's syndrome, etc.) can be detected initially by physical appearance.

B. Eyes, Ears, Nose, and Throat

Have the child's eyes and ears been examined recently? Does the child have chronic sniffing that could actually be a vocal tic? Have there been any complaints of blurred vision? Most psychotropic medications can affect vision, though this is an uncommon complaint in children.

C. Respiratory

Is there any history of wheezing, asthma, chronic use of sympathomimetic medications, or frequent cough? This is important for drug interactions, especially stimulants (see Chapter 8) and antidepressants (see Chapter 9), which exaggerate the effect of antiasthma drugs. For instance, propranolol (Chapter 15), a subadrenergic blocker effective against many peripheral somatic manifestations of anxiety, is contraindicated for children with asthma.

D. Cardiovascular

Is there a history of heart murmur, chest pain (even for prepubertal children), fainting, or dizziness upon standing? If the child is participating in athletics, are there any complaints (shortness of breath, chest pain, or dizziness) suggestive of cardiac dysrhythmias? This is vital information since stimulants, antidepressants, and neuroleptics all have important effects on heart rate, blood pressure, and cardiac conduction and excitability (see Chapters 8–10). Indeed, in recent years, concern about the cardiac safety of tricyclic antidepressants (TCAs) for children has steadily increased as a result of reports of sudden death in at least four children receiving TCAs at usual therapeutic doses.[1-5] Careful monitoring is essential, and a pretreatment electrocardiogram (ECG) is now strongly recommended prior to treatment with TCAs (see Section IX.A).

E. Gastrointestinal

Given the common occurrence of gastrointestinal (GI) side effects from psychoactive medications such as neuroleptics (constipation) and stimulants (stomachache), a complete review of any history of nausea, vomiting, diarrhea, constipation, stomachache, or jaundice is needed. The GI system is commonly involved in affective illnesses (constipation) and anxiety disorders (diarrhea), and drug choice may be governed by side-effect profiles of medications.

F. Urinary Tract

Although preexisting problems or medication-related complications to the urinary tract are less common in children compared with the elderly, psychotropic medications may exacerbate or ameliorate urinary tract symptomatology. It should be ascertained that an individual has no renal disease, given the fact that most psychotropic medications are eliminated by the kidneys. This is especially critical for lithium treatment (see Chapter 9). Furthermore, some medications may exacerbate preexisting problems with enuresis (e.g., thioridazine), whereas others (tricyclic antidepressants) have been well documented to reduce or eliminate enuresis (see Chapter 9).

G. Genital and Reproductive Systems

Perhaps more critical for pubescent minors, the possibility of pregnancy is always a consideration before initiating trials of medication. Proper referral to a family physician or planned-parenthood organization might be considered. Teenagers need to be queried alone since they may be reluctant to admit to sexual activity or contraceptive use in front of their parents. The birth control pill has a myriad of side effects and may be the sole cause of affective illness. Similarly, neuroleptics and selective serotonin reuptake inhibitors (SSRIs) can interfere with sexual functioning and cause some mature adolescents to experience complications such as menstrual disturbances and galactorrhea (see Chapter 10).

H. Musculoskeletal System

Although a classic disease of the musculoskeletal system is rare in minors, any history of multiple complaints of joint aches, muscle pains, or weakness is important to obtain. Also, there are important musculoskeletal side effects of certain psychoactive drugs, notably stimulants (tics) and neuroleptics (dystonias, parkinsonism), so that predrug assessments will show these to be drug-emergent.

I. Integument (Skin)

The skin is a common target for side effects of psychoactive drugs. Photosensitivity is sometimes seen with neuroleptics, especially with chlorpromazine. A prior history of skin sensitivity or medication allergy would be important in guiding parents, particularly in hot and sunny climates. Any skin disorder that interferes with heat dissipation would be critical to assess, particularly for children treated with neuroleptics, which can interfere with temperature regulation, or lithium, where disturbances of fluid and electrolyte balance can be fatal.

J. Endocrine System

A review of the endocrine system is important especially in affective illnesses and ADHD. Symptoms of hypothyroidism or a family history of hypothyroidism in a hyperactive child would warrant the diagnostic evaluation of generalized resistance to thyroid hormone.[6] A positive history of hot or cold intolerance, dry skin, rapid or slow heart rate, increased fluid intake, or growth abnormalities would suggest the need for baseline thyroid studies and a careful physical exam.

K. Central Nervous System

Clearly, the review of the central nervous system is crucial in ruling out other neurological syndromes and clarifying baseline state. Questions should be asked about any history of seizures, staring spells, absences, fainting, dizziness, headaches, numbness, tingling, tremor, weakness, clumsiness, speech problems, pain, and motor or vocal tics. An electroencephalogram (EEG) should be considered only if the history is suggestive of absences, seizures, or dyscontrol syndromes consistent with any form of epilepsy. Also, since most psychotropic drugs can cause neurological-type symptoms, it is important that a baseline be established.

IV. PSYCHIATRIC REVIEW

A brief psychiatric review of systems often adds further information of critical value. For example, regardless of the nature of the initial complaint or presenting symptoms, the clinician should inquire about such other symptoms as hallucinations, anxiety states, affective state, thinking problems, delusions, and compulsions. Baseline observations by the clinician as well as those reported by other reliable observers in other locations, such as the home and school, should be described both qualitatively and quantitatively and noted in terms of the circumstances in which they occur. It is important to include usual eating and sleeping patterns because these may be altered by many drugs. A thorough psychiatric review of systems is important in developing the most complete differential diagnosis and avoiding the difficulties of starting a psychotropic medication (e.g., stimulants) only to later learn that the patient has had auditory or visual hallucinations for some years.

V. PHYSICAL AND NEUROLOGICAL EXAM

No clear-cut guidelines exist for the role of either a physical or neurological exam in the use of psychotropic medications in children. Only on a case-by-case basis can a prescribing physician decide whether to rely on a nine-month-old brief "school" physical exam administered by a busy pediatrician at one extreme or to require a recent pediatric neurological evaluation at the other extreme. One's level of suspicion should be dictated by the nature of the presenting complaint and history.

However, in general, it is prudent for children and adolescents to have a physical examination prior to initiation of psychoactive medication therapy, which should include a record of baseline temperature, pulse, heart and respiration rates, and blood pressure. Many psychoactive medications will alter blood pressure and pulse, so it is prudent to record these parameters (such as standing and supine measurements) before starting medication in the event that orthostatic difficulties occur. Height and weight measurements at regular intervals before and during medication therapy not only are good practice in view of side effects of certain drugs (stimulants, weight loss; neuroleptics, weight gain) but also reassure both clinicians and parents that growth is not being affected. Weight can also be a good indicator of therapeutic effects on severe depression. Height and weight should be entered on standardized growth charts so that serial measurements and percentiles may be plotted over time. Whenever dosage is increased, it is important to check blood pressure, pulse, height, and weight. A pregnancy test and evaluation for adequate contraceptive use should also be considered for any adolescent who might be pregnant, because drugs may have known or unknown adverse effects on the developing fetus. Since many teens may be reluctant to discuss sexual activity, obtaining a history of date of last menstrual period (normal or abnormal) is critical.

A simple neurological exam can be easily incorporated into the office practice of child and adolescent psychiatry, or this may be delegated to another physician on occasion. However, documentation may be critical regarding when this was performed and by whom. For children who may receive either stimulant medication or neuroleptic medication, a baseline screen for abnormal involuntary movements, including motor and vocal tics, should be performed and documented in the medical record. Spontaneous, stereotyped muscular movements are common in children. In children being considered for neuroleptic treatment, symptoms of tardive dyskinesia (lip licking, tongue thrusting, puffing or pouting of the lips) should be documented, since these medications may produce this neurological disorder. For assessing abnormal movements or tardive dyskinesia, the use of a rating scale such as the Abnormal Involuntary Movement Scale (AIMS) is strongly recommended (see Section VIII.C.1).

VI. BASELINE BIOCHEMICAL ASSESSMENT OF BLOOD AND URINE

The use of indiscriminate measurements of complete blood counts and blood chemistries for the purpose of defensive medicine either before starting medications or following medications is to be discouraged. Laboratory studies should be ordered (1) for specific diagnostic considerations (e.g., thyroid studies to evaluate depression), (2) for baseline assessment where proposed medications could alter organ systems [e.g., assessments of thyroid function before lithium is instituted and of liver function for patients treated with pemoline (Cylert®)], and (3) where there is suspicion of physical disease. Clearly, the prescribing physician must be familiar with each psychotropic medication prescribed and its effect on clinical chemistry and blood elements.

The routine ordering of blood work for no other reason than the fact that a child is on medication is not warranted. For instance, in a routine case of ADHD with an endocrine review of systems and a negative family history for endocrine disease, no blood work is necessary for the use of methylphenidate (Ritalin®) or dextroamphetamine (Dexedrine®) (see also Chapter 8). Additionally, if a social history of an ADHD child reveals little chance of ingestion of lead products, measurement of blood lead levels is unnecessary. However, a complete blood count should be performed in young patients on neuroleptic medication or carbamazepine if any signs of fever, sore throat, or infection develop because of the documented effect that these drugs can produce a suppression of white blood cell count.

VII. SPEECH AND LANGUAGE ASSESSMENT

Given the potential of psychotropic medications to alter speech and language skills, some baseline assessment is desirable. A large overlap exists between children with speech and language problems and children with behavior difficulties who require medication.[7]

Screening children for problems with speech and language is achieved by obtaining an accurate history and by informally interacting with the child, noting speech and language. There is no single speech and language screening test that serves all ages.

The history should look for particular items that may indicate dysfunction in this area, such as problems with articulation, recurrent otitis media, or delayed acquisition of clear speech. The history should also screen out any genetic or environmental causes. Parental concerns can often alert the clinician to determine if further evaluation is warranted by comparing the child's observed speech and language ability to normative data.

In addition to evaluating intelligibility of speech and articulation, the clinician should look out for items such as abnormal voice quality and pitch, limited syntax, failure to comprehend language as expected, sparsity of speech, narration difficulties, inability to develop complex language structures, and perceptive language problems. If there are any doubts, a full-scale evaluation of speech and language should be conducted through referral to a qualified speech and language pathologist.

The literature regarding drug effects on speech and language in the pediatric population is sparse, and it is suggested[8] that there is no established psychopharmacological treatment for speech and language disorders in children. Psychoactive drugs such as neuroleptics, stimulants, and tricyclic antidepressants can alter speech production, rate, volume, and coherence. The precipitation of mania by tricyclic antidepressants is often characterized initially by pressured or very rapid speech production. At a minimum, the mental status exam should include notation of speech and language function at presentation.

VIII. MONITORING SIDE EFFECTS

A. General Principles

This section will review various methods of measuring and monitoring physical side effects in the area of pediatric neuropharmacology. Side effects may involve the systems that are listed in Table 4. Expected physiological effects and specific side effects of different classes of drugs (e.g., stimulants, antidepressants, antipsychotics) are discussed in the chapters on those drugs and so will not be discussed here.

1. *Expect side effects and look for them.* With the increasing use and diversity of psychoactive drugs for the treatment of children and adolescents, it is essential that clinicians actively screen for potential adverse reactions.

2. *Children and adolescents are developing rapidly.* Thus, they are potentially more vulnerable to pharmacotherapy. Particular attention therefore needs to be directed toward physical development, especially where medication is given for long periods (e.g., stimulants in ADHD). Most unwanted side effects in the child are similar to those in the adult, yet they differ in terms of severity and response to changes in medication.

3. *Children don't complain.* Children are often poor informants in verbalizing subjec-

**TABLE 4. General Systems and Medical Tests
Affected by Psychoactive Drugs**

1. Behavior (behavioral toxicity)
   (a) Gross behavior, mood, and personality
   (b) Cognition, psychomotor behavior, and learning
2. Behavioral and other withdrawal effects and supersensitivity psychosis
3. Central nervous system
   (a) Extrapyramidal (acute dystonic reactions, parkinsonian reactions, akathisia, dyskinesias)
   (b) Other (e.g., seizures)
   (c) Tardive and withdrawal dyskinesias
4. Autonomic nervous system
5. Laboratory (endocrine and metabolic)
6. Intelligence (IQ)
7. Linear growth and weight
8. Cardiovascular system [including electrocardiogram (ECG)]
9. Electroencephalogram (EEG)
10. Ophthalmologic (pupil size, reactivity, accommodation)
11. Dermatologic (rashes, photosensitivity)
12. Allergic

tive feelings. Therefore, the importance of actually monitoring drug response cannot be overemphasized.

4. *What one knows one sees.* The clinician must be thoroughly acquainted with the possible side effects of the drug, keeping in mind the range of possible variations of response between individuals.

5. *Maintain an index of suspicion.* Even if the indication for the use of a medication is well established, periodic baseline information (detailed history, blood pressure, body weight, pulse rate, lab data, etc.) should be acquired on any organ system that might be adversely affected by the drug. Careful monitoring of the patient is required especially during dosage regulation in order to recognize side effects.

6. *Use parents as assessors.* Another vital procedure in monitoring side effects is to alert and educate parents and teachers regarding the potential side effects of the chosen drug as well as the therapeutic benefits so that parents may form realistic expectations.

7. *Educate the child and get him or her on side.* Knowledge should be shared with the child depending on the child's age. Adolescents and older children or children who are not resistant to pharmacotherapy should be told why they are receiving medication in a language suitable to their cognitive level. Very young children, highly suggestible children, or children who are opposed to or react negatively to medication would most likely not benefit from a detailed discussion of the above. Sensitive counseling can usually help overcome any fears that the child may have.

8. *Be active and systematic.* Since this young age group will usually provide information less readily than adults, it is important that the child or adolescent be systematically questioned about compliance and the development of any side effects. In addition to regular observations of the child by the clinician to determine the optimal dose, supplemental reports from parents and teachers are often invaluable sources of information.

9. *Do a screen before starting medication.* This will help to prevent false attributions of effects to drugs.

10. *If possible, begin with placebo for one week and rescreen.* This will deal with anxiety and expectancy-generated "side effects."

B. Types of Measures

The following measures are utilized for the assessment of side effects[9]:

1. Rating scales
2. Checklists (developed for specific drugs)
3. Physical and neurological exam
4. Laboratory studies
5. Electrophysiological studies (EEG and ECG)

C. Formal Side-Effects Rating Scales

As it is not possible to explore the physical measurements of drug effects in great depth here, a 1985 special issue of the Psychopharmacology Bulletin,[10] published by the National Institute of Mental Health (NIMH), is strongly recommended for a more comprehensive and informative review of assessment techniques for use in children and adolescents. One of the most influential publications concerning rating scales and psychopharmacological research in children, this special issue includes items such as forms for documenting demographic and family data, psychiatric assessment scales, neurological exams, and instruments for measuring adverse effects, as well as a review of pediatric drug compliance. Some of these topics will be highlighted in the subsequent discussion of medication compliance, measurement of neurological functioning level using the revised PANESS scale, and an overview of rating scales and other available assessment methods for documenting adverse changes resulting from drug treatment. In addition, this special issue of *Psychopharmacology Bulletin* describes scales for potential use in monitoring drug effects in children with specific disorders, including schizophrenia, tic disorder and Tourette syndrome, mental retardation, and autism. These types of scales are covered in Chapter 5.

Although rating scales are an essential component of psychopharmacological research and tend to be used less in clinical practice, perhaps those most frequently used are Conners' Parent Rating Scale (CPRS), Conners' Teacher Rating Scale (CRS), and the Child Behavior Checklist (CBCL). For a more detailed description of these specific rating scales, see Chapter 5.

1. Side-Effects Rating Scales

The use of subjective rating scales as a means of assessing side effects in pediatric psychopharmacology is important to the clinician in terms of charting an individual patient's progress on a specific drug as well as in comparing drugs. Although such rating scales are probably not commonly used in practice for the assessment of side effects, their use is to be encouraged since they may elicit medication-induced symptoms that the patient or family might not have reported.

One inherent difficulty with this idea has been a lack of consensus on instruments that systematically evaluate side effects and drug efficacy among children. This has led to confusion and slow progress in the field of pediatric psychopharmacology. Indeed, it should be noted that there is still a remarkable absence of psychometrically validated side-effect measures for use by parents and teachers in the field. For practitioners, the development of techniques for determining the presence of side effects in children has also been hindered by the inherent difficulties in effective communication on such a technical subject between practitioners and young patients. However, a number of general rating scales have been developed that can be used by practitioners and applied to the pediatric population. Some of these scales are still in an early stage of development; much more needs to be learned about their reliability, validity, and appropriateness for pediatric populations. [Drug-specific scales such as Barkley's for stimulants (see Chapter 8) are not considered here but in the relevant chapters.]

Dosage Record and Treatment Emergent Symptom Scale (DOTES).[11] The DOTES, published by the Early Clinical Drug Evaluation Unit (ECDEU) of the NIMH, is a general rating scale that has been clinically useful in both children and adults to assess the presence and intensity of psychotropic medication side effects (see Table 5). The DOTES involves a systematic review of all body systems through both inquiry and simple physical exam. Judgments on intensity, relationship of symptoms to the medication, and action taken for each symptom occurrence are required. Daily drug dosages, ratings of symptom severity and subjective distress, and various adverse effects may also be recorded. In order to prevent the appearance of "false" side effects, it is important to establish baseline symptomatology by administering the DOTES before the initiation of drug treatment.

The DOTES can also be used in conjunction with the NIMH-developed *Treatment Emergent Symptoms Scale* (TESS),[12] a separate six-item scale that allows the rater to record any symptoms not listed on the DOTES.

Subjective Treatment Emergent Symptom Scale (STESS).[13] The STESS, also developed by the ECDEU, is a 32-item, five-point scale suitable for children up to age 15. Designed to acquire information on the existence of physical complaints, the STESS may be completed by the child, parent, or other rater. The rater is not asked to judge the relationship between symptoms and drug. In addition, the scale may be used by the clinician as a screening device for treatment-emergent symptoms. Once again, it is essential that the scale be administered once during the baseline period (pretreatment) and at least once posttreatment.

TABLE 5. Side Effects Assessed Using the Dosage Recorded Treatment Emergent Symptom Scale (DOTES)[a]

1. Headache	11. Diarrhea	20. Nasal congestion
2. Nausea/vomiting	12. Dermatologic changes	21. Drowsiness
3. Blurred vision	13. Tremors	22. Insomnia
4. Excitement/agitation	14. Rigidity	23. Toxic confusional state
5. Depressive affect	15. Dystonia	24. Tachycardia
6. Dizziness	16. Increased motor activity	25. Hypertension
7. Akathisia	17. Dry mouth	26. Hypotension
8. Weight loss	18. Increased salivation	27. Anorexia/decreased appetite
9. Weight gain	19. Sweating	28. Abnormal liver enzymes
10. Constipation		

[a]Reprinted with permission from Garvey *et al.*[55]

STUDY	PATIENT	FORM	PERIOD	RATER	HOSPITAL
(1-6)	(7-9)	(10-12) 117	(13-15)	(16-17)	(79-80)

PATIENT'S NAME

RATER

DATE

DEPARTMENT OF HEALTH, EDUCATION, AND WELFARE
PUBLIC HEALTH SERVICE
ALCOHOL, DRUG ABUSE, AND MENTAL HEALTH ADMINISTRATION
NATIONAL INSTITUTE OF MENTAL HEALTH

ABNORMAL INVOLUNTARY MOVEMENT SCALE (AIMS)

INSTRUCTIONS: Complete Examination Procedure (reverse side) before making ratings.
MOVEMENT RATINGS: Rate highest severity observed. Rate movements that occur upon activation one *less* than those observed spontaneously.

Code:
0 = None
1 = Minimal, may be extreme normal
2 = Mild
3 = Moderate
4 = Severe

(Circle One)   CARD 01 (18-19)

FACIAL AND ORAL MOVEMENTS:

1. Muscles of Facial Expression
e.g., movements of forehead, eyebrows, periorbital area, cheeks; include frowning, blinking, smiling, grimacing
0 1 2 3 4   (20)

2. Lips and Perioral Area
e.g., puckering, pouting, smacking
0 1 2 3 4   (21)

3. Jaw
e.g., biting, clenching, chewing, mouth opening, lateral movement
0 1 2 3 4   (22)

4. Tongue
Rate only increase in movement both in and out of mouth, NOT inability to sustain movement
0 1 2 3 4   (23)

EXTREMITY MOVEMENTS:

5. Upper (*arms, wrists, hands, fingers*)
Include choreic movements, (i.e., rapid, objectively purposeless, irregular, spontaneous), athetoid movements (i.e., slow, irregular, complex, serpentine).
Do NOT include tremor (i.e., repetitive, regular, rhythmic)
0 1 2 3 4   (24)

6. Lower (*legs, knees, ankles, toes*)
e.g., lateral knee movement, foot tapping, heel dropping, foot squirming, inversion and eversion of foot
0 1 2 3 4   (25)

		0	1	2	3	4	
TRUNK MOVEMENTS:	7. Neck, shoulders, hips e.g., rocking, twisting, squirming, pelvic gyrations						(26)
	8. Severity of abnormal movements	None, normal 0	Minimal 1	Mild 2	Moderate 3	Severe 4	(27)
GLOBAL JUDGMENTS:	9. Incapacitation due to abnormal movements	None, normal 0	Minimal 1	Mild 2	Moderate 3	Severe 4	(28)
	10. Patient's awareness of abnormal movements Rate only patient's report	No awareness 0	Aware, no distress 1	Aware, mild distress 2	Aware, moderate distress 3	Aware, severe distress 4	(29)
DENTAL STATUS:	11. Current problems with teeth and/or dentures	No 0	Yes 1				(30)
	12. Does patient usually wear dentures?	No 0	Yes 1				(31)

MH-9-117

FIGURE 1. Abnormal Involuntary Movement Scale (AIMS).

EXAMINATION PROCEDURE

Either before or after completing the Examination Procedure observe the patient
unobtrusively, at rest (e.g., in waiting room).

The chair to be used in this examination should be a hard, firm one without arms.

1. Ask patient whether there is anything in his/her mouth (i.e., gum, candy, etc.)
   and if there is, to remove it.

2. Ask patient about the current condition of his/her teeth. Ask patient if he/she
   wears dentures. Do teeth or dentures bother patient now?

3. Ask patient whether he/she notices any movements in mouth, face, hands, or feet.
   If yes, ask to describe and to what extent they currently bother patient or interfere
   with his/her activities

4. Have patient sit in chair with hands on knees, legs slightly apart, and feet flat on
   floor. (Look at entire body for movements while in this position).

5. Ask patient to sit with hands hanging unsupported. If male, between legs, if female
   and wearing a dress, hanging over knees. (Observe hands and other body areas.)

6. Ask patient to open mouth. (Observe tongue at rest within mouth.) Do this twice.

7. Ask patient to protrude tongue. (Observe abnormalities of tongue movement.)
   Do this twice.

■ 8. Ask patient to tap thumb, with each finger, as rapidly as possible for 10—15 seconds;
   separately with right hand, then with left hand. (Observe facial and leg movements.)

9. Flex and extend patient's left and right arms (one at a time.) (Note any rigidity
   and rate on DOTES.)

10. Ask patient to stand up. (Observe in profile. Observe all body areas again, hips
    included.)

■ 11. Ask patient to extend both arms outstretched in front with palms down. (Observe
    trunk, legs, and mouth.)

■ 12. Have patient walk a few paces, turn, and walk back to chair. (Observe hands and
    gait.) Do this twice.

■ Activated movements

MH-9—117 (Back)
11-74

FIGURE 1. *(Continued)*

Abnormal Involuntary Movement Scale (AIMS).[14] The prevalence of tardive dyskinesia as a side effect in patients with long-term exposure to neuroleptic medication has become a serious concern to clinicians. Characterized by abnormal involuntary movements of the tongue, lips, jaw, face, trunk, or extremities, tardive dyskinesia is often considered to be a debilitating and often irreversible adverse reaction from the clinical as well as legal standpoint. Thus, the importance of early detection and routine screening of patients for the presence of abnormal involuntary movements cannot be understated.

Perhaps the most widely used standardized rating instrument in the assessment of dyskinetic movements is the AIMS (see Fig. 1) developed by the Psychopharmacology Research Branch of the NIMH. Though initially developed for adults, it is also appropriate for children. This global 12-item scale consists of dyskinetic ratings of the face, lips, jaw, tongue, upper and lower extremities, and trunk. Abnormal involuntary movements are rated on a five-point scale from 0 to 4, with 0 being none, 1 being minimal or extreme normal, 2 being mild, 3 being moderate, and 4 being severe. In addition, ratings for global severity, incapacitation, patient awareness, and dental status are recorded. Knowledge of a baseline and subsequent AIMS ratings is most helpful to the clinician in assessing any changes in baseline abnormal involuntary movements—increases, decrements, or changes in topography—during the course of active treatment with psychoactive medication, as well as during periods of withdrawal from medication. These ratings are often essential to differentiate preexisting abnormal involuntary movements from withdrawal dyskinesias. For instance, a baseline assessment of abnormal movements is recommended in children with developmental disabilities in order to distinguish commonly seen stereotypies and mannerisms from subsequent tardive or withdrawal dyskinesias if they occur.[15] The clinician should keep in mind that the AIMS is a global rating scale and has good validity.[16]

It is optimal to perform the AIMS exam procedure prior to chronic neuroleptic treatment and at regular intervals thereafter while the patient remains on drug therapy. The neurological exam should be concerned only with abnormal involuntary movements, specifically those characteristic of tardive dyskinesia. Neurological systems such as sensory or pyramidal should not be involved. Videotaping subjects may also assist in assessing dyskinetic movements. If early signs of abnormal involuntary movements are detected, the clinician should consider lowering the dose of the antipsychotic drug or discontinuing the medication.

Other side-effects rating scales* that have been found to be appropriate and reliable in children and adolescents include *Withdrawal Emergent Symptom Checklist* (WESC), which measures behavioral and other withdrawal effects on a 13-item scale, the *Simpson–Angus Scale for Extrapyramidal Symptoms* (SASEPS), which measures parkinsonian side effects, and the *NIMH Systematic Assessment for Treatment Emergent Events* (SAFTEE-GI), an 11-page form which includes 68 adverse effects, laboratory/physical findings, and dosage record.[9] In addition, Barkley[17] has created a side-effects rating scale for the stimulant drugs and has found it to be quite sensitive to the behavioral side effects of these compounds in drug research.[17] Similar rating scales should be developed for other psychoactive medications and used along with the more traditional behavior rating scales in future drug research with children.

This in no way comprises a comprehensive list of rating scales that are currently available to assess the side effects of psychoactive medication in children and adolescents. For a more thorough review of techniques and ratings used for the assessment of adverse

---

*All scales appearing in the special feature on rating scales and assessment instruments of *Psychopharmacology Bulletin* (1985) may be obtained from NIMH, 5600 Fishers Lane, Room 18C-06, Rockville, MD 20857.

effects, the *Psychopharmacology Bulletin*[9] and a monograph by Campbell et al.[16] are suggested.

"Customized Target Symptoms" and Side Effects. Much of the evidence (except in the case of stimulants) on the development of assessment instruments used for the treatment of the pediatric population is based on research involving adult populations.[9] Thus, for the young patient, the practicing clinician may find it useful to select specific target symptoms (such as impulsivity rather than fidgetiness in the hyperactive child) at which drug treatment should be directed and then "customize" side-effect and target-symptom checklists for that specific drug by listing expected side effects.

2. Physical and Neurological Exam for Soft Signs

A standard neurological exam for children primarily involves developmental assessment and observation of motor function as well as screening for minor physical anomalies. Since it has been suspected that various pediatric disorders might be associated with an increased frequency of neurological "soft signs," the quest for quantifying subtle central nervous system (CNS) disturbances as well as standardizing a large battery of "soft signs" in children was facilitated by the development of the *Physical and Neurological Examination for Soft Signs* (PANESS)[18] in 1976.

The ECDEU's original PANESS consists of a 15-item physical exam and a 43-item scored neurological exam designed specifically to evaluate the presence of soft signs in children up to the age of 15 for drug studies. It has been suggested that the PANESS be administered once before pharmacological intervention and at least once posttreatment. In 1985, a revised PANESS[19] was published after intensive research in various pediatric populations had questioned the clinical validity, reliability, and diagnostic power of certain individual items on the 1976 PANESS. Methodological problems in administering and scoring the exam also highlighted the need for further changes and refinement of the original exam.

The Physical Examination section, while self-explanatory for physicians, includes the following recordings: Age, Height, Weight, Head Circumference, Pulse, Blood Pressure, Visual Acuity, Ophthalmoscopic, Audiogram, Handedness, Physical Examination (cardiovascular, pulmonary, liver, kidney, musculoskeletal, etc.), Past Medical History, Abnormal Physical Findings, and Diagnosis (using ICD-8 terminology). This section of the PANESS may be used independently or in conjunction with the neurological exam.

The revised Neurological Examination for Subtle Signs contains a number of motor and sensory clinical procedures, divided into clusters, that include the following test areas: Lateral Preference Pattern, Gait and Balance, Impersistence, Involuntary Movements, Repetitive Movements (timed coordination), Sequenced/Patterned Movements (timed coordination), and Asymmetry. Extraneous "overflow" movement is also coded. Though the rater does not have to be a physician, the nature of the exam (emphasis on proper instruction and clear demonstration to the patient) dictates that the examiner be thoroughly familiar with the procedures for administering the exam, which may require additional training. A positive and encouraging atmosphere throughout the exam is of high importance. For detailed procedures on how to conduct and score the revised exam, the ECDEU Assessment Manual should be consulted.

Despite the interest in child psychiatry and developmental pediatrics in "soft signs," no clear role for the PANESS as a diagnostic or predictive instrument has yet been demonstrated in pediatric psychopharmacology. However, particularly with agents that clearly alter motor function (e.g., neuroleptics or anticonvulsants), some assessment of neurological systems is advisable before initiating therapy, and parts of a well-standardized neurological exam might be clinically useful.

D. Compliance (Adherence) with Medication

The issue of noncompliance (nonadherence) is a serious problem in pediatric psycho-pharmacological treatment that has not been recognized by most investigators[20] (see also Chapter 1). Obviously, for psychopharmacotherapy to be effective in the disorder for which it is prescribed, the drug must be taken following the prescribed directions. Indeed, failure of the child to take medication as properly prescribed is probably the most likely explanation for a child's lack of response, unexpectedly poor response, or increased variability in response to a given drug. Noncompliance can range from altering the prescribed system in terms of number of doses or length of treatment to completely failing to take the drug. Clearly, a child will not experience any beneficial drug effects if a drug is not taken. As mentioned previously, close monitoring of treatment response is required should any unexpected side effects emerge.

Many factors may interfere with compliance. Some parents will at times withold medication if their child appears to be doing well or, conversely, increase the medication without the clinician's approval if behavior worsens. Some may even administer the drug to the child as a punishment. At times, some children and adolescents may actively try to avoid ingesting medication. Another factor that influences compliance, particularly in older children and adolescents, is related to side effects. For example, if they feel "funny" or develop a stomachache, they may be more reluctant to take medication. The more responsible a child is for administering his or her own medication, the more likely it is, in general, that unpleasant, untoward effects will interfere with compliance.

Direct and objective measures of compliance (i.e., laboratory testing—measuring serum or blood levels of the drug, testing for urinary excretion of the drug itself or a metabolite, etc.) as well as indirect measures (i.e., interviews, pill counts) are reviewed in detail in the special issue of *Psychopharmacology Bulletin*[20] and should be consulted for details.

Because children are less likely to verbalize their feelings and state whether they are properly adhering to their medication, clinicians should take special caution not to over-estimate compliance in their young patients. Unlike adult compliance, pediatric compliance involves the decisions of two people: the child and the parent. Simple medication error (misunderstanding of instructions, carelessness) needs to be differentiated from intentional noncompliance on either the child's or the parent's part. Counseling and education can often improve patient compliance if the problem is the former, whereas the latter problem requires a more detailed and sensitive approach. Establishing a trusting clinician–patient relationship is of key importance in pediatric drug compliance. This is especially true in the adolescent population, as adolescents are often entrusted to make decisions on their own. It is also essential to carefully assess the attitude and reliability of the persons who will be responsible for administering the medication in order to make a reliable assessment of drug efficacy and compliance. Noncompliance may be reduced sometimes if an adequate, understandable explanation of the simple pharmacokinetics of the drug is given to parents and patients when initially discussing medication; for example, the importance of keeping blood levels fairly constant by taking the medication as prescribed can be emphasized and reviewed again if lack of compliance becomes important. Side effects should be explained so that the child or adolescent understands them. In highly resistant children or adolescents or "somatizers,"too complete a discussion of rare and unusual side effects can complicate side-effects monitoring. The dangers of sudden discontinuation should be discussed, particularly for clonidine as well as for tricyclic antidepressants, as significant GI symptoms can result from rapid discontinuation of these drugs. Prior knowledge can help increase a child's sense of control and decrease fear of some untoward effects.

IX. LABORATORY MEASURES AND MONITORING

The role of the laboratory in the evaluation of children and adolescents with behavioral problems has become increasingly prominent as a supplement to the crucial clinical history and physical exam. A wide array of laboratory measures is available to the clinician for the diagnosis and management of behavioral difficulties in children. Rapid advances such as the development of highly technical instruments for imaging the brain as well as measuring endogenous and exogenous biologically active substances have also provided major contributions to the field of pediatric neuropharmacology.

This section will focus only on the utility of the more commonly considered laboratory measures in evaluating behavioral problems in the pediatric population. Many of these tests will be addressed more specifically under each class of medications or, if appropriate, for specific drugs later in this book. Obviously, the premedication workup will be influenced by and should be modified to accommodate any particular abnormal findings in the medical history or examination, such as renal, thyroid, and cardiac abnormalities, or any initial abnormal findings in the laboratory results themselves. The clinician should be aware that much of the information in child and adolescent psychiatry is extrapolated from research in adult populations with a few exceptions as outlined below.

A. Electrocardiogram

The use of tricyclic antidepressants (TCAs) in the pediatric population has become the subject of considerable controversy[21] since the reports of additional cases of sudden death in children treated with presumably therapeutic doses of desipramine[1–5,22] and the combination of clonidine and methylphenidate.[23] These reports highlight the need for careful consideration of the use of ECG in children treated with TCAs.

In a recent review of the cardiovascular effects of TCAs, Wilens et al.[24] state:

> In summary, the TCA treatment in children and adolescents appears to produce predictable and generally minor cardiovascular changes. We recommend routine monitoring of the ECG at baseline and the use of TCA assay and repeat ECG after significant dose increases and routinely when robust daily doses are administered. By the nature of infrequent serious adverse events, it is unclear if stringent monitoring of TCA treatment can reduce the risk of sudden death during TCA treatment and indeed the contribution of the TCAs to such dire events remains unclear.

They further state that "there are inadequate data on cardiovascular risk factors to support or reject the notion of clinically significant differences between TCAs in rates of adverse cardiac effects with therapeutic dosing." Of particular concern is delayed cardiac conduction as reflected on the ECG by increases in PR and QRS intervals, cardiac arrhythmias, and tachycardia. In overdose, delayed conduction may lead to a complete heart block or ventricular reentry arrythmias.

For those clinicians who, despite the controversy, continue to use desipramine or other tricyclics in children and adolescents, a recent brief review of published guidelines[25] for the monitoring of ECG parameters exists. Data are based on established age-dependent normative values[25,26] coupled with parameters adapted from ongoing pharmacological trials, as well as from clinical experience with large numbers of children and adolescents. What the critical reader must appreciate is that experts do not agree on ECG parameter monitoring, given the inherent ethical and safety issues in studying this area.

B. Blood Levels

As covered in Chapter 2 and in chapters on specific medications, it is clear that laboratory measurement of serum concentrations of medications plays a crucial role in neuropharmacology. Indications for measuring drug levels include checking for compliance as well as monitoring for toxicity, since modest to good correlations do exist between ECG changes and blood levels, particularly for nortriptyline, and less so for desipramine.[27] A problem of note is that there can be up to a 7-fold difference in plasma levels between individuals on comparable doses of TCA and even higher differences among those on neuroleptics.

Monitoring blood levels has become more of an issue with the more widespread use of the new serotonin reuptake inhibitors. These new classes of medications have profound effects on the cytochrome P450 enzyme system and thus alter blood levels of a wide array of other medications commonly used in psychiatry. For a review of this topic, see Ciraulo and Shader[28,29] and Chapter 2.

C. Dexamethasone Suppression Test

Though nonsuppression of cortisol secretion during the dexamethasone suppression test (DST) has been statistically correlated with the diagnosis of major depression with melancholia[30] or endogenous depression, the DST has not proven to be clinically useful in children[31] or adolescents.[31,32] It may support a diagnosis of a psychiatric disorder, but it does not exclude one. Problems with the DST include inability to predict prognosis and assist in the choice of medication, as well as the high frequency of false-positive results that confound its interpretation.

D. Thyroid Function Tests

Laboratory tests of thyroid function, including serum thyroxine (T4), triiodothyronine resin uptake, thyroid-stimulating hormone (TSH), and serum triiodothyronine (T3) levels, are beneficial in evaluating psychiatric symptoms. Symptoms that may be associated with abnormal thyroid function include anxiety, depression, mental retardation, dementia, restlessness, mental status change, and psychosis. If thyroid disease is suspected to be contributing to a disorder, screening tests of thyroxine and triiodothyronine resin uptake should be conducted. Thyroid-stimulating hormone levels should be determined if results are abnormal or barely normal. A thyrotropin-releasing hormone stimulation test may be considered if initial studies are ambiguous. However, this test has not shown clinical utility in the diagnosis or treatment of depression in adolescents.[30]

A report by Hauser et al.[6] documented an association between ADHD and a rare condition known as resistance to thyroid hormone (RTH) caused by a mutation in the thyroid receptor gene (hTRB) on chromosome 3. The syndrome is characterized by peripheral resistance to thyroid hormone action and should be suspected in children with goiter, low weight, short stature, and hearing or speech abnormalities.[33] The biochemical profile is characterized by the association of a high free T4 and a detectable TSH (usually in the normal range). This defines an inappropriate secretion of TSH, for which RTH is by far the main diagnosis in childhood.

Confirmation of resistance comes clinically after T3 suppression test. For an excellent review, see Retoff and Weiss[33]. Because RTH is a rare condition, routine screening for RTH is not warranted in ADHD, except for children or adults with a family history suggestive of thyroid disorder or with other indicators of RTH. The use of thyroid function tests for those to whom lithium will be administered is discussed in Chapter 9.

E. Electroencephalography

An EEG may be considered for patients to whom antipsychotics, tricyclic antidepressants, or lithium will be administered, because all of these drugs have been associated with either lowered threshold for seizures or other EEG changes. Indications would include patients who have a history of seizure disorder, who are on an antiepileptic drug for a seizure disorder, or who may be at risk for seizures (e.g., following brain surgery or head injury). A complete EEG and neurologic consultation should be obtained when the physical exam and history indicate gross motor seizures, absences, complex partial seizures, temporal lobe epilepsy, or dyscontrol syndromes. However, the routine use of the EEG as a baseline workup for normal, healthy youngsters is not necessary given the high prevalence of abnormal EEG findings in the general population[34] and the difficulty of their interpretation. Nevertheless, if a seizure disorder or EEG abnormalities are known to exist, a baseline EEG should be obtained and the EEG periodically monitored.

F. Catecholamine and Enzyme Assays

In evaluating young patients for anxiety, catecholamines (homovanillic acid, vanillyl-mandelic acid, metanephrines) are assayed in a 24-hr urine collection for the presence of pheochromocytoma. It is suggested that only patients with accompanying abnormal levels of autonomic function be screened for pheochromocytoma, rather than all anxiety patients.[35] Research studies measuring urinary and serum catecholamines in hyperactive patients have no clinical application at present.[36]

Though enzyme measurements are common in research settings,[37] they have not been applied clinically to children and adolescents with behavioral disorders. Enzymes measured include monoamine oxidase, catechol-O-methyltransferase, dopamine β-hydroxylase, and adenylate cyclase.

For children treated with neuroleptics, the development of neuroleptic malignant syndrome (NMS) is characterized by fever, muscle rigidity, stupor, and autonomic dysfunction. Blood levels of creatine phosphokinase and white cell counts can be crucial in diagnosing this rare complication, but routine measurement is not necessary.

G. Lumbar Punctures

Much of the data on the use of lumbar punctures to measure cerebrospiral fluid (CSF) in pediatric psychopathology is from research studies,[38–40] with the central focus being on the concentration of the serotonin metabolite 5-hyroxyindoleacetic acid (5-HIAA). Lower CSF 5-HIAA concentrations have been reported in children and adolescents with histories of aggression,[38,40] offering further support for analogous studies in adults. However, the impact of an abnormal 5-HIAA concentration on treatment is still unestablished, and further documentation in childhood psychiatric disorders is needed. Clearly, clinical pictures of altered mental status consistent with CSF infection warrant examination of CSF with lumbar puncture, but routine screens do not.

H. AIDS Screening

Screening for sexually transmitted disease agents such as HIV and *Treponema pallidum* (using the Venereal Disease Research Laboratory test) should be done in children and adolescents who present a history of sexual abuse or sexual activity and are being evaluated for symptoms of depression or changes in cognitive function.[41] Positive results should be followed with the fluorescent treponemal antibody absorption test (FTA-ABS) and the possibility of an infectious disease consultation dependent on subsequent results. Children and adolescents considered to be at risk should be screened for HIV.

I. Toxicology

For adolescents with new-onset psychosis or behavioral changes, testing for drugs of abuse may be helpful (see Chapter 11). For those in a substance-abuse treatment program, continuous monitoring of compliance with drug abstinence is recommended. If substance abuse is known or suspected, screening of urine and/or blood for toxic substances may be indicated. Lead ingestion, though rare, can also be measured as a potential cause of behavioral difficulty. Cardiovascular toxicity of TCAs is of concern in all age groups but especially in children and younger adolescents. Monitoring TCA blood levels should be done whenever the dose is increased to ensure that blood levels remain safely below toxic levels. In addition, careful clinical observation and concentration monitoring are crucial when combination overdoses (e.g., MAO inhibitors and TCAs) are suspected (see subsequent chapters on specific classes of drugs).

J. Genetic Studies

Genetic studies of childhood psychopathology have provided evidence for relationships between specific chromosomal abnormalities and psychopathology. Twin studies have supported a higher concordance for a particular disorder among monozygotic (rather than dizygotic) twins. In addition, family studies have revealed a greater occurrence of certain disorders in at-risk family members.[42] In child and adolescent psychopathology, the most common form of genetic assessment is karyotyping, which determines chromosome number and morphology. Though physical evidence that would lead clinicians to suspect sex-chromosome abnormalities may not be readily visualized in prepubertal children, it has been suggested that deficits in cognitive development and functioning are influenced by abnormal numbers of X chromosomes.[43]

There have also been associations between increased numbers of Y chromosomes and increased risks of behavioral problems, most notably impulsivity and immaturity.[44] Childhood karyotyping can provide support for certain medical interventions, such as testosterone replacement for patients with Klinefelter's syndrome, leading to improved social functioning.[45] The identification of Wilson's disease, a recessively inherited disorder of copper metabolism, is important in adolescents with incongruous behavior, personality change, cognitive impairment, anxiety, and depression.[46] Though it is not diagnosable by genetic measures, its identification (low serum ceruloplasmin level, low total serum copper level, and raised urinary copper excretion) is critical because it is a treatable metabolic disorder.

Fragile X syndrome, so named because of the propensity for breakage on the long arm of the X chromosome under certain conditions, is the most common inherited form of mental retardation[47] after Down's syndrome. It accounts for 8% of all children with learning disability and carries with it an increased risk of psychopathology[48] including hyperactivity, short attention span, social skills deficits, anxiety, and depression. Irritability, aggressiveness, and tantrums are also reported to be characteristics, and hyperactivity and aggression are considered to be more controversial components of the disorder.[47,49] Clinical indications for fragile X screening include distinctive physical features such as large or prominent ears, a long face, and postpubertal testicular enlargement, which is found in 80% of affected adult males. These typical features are often not found in prepubertal males. Female carriers have more subtle facial abnormalities, including high broad forehead, prominent ears, and a long narrow face. These features are more common in females with learning disabilities. Extreme shyness, anxiety and social avoidance, withdrawal, and poor eye contact are also commonly reported in females with fragile X. For a complete review of the fragile X syndrome, see Reiss.[47]

K. Brain Imaging

The various types of instrumentation currently available for brain imaging—computed tomography (CT), magnetic resonance imaging (MRI), EEG spectral tomography, positron-emission tomography (PET), and cerebral blood flow—have all been utilized in studying clinical problems in child psychopathology. Despite the extensive use of CT and significant findings with MRI in autism and ADHD patients,[50] the routine use of imaging studies is not indicated in children with behavioral disorders. PET measurements of brain glucose metabolism (using fluoro-2-deoxy-D-glucose) or of blood flow (using radioactive water as a tracer) have not found a permanent place outside research studies and are not clinically indicated as of yet, except perhaps in the presurgical evaluation of children with intractable epilepsy.[51] However, MRI or CT (with or without contrast) is considered clinically useful for ruling out brain tumors and for mapping signs of increased intracranial pressure, changing or degenerative neurological signs, craniofacial malformations, suspected syndromes, or inherited syndromes that include CNS structures. The clinical utility of EEG spectral tomography (mapping of brain electrical activity) in children and adolescents has not been supported by any studies.

L. Routine Liver, Kidney, and Serum Measures

Complete blood counts, assays of liver enzymes, and assessment of kidney function and frequent urinalysis are important in the routine use of psychoactive medications only if particular medications may alter organ functioning or if there is some question as to the integrity of the liver or kidney to handle the metabolism of the drug. An example is lithium, which can affect kidney function. Because of reported adverse effects of lithium carbonate on the kidney, baseline evaluation of kidney function should be determined. It would also be mandatory to obtain regular complete blood counts for following children on newer drugs such as clozapine. Tests for serum amylase and electrolyte values may be useful in assessment and follow-up of bulimic patients.[52]

X. CONCLUSIONS

The importance of a thorough predrug physical assessment and the monitoring of side effects once psychoactive medication has been prescribed cannot be overemphasized in children and adolescents. Because different symptoms or side effects may mimic other illnesses, the clinical history and physical exam are crucial in making a differential diagnosis that directly impacts on the nature and course of medication to be prescribed. Laboratory tests should not be used as a substitute. Indeed, laboratory measures should have only a peripheral value in making a diagnosis and should be targeted to any existing or suspected disease and to more common side effects. Judicious use of laboratory parameters may thus be valuable to the clinician in answering specific questions of evaluation and medical management of young patients treated with psychoactive medications.

REFERENCES

1. Abramowicz M: Sudden death in children treated with a tricyclic antidepressant. *Med Lett Drugs Ther* 32:53, 1990.
2. Riddle MA, Nelson JC, Kleinman CS, et al: Sudden death in children receiving Norpramin: A review of three reported cases and commentary. *J Am Acad Child Adolesc Psychiatry* 30:104–108, 1991.
3. Riddle MA, Geller B, Ryan, ND: Another sudden death in a child treated with desipramine. *J Am Acad Child Adolesc Psychiatry* 32:792–797, 1993.
4. Biederman J: Sudden death in children treated with a tricyclic antidepressant. *J Am Acad Child Adolesc Psychiatry* 30:495–498, 1991.
5. Biederman J, Thisted RA, Greenhill LL, Ryan ND: Estimation of the association between desipramine and the risk for sudden death in 5- to 14-year-old children. *J Clin Psychiatry* 56(3):87–93, 1995.
6. Hauser P, Zametkin A, et al: Attention deficit hyperactivity disorder in people with generalized resistance to thyroid hormone. *N Engl J Med* 328:997–1001, 1993.
7. Cantwell DP, Baker L: Psychiatric disorder in children with speech and language retardation: A critical review. *Arch Gen Psychiatry* 34:583–591, 1977.

8. Gittelman-Klein R, Spitzer RL, Cantwell D: Diagnostic classifications and psychopharmacological indications, in Werry JS (ed): *Pediatric Psychopharmacology: The Use of Behavior Modifying Drugs in Children.* New York, Brunner/Mazel, 1978, pp 136–167.

9. Campbell M, Palij, M: Measurement of side effects including tardive dyskinesia, in special issue of *Psychopharmacology Bulletin: Rating Scales and Assessment Instruments for Use in Pediatric Psychopharmacology Research.* Published by the National Institute of Mental Health. *Psychopharmacol Bull* 21(4):1063–1066, 1985.

10. Special issue of *Psychopharmacology Bulletin: Rating Scales and Assessment Instruments for Use in Pediatric Psychopharmacology Research.* Published by the National Institute of Mental Health. *Psychopharmacol Bull* 21(4), 1985.

11. Guy W: Dosage Record and Treatment Emergent Symptoms Scale, in: *ECDEU Assessment Manual for Psychopharmacology (Revised).* US Department of Health, Education and Human Welfare publication (ADM) 76-338, 1976, pp 223–244.

12. Guy W: Treatment Emergent Symptoms Scale—Write-In, in: *ECDEU Assessment Manual for Psychopharmacology (Revised).* US Department of Health, Education and Human Welfare publication (ADM) 76-338, 1976, pp 341–345.

13. Guy W: Subjects Treatment Emergent Symptoms Scale, in: *ECDEU Assessment Manual for Psychopharmacology (Revised).* US Department of Health, Education and Human Welfare publication (ADM) 76-338, 1976, pp 347–350.

14. Guy W: Abnormal Involuntary Movement Scale, in: *ECDEU Assessment Manual for Psychopharmacology (Revised).* US Department of Health, Education and Human Welfare publication (ADM) 76-338, 1976, pp 534–537.

15. Meiselas KD, Spencer EK, Oberfield R, Peselow ED, Angrist B, Campbell M: Differentiation of stereotypies from neuroleptic-related dyskinesias in autistic children. *J Clin Psychopharmacol* 9:207–209, 1989.

16. Campbell M, Green WH, Deutsch SI: *Child and Adolescent Psychopharmacology.* Beverly Hills, Calif, Sage Publications, 1985, pp 11–42.

17. Barkley RA:, 1981.

18. Guy W: Physical and Neurological Examination for Soft Signs, in: *ECDEU Assessment Manual for Psychopharmacology (Revised).* US Department of Health, Education and Human Welfare publication (ADM) 76-338, 1976, pp 383–406.

19. Denckla MB: Revised neurological examination for subtle signs, in special issue of, *Psychopharmacology Bulletin: Rating Scales and Assessment Instruments for Use in Pediatric Psychopharmacology Research.* Published by the National Institute of Mental Health, *Psychopharmacol Bull* 21(4):773–789, 1985.

20. Sleator EK: Measurement of compliance, in special issue of *Psychopharmacology Bulletin: Rating Scales and Assessment Instruments for Use in Pediatric Psychopharmacology Research.* Published by the National Institute of Mental Health, *Psychopharmacol Bull* 21(4):1089–1093, 1985.

21. Werry JS: Resolved: Cardiac arrhythmias make desipramine an unacceptable choice in children. *J Am Acad Child Adolesc Psychiatry* 34:1239–1241, 1995.

22. Popper C, Elliot, GR: Postmortem pharmacokinetics of tricyclic antidepressants: Are some deaths during treatment misattributed to overdose? *J Child Adolesc Psychopharmacology* 3:10–12, 1993.

23. Maloney MJ, Schwam JS: Clonidine and sudden death [letter]. *Pediatrics,* 96:1176–1177, 1995.

24. Wilens TE, Biederman J, Baldessarini, RJ, et al: Cardiovascular effects of therapeutic doses of tricyclic antidepressants in children and adolescents. *J Am Acad Child Adolesc Psychiatry,* 35(11):1491–1501, 1996.

25. Johnston HF, Fruehling, JJ: Experts do not agree on monitoring EKGs. *Just the Fax,* 1(1):1–3, 1994.

26. Park, M: *Pediatric Cardiology for Practitioners.* Chicago, Year Book Medical Publishers Inc., 1988.

27. Wilens T, Biederman J, Spencer T: A retrospective study of serum levels and electrocardiographic effects of nortriptyline in children and adolescents. *J Am Acad Child Adolesc Psychiatry* 32:270–277, 1993.

28. Ciraulo DA, Shader RL: Fluoxetine drug–drug interactions: I. Antidepressans and antipsychotics. *J Clin Psychopharmacol* 10:48–50, 1990.

29. Ciraulo DA, Shader RL: Fluoxetine drug-drug interactions: II. *J Clin Psychopharmacol* 10:213–217, 1990.

30. Khan AU: Biochemical profile of depressed adolescents. *J Am Acad Child Adolesc Psychiatry* 6:873–878, 1987.

31. Doherty M, Madansky D, Kraft J, et al: Cortisol dynamics and test performance of the dexamethasone suppression test in 97 psychiatrically hospitalized children aged 3–16 years. *J Am Acad Child Psychiatry* 25:400–408, 1986.

32. Klee S, Garfinkel B: Identification of depression in children and adolescents: The role of the dexamethasone suppression test. *J Am Acad Child Psychiatry* 23:410–415, 1984.

33. Retoff S, Weiss S: The syndromes of resistance to thyroid hormone. *Endocr Rev* 34:348–399, 1993.
34. Kinsbourne M: Disorders of mental development, in Menkes JH (ed): *Textbook of Child Neurology*, ed 3. Philadelphia, Lea & Febiger, 1985, pp 764–801.
35. Raj A, Sheehan D: Medical evaluation of panic attacks. *J Clin Psychiatry* 48:309–313, 1987.
36. Zametkin A, Rapoport J: Neurobiology of attention deficit disorder with hyperactivity: Where have we come in 50 years? *J Am Acad Child Adolesc Psychiatry* 26:676–686, 1987.
37. Bowden CL, Deutsch CK, Swanson JM: Plasma dopamine beta hydroxylase and platelet monoamine oxidase in attention deficit disorder and conduct disorder. *J Am Acad Child Adolesc Psychiatry* 27:171–174, 1988.
38. Kruesi MJP: Cruelty to animals and CSF 5-HIAA. *Psychiatry Res* 28:115–116, 1989.
39. Kruesi MJP, Linnoila M, Rapoport JL, et al: Carbohydrate craving, conduct disorder and low CSF 5-HIAA. *Psychiatry Res* 16:83–86, 1985.
40. Kruesi MJP, Rapoport JL, Hamburger S, et al: CSF monoamine metabolites, aggression and impulsivity in disruptive behavior disorders of children and adolescents. *Arch Gen Psychiatry* 47:419–426, 1990.
41. Diederich N, Ackerman R, Jurgens R, et al: Early involvement of the nervous system by human immune deficiency virus (HIV): A study of 79 patients. *Eur Neurol* 28:93–103, 1988.
42. Leckman JF, Weissman MM, Pauls DL: Family-genetic studies and identification of valid diagnostic categories in adult and child psychiatry, *Br J Psychiatry* 151:39–44, 1987.
43. Walzer S, et al: A method for the longitudinal study of behavioral development in infants and children: The early development of XXY children. *J Child Psychol Psychiatry* 19:213–229, 1978.
44. Ratcliffe SG, Field MAS: Emotional disorder of XYY children: Four case reports. *J Child Psychol Psychiatry* 23:401–406, 1982.
45. Nielsen J, Pelsen B, Sorenson K: Follow-up of 30 Klinefelter males treated with testosterone. *Clin Genet* 33:262–269, 1988.
46. Dening T, Berrios G: Wilson's disease: Psychiatric symptoms in 195 cases. *Arch Gen Psychiatry* 46:1126–1134, 1989.
47. Reiss A: Fragile X syndrome, in Obrien G, Yule, W (eds): *Clinics in Developmental Medicine*, vol. 138. Keith Press, London, 1995, pp 115–120.
48. Hagerman R, Silverman A (eds): *Fragile X Syndrome: Diagnosis, Treatment, and Research*. Baltimore, Johns Hopkins University Press, 1991.
49. Turk, J: The fragile X syndrome: On the way to a behavioral phenotype. *Br J Psychiatry* 160:24–35, 1992.
50. Courchesne E, Yeung-Courchesne R, Press G, et al: Hypoplasia of cerebellar vermal lobules VI and VII in autism. *N Engl J Med* 318:1349–1354, 1988.
51. Chugani H: Personal communication.
52. Gwirtsman HE, Kaye WH, George DT, et al: Hyperamylasemia and its relationship to binge–purge episodes: Development of a clinically relevant laboratory test. *J Clin Psychiatry* 50(6):196–204, 1989.
53. Schoonover SC: Introduction: The practice of pharmacotherapy, in Bassuk EL, Schoonover SC, Gelenberg AJ (ed): *The Practitioner's Guide to Psychoactive Drugs*, ed 2. New York, Plenum Press, 1983, pp 10–11.
54. Garvey CA, Gross D, Freeman L: Assessing psychotropic medication side effects among children. *J Child Adolesc Psychiatr Ment Health Nurs* 4(4):127–131, 1991.

5

Monitoring and Measuring Drug Effects. II. Behavioral, Emotional, and Cognitive Effects

MICHAEL G. AMAN, Ph.D., and DEBORAH A. PEARSON, Ph.D.

I. INTRODUCTION

This chapter surveys methods of assessment that have been and can be used by practitioners clinically for assessing drug effects. The authors have assumed that most practitioners will have limited resources, and therefore decisions had to be made in choosing two or three of the best approaches for assessing a given behavior or function. This does not mean that there are not other good tests and scales available—simply that a line had to be drawn to offer clinicians a practical number of alternatives. While the emphasis is on the practitioner's need, hopefully the information presented will also aid in clinical trials and the interpretation of their results.

Evaluations are set out in two tiers: (1) an elemental core that may be used in a small practice and (2) a larger battery that might be employed in a larger setting, such as a hospital-based clinic. Practitioners are encouraged to use as many elements as make sense in the given situation in order to derive as complete and balanced a picture of treatment effects as possible.

The chapter is organized into three areas as follows: (1) rating scales, (2) direct observations of behavior, and (3) performance, IQ, and achievement tests. There have been relatively few previous general reviews of assessment techniques for evaluating drug effects in children, but clinicians wanting to set up an assessment package may wish to

MICHAEL G. AMAN, Ph.D. • The Nisonger Center for Mental Retardation and Developmental Disabilities, Ohio State University, Columbus, Ohio 43210-1296. **DEBORAH A. PEARSON, Ph.D.** • Department of Psychiatry and Behavioral Sciences, University of Texas Health Science Center, Houston, Texas 77030.

Practitioner's Guide to Psychoactive Drugs for Children and Adolescents (Second Edition), Werry and Aman, eds. Plenum Publishing Corporation, New York, 1999.

consult Refs. 1 and 2. There are two excellent specialized texts on assessment[3,4] and a useful special issue of *Psychopharmacology Bulletin*.[5] Readers who want more details on the instruments discussed here (as well as numerous measures not discussed) are urged to consult these.

Recently, Hogg, Rutter, and Richman[6] published a workbook that contains the revised Rutter (formerly Isle of Wight) scales. It contains parent and teacher instruments for preschool and school-age children (four instruments). Also included are the Behavioural Screening questionnaire, the Behavioural Checklist, and the Werry–Weiss–Peters Activity Rating Scale. The instruments come in a manual with instructions and a strong plastic overlay for scoring. Once the workbook is purchased, the buyer can copy the forms as necessary.[6] Some, but not all, of these scales are discussed here. The instruments are widely used outside the United States (especially in the United Kingdom) and are primarily diagnostic/epidemiological instruments and have not to our knowledge been used much as measures of drug effects. The workbook arrived too late for review, but workers should be aware of it.

II. MEASUREMENT

A. Purposes

Throughout this monograph, it is made clear that there are two main classes of indication for pharmacotherapy: (1) behavioral/symptomatic (e.g., aggressiveness) and (2) disorder/cluster/dimension (e.g., ADHD, Tourette syndrome). While this distinction can be rather artificial at times, in some circumstances it is very real. A good example is provided by the pharmacotherapy of schizophrenia or major depression: medication has both *disorder-specific* actions (antipsychotic or antidepressant) and *symptomatic* indications (insomnia, anxiety, agitation) which differ in dosage, time frame of response, and even, at times, type of medication. While, as noted in Chapter 1, pediatric psychopharmacology began as largely symptomatic, as in adults indications are increasingly becoming those of disorders (e.g., ADHD). Not only are there two classes of indications but also two purposes of measurement: (1) for diagnosis (see Chapter 7) and (2) for assessing success of pharmacotherapy. This chapter emphasizes the measurement of outcome or drug-related changes. Side effects are covered in Chapter 4 as well as in chapters on particular drugs. Because of the range of defining symptoms, diagnostic determinations will ordinarily require a broader assessment than what is needed to monitor therapeutic drug changes, which will be more problem-oriented.

B. Diagnosis

Here only disorders will be addressed, as dimensions are covered later. The traditional way to approach this has been through the medical methods of a history and examination interview. Before the appearance of the fourth edition of the *Diagnostic and Statistical Manual of Mental Disorders* (DSM-IV),[7] necessary and sufficient criteria for diagnosis of child psychiatric disorders were mostly ill defined. This has now changed, and even the 10th revision of the World Health Association diagnostic system (ICD-10), published in 1991, has become much more exact, although not as legalistically so as DSM. With this shift has come more attention to the data-gathering or diagnostic interview. Ambrosini[8,9] has pointed out that there are three main types of interview, to which a fourth will be added here.

1. Unstructured Interview

The traditional interview in child psychopathology is a free-floating interview that is conducted more as a kind of human transaction than a technical data-capture process. Of course, no professional ever approaches an interview without some preconceptions and theoretical constructs as guides, so that "unstructured" is always a relative term. There has been very little research on this type of interview or on how it differs from one training center or one profession to another.[10] There has simply been an assumption that all diagnoses are derived from the same data and are thus comparable. The existing research suggests that clinicians who work together can thus achieve modest reliability—but only for some diagnostic categories.[9,11] It has been assumed that the lack of reliability in some categories is a function of the diagnostic criteria, but it could just as well be due to the imperfections of the diagnostic process. Clinicians who do not work together may show lower interdiagnoser reliability, but research of this type is rare.

2. Structured Interview

The structured interview is the exact opposite of the unstructured interview and, as the name suggests, usually consists of a series of questions, observations, or tests that must be carried out exactly as specified. Intelligence tests are good examples. DSM-IV is ideally suited to this type of interview, and, not surprisingly, several structured interviews have emerged since its appearance. One is the Diagnostic Interview Schedule for Children (DISC), modeled on the adult DIS used in the U.S. National Institute of Mental Health's Epidemiological Catchment Area (ECA) Study.[12] Structured methods have advantages (e.g., ensuring that the domain of diagnostic symptoms is properly covered, minimization of variations in how questions are asked, and leaving little to individual interpretation) and disadvantages (rigidity, cumbersomeness, user-unfriendliness). They are particularly suited to lay interviews and to research but are not likely to suit busy, experienced clinicians used to homing quickly in on the problem. Structured interviewers can achieve good reliability,[9] but they may have other problems. For example, the DISC has taken much longer to develop than expected because of problems in determining necessary thresholds to establish the presence of a disorder.[9]

3. Semistructured Interview

Semistructured interviews are a compromise between the two types of interview considered above. They provide for flexibility and brevity, but they require that the interviewer be trained and experienced enough to make some degree of judgment and interpretation of the child's or parent's response.[8,9] Good examples of such interviews that have shown satisfactory reliability are the Isle of Wight Parent and Child Interviews,[13] the Kiddie Schedule for Affective Disorders and Schizophrenia (K-SADS),[8,9,14] the Diagnostic Interview for Children (DICA),[15] and the Interview Schedule for Children (ISC).[16,17]

4. Symptom Checklists

Symptom checklists differ from the above in that, while there is no structure to the interview, the clinician can go through a symptom checklist rather similar to the systems inquiry in physical examination as a kind of aide-mémoire to prompt the interviewer to make sure all relevant areas have been covered. One example is the Child Symptom Inventory version 4,[18] which has good correlation with results from the K-SADS.

5. Adolescents

It is only recently that adolescence has come firmly within the purview of child health and allied disciplines. This has exposed a no-man's-land in diagnosis and assessment. Few scales specifically for adolescents exist. Usually, a choice must be made between child and adult scales depending on the disorder and the maturity of the subject. Many of the interviews recommended here have adult equivalents (e.g., SADS, DIS), and these are probably more suitable for older adolescents.

6. Summary

The current widely used unstructured clinical diagnostic interview is of unknown but probably variable reliability, although some disorders seem more robust than others to this method.[9,11] However, although more thorough and more reliable and increasingly used in research, structured and semistructured methods need further development (most notably shortening) before they are likely to be used by most clinicians.[9] They also (mostly) have yet to show their sensitivity and specificity in diagnosing, although to some extent this is tied to the uncertain validity of many childhood diagnoses. This should not stop those who wish to learn about them from doing so, but the real challenge lies with directors of training in child psychiatry and allied disciplines who have the power to change things radically within a few years. In the meantime, the type of interview is a matter of personal choice, but the increasing revelation of comorbidity in studies using more formalized methods of diagnosis and the rapidly developing disorder-specific focus of pharmacotherapies should make clinicians more interested in improving their interviewing. In this process, they are likely to be helped by the increasing use of the microcomputer. Computer algorithms for the DICA* and the DISC† are already available commercially as are other more focused interviews such as for depression. These computer-based systems have the advantages of both diagnostic precision and the simultaneous compiling of standard, comprehensive, and legible patient files that can also be aggregated to provide statistics across patients. There is no doubt where the future lies; the problem is the present.

In pediatric psychopharmacology, the interview has two functions—to diagnose and to assess treatment. In these functions, the interview can be buttressed by appropriate, standardized scales discussed in the sections that follow.

III. RATING SCALES

Rating scales of various types have traditionally formed the mainstay of clinical assessment in pediatric psychopharmacology. Here, available scales have been grouped as

*Marketed by Multihealth Systems Inc., 908 Niagara Falls Blvd., North Tonawanda, NY 14120-2060.
†Available from Division of Child and Adolescent Psychiatry, New York State Psychiatric Institute, 722 W. 168th Street, New York, NY 10032.

follows: (1) general-purpose scales, (2) scales for a specific diagnosis, symptom, or problem behavior: (a) hyperactivity (ADHD), (b) conduct and oppositional disorders, (c) depression, (d) bipolar mood disorder, (e) anxiety, (f) tic disorders, (g) mental retardation with associated behavior disorders, and (h) autism, and (3) preschool rating scales.

A. Some General Considerations

Rating scales have a number of features that make them attractive for assessing the effects of psychoactive drugs:

1. They are generally economical, as they can typically be completed in a few minutes, usually by caregivers or teachers.
2. Unlike certain indices (such as direct observations of behavior), rating scales enable raters to aggregate behaviors across a wide range of settings and over time. Hence, infrequently occurring behaviors and problems can be detected and recorded.
3. Behavior rating scales usually comprise behavioral items of importance to caregivers and hence tend to be clinically relevant and consumer-oriented.
4. Most good rating scales have norms, which assist clinicians in determining how "abnormal" the problem is.
5. Many rating scales have been shown to be highly sensitive to pharmacological treatment.

Although rating scales are an extremely efficient and inexpensive way of assessing treatment effects, they also have some limitations. First, there is the problem of rater subjectivity in determining whether a given behavior constitutes a problem and, if so, how serious the problem is. As a way of minimizing this, whenever possible the same rater (e.g., parent, teacher) should always repeat the ratings on a given child.[19] In this way, changes occurring across time and treatments can be attributed largely to changes in the child's behavior rather than changes in standards across raters. Second, there is a tendency for raters to score extreme children as less severe over successive ratings, especially between the first and second ratings. This phenomenon occurs with many different types of scales.[20] It has been likened to a practice effect,[21] but it may be more accurately characterized as regression to the mean.[22] The best way to minimize this phenomenon is to ensure that each child is assessed at least twice during baseline, before instituting any form of therapy. The critical comparison then would be between the second rating and subsequent ratings obtained during treatment. Third, there is the problem of "halo effects," which may be described as the tendency of some raters to score the child in terms of the rater's overall impression of the child, regardless of the content of various items and their contribution to different domains or subscales. The best way to check for this is to scan the scale or subscales for peaks and troughs. The appearance of consistently high scores, irrespective of behavioral domain, may cause the clinician to question a rater's judgment and seek a replacement. One way of obviating this problem is to employ more than one rater whenever possible. Finally, another important issue relates to the type of problem being assessed. Informants are fairly reliable in reporting acting-out problems and disorders (e.g., hyperactivity, fighting, conduct disorders) but appear less so with internalizing or emotional problems (e.g., anxiety, dysphoria, depression), which create discomfort for the child but little disruption for society.[23–26] At least one study indicated a tendency for children to report more phobic, anxiety, obsessive, and depressive symptoms than their mothers, suggesting that these may be areas in which children may be the best or only source of

CLINICAL GLOBAL IMPRESSIONS

Patient's Name:_____ Date: _____

---

1. SEVERITY OF ILLNESS

Considering your total clinical experience with this particular population, how mentally ill is the patient at this time?

0 = Not assessed	4 = Moderately ill
1 = Normal, not at all	5 = Markedly ill
2 = Borderline mentally ill	6 = Severely ill
3 = Mildly ill	7 = Among the most extremely ill patients

THE NEXT TWO ITEMS MAY BE OMITTED AT THE INITIAL ASSESSMENT BY MARKING "NOT ASSESSED" FOR BOTH ITEMS

---

2. GLOBAL IMPROVEMENT–Rate total improvement whether or not, in your judgement, it is due entirely to drug treatment.

Compared to his condition at admission to the project, how much has he changed?

0 = Not assessed	4 = No change
1 = Very much improved	5 = Markedly ill
2 = Much improved	6 = Much worse
3 = Minimally improved	7 = Very much worse

---

3. EFFICACY INDEX – Rate this item on the basis of DRUG EFFECT ONLY.

Select the terms which best describe the degrees of therapeutic effect and side effects and record the number in the box wherethe two items intersect.

EXAMPLE: Therapeutic effect is rated as "Moderate" and side effects are judged "Do not significantly interfere with patient's functioning". Record 06 in rows 40 and 41.

THERAPEUTIC EFFECT	SIDE EFFECTS			
	None	Do not significantly interfere with patient's functioning	Significantly interferes with patient's functioning	Outweighs therapeutic effect
MARKED - Vast improvement. Complete or nearly complete remission of all symptoms.	01	02	03	04
MODERATE - Decided improvement. Partial remission of symptoms.	05	06	07	08
Minimal - Slight improvement which does not alter status of care of patient.	09	10	11	12
UNCHANGED OR WORSE	13	14	15	16
Not Assessed = 00				

information about symptoms.[25] This differential sensitivity is responsible for the prominence of self (versus informant) rating scales for internalizing disorders.

B. "General-Purpose" Rating Scales

Not all practices will be able to use the array of instruments for particular disorders/problems discussed below. Therefore, general instruments suitable for most young persons seen in most practices will now be described.

1. Clinical Global Impressions (CGI)

The CGI Scale[5] is the simplest and best known of all scales in the field. It was developed to formalize and quantify the usual way judgments of drug efficacy are made clinically by physicians and others by amalgamating all available information from a multitude of sources, such as the physician's examination of the patient, parent's reports, and teacher's reports. The practitioner records this information onto three subscales: (1) Severity of Illness [coded on a scale ranging from 1 (Normal) to 7 (Extremely ill)], (2) Global Improvement, and (3) an Efficacy Index. Severity of Illness is rated at each assessment, whereas Global Improvement is scored only after treatment has begun. Finally, the Efficacy Index is rated on a two-way scale in which Therapeutic Effect (unchanged, minimal, moderate, or marked) is pitted against Side Effects ("none" through "outweighs therapeutic effect," four-point scale) (see Fig. 1).

The biggest drawback with the CGI is its unknown psychometric characteristics, as they vary across clinical populations, physicians, and types of drugs. Another problem is that it is not always clear what criteria are being brought to bear when a given clinician evaluates a child. Nevertheless, the CGI provides a useful, simple, quick, and easy way for the practitioner to systematize his or her overall impressions of how well a given patient fared with each treatment.

2. Customized Scales

One practical all-purpose approach to assessing treatment effects is to tailor-make instruments that reflect the principal target symptoms of a given child or adolescent. In one such example of this approach in the treatment of hyperactive children,[27] parents were asked to list the four or five things about their child's behavior that they found most worrisome. These symptoms were then written down for subsequent rating by the parents each time they returned for the study. A similar approach might be to adapt DSM diagnostic criteria that are relevant for a given child and ask parents and teachers to assess the child on these for each treatment condition.

Another approach is to use the Maladaptive Behavior Scale (MABS),[28] which requires the rater to estimate both the frequency of the behavior and its intensity. Frequency is rated on a six-point scale ranging from "Did not occur during preceding 8 hours" to "More than 12 times during the preceding 8 hours." Intensity is coded on a similar six-point scale,

---

FIGURE 1. Clinical Global Impressions Scale developed by the U.S. National Institute of Mental Health. [See *Psychopharmacol Bull.* 21(4): 839–843, special issue on "rating scales and assessment instruments for use in pediatric psychopharmacology research."] Reproduced by permission of editorial management, *Psychopharmacology Bulletin.*

which describes various degrees of severity. Each MABS form allows for the rating of three target symptoms. The MABS was developed for use in residential-type settings, and the frequency and intensity scales may not be suited to outpatients although variations to suit them could easily be made.

3. Child Behavior Checklist and Its Analogues

Probably the most extensively researched behavior rating scale for youngsters is the Child Behavior Checklist (CBCL),[29] designed as a parent–rating instrument for assessing children aged 4 to 16 years. It comprises two main sections: (1) Social Competence has 20 items on amount and quality of the child's involvement in sports, hobbies, organizations, jobs, friendships, etc., scored on three-point scales corresponding to "below average" to "above average"; (2) a Behavior Problem scale comprises 112 specified items plus one for the parent to write in additional difficulties. Items are rated on a three-point scale.

Although different item pools were formerly used depending on age and sex group, the CBCL now has the same eight factor-analytically derived subscales, regardless of the child's age or gender: (1) Aggressive behavior, (2) Anxious–depressed, (3) Attention problems, (4) Delinquent behavior, (5) Social problems, (6) Somatic complaints, (7) Thought problems, and (8) Withdrawn. This new uniform factor structure can now be used to follow the same child over time without the complications that formerly occurred when the child reached a given age or when boys and girls were to be compared. Although some of the factor labels are similar to ones used in diagnostic systems like the DSM-III-R, they are not intended to imply that such a diagnosis would be appropriate for a child who scores high on the dimension. As well as these subscales, there are two broad-band factors labeled as Internalizing and Externalizing, based on second-order factor analysis.

There is a large volume of psychometric data on the CBCL.[26,29] Test–retest agreement has been found to be high, and interrater agreement (between parents) moderately high. The CBCL appears to have good content validity, moderately high convergent validity (agreement with other rating scales), and satisfactory-to-good criterion-group validity (i.e., differences between clinical and control groups).

A close relative of the CBCL is the Teacher Report Form (TRF).[30] The first two pages of the TRF request information about the child's background, academic performance, and adaptive functioning. The remainder of the form contains behavior-problem items, most of which are the same or analogous to those in the CBCL. The TRF is scored in a similar fashion to the CBCL, and it results in a similar set of subscales. The major differences are that the TRF was designed for children aged 5 to 18 years (instead of 4 to 18), and certain behaviors not readily observed in the classroom (e.g., "bowel movements outside toilet") have been replaced with unrelated items that may be salient in school.

There is also a Youth Self-Report (YSR)[31] (one of the rare adolescent scales), which allows youngsters aged 11 to 18 years to rate themselves. The behavior-problem items are generally the same as those in the CBCL except that they have been worded in the first person. The YSR may prove to be especially helpful in assessing internalizing disorders, where the level of agreement between the child and significant adults is often very poor[32] and where personal discomfort is often the principal target of treatment. McConaughy[26] has also summarized other assessments that are part of the "CBCL package," including a standardized Direct Observation Form for recording a child's behavior in group or classroom situations and a Semistructured Clinical Interview for Children.

Although the CBCL and related scales are suggested as general-purpose instruments in assessing drug effects, several issues should be kept in mind. First, the length of these scales is an asset in that it may help in formulating a diagnosis but disadvantageous in that it may raise opposition, especially if several ratings are requested. One way around this may be to request ratings on only the internalizing or externalizing items (as appropriate) on subsequent ratings or even to request ratings only on the most relevant subscale(s). Second, the drug sensitivity is largely unknown, as the CBCL has been used in only a few drug investigations. The best policy may prove to be to use diagnosis-specific instruments discussed later in this chapter, whenever possible. However, when this proves to be unfeasible for practical reasons, the CBCL and its variants are worthy of serious consideration.

In summary, the international popularity and supporting data make the CBCL worth considering as a general-purpose assessment instrument, but the movement in pediatric psychopharmacology toward diagnosis-based pharmacotherapy may make the CBCL less suitable over time.

4. Conners' Rating Scales—Revised

A major restructuring and restandardization of the Conners scales (originally developed for drug studies around 1970) took place in 1997.[33] A summary of the new Conners system (referred to as Conners' Rating Scales—Revised) is presented in Table 1. In brief, the Conners package includes four units or modules, which can be broken down further

TABLE 1. Summary of Conners' Rating Scales—Revised[a,b]

Conners' Parent Rating Scale (CPRS)	Conners' Teacher Rating Scale (CTRS)
1. *Oppositional* (12/6)	1. *Oppositional* (6/5)
2. *Cognitive Problems* (10/6)	2. *Cognitive Problems* (7/5)
3. *Hyperactivity* (9/6)	3. *Hyperactivity* (7/7)
4. Anxious–Shy (8)	4. Anxious–Shy (8)
5. Perfectionism (7)	5. Perfectionism (6)
6. Social Problems (5)	6. Social Problems (5)
7. Psychomatic (6)	*ADHD Index* (12/12)
ADHD Index (12/12)	Conners' Global Index (10)[c]
Conners' Global Index (10)[c]	DSM-IV Symptoms (18)
DSM-IV Symptoms (18)	Total number of items: Long version, 59; short
Total number of items: Long version, 80; short version, 27	version, 28
Conners–Wells' Adolescent Self-Report Scale (CASS)	Conners ADHD/DSM-IV Scales—Parent/
1. Family Problems (12)	Teacher/Adolescent (CADS-P/T/A)
2. Emotional Problems (12)	1. ADHD Index (12/12/12)
3. *Conduct Problems* (12/6)	2. DSM-IV Symptoms (18/18/18)
4. *Cognitive Problems* (12/6)	Total number of items: CADS-P, 26; CADS-T,
5. Anger Control Problems (8)	30; CADS-A, 30
6. *Hyperactivity* (8/6)	
ADHD Index (12/12)	
DSM-IV Symptoms (18)	
Total number of items: Long version, 87; short version, 27	

[a]With the exception of the CADS-P, CADS-T, and CADS-A (lower right quadrant), all scales are available in a long and short version. Subscales listed in *italics* are present in both the long and short versions.
[b]Numerals in parentheses indicate the number of items on the subscales. The second numeral after each italicized subscale indicates the number of items on the short version.
[c]The Conners Global Index is available as a brief scale in its own right.

still. These are Conners' Parent Rating Scale—Revised (CPRS-R) (with separate long and short versions), Conners' Teacher Rating Scales—Revised (CTRS-R) (long and short versions), Conners—Wells' Adolescent Self-Report Scale (CASS) (long and short versions), and the Conners' ADHD/DSM-IV Scales (CADS), which are available in parent, teacher, and adolescent (self-report) forms (see Table 1). In general, the long versions of the scales are about twice as long as the short versions, and they include subscales for both externalizing and internalizing behavior problems. Conversely, the short forms typically include only subscales relevant to acting-out problems and hyperactivity, and they contain only the most robust subscale items. The parent and teacher scales were developed for children and adolescents aged 3 to 17 years, inclusive, whereas the CASS was developed for adolescents aged 12 to 17 years, inclusive.

With the exception of Conners' ADHD/DSM-IV Scales (described later), all of the items on the revised Conners scales were derived from their predecessors and/or DSM ADHD content. All except the CADS were empirically derived using factor analysis with cross validation. The standardization samples for the CPRS-R and CTRS-R totaled slightly under 2000 each, whereas the standardization samples for the self-rating scales totaled around 3400 adolescents. In general, psychometric work on the Conners' Rating Scales— Revised was comprehensive. Internal consistency (coefficient alpha) and test–retest reliability data generally look good, whereas ratings between raters having different roles (e.g., parent/teacher) was modest[33] as is usually found with all rating scales. A wealth of validity data are presented on all versions of the revised scales, including factorial validity, convergent validity, and discriminant validity (e.g., ability to differentiate ADHD and nondiagnosed children). As would be expected, the new CPRS and CTRS correlate well with their respective predecessors. At the time of this writing, data are not available on the sensitivity of these instruments to drug effects. However, given that their predecessors were all sensitive to the effects of medication (especially to stimulants in ADHD children) and given that the development procedures and items are very similar, it would be surprising if the Conners' Rating Scales—Revised are not also very sensitive to medication effects.

The long versions of the CPRS-R, CTRS-R, and CASS would all appear to be good "general-purpose" instruments for assessing medication effects in a wide array of conditions. The remaining scales would more appropriately be reserved for acting-out conditions, as discussed later.

5. Revised Behavior Problem Checklist (RBPC)

The RBPC[34] is an 89-item revised version of the extensively investigated and used 51-item Behavior Problem Checklist.[35] It comprises six factor-analytically derived subscales, as follows: (I) Conduct Disorder (22 items), (II) Socialized Aggression (17 items), (III) Attention Problem–Immaturity (16 items), (IV) Anxiety–Withdrawal (11 items), (V) Psychotic Behavior (6 items), and (VI) Motor Excess (5 items). Interrater reliability appears to be adequate for the RBPC,[35] and internal consistency moderately high,[34,36] and clinical and nonclinical samples have shown marked differences.[36,37] The RBPC can be filled in by any adult having a good knowledge of the youngster, and it is a well-established instrument and a good "general-purpose" rating scale. It is no longer in the public domain.

Scales that are recommended for general-purpose applications in monitoring drug effects are listed in Table 2, which also presents recommendations for the major disorders discussed in this chapter.

C. Hyperactivity (ADHD)

There are a large number of scales for assessing hyperactivity, but only a few can be discussed here.

1. Teacher Rating Scales

Two abbreviated (single-domain) scales and two multidomain instruments are recommended. Depending on the clinical context and available resources, the clinician may want to adopt just one of these or one from each category. The most popular scales for hyperactivity have been the Conners Questionnaires. As noted above, these have been revised and re-normed, and, given their history, they will probably continue to be among the most frequently used assessment instruments for ADHD.

a. ADHD-Only Instruments

Either the CADS, the ADHD Rating Scale,[38,39] or the Childhood Attention Problems (CAP) Scale,[40] is suggested whenever repeated ratings are required in a relatively brief time period (e.g., during dosage adjustment) when the clinician does not want to alienate the rater.

i. Conners' ADHD/DSM-IV Scales and Conners' Global Index. These render two measures, the *ADHD Index* and the *DSM-IV Symptoms Subscale*. Although 12-item ADHD Indices are available for parent, teacher, and self ratings, the item content is not identical across types of rater. The ADHD Index was developed as a measure of "risk" for having ADHD. Essentially, the items were selected for their ability to discriminate ADHD from non-ADHD children, and all three versions (parent, teacher, self-rating) are quite effective in identifying or "classifying" children as having ADHD or not.[33] We see no reason why the measure will prove insensitive to drug effects.

The *DSM-IV Symptoms Subscale* is really a misnomer in that it contains only the 18 DSM symptoms for ADHD. It provides a Total score and separate Inattentive and Hyperactive–Impulsive subscores. The psychometric characteristics for both the ADHD Index and the DSM-IV Symptoms Subscale are quite favorable and often appeared slightly better than those for the Hyperactivity subscales on the CPRS, the CTRS, and the CASS.[33]

Finally, a note is in order about the 10-item *Conners' Global Index*. This was previously referred to variously as "Conners Abbreviated Symptom Scale" and the "Hyperactivity Index."[41] The Index was developed as a general index of disruptive behavior, but it was often misused in clinical research to identify or define groups of ADHD children. We feel that Conners has correctly renamed the scale to avoid confusion, as the scale also measures emotionality. The new manual provides norms for the total Global Index, as well as the Restless–Impulsive and Emotional Lability subscores. Although clinicians no doubt will continue to use this scale to monitor treatment, we feel that the ADHD Index and the DSM-IV Symptoms Subscale are better.

ii. The ADHD Rating Scale. This is an 18-item instrument based on the symptoms specified in the DSM-IV. Nationally representative samples were derived for approximately 1900 children for the Teacher version[38] and for nearly 2000 children for the Parent version.[39] Factor analysis indicated that the ADHD Rating Scale has two factors of nine items each: the Inattention subscale and the Hyperactivity–Impulsivity subscale. The ADHD Rating Scale has good internal consistency and good test–retest reliability, and its

TABLE 2. Recommended Assessment Tools Presented by Problem Condition[a,b]

Condition	Strongly recommended	Recommended
General purpose (most conditions)	Clinical Global Impressions (D) Custom-Made Scales (P,T) Youth Self-Report (S) *or* Child Behavior Checklist (P) Teacher Report Form (T) Conners–Wells' Adolescent Self-Report Scale (S)	Conners' Parent Rating Scale—Revised (long) (P) Conners' Teacher Rating Scale—Revised (long) (T) Conners–Wells' Adolescent Self-Report Scale (S)
Hyperactivity (ADHD)	Clinical Global Impressions (D) Conners' ADHD Index (brief) (P, T, S) *or* DSM-IV Symptoms Subscale (brief) (P, T, S) *or* Conners' Parent Rating Scale—Revised (P) Conners' Teacher Rating Scale—Revised (T) Conners–Wells' Adolescent Self-Report (S)	ACTeRS (P, T) *or* ADHD Rating Scale (P, T) *or* Halperin Continuous Performance Task (A) *or* Conners' Continuous Performance Task (A)
Oppositional, conduct, and aggression problems[c]	Clinical Global Impressions (D) Conners' Parent Rating Scale (P) *or* Peer Conflict Scale (P) New York Teacher Rating Scale (T)	Revised Behavior Problem Checklist (P) *or* Child Behavior Checklist (P) Conners' Teacher Rating Scale—Revised (T) *or* Revised Behavior Problem Checklist (T) *or* Teacher Report Form (T) Conners–Wells' Adolescent Self-Report Scale (S) *or* Youth Self Report (S) *or* Children's Inventory of Anger (S)

Disorder		
Depressive disorders	Children's Depression Rating Scale—Revised (D) *or* Bellevue Index of Depression (D) Children's Depression Scale (S) *or* Children's Depression Inventory (S) Children's Depression Scale (P, T) *or* Bellevue Index of Depression (P, T)	Reynold's Adolescent Depression Scale (S) Children's Depression Inventory (Parent Version) (P) *or* Emotional Disorders Rating Scale (P, T, C)
Bipolar disorder (mania)	Mania Rating Scale (D) Self-Report Manic Inventory (S)	Manic-State Rating Scale (D)
Anxiety and anxiety disorders	Childhood Anxiety Sensitivity Index (S) *or* State Trait Anxiety Inventory for Children (S) *or* Revised Children's Manifest Anxiety Scale (S) Emotional Disorders Rating Scale (P, T, C)	DSM-derived scales (S, P, T, C, D) *or* Fear Survey Schedule for Children—Revised (S) *or* Child Anxiety Frequency Checklist (S) Louisville Fear Survey for Children (P, T)
Obsessive–compulsive disorder	Leyton Obsessional Inventory—Child (C) Yale–Brown Obsessive–Compulsive Scale (P, S)	
Tic and Tourette disorders	Yale Global Tic Severity Scale (D) Tourette Syndrome Severity Scale (P) *or* Tourette Syndrome Symptom List (P) MOVES[d] (S)	Tourette Syndrome Global Scale (D) Percentage reduction estimates (S) Tic counts with videotapes (O)
Mental retardation	Clinical Global Impressions (D) Aberrant Behavior Checklist (P, T, C) *or* Nisonger Child Behavior Rating Form (P, T) (Plus other scales contingent on specific behavior problems) →	Developmental Behaviour Checklist (P, T, C) Behavior Problems Inventory (Aggression/Self Injury) (P, T, C) Emotional Disorders Rating Scale (C, P?, T?) Maladaptive Behavior Scale (P, T, C) Attention Checklist (T) Self-Injurious Behavior Questionnaire (P, T, C)

TABLE 2. (*Continued*)

Condition	Strongly recommended	Recommended
Childhood autism	Clinical Global Impressions (D)	Conners' ADHD Index (P, T, S)
	or	*or*
	Children's Psychiatric Rating Scale (D)	Conners' DSM-IV Symptoms Subscale (P, T, S)
	Aberrant Behavior Checklist (P, T, C)	Timed Stereotypies Rating Scale (D, O)
	or	Real Life Rating Scale (O)
	Nisonger Child Behavior Rating Form (P, T)	Developmental Behavior Checklist (P, T, C)
	(Other scales contingent on specific behavior problems) →	
Preschool-age children	CBCL/2–3 or CBCL/4–18, as appropriate (P)	Behavioural Screening Questionnaire (T)
	Preschool Behavior Questionnaire (T, P?)	*or*
		Symptom Checklist (T)
		Behavior Check List (P)

[a]Tools are categorized as follows: D, doctor; P, parent; T, teacher, C, other care provider; S, self, O, other; A, automated/computer test.

[b]Note: In general, practitioners should strive to obtain data from as many sources as possible when monitoring treatment. Hence, it is desirable to have one instrument from each of the following categories: D, T, P, S.

[c]For inpatient settings, the following instruments may be helpful: Overt Aggression Scale (C), Staff Observation Aggression Scale (C), Social Dysfunction and Aggression Scale (D).

[d]MOVES, *Motor Tic, Obsessions and Compulsions, Vocal Tic Evaluation Survey.*

validity is generally supported.[42] The Parent version of the ADHD Rating Scale is presented in Fig. 2, and it may be reproduced by readers, *provided that they do not alter its format or wording*. As indicated in the caption to Fig. 2, the wording of the Teacher version is identical, although the instructions differ slightly. The ADHD Rating Scale is brief, it is free, its psychometric characteristics are good, it has a good normative base, and it is grounded in the DSM-IV.

iii. The CAP Scale. The CAP Scale (Fig. 3) was derived from the TRF[30] by extracting items that consistently loaded heavily on the Hyperactivity factor of the TRF and that were consistent with DSM-III-R criteria for ADHD. There are two factor-analytically derived subscales obtained by adding item scores: Inattention (items 1, 2, 5, 7, 9, 10, and 12) and Hyperactivity (items 3, 4, 6, 8, and 11). The normed cutoff scores corresponding to 1.5 standard deviations above the mean (93rd percentile) are 9 and 7 (for boys and girls, respectively) for Inattention, 6 and 5 for Overactivity, and 15 and 11 for the summed Total Score. There are no age differences for norms. The full set of norms is available in a publication by Barkley.[43]

Edelbrock[40] has presented some preliminary data on the psychometric characteristics of the scale, and, in brief, it is adequately reliable and valid.[44,45] In summary, at 12 items, the CAP Scale is easy to administer, its structure makes sense in light of current concepts of hyperactivity, and early indications are that it has good psychometric characteristics. The CAP Scale is drug-sensitive, but unfortunately *there is no parent companion version*.

b. Scales for ADHD plus Other Symptoms

i. Conners' Teacher Rating Scale—Revised.[33] This was described earlier under General Rating Scales. The long version has six subscales (1. Oppositional, 2. Cognitive problems, 3. Hyperactivity, 4. Anxious–shy, 5. Perfectionism, and 6. Social problems), plus the ADHD Index, Conners' Global Index, and the DSM-IV Symptoms score. The short version has three subscales (1. Oppositional, 2. Cognitive problems, and 3. Hyperactivity), plus the ADHD Index. The long version has 59 items, and the short version has 28 items.

ii. The ACTeRS (2nd Edition). Although originally called the ADD-H Comprehensive *Teacher* Rating Scale, the manual and published scales now simply refer to this instrument as the ACTeRS. The reason is that a parallel parent version has been added to the available package. The ACTeRS was empirically derived and specifically designed for clinical management and research with ADHD children.[46,47] The teacher version has 24 items that score onto four factor-analytically derived subscales designated as follows: (1) Attention, (2) Hyperactivity, (3) Social Skills, and (4) Oppositional. The ACTeRS is relatively pure factorially, has good interrater reliability, and is sensitive to psychostimulant treatment.[47-49] The teacher norms are based on ratings of some 3600 children.[47] A recent development is the *parent* version of the ACTeRS, which contains the same empirically derived subscales as the teacher version, plus a fifth subscale called Early Childhood. This subscale gives details about early-childhood behavior. It is not clear from the manual what the data base is for the parent norms. The parent version is available in both English and Spanish and has 25 items. Children from ethnic minorities appeared to score worse on the ACTeRS teacher scale, but the differences were small and standardized mean differences were minor.[50] Both versions can be administered and/or scored by microcomputer. Like the Conners scales, the ACTeRS is copyrighted and commercially available.[47] The ACTeRS is convenient, relatively brief, and easy to score and interpret and should be regarded as one of a handful of proven ADHD assessment instruments.

ADHD Rating Scale—IV—Home Version

Child's Name _____

Child's Age _____ Sex: M   F   Grade _____ Child's Race: _____

Completed by: ____Mother ____Father ____Guardian ____Grandparent

Circle the number that *best describes* **your child's home behavior over the past 6 months.**

		Never or Rarely	Some-times	Often	Very Often
1.	Fails to give close attention to details or makes careless mistakes in schoolwork.	0	1	2	3
2.	Fidgets with hands or feet or squirms in seat.	0	1	2	3
3.	Has difficulty sustaining attention in tasks or play activities.	0	1	2	3
4.	Leaves seat in classroom or in other situations in which remaining seated is expected.	0	1	2	3
5.	Does not seem to listen when spoken to directly.	0	1	2	3
6.	Runs about or climbs excessively in situations in which it is inappropriate.	0	1	2	3
7.	Does not follow through on instructions and fails to finish work.	0	1	2	3
8.	Has difficulty playing or engaging in leisure activities quietly.	0	1	2	3
9.	Has difficulty organizing tasks and activities.	0	1	2	3
10.	Is "on the go" or acts as if "driven by a motor."	0	1	2	3
11.	Avoids tasks (e.g., schoolwork, homework) that require sustained mental effort.	0	1	2	3
12.	Talks excessively.	0	1	2	3
13.	Loses things necessary for tasks or activities.	0	1	2	3
14.	Blurts out answers before questions have been completed.	0	1	2	3
15.	Is easily distracted.	0	1	2	3
16.	Has difficulty awaiting turn.	0	1	2	3
17.	Is forgetful in daily activities.	0	1	2	3
18.	Interrupts or intrudes on others.	0	1	2	3

CAP Rating Scale

Child's Name: _____   Child's Age: _____
Filled out by: _____   Child's Sex: [ ] M [ ] F

Directions:
Below is a list of items that describes pupils. For each item that describes the pupil now or within the past week, check whether the item is **Not True, Somewhat or Sometimes True, or Very or Often True.** Please check all items as well as you can, even if some do not seem to apply to this pupil.

		Not True	Somewhat or Sometimes True	Very or Often True
1.	Fails to finish things he/she starts	[ ]	[ ]	[ ]
2.	Can't concentrate, can't pay attention for long	[ ]	[ ]	[ ]
3.	Can't sit still, restless, or hyperactive	[ ]	[ ]	[ ]
4.	Fidgets	[ ]	[ ]	[ ]
5.	Daydreams or gets lost in his/her thoughts	[ ]	[ ]	[ ]
6.	Impulsive or acts without thinking	[ ]	[ ]	[ ]
7.	Difficulty following directions	[ ]	[ ]	[ ]
8.	Talks out of turn	[ ]	[ ]	[ ]
9.	Messy work	[ ]	[ ]	[ ]
10.	Inattentive, easily distracted	[ ]	[ ]	[ ]
11.	Talks too much	[ ]	[ ]	[ ]
12.	Fails to carry out assigned tasks	[ ]	[ ]	[ ]

Please feel free to write any comments about the pupil's work or behavior in the last week.

FIGURE 3. Childhood Attention Problem (CAP) Scale, developed by Craig Edelbrock (1978). Reproduced by permission from Barkley R: *Attention-Deficit Hyperactivity Disorder: A Clinical Workbook.* New York, Guilford Press, 1991.

iii. The IOWA Conners Teacher's Rating Scale. Loney and Milich[51] concluded that the Conduct (Aggression) and Hyperactivity subscales were not helpful in separating patients clinically because of cross-loading of items. They constructed "pure" measures of aggression and hyperactivity by using items (five of each) that correlated only on Hyperactivity (which they named Inattention–Overactivity) or Conduct Problem (named Aggression).

← ───

FIGURE 2. ADHD Rating Scale. Reproduced by permission of the authors, George DuPaul et al. Readers may reproduce this form but are asked not to alter its format without the permission of its developers Dr. George DuPaul and his colleagues. ©G. DuPaul, A. Anastopoulos, T. Power, R. Reid, M. Ikeda, and K. McGoey. Dr. DuPaul's address is College of Education, Lehigh University, 111 Research Drive, Bethlehem, PA 18015. The ADHD Rating Scale-IV—School Version is identical except that teachers are asked to circle the number that best describes *this student's school behavior* over the past 6 months (*or since the beginning of the school year*).

These two subscales have been shown to be reliable to test–retest, internally consistent, and drug-sensitive.[51–53] The IOWA Conners Teacher's Rating Scale was normed on a large group of children in kindergarten through fifth grade.[54] It has the advantages of being brief and soundly derived, but the small numbers of items and the fact that it was derived solely with teacher ratings may limit its application.

2. Parent Rating Scales

a. ADHD-Only Instruments

Conners' ADHD, Conners' DSM-IV, and Conners' Global Index, which were described under the teacher instruments, all have companion parent versions (see Table 1). The ADHD Index has 12 items, the DSM-IV has 18, and Conners' Global Index has 10 items. Any of these can be used individually to monitor drug effects, especially where frequent reassessments are required. The 18-item ADHD Rating Scale discussed earlier under teacher instruments can be used by parents as well as teachers.

b. Scales for ADHD plus Other Symptoms

i. Conners' Parent Rating Scale—Revised.[33]   This was described earlier under "General-Purpose" Rating Scales (see also Table 1). The subscales on the long version are designated as follows: 1. Oppositional, 2. Cognitive problems, 3. Hyperactivity, 4. Anxious–shy, 5. Perfectionism, 6. Social problems, and 7. Psychosomatic, plus the ADHD Index, the DSM-IV Symptoms score, and Conners' Global Index. The short version has subscales 1–3, plus the ADHD Index. The long version has 80 items, whereas the short version has 27. Unless there is ongoing concern about internalizing symptoms, the short form appears to be more time-effective.

3. Self-Rating Hyperactivity Scales

Conners and Wells[33,55] developed Conners–Wells' Adolescent Self-Report Scale (CASS), which was designed for adolescents aged 12 to 17 years inclusive. The long version of the CASS has the following subscales: 1. Family problems, 2. Emotional problems, 3. Conduct problems, 4. Cognitive problems, 5. Anger control problems, and 6. Hyperactivity, plus the ADHD Index and the DSM-IV Symptoms score. The short version of the CASS contains subscales 3, 4, and 6 from the above, plus the ADHD Index. The long version has 87 items, whereas the short version has 27 (see Table 1). Once again, unless there is concern about internalizing symptoms, we recommend use of the short version.

4. Situation-Specific Scales

Situation-specific scales differ from all of the above in that they ask questions about behavior in specific situations (e.g., meals) rather than providing more global ratings.

The Werry–Weiss–Peters Activity Scale[56] was designed for use by parents and other domestic caregivers. The scale is widely used, is drug-sensitive, but is only lightly researched. It correlates as much with conduct problems as with attentional–overactivity problems.[1,57] It is in the public domain.

The Home Situations Questionnaire (HSQ) and the School Situations Questionnaire (SSQ) are parallel instruments.[58] There are 16 situations in the HSQ and 12 in the SSQ, each of which yields two scores: (1) Number of situations and (2) Mean severity score. Test–retest reliability is moderately high, but interrater reliability is unknown. Both instruments appear to be sensitive to stimulant medication.[58]

5. Summary

To conclude, because Conners' Rating Scales—Revised and the ACTeRS cover more areas, they are recommended for assessing drug effects. Where time is limited or where multiple ratings will be required, the single-domain instruments like the Conners' ADHD Index, Conners' DSM-IV Symptoms scale, the CAP Scale, or the ADHD Rating Scale may be preferred (see Table 2).

D. Oppositional, Conduct, and Aggressive Problems

1. Introduction

Available tools for assessing oppositional, conduct, and aggressive problems have been reviewed more extensively elsewhere.[59,60] Aggression is a complex behavior and may be (a) physical or verbal, (b) adult-directed or peer-directed, (c) reactive and retaliatory or planned and proactive, and (d) eruptive or antisocial/hostile.[61] It may be covert (as in the case of stealing) or overt (as in fighting). Hence, comprehensive coverage with a single instrument is difficult. Several instruments are available that either have been used for assessing drug effects on hostility in children or have obvious potential in that regard. As with most externalizing behavior, the majority of these instruments are for use by the child's significant adults, such as parents, teachers, or care workers.

2. Informant Instruments

a. New York Teacher Rating Scale (NYTRS)

A major recent development for the assessment of disruptive and aggressive behavior is the New York Teacher Rating Scale (NYTRS) for Disruptive and Antisocial Behavior.[62] The NYTRS is a 36-item instrument that was derived by factor analysis from a large population of first through tenth-graders in Westchester County, New York, and Staten Island, New York. The NYTRS provides scores on four subscales: Defiance (14 items), Physical Aggression (5 items), Delinquent Aggression (4 items), and Peer Relations (7 items). In addition, there are four items that did not load sufficiently to be grouped with a subscale but were retained because of their face validity. Besides the four subscales, two composite scales can also be derived: Antisocial Behavior Scale is made up of the Physical Aggression and Delinquent Aggression subscale items (plus the four nonloading items), and the Disruptive Behavior Scale comprises all items except those on the Peer Relations subscale.

DSM-IV criteria for Oppositional Defiant Disorder and Conduct Disorder are well represented on the NYTRS. It provides a broad-band measure of disruptive behavior, but it also contains narrow-band subscales that enable the clinician to assess specific areas of change. Validity data are good, internal consistency is moderate to excellent, and test–retest reliability appears to be good, but preliminary data on interrater reliability are variable.[62] In our opinion, this is the best available teacher scale for assessing hostility and aggression.

b. The Conners Scales

Conners' Teacher Rating Scale—Revised and Conners' Parent Rating Scale—Revised[33] have obvious potential for assessing aggression and other forms of hostility. Both versions have subscales relevant to aggression and conduct problems, including the Oppositional and Conduct problem subscales.

Unlike the assessment of pharmacological effects on hyperactivity, that of effects on aggression is not extensive, but growing. The Conduct subscales of the forerunners to Conners' Rating Scales–Revised (namely, Conners' Teacher Rating Scale and Conners' Parent Rating Scale) were usually sensitive to methylphenidate in hyperactive/aggressive youngsters.[45,63,64] The sensitivity of the forerunner to Conners' Global Index (namely, Conners' Hyperactivity Index) was more variable, especially with parents.[45,52] The IOWA Conners Teacher's Rating Scale (discussed above) may also be a good choice if a brief index is to be used. It has been shown to be drug-sensitive in aggression.[52,53]

c. The Peer Conflict Scale

The Peer Conflict Scale[65] was developed to assess physical and verbal interactions between the patient and other children. It comprises 10 items, rated on a four-point scale, that were derived from a behavior observation code for assessing social and aggressive behavior.[66] The Peer Conflict Scale is reproduced in Fig. 4. Published psychometric data available on the Peer Conflict Scale are limited.[67] Its relation to direct observations of noncompliance was quite high, test–retest reliabilities were moderately high, and it was partially drug-sensitive in one study.[52]

d. Child Behavior Checklist (CBCL) and Teacher Report Form (TRF)

The CBCL and TRF, described earlier, have two subscales relevant to assessing hostility, namely, a Delinquent Behavior subscale and an Aggressive Behavior subscale. One study found parent ratings of Delinquency to be sensitive to methylphenidate in aggressive boys, and teacher ratings on the Aggression subscale to be less so.[45] The CBCL and TRF certainly warrant consideration for use in monitoring drug effects on conduct problems and aggressive behavior though their definitive value needs clarification.

e. Revised Behavior Problem Checklist

The RBPC, discussed above, places a heavy emphasis on conduct problems, aggression, and hostility, with 39 of its 89 items scoring on either Conduct Problem or Socialized Aggression subscales. As such, it has considerable relevance to the assessment of aggressive types of disorders. However, the lack of drug studies with this instrument makes it difficult to judge its usefulness.

f. Inpatient Rating Scales

Three other instruments deserve mention. Though these have been used primarily with adult psychiatric inpatients, they should be useful with minor adaptations for those severely aggressive children who may be in an inpatient setting.

The first scale, the Overt Aggression Scale,[68] calls for each episode of aggression to be rated on four categories of (1) Verbal aggression, (2) Physical aggression against objects, (3) Physical aggression against self, and (4) Physical aggression against other people. Staff intervention is also rated. Interrater reliability appears to be adequate, although data are sparse. The second is the Staff Observation Aggression Scale (SOAS),[69] which was designed to assess the severity and frequency of assaultive acts by psychiatric and psycho-

PEER CONFLICT SCALE

Child's Name: _____

Instructions:

Beside each item below, indicate the degree of the problem with a checkmark (✓). Please respond to all items. Evaluate the child's behavior on the following days:

_____

Item	Not at all	Just a little	Pretty much	Very much
1. Grabs things from other children				
2. Throws things at other children				
3. Smashes or destroys things				
4. Gives dirty looks or makes threatening gestures to other children				
5. Curses at or teases other children to provoke conflict				
6. Damages other children's property				
7. Hits, pushes, or trips other children				
8. Threatens to hurt other children				
9. Engages in physical fights with other children				
10. Annoys other children to provoke them				

Comments: _____

_____

_____

Name of person completing this form: _____

Dated: _____

FIGURE 4.   Peer Conflict Scale. Readers wishing to use this instrument should contact K. D. Gadow, Department of Psychiatry and Behavioral Science, Putnam Hall, South Campus, State University of New York at Stony Brook, Stony Brook, NY 11794–8790. ©K. D. Gadow.

geriatric inpatients. Incidents are reported in five categories: (1) Type of provocation, (2) Means used by the patient, (3) Aim of the aggression, (4) Consequence(s) for the victim, and (5) Measures taken to stop the aggression. Categories 2–4 contribute to a Global Severity score. Preliminary interrater reliability data appeared to be good, and the SOAS was capable of discriminating between different adult diagnostic groups. The Social Dysfunction and Aggression Scale (SDAS)[70] includes milder forms of aggressive behavior than might be captured in the two just described. The SDAS is similar in format to the

Hamilton Depression Scale and is completed by the clinician for the previous 3–7 days. It has 11 items, 9 of outward aggression and 2 of inward aggression. Interrater reliability appears high.

All of these scales have potential utility for assessing aggression in an inpatient setting, although much of the data is from adult samples; two focus only on severe aggression, and drug sensitivity is largely untested.

3. Self-Rating Scales

Self-rating scales may be problematic for externalizing behavior because of under-reporting, especially with delinquency. They may, however, give some perspective on the child's view of his or her problems.

a. The Youth Self-Report (YSR)

The YSR has been described above and is designed for 11- to 18-year-olds.[31] Like the associated CBCL and TRF, it also has a Delinquent behavior subscale (11 items) and an Aggressive behavior subscale (19 items). Its utility for assessing aggression in youth is unknown but, given the popularity of the CBCL and the TRF, its use is likely to increase.

b. Conners–Wells' Adolescent Self-Report Scale

The longer version of the CASS[33] has a Conduct Problems and an Anger Control Problems subscale, whereas the latter does not appear on the short version. Although the CASS has obvious potential for assessing drug effects, research data are not yet available to judge it.

c. Children's Inventory of Anger

The Children's Inventory of Anger is an instrument for measuring self-perceived anger in children.[71] It was drug-sensitive in one study.[72] Scales of this type are worth considering in assessing children having aggressive disorders, although their rightful place is unknown.

4. Conclusions

It is clear that there are a multitude of choices for assessing aggressive behavior in children and adolescents. As it was specifically designed for assessing aggression, the New York Teacher Rating Scale must be recommended the most strongly of those cited. Because of the favorable data (indicating reasonable sensitivity to treatment effects) from drug studies with the forerunners of the Revised Conners' Teacher and Parent Rating Scales, the conduct subscales from the Conners scales can be recommended. For clinicians seeking a very brief instrument, the IOWA Conners Teacher's Rating Scale is recommended. Gadow's Peer Conflict Scale is also suggested. The aggression scales in the RBPC, the CBCL, and the TRF are also suggested for use in outpatient settings, even though their sensitivity to drug effects is as yet untested. Self-rating scales are an unknown quantity at this stage. However, it may be informative to obtain a measure of the young-ster's perceptions of any changes resulting from pharmacotherapy, a greatly neglected area in psychopharmacology. Instruments that are recommended for the assessment of drug effects on aggression in children and adolescents are listed in Table 2.

E. Depression

Depression is a confusing term since it can be a symptom, a personality trait, or a group of different DSM-IV or ICD-10 disorders (e.g., major depression, dysthymia). However, apart from diagnosis, it is likely that any scale that addresses a good range of depressive symptoms and is able to be given repetitively might be helpful for assessing relevant drug effects.

Kazdin[73] has traced the concept of depression in children from early psychoanalytic thinking (when depression was believed not to occur in youngsters), through an era when it was widely thought to be expressed in altered form (masked depression), to the currently prevalent position that depression in children and adolescents shares the same essential features that occur in adults. Despite this agreement, there are a number of problems that differentiate child depression from the adult syndrome: relative lack of response to anti-depressants (see Chapter 9) and high comorbidity, making primary diagnosis difficult.[32,74] However, Emslie[75] has recently provided evidence that fluoxetine is effective in treating childhood depression, as least as measured using clinician-based assessment indices. There has been a proliferation of instruments for assessment of child and adolescent depression in the last decade, although there is only room here to assess a few. More detailed information is available elsewhere.[73,76–79]

Many of the issues in assessing depression in children are similar to those in assessing anxiety (see below). (1) Children and adolescents may lack sophistication in recognizing, labeling, and characterizing their emotions. (2) As with most rating scales (see above), there is "instrument decay," a tendency for self and informant ratings to improve irrespective of the presence or success of intervention with repeated administration.[80] (3) There is almost no literature on the utility of existing instruments for monitoring therapeutic change.[81] Most of the literature concerns their reliability and validity in classifying children as depressed or not. (4) There is confusion in the use of the term depression as a symptom, a personality trait, and a disorder and to designate different disorders (e.g., major depression, dysthymia). These problems and the high level of current research activity in childhood depression mean that recommendations are necessarily tentative.

1. Self-Rating Scales for Depression

Not surprisingly, there has been more interest in self-rating scales in depression (given its internalizing nature) than in hyperactivity or aggression. Numerous self-rating scales exist, but only the better established ones are discussed here.

a. Children's Depression Inventory (CDI)

The CDI[82,83] is the most frequently used self-rating scale for depression, although that alone does not make it the best suited for drug assessment. The development of the CDI was based on the Beck Depression Inventory for adults,[84] with items added relating to school and peer functioning. The CDI has a manual,[83] standardized norms (based on 1266 Florida students, aged 7–16 years old), and five factors related to child and adolescent depression (Negative Mood, Interpersonal Problems, Ineffectiveness, Anhedonia, Negative Self Esteem), in addition to the Total CDI Score. The CDI is composed of 27 items, which are scored 0 (absence of symptom), 1 (mild symptom), or 2 (definite symptom). The child chooses one of three sentences (normal through depressive) that describes himself or herself over the previous two weeks. Usually, the examiner reads the instructions and items aloud while the youngster marks the answers, although group administration is also permitted. Normative data are available for the CDI Total Score and for each of the factors. Scores are not affected by age but are affected by gender (sometimes boys score higher, sometimes girls, depending on subscale and study)[83,85,86] and ethnicity (Hispanic, Japanese, and Egyptian samples have been found to score higher).[87–89] CDI scores have been found to remain fairly stable across several years of data collection and to also predict young adult functioning.[90] The new CDI features a paper-and-pencil "QuikScore" template; PC-based scoring (and administration) is also available.

The CDI now includes a "CDI Short Form," which consists of 10 items. The short form yields only a total score and is appropriate for general screening. It does not include the suicidal ideation question, seemingly an important omission. There are no age or gender effects for the Short Form.

Internal consistency is high, and test–retest reliability variable (0.38–0.82, with the highest test–retest reliability figures occurring between 2-to 3-week readministrations of the test, as would be expected of an index that measures state characteristics).[83] There are moderate intercorrelations among the factors (0.24–0.59), and they also have moderate correlations with the total CDI score (0.55–0.82). There is variable agreement between adult and child ratings.[91–93] In terms of validity, the CDI discriminates between depressed and nondepressed samples of children,[82,92] although there is considerable overlap. Scores on the CDI appear to correlate moderately highly with those on anxiety and on self-esteem inventories,[82] and with other depression scales.[91] It has been used in at least two drug studies[74,94] and was found sensitive, although Emslie[75] did not find it to be sensitive to fluoxetine treatment.

It is difficult to know how strongly to recommend this instrument for drug monitoring. Psychometric data are more extensive for this than for other similar instruments, but the narrow three-point scale may make the CDI relatively insensitive. Although the CDI warrants consideration for drug monitoring, it may not be as sensitive as other scales. However, it appears to be a solid measure of severity of depression,[95] and provides excellent clinical information.

b. Children's Depression Scale (CDS)

The CDS[96] is probably the second most studied rating scale for depression in children. The CDS comprises 66 items printed on color-coded cards; 48 of the items are depressive in content and 18 euthymic. Boxes, identified with the words "Very wrong" through "Very right" are arrayed before the child, and the youngster inserts each card into the appropriate box. Higher scores on the depressive items indicate greater severity of depression. The CDS has eight subscales: (1) Affective response, (2) Social problems, (3) Self esteem, (4) Preoccupation with sickness, (5) Guilt, (6) Miscellaneous D (Depression) items, (7) Pleasure and enjoyment, and (8) Miscellaneous P (Positive). The first six are combined into a Total Depression Score, and the last two into a Total Positive Score. However, factor analysis has failed to validate these intuitive subscales.[97] The CDS has acceptable internal consistency,[97] and test–retest reliability, and it discriminates between children with and without depressive disorder.[92,97,98] Depression scale totals were correlated positively with neuroticism scores on the Eysenck Personality Questionnaire,[98,99] and with scores on the CDI.[92] Parent and child ratings showed moderate agreement.[92] Because a number of difficulties have been associated with the CDS (e.g., excessive length, redundancy among test items), this index has been revised recently.[100] The CDS-R retains 19 of the original 66 items, which are organized into four subscales: Loneliness/Death, School-Related Depression, Positive Self-Esteem, and Self-Downing. The internal consistency of the revised scale is fairly high ($\alpha = 0.86$). The authors point out that although the original CDS subscale structure is useful for clinical assessment, further refinement of the CDS-R will be necessary for its use as a research tool in nonclinical populations. However, to date, we are unaware of any medication studies that have used the CDS-R.

Because of its five-point scoring, the CDS may prove more sensitive than the CDI to treatment effects, although relevant data are not yet available. Where time allows for completion of a 66-item scale, the CDS would certainly warrant serious consideration as an evaluation tool. The scale's developers support the use of the scoring boxes because of their "gamelike quality," although a modified paper-and-pencil format may be more practical in an office setting. As with the CDI, the CDS may have a problem of lack of conceptual clarity in that the type of "depression" (disorder, trait, or symptom) being assessed is not specified.

c. Depressive Self-Rating Scale

This 18-item (scored 0–2) scale has the virtue of brevity.[101] Test–retest and split-half reliability are high, but drug sensitivity is unknown.[101]

d. The Reynolds Scales

There are two related instruments, the 29-item Reynolds Child Depression Scale (RCDS)[102] and the 30-item Reynolds Adolescent Depression Scale (RADS).[103] The RCDS, for grades 3 through 6, ages 8–12 years, comprises 29 items tapping symptoms of depression that the child has experienced in the last 2 weeks. The 29 depression items are scored using a Likert-type four-point scale, while the last item consists of five faces ranging from happy to sad (scored 1–5). The RCDS total score is the summation of the 30 items. The RCDS can be administered individually or in a group format; it is given orally to children under 10 years old and is read by older children. It takes approximately 10 minutes to complete. Scores correlate well with those from the CDI as well as measures of anxiety and self-esteem, and internal consistency is high.[95] However, self-ratings do not correspond well with parent and teacher ratings of depression.[104]

The RADS[103] comprises 30 items tapping depressive symptomatology that are rated using a four-point scale. It is designed to be used for adolescents aged 13–18, although it can be given to any adolescent who is in a junior high or high school setting. The RADS takes approximately 5–10 minutes to complete and can be administered individually, in small groups, or even in large groups [there is an optical character recognition (OCR) scoring format available]. The RADS is also available in a computerized administration format; although individuals in the general population show no preference between clinician- and computer-administered versions, psychiatric patients prefer the clinician-administered version.[105] The RADS total score is derived by summing individual test items, with scores of 77+ being considered to be indicative of clinical depression. Internal consistency and test–retest reliability are high,[106] especially over shorter intervals, e.g., less than 3 months.[103] There is high convergent validity between the RADS and the Beck Depression Inventory, the Center for Epidemiological Studies Depression Scale, the Zung Self-Rating Depression Scale,[107] and the Hamilton Rating Scale.[103] Recent studies have found that the RADS can successfully identify depression in Latino samples[108] and that adolescent girls consistently have higher RADS scores, consistent with higher levels of depression, than adolescent boys.[103,109]

There are obvious similarities between the two Reynolds scales, which may be a strength, as they presumably could be used as parallel tools for assessing children and adolescents. The psychometric characteristics of both scales appear to be very good, and data are available on hundreds of subjects. Unlike most instruments for assessing affective symptomatology, the Child Depression Scale and the RADS used DSM-III-R symptoms, as well as additional symptoms from the Research Diagnostic Criteria (RDC) and the Schedule for Affective Disorders and Schizophrenia (SADS) (child and adult versions),[103] which makes its concept of "depression" clearer than for many of the other depression scales. Also, it uses a refined four-point scoring format that should be sensitive to modest or subtle treatment effects. However, many items were selected for relevance to a school setting, which may reduce its applicability in clinical practice.[77] Also, in one treatment study, the RADS proved to be less sensitive than the Beck Depression Inventory or the Bellevue Index of Depression.[106]

e. Conclusion

Sufficient data do not exist to make a recommendation on which self-rating scale is best for monitoring drug effects. Because the CDS has more items (which tends to increase relability) and a five-point scale, it would appear to have potential, and availability of a parallel informant version is an added strength. On the other hand, its length may make it somewhat unwieldy in clinical practice. The CDI and Depressive Self-Rating Scale appear to be much the same in terms of their structure. The fact that there are substantial psychometric data on the CDI makes it attractive. Finally, the Reynolds scales also appear to have potential, being centered on DSM criteria, although they do not seem to have been used in clinical research to the extent that some of the others have. The recommended self-rating scales are listed in Table 2.

2. Informant (Parent and Teacher) Scales

a. Children's Depression Inventory

Several authors have developed informant versions of the CDI by rewording the items in the third person.[92,110,111] Studies have shown variable agreement between children's and parents' ratings on the two versions, ranging from low to quite high.[92] The arguments for and against the informant version appear to be similar to those for the self-rating format.

b. Children's Depression Scale

The CDS contains both a self-rating and an informant version. Unlike the ballot-box format employed with children, the adult version is purely a paper-and-pencil instrument.

c. Bellevue Index of Depression (BID)

The BID[112] can be used both as a paper-and-pencil (informant) instrument and as the basis for a semistructured interview. The BID consists of 40 items that are scored on a severity scale (0–3) and on duration ("less than one month" to "always"). In order to be scored as a symptom of depression, a given item must be present for longer than a month but not more than 2 years. This is a unique feature of the BID and clearly ties it to depression as a disorder that usually lasts from a few weeks to 2 years. The BID has been used to assess depression in adolescents with mental retardation,[113] and it has been found to correlate with other widely used measures of depression (CDI, Reynolds CDS).

d. Emotional Disorders Rating Scale (EDRS)

The EDRS is a 59-item scale for assessing disorders of mood and emotion in children and adolescents.[114] Like those in the BID, the items (except those in Hostility/Anger and the Irritability subscales; see below) were based on DSM-III-R symptoms. Assignment of items to scales was on clinical grounds, and each item is rated for frequency and severity. As there is a strong correlation between the two, severity ratings alone may suffice.[114] Although based on the DSM-III-R, the EDRS does not yield diagnoses as such. The EDRS has 59 items and eight component subscales: Anxiety, Hostility/Anger, Psychomotor Retardation, Depressed Mood Verbal, Depressed Mood Nonverbal, Somatic Vegetative, Sleep Disturbance, Irritability, and Elated/Manic Mood. The psychometric characteristics of the EDRS (and its close relative, the EDRS-DD) are variable, but on average test–retest reliability is low and interrater reliability is moderately high.[115] Validity data are available only for the depression scales and tend to be supportive.

The EDRS is fairly new, but the Psychomotor Retardation, the Depressed Mood Nonverbal, and the total depression subscales have been found to be sensitive to antidepressant medications such as tricyclic antidepressants and SSRIs.[116] It also has the advantages of being a nonobtrusive observational instrument and of simultaneously assessing anxiety, which often occurs with depression.[32]

e. Rating Scale of Dysphoria (RSD)

The RSD is both a self-report and an informant scale developed by rewriting items in the Peer Nomination Inventory of Depression.[117] The RSD includes 12 items rated on a five-point scale. It does not appear to be psychometrically robust: ratings between parents agree at low/moderate levels, there is poor mother–child agreement, and congruence with the Center for Epidemiological Studies Depression Scale for Children (CES-DC) is poor.[117] Further, the items of the RSD have a poor relationship with dysthymia.

f. Conclusion

With the probable exception of the RSD, all of the scales discussed are worthy of consideration for monitoring treatment effects. The most highly recommended are the CDS and the BID informant scale (see Table 2). The CDI and the EDRS are also recommended (especially the latter, which includes an anxiety subscale).

3. Interviews

There are several good interview systems for assessing childhood depression, but only two will be discussed here because of their relative brevity and hence suitability for practice.

a. Children's Depression Rating Scale—Revised (CDRS-R)

The CDRS-R is a clinically derived scale for practitioners to assess severity of depression in children aged 6 to 12 years by integrating information from all available sources.[118] It has 17 items (scored 1–7), 14 based on verbal responses and 3 on behavior (e.g., hyperactivity). The scoring of all behavioral items is described to minimize subjectivity. The scale takes 20–30 min to complete.[118] Interexaminer reliability is high,[118,119] item–total correlations are respectable,[119] and test–retest reliability (over 4 weeks) is high.[118] Though data on the CDRS-R are limited, those that exist are positive. Given its relative brevity, the CDRS-R could be a good monitoring tool if it can be shown to be drug-sensitive.

b. Bellevue Index of Depression (BID)

The BID[112] was described earlier. In addition to its paper-and-pencil format, the BID can also be used to guide semistructured interviews with youngsters and their parents. It takes 15–30 min to work through all 40 questions,[112] although a shortened version of the BID also exists.[120] It could become a popular assessment tool, especially since it has been shown to be sensitive to fluoxetine treatment in children and adolescents.[75]

c. Other Interview Schedules

The *Diagnostic Interview for Depression in Children and Adolescents* (DIDCA)[121] is a semistructured interview to diagnose and assess Major Depressive Episode in youngsters. It covers 10 key symptoms (e.g., sad/dysphoric mood, appetite disturbances), and each is further broken down with several specific examples. There is one version for interviews with the child (DIDCA-C) and one for interviews with the primary caretaker (DIDCA-P). Items are rated for presence over the last 4 weeks. In addition, there are follow-on questions to determine whether the symptom ever occurred in the child's lifetime. The DIDCA appears to be quite brief, making it suitable for clinical use.

Other interview systems for assessing depression in children and adolescents include all the structured diagnostic interviews discussed earlier (DISC, DICA, ISC, and K-SADS) and the School Age Depression Listed Inventory (SADLI).[122] The SADLI is the only one of these that was devised solely as an assessment instrument for depression.

4. Other Instruments

There are numerous other instruments for assessing depression in youngsters.[73,77,79] One that has attracted attention is the Peer Nomination Inventory of Depression (PNID)[123,124] in which children are asked to name classmates who fit 20 questions (e.g., "Who plays alone?"). It is unlikely that such a complicated procedure would be feasible in most clinical settings.

5. Conclusions

Depression is difficult to assess in children because they may have problems in recognizing or describing depressive symptoms and because of the lack of conceptual clarity and the tendency of depression to occur with other (especially anxiety) disorders. Several sources (child, parents, teachers) should be used in diagnosis and when assessing treatment response. As with other scales, there is a tendency for scores to decline over time. There are insufficient data to recommend specific instruments with confidence, although on the basis of psychometric characteristics and practical considerations (e.g., time to complete), some appear to be better than others (see Table 2 for listing). In addition, the choice of instrument will depend on whether the child is thought to have a disorder (major depression, dysthymia), depressive personality trait, or merely depressive symptoms.

F. Bipolar (Manic–Depressive) Mood Disorder (Mania)

As assessment of depression has already been discussed, this section will be confined to mania. This usually does not begin until adolescence and in childhood may take an atypical form, though this is controversial (see Chapter 9).[125] Recently, Kovacs[126] suggested that children who have unipolar depression convert more frequently to bipolar illness than do adults, indicating that manic-depressive disorder during childhood can be a serious affective disorder. Mania is ordinarily diagnosed by using a DSM-IV (or ICD-10) oriented interview such as DICA or K-SADS or, more usually, an unstructured clinical interview. When mania has been diagnosed, there are a number of scales that could be used to assess response to pharmacotherapy, but only one, the Manic-State Rating Scale,[127,128] seems to have adequate psychometric data. It has 26 items, of which 11 are considered "core" manic behaviors. It is designed for inpatients and is to be based on nurses' observations, requires training, and is reliable and valid, but it is rather cumbersome and somewhat ill defined.[128] Inspection suggests it would be suitable for adolescents.

As has been noted elsewhere,[129] few double-blind-placebo controlled medication treatment studies of mania have been done. The Self-Report Manic Inventory (SRMI) has been found to reliably diagnose bipolar disorder and to be sensitive to clinical improvements during general inpatient treatment.[130] Another promising measure of bipolar illness in children and adolescents is the Mania Rating Scale (MRS).[131] This 11-item instrument (originally developed for use in adults with bipolar illness) features seven items that are rated 0 to 4 and four items that are rated 0 to 8 (depending upon the weighting of the item), with higher scores indicating more severe bipolar symptomatology. Fristad and her colleagues,[132,133] using clinician-completed versions of the MRS, have recently shown that the instrument correlates highly ($r = 0.82$) with the Clinical Global Impression—Mania (CGI-M), an index measuring severity of bipolar symptoms which mirrors DSM-III-R criteria;[134] it is able to differentiate reliably between children with bipolar disorder and inpatient and outpatient children with ADHD, and has acceptable internal consistency ($\alpha = 0.80$). Given its brevity, and its correlation with DSM criteria, it would appear that this instrument is a helpful measure for diagnosis. Furthermore, a Modified Mania Rating Scale (MMRS) has been found to be sensitive to divalproex sodium (Depakote®) treatment for mania in a small ($n = 6$) study of older adolescents and young adults with bipolar disorder.[135] However, it remains to be seen if the MRS is sensitive to medication treatment in larger studies of children and adolescents with bipolar illness.

Among scales for assessing depression in children and adolescents, the Emotional Disorders Rating Scale[114] was discussed above. With the marked rise in interest in bipolar disorder in children and adolescents, there is a need for a good drug-sensitive mania scale.

G. Anxiety Disorders

Although there has been an increase in studies of anxiety and its disorders in recent years, there has not been much drug research and much of what there is, is unsophisticated and of considerable antiquity.[136] There are several good reviews of assessment of anxiety disorders in children.[74,137–141]

Anxiety is classified in a number of ways:

(1) *Global versus specific.* This classification is one of the more common. Global anxiety is presumed to be consistent across situations and time, while specific anxiety is regarded as dependent on a specific stimulus or situation.[136,141]

(2) *State and trait anxiety.* The first is regarded as relatively transitory and in response to a given stressor, while the latter is presumed to reflect a stable characteristic of the child's personality.[141] As Klein[140] notes, it is probably judicious to attempt to assess both state and trait anxiety when anxiety is the target of treatment.

(3) *Anxiety as a disorder*. DSM-IV lists one specific anxiety disorder associated with childhood and adolescence (separation anxiety), but children may also have most of the adult anxiety-related disorders, e.g., generalized anxiety disorder (includes the former overanxious disorder of childhood), panic, phobic, and obsessive–compulsive (see below).

Much of the research on anxiety is on the nondisorder type, but most of the pharmaco-therapeutic interest so far is on the disorders (see Chapter 7).

1. Self-Rating Scales

There is a general lack of data concerning the validity of child versus adult informant ratings of children's anxiety (which have low agreement with each other). With this in mind, it is wise to use both the child's appraisal of his or her internal state as well as that of significant others when assessing anxiety.

a. Fear Survey Schedule for Children (FSSC-R)

Sherer and Nakamura[142] adapted the adult Fear Survey Schedule for use with children, and the 80-item instrument was subsequently revised to simplify scoring (three-point scale).[143] Internal consistency is moderate to high,[143,144] test–retest reliability is good, especially in the short term,[143] it correlates moderately highly with trait anxiety on the State–Trait Anxiety Scale for Children,[143–145] and girls score higher than boys.[143,146,147] The FSSC-R has recently been updated to the FSSC-II,[148] but the factor structure remains similar to that of the FSSC-R. The FSSC-II factors are: (1) Fear of Death and Danger, (2) Fear of the Unknown, (3) Fear of Failure and Criticism, (4) Animal Fears, and (5) Psychic Stress–Medical Fears. The internal consistency is very high (0.96), as is the one-week test–retest reliability (0.90). The new FSSC-II is modestly correlated with the Revised Children's Manifest Anxiety Scale (RCMAS) ($r = 0.42$) and the Trait Anxiety Scale from the Spielberger State-Trait Anxiety Inventory for Children, ($r = 0.39$). Children having diagnoses of separation anxiety had modestly higher scores in one study,[143] but in another, children with various anxiety disorders did not differ from each other.[149] However, the pattern of intense fears did reveal qualitative differences between the groups. In general, girls have been found to have higher anxiety scores than boys, and younger children have been found to be more anxious than older children.[147,148,150,151] Despite this decline over time in anxiety levels, the most common fears appear to remain fairly constant over the early to mid-elementary school years and include fears of injury, death, and danger.[147] Children with intellectual disabilities have also been shown to have higher levels of fearfulness than children without developmental disabilities, perhaps reflecting a mental-age-related phenomenon.[151,152] However, children with mental retardation did not have age-related declines in anxiety in at least one study.[153] Interestingly, although the FSSC-R differentiates boys with high anxiety levels from boys without psychiatric diagnosis, it does not differentiate boys with anxiety from boys with ADHD.[154] In recent years, the FSSC-R has been translated to Chinese[155] and Turkish,[156] and has been found reliably to identify anxiety in these cultures.

To our knowledge, the FSSC-R has not been used for drug research, so its sensitivity to pharmacotherapy cannot be assessed at this stage. The FSSC-R may prove useful in treatment for pinpointing sources of fear in a given child and possibly for monitoring the effects of treatment on these fears, but treatment is not often likely to be pharmacologic (see Chapter 7).

b. Revised Children's Manifest Anxiety Scale (RCMAS)

The original Children's Manifest Anxiety Scale[157] and the revised version were adaptations of a popular adult scale.[158] The RCMAS comprises 37 statements to which the child is asked to respond "true" or "false." There are 9 lie-scale items, and the remainder load on one of three empirically derived subscales: (1) Physiological, (2) Worry and oversensitivity, and (3) Concentration;[159,160] in addition, there is a total score. Reliability appears to be adequate.[115] The RCMAS correlated highly with trait but not state scores from the State–Trait Anxiety Scale for Children (STAIC),[145] suggesting that it assesses stable (personality) characteristics.[161] One study failed to show RCMAS differences between children with and without anxiety disorders, although those with depressive disorders scored significantly higher than those without.[162] One recent study[163] demonstrated that although the RCMAS reliably differentiated children with anxiety disorders from a group of children without psychiatric diagnoses, no differences existed between children with anxiety and children with externalizing disorders. Similarly, children with anxiety and ADHD have also been found to score similarly on this scale.[154] The RCMAS has also demonstrated efficacy in identifying elevated anxiety levels that are related to physical illness of family members.[164] The RCMAS or its predecessor has been used in only two drug studies,[165,166] and sensitivity was not impressive, but more data are needed. Indirect evidence for sensitivity to medication response comes from a recent study showing the RCMAS to be sensitive to change over time in adolescents who were hospitalized in a psychiatric setting.[167]

Interestingly, a new revision of the original Children's Manifest Anxiety Scale[157] has recently been reported.[168] Preliminary results using this scale were not suggestive of age-related differences in anxiety levels but were suggestive of higher levels of anxiety in girls than in boys.

c. Childhood Anxiety Sensitivity Index (CASI) and Child Anxiety Frequency Checklist (CAFC)

One interesting development in the child-anxiety literature is the creation of instruments that attempt to disentangle the existence of anxiety itself from the perception of anxiety as harmful or aversive. The CASI[169] (Fig. 5) is an 18-item modification of the adult instrument[170] and assesses sensitivity to anxiety (i.e., perceptiveness to anxiety) by asking children to rate how aversively they view 18 anxiety symptoms on a three-point scale. The CAFC, adapted from the adult AFC,[170] evaluates the frequency of eight anxiety symptoms, such as rapid heartbeat, shakiness, and trouble catching one's breath. Test–retest reliability of the CASI was moderate to high, and internal consistency was moderate, whereas for the CAFC both were moderate.[169] Children with diagnosed anxiety disorders have been shown to have higher scores on the CASI relative to children without any psychiatric diagnoses; however, no significant differences emerged between children with anxiety disorders and children with ADHD or externalizing disorders in general.[154,163]

The CASI and CAFC are only weakly correlated, indicating that they assess different attributes. Both the CASI and the CAFC correlate significantly with the FSSC-R and trait scores on the STAIC, though CASI scores accounted for most of the variance in FSSC-R and STAIC ratings. It was also highly correlated with the RCMAS (0.62).[171] It may be the case that the CASI is more appropriate for use with children aged 12 years and older— beyond this age, the CASI appears to predict more than just trait anxiety. It may be the case

CASI

Name: _____   Age: _____   Dated: _____

Directions: A number of statements which boys and girls use to describe themselves are given below. Read each statement carefully and put an X in the box in front of the words that describe you. There are no right or wrong answers. Remember, find the words that best describe you.

1. I don't want other people to know when I feel afraid.	____None	____Some	____A Lot
2. When I cannot keep my mind on my schoolwork I worry that I might be going crazy.	____None	____Some	____A Lot
3. It scares me when I feel "shaky".	____None	____Some	____A Lot
4. It scares me when I feel like I am going to faint.	____None	____Some	____A Lot
5. It is important for me to stay in control of my feelings.	____None	____Some	____A Lot
6. It scares me when my heart beats fast.	____None	____Some	____A Lot
7. It embarrasses me when my stomach growls (makes noise).	____None	____Some	____A Lot
8. It scares me when I feel like I am going to throw up.	____None	____Some	____A Lot
9. When I notice that my heart is beating fast, I worry that there might be something wrong with me.	____None	____Some	____A Lot
10. It scares me when I have trouble getting my breath.	____None	____Some	____A Lot
11. When my stomach hurts, I worry that I might be really sick.	____None	____Some	____A Lot
12. It scares me when I can't keep my mind on my schoolwork.	____None	____Some	____A Lot
13. Other kids can tell when I feel shaky.	____None	____Some	____A Lot
14. Unusual feelings in my body scare me.	____None	____Some	____A Lot
15. When I am afraid, I worry that I might be crazy.	____None	____Some	____A Lot
16. It scares me when I feel nervous.	____None	____Some	____A Lot
17. I don't like to let my feelings show.	____None	____Some	____A Lot
18. Funny feelings in my body scare me.	____None	____Some	____A Lot

FIGURE 5. Children's Anxiety Sensitivity Index, Reproduced by permission of Dr. W. K. Silverman. Readers may reproduce this form but are asked not to alter its format or content without the permission of Dr. W. K. Silverman. ©Copyright Wendy K. Silverman, Department of Psychology, Florida International University, University Park, Miami, Florida.

that cognitive development in children younger than 12 years is insufficient for them to have truly developed anxiety sensitivity, because they may be unable to reason about abstract negative events in the future[171] or to express anxiety. To date, there are no tests of the drug sensitivity of these instruments. However, given the relative dearth of anxiety instruments, the CASI and CAFC warrant consideration, particularly since psychotropic medications may affect the cognitive appraisal of anxiety tapped by the CASI rather than rate or frequency of anxiety.

d. State–Trait Anxiety Scale for Children (STAIC)

The STAIC is a self-report inventory that can be administered singly or in groups.[145] It was developed for children of elementary-school age and is in two parts, Anxiety-State and Anxiety-Trait scales, both of which are 20 items long and take about 7–10 min to complete. The Anxiety-State scale asks the child to respond as to how he or she feels right now, and the Anxiety-Trait scale how he or she usually feels. Both use a three-point scale for items. Norms are available only for fourth- to sixth-grade children. Eight-week test–retest reliabilities are moderately high on the Trait scale and, as would be expected, lower on the State scale.

Emotionally disturbed children have higher scores than normal on both parts.[169,172] Specificity for anxiety disorders is good, but sensitivity (detecting true positives) is poor.[162] The STAIC correlates variably with the RCMAS (or its predecessor, the CMAS), although most correlations are moderately high or better.[161,165,173] The scale has received widespread endorsement; for example, it is frequently used as a validating measure for other instruments, it discriminates between anxiety and control groups, and it provides separate measures of state and trait anxiety. Intriguingly, a recent study[174] has found an intergenerational link in trait anxiety: higher levels of trait anxiety in children were associated with higher levels of trait anxiety in mothers and fathers. High levels of anxiety, as measured by the STAIC, have also been associated with eating disorders.[175] Though the STAIC has not been used in drug studies, it is a measure worth considering.

An interesting finding that emerged in several of the studies listed above is that these questionnaires appear to differentiate children with anxiety disorders from non-diagnosed children fairly reliably, but there is less specificity between children with anxiety disorders and other clinic-referred children (e.g., children with ADHD or disruptive behavior disorders in general). As Perrin and Last[154] point out, it may be the case that our current crop of measures are simply insufficient. Or it may be the case that there is a greater degree of overlap in symptomatology between children with anxiety and those with ADHD than has been described in the literature.

2. Specific Anxiety Disorders

a. Obsessive–Compulsive Disorder (OCD)

OCD is marked by repetitive intrusive thoughts [e.g., of contamination and/or rituals (such as hand washing)] that are recognized by the patient as unfounded. It is both distressing and often relapsing or chronic,[176] and pharmacotherapy, especially with serotonergic antidepressants (see Chapter 9), is now an accepted part of treatment. In about 50% of adult cases, OCD begins in childhood. In diagnosis of OCD in children and adolescents, much work has been done with the self-report Leyton Obsessional Inventory—Child version, which is an adaptation of the adult scale.[177] There are two versions: a 44-item scale (for diagnosis) and a short 20-item scale (for surveys),[178] and items are scored for resistance, interference, and presence versus absence. It has good test–retest reliability and discriminates patients from normals but has only modest specificity for OCD.[179–181] Most importantly, it is drug-sensitive.[177] Full details, including the scale itself and how to administer it, are readily available,[177] and it is strongly recommended.

The Yale–Brown Obsessive Compulsive Scale (Y-BOCS) is a 19-item rating scale that is typically administered in a semistructured interview format by a clinician, who then completes the questionnaire.[182,183] It can also be used as a self-report instrument. Of the 19 items, there are 10 critical items that contribute to the total score: 5 tapping obsessions and 5 tapping compulsions. In general, clinical subjects report more symptomatology using the self-report format than they do in an interview format.[184] Interrater reliability of the interview format has been shown to be excellent. Internal consistency was acceptable, and convergent validity with other OCD measures was good, but stability over 7 weeks was disappointing as was divergent validity (e.g., it showed a tendency to correlate with depression).[185] There is also a child and adolescent version (the CY-BOCS), which has been shown to be sensitive to risperidone treatment[186] and behavioral psychotherapy.[187]

b. Panic Disorder

Panic disorder is characterized by short episodes of a fulminating sense of impending death accompanied by objective signs of terror, all appearing suddenly and without apparent cause. It is treated pharmacologically with antidepressants (see Chapter 9). Its occurrence in children is disputed; and typically, it begins in late adolescence.[74] It is likely that the DIS scales developed for the International Study of Panic Disorder[188] would serve for children and adolescents, but for routine diagnosis the DSM-IV based interviews like DICA and K-SADS, discussed earlier, have limited (and inadequate) screening sections on panic disorder.[74] To assess change, simple frequency recordings and general-purpose instruments like the CGI can be used. Adolescents with panic attacks were found to have higher levels of anxiety, as assessed by the RCMAS, than adolescents who had never experienced a panic attack.[189]

c. Separation Anxiety Disorder

Separation anxiety self-explanatory disorder often presents as school refusal. While this disorder has been the subject of a few pharmacological studies (Chapter 7),[74] only ad hoc or general-purpose diagnostic or anxiety instruments already described seem to have been used in diagnosis and assessment of change. One such instrument is the DISC, which has been shown to be an effective instrument for parental report of separation anxiety disorder.[190] Separation anxiety has been identified as one of the avenues by which children progress to panic disorders, although many other pathways also lead to panic.[191]

d. Phobic Disorders

Phobic disorders are best diagnosed and any change evaluated using the FSS (see above).[74] The Schedule for Affective Disorders and Schizophrenia for School-Age Children and the Children's Global Assessment Scale have also been used to study phobias in adolescents.[192]

e. Posttraumatic Stress Disorder (PTSD)

PTSD attained interest as a consequence of the Vietnam War and has subsequently been diagnosed in children and adolescents who have experienced sexual and physical abuse, disasters, or kidnapping. While ordinarily it would be diagnosed using DSM-IV-oriented interviews or checklists, there is at least one specific technique, the PTSD Reaction Index, which evaluates 16 PTSD symptoms[193] following a special semistructured interview. The PTSD Reaction Index has identified children with PTSD following natural disasters such as hurricanes.[194,195] No information was obtainable on drug sensitivity or psychometric characteristics other than that the index correlates well with adolescent and clinician diagnoses of PTSD. The PTSD module of the DICA has been used to identify this disorder among Cambodian refugee youths.[196]

3. Personality Scales

Some of the best known personality scales are relatively old self-rating instruments, namely, the California Test of Anxiety, the Eysenck Personality Questionnaire (the neuroticism dimension), and the Cattell Scales.[140] These instruments do not assess various types of anxiety (e.g., separation, panic), most assume a high level of reading skills (or must be read to the child), and they fail to address how the fear affects the child's life.[140] However, other instruments such as the Personality Inventory for Children[197] (under revision as of this writing) do measure anxiety, along with a number of other behavioral and developmental factors. Some of these instruments, therefore, have very limited utility for assessing anxiety in children,[140] and, by extension, any role for assessing drug effects cannot be recommended.

4. Behavior Rating Scales for Anxiety

Behavior rating scales completed by significant other figures in the child's life, such as parents and teachers, could also be useful in monitoring drug effects.

a. Louisville Behavior Check List

In the revised version of the Louisville Behavior Check List,[198] there is an 18-item Fear subscale containing items referring to specific fears such as fear of the dark and death. Some reflect difficulty in coping alone, and others reflect worrying behaviors that are general and repetitive. There is also a 15-item (17 for girls) Sensitivity subscale relating to internal and external cues and inappropriate reactions to stress (e.g., cries easily, feels more pain than normal). Both subscales discriminated between children with phobias and control subjects, and split-half reliabilities were quite high for both the phobic and normal samples.[198] There is no reason that the anxiety subscales of the Check List could not be used without the remainder of the instrument for assessing treatment outcome in high-anxious children, though the check list has not been used in drug studies.

b. Louisville Fear Survey for Children

This clinically derived scale has 81 items (each scored 1–3) covering many fears in children aged 4 to 18 years[199] and can be completed by children or adult informants, although published data are only available from parents. There is good split-half reliability, and there are three factor-analytically derived subscales: (I) Fear of physical injury, (II) Fear of natural events, and (III) Fear of psychic stress (taking tests, being criticized, etc.). It has not been used in drug studies.

5. Structured Interviews

There is no reason to suggest that the anxiety disorders portions of structured interviews discussed above (such as the DICA, K-SADS, or ISC) could not be repeated to assess drug effects on anxiety. There is also a specialized Anxiety Disorders Interview Schedule (ADIS), developed to permit differential diagnoses among the childhood anxiety disorders in children 6 to 18 years of age.[200]

6. Conclusions

Several conclusions should now be obvious. (1) There is not a large selection of instruments from which to choose in assessing anxiety, and in those that do exist, there is not much research from drug studies to indicate which instruments are the most promising for practitioners wishing to monitor treatment effects. (2) The common use of a Yes/No dichotomy restricts the possibility of detecting less than complete "cure" of a symptom, although clinicians could alter instruments when appropriate and use graduated scoring.[140] However, this would limit the use of any norms. (3) It may be desirable to reword some of the better self-rating instruments in the third person for use by informants such as parents and teachers. (4) Practitioners may do better to place reliance on behavioral indicators such as days of school absences, degree of approach to feared stimuli (e.g., dogs, enclosed places, elevators), and behavior during clinical examination or tests.* (5) As with depression, there is a need to distinguish between anxiety as a symptom, as a personality trait, and as one of the several particular anxiety disorders such as panic, obsessive–compulsive, or phobic disorder. Some instruments, such as the ADIS, ISC, and DISC, are designed to assess disorders, but most were constructed prior to 1980 and are not disorder-specific. Since pharmacotherapy is increasingly becoming disorder-oriented (e.g., OCD, panic disorder), the older or more general anxiety/fear schedules may be less suited to diagnosis but might still be useful in assessing anxiolytic drug effects.

Recommendations

Faced with little empirical data on drug sensitivity, it is possible only to be tentative: (1) *Brief assessments* tailored to the particular anxiety symptoms can be custom-made for each child when the anxiety is not a defined disorder like OCD. The strategy would be similar to that described earlier under "general-purpose" scales. (2) When the child has a specific anxiety disorder, an appropriate instrument, such as the Leyton Obsessional Scale, should be used. The new ADIS is also worth a trial, although it covers all anxiety disorders, and the sections on the relevant disorders in the K-SADS, DICA, or ICS can be considered. When no appropriate instrument exists, DSM-IV symptoms such as separation anxiety disorder and panic disorder could be (and in some cases have been)[74] constructed in questionnaire format. (3) Among nonspecific anxiety standardized instruments, the CASI would seem to warrant clinical trials, because it assesses the child's reaction to his or her anxiety. Among the older standardized instruments, both the STAIC and the RCMAS also deserve consideration.

H. Other Disorders

1. Schizophrenia

Schizophrenia is rare in children but peaks in late adolescence. For diagnosis, a DSM-IV or ICD-10 oriented interview is needed, where possible, using one of the recommended semistructured interviews, either child (e.g., K-SADS, DICA, ISC) or, for older adolescents, adult types (SADS, DIS, etc). If these are thought too cumbersome, a symptom checklist such as the Child Symptom Inventory–4[18] may be used instead. The K-SADS, in particular, and a derivative covering the psychosis section, the Interview for Childhood Disorders and Schizophrenia (ICDS),[201] have shown promising reliability (interrater, test-retest) for child schizophrenia, though more data are needed.[201] In assessing treatment, in addition to the usual CGI and other general-purpose scales, there are some disorder-specific scales such as the ICDS, the Kiddie Formal Thought Disorder Scale, and the Kiddie Positive and Negative Symptom Scales for Children and Adolescents,[202] which are adaptations of their adult namesakes. While psychometrically promising, none of these has yet been used in drug studies, but this reflects the dearth of such studies and a real need in child/adolescent schizophrenia (see Chapter 10).

2. Tic and Tourette Disorders

Although externally observable, tic symptoms can be surprisingly difficult to assess. This is because (a) they can run the gamut from barely discernible to highly intrusive, (b) they can vary markedly from patient to patient, (c) they can change within patients from one time to the next, and (d) they are influenced by environmental stressors.[203] There are several scales available for assessing tics,[203,204] but we will emphasize practitioner instruments here.

The Yale Global Tic Severity Scale (YGTSS)[205] is an inventory of motor and phonic tics, both simple and complex. The clinician rates each type of tic (motor and phonic) on separate six-point scales for number, frequency, intensity, complexity, interference, and overall impairment. These are then summed onto a *total motor* and a *total phonic* score, and the clinician makes an *overall impairment rating*. Finally, all three of these are added to compute the Global Severity Score. The YGTSS has established construct validity, good interrater reliability, and concurrent validity with other tic scales,[203] and it is drug-sensitive.

The Tourette Syndrome Global Scale (TSGS)[206] comprises separate tic and social functioning sections that are weighted equally in calculating a Global Score. The tic domain includes simple motor tics, complex motor tics, simple phonic tics, and complex phonic tics. Each of these is rated for frequency and disruption to the patient's functioning on scales ranging from 0 to 5. The social functioning domain comprises clinician ratings of disruptive behavior, motor restlessness, and school/work problems to render scores in the range of 0 to 50. The TSGS appears to have adequate to good interrater reliability and it is drug-sensitive.[203] However, it seems to us that, if one looks solely at the total score, there is an unnecessary confusion of tic symptomatology with potentially separable social–emotional problems. This may be rectified by treating the tic and social functioning domains separately or by using only the tic domain.

The Tourette Syndrome Severity Scale (TSSS) gives a measure of the severity of Tourette symptoms.[204,207] The patient and informants living with the patient are asked to rate the tics on four attributes: (a) noticeable to others, (b) tendency to elicit comments or curiosity, (c) leading to the patient being considered odd or bizarre, and (d) interference with patient functioning. The ordinal ratings on these attributes are summed to give a qualitative description of severity. The TSSS is reliable across raters and is consistent with patient's self-ratings, and it is sensitive to medication.[207]

A recent addition to the tic assessment instruments is the *Motor Tic, Obsessions and Compulsions, Vocal Tic Evaluation Survey* (MOVES), which is a self-rating tool designed for completion by children (7 years and older), adolescents, and adults.[208] The MOVES has four items each for assessing motor tics, vocal tics, obsessions, and compulsions and one each for copropraxia, echolalia, echopraxia, and palilalia (20 items total). The motor and vocal tic items are combined to produce a Tic Subscale, the Obsessive and Compulsive items form an Obsessive–Compulsive Subscale; all 20 items contribute to a Total Score. Each item is scored 0 to 3 (*never* to *always*), respectively. The MOVES appears in Fig. 6.

Psychometric work indicates that the MOVES differentiates Tourette syndrome patients from controls and related clinical groups, and there is substantial agreement between relevant MOVES subscales and other instruments designed to assess tics, compulsions, obsessions, and OCD.[208] Test–retest reliability was only moderate; the MOVES showed a

MOVES Survey

Answer the questions below for the past ____ week(s).	NEVER	SOMETIMES	OFTEN	ALWAYS
1. I make noises (like grunts) that I can't stop.				
2. Parts of my body jerk again and again, that I can't control.				
3. I have bad ideas over and over, that I can't stop.				
4. I have to do things in certain order or certain ways (like touching things).				
5. Words come out that I can't stop or control.				
6. At times I have the same jerk or twitch over and over.				
7. Certain bad words or thoughts keep going through my mind.				
8. I have to do exactly the opposite of what I'm told.				
9. The same unpleasant or silly thought or picture goes through my mind.				
10. I can't control all my movements.				
11. I have to do several movements over and over again, in the same order.				
12. Bad or swear words come out that I don't mean to say.				
13. I feel pressure to talk, shout, or scream.				
14. I have ideas that bother me (like germs or like cutting myself).				
15. I do certain things (like jumping or clapping) over and over.				
16. I have habits or movements that come out more when I'm nervous.				
17. I have to repeat things that I hear other people say.				
18. I have to do things I see other people do.				
19. I have to make bad gestures (like the finger).				
20. I have to repeat words or phrases over and over.				

FIGURE 6. *Motor Tic, Obsession and Compulsion, and Vocal Tic Evaluation Scale* (MOVES). Reproduced by permission from Gaffney GR, Sieg K, Hellings J: The MOVES: A self-rating scale for Tourette's Syndrome. *Journal of Child and Adolescent Psychopharmacology* 4:269–280, 1994.

mean reduction of 33% in total scores in 16 patients initiating pharmacotherapy. Given that patient dissatisfaction with treatment and/or side effects is a major reason for failure of pharmacotherapy, a measure of the patient's perception may be very helpful in making treatment decisions.

Leckman et al.[203] also described a scale that they developed to help *parents* document changes in tics over time. The Tourette Syndrome Symptom List divides tics into simple motor (9 symptoms), complex motor (9 symptoms), simple phonic (4 symptoms), and complex phonic tics (5 symptoms) and behavior problems (4 generic categories). Each symptom is simply rated on a six-point ordinal scale from 0 (not at all) to 5 (almost always).

Finally, investigators have employed videotapes of tics recorded while the patient is engaged in standard activities (arithmetic computation, reading passages, and while at rest). Such measures of tic counts have proven to be reliable and sensitive to medication effects, but they do not appear to be as valid as practitioner ratings on standardized scales.[204] Workers have also used adult patients' estimates of percentage reduction in tic severity, and these were highly sensitive to medication effects.[207]

I. Mental Retardation

Mental retardation is a nonspecific label, applied to a heterogeneous population, that does not necessarily signify the presence of psychopathology. However, rates of various psychiatric disorders and symptoms are higher in this population than in the general population.[115] Scales already described for assessing specific symptoms and disorders in other groups of children can often be applied with children and adolescents who are mentally retarded, but limitations in self-expression and developmental variations may make these instruments unacceptable. In this section, selected instruments developed specifically for children with mental retardation will be discussed briefly. Comprehensive reviews of methods of assessing psychopathology in mentally retarded patients[115] and drug effects[7] are available elsewhere.

1. The Aberrant Behavior Checklist (ABC)

The ABC is the only empirically derived instrument that was specifically developed for assessing treatment effects in patients with mental retardation.[209] The ABC has 58 items that divide into five factor-analytically derived subscales: (I) Irritability/Agitation/Crying (15 items), (II) Lethargy/Social Withdrawal (16 items), (III) Stereotypic Behavior (7 items), (IV) Hyperactivity, Noncompliance (16 items), and (V) Inappropriate Speech (4 items). It has good test–retest reliability,[209,210] adequate interrater reliability,[211,212] and good criterion group validity, and subscale scores correlate moderately highly with similar dimensions from other scales.[115,212] Its factor structure has been replicated with adolescents and adults in institutional settings[213–215] and with children in the community[216,217] and in inpatient settings.[210,218] To date, the ABC has been used in approximately 70 studies and is by far the most used instrument for assessing drug effects in mental retardation and autism.[210]

The ABC has been used to assess drug effects, both in institutions[2] and in the community, in children and adolescents,[219–222] and it is among the most sensitive measures of drug effects in this population.[222] It can be completed by parents, teachers, and other care providers and is available in a community version (i.e., without any references to an institutional setting).[222]

2. The Nisonger Child Behavior Rating Form (N-CBRF)

The N-CBRF[223] is a very recent scale that was developed at Ohio State University's Nisonger Center, for children with developmental disabilities. The N-CBRF was empirically derived by factor analysis from ratings by parents and teachers on children seeking assessment for cognitive, behavioral, or other problems. The N-CBRF comprises similar parent and teacher versions with five problem behavior subscales in common and a sixth that differs. The first five subscales were labeled as follows: 1. Conduct problem, 2. Insecure/anxious, 3. Hyperactive, 4. Self-injury/stereotypy, and 5. Self-isolated/ritualistic. The sixth subscale on the parent version is called *Overly sensitive*, whereas on the teacher version it is

Irritable. There are 60 items on both versions of the N-CBRF. Both scales also have a *Positive/Social* section, encompassing 10 items, that score onto a *Compliant/calm* and an *Adaptive/social* subscale. Psychometric characteristics appeared to be very satisfactory, as assessed by internal consistency, interrater reliability, and correspondence of scores with the ABC.[223]

Norms are available for the developmental sample in the form of percentiles, T scores, and means and standard deviations.[224] At the time of writing, the N-CBRF is being used in several drug studies in the United States and Canada and across Europe, and its sensitivity to medication effects should be known soon. The N-CBRF is in the public domain and can be obtained from Michael Aman, one of its developers.

3. Behavior Problems Inventory (BPI)

The BPI was developed to assess various types of destructive behavior in epidemiological surveys of mentally retarded children and adults.[225] The instrument has 29 items rated on a six-point scale, with three clinically derived subscales of self-injurious behavior (15 items), stereotypic behavior (5 items), and aggression (9 items). Reliability varies from mediocre to excellent,[115] but until recently the BPI has not been used in drug assessment. Like the N-CBRF, the BPI was being used in several multisite trials across North America and Europe at the time of writing. For monitoring medication effects, the frequency scheme for scoring items might need to be modified in scoring to suit the characteristics of the patient(s) concerned.

4. Emotional Disorders Rating Scale for Developmental Disabilities (EDRS-DD)

The EDRS-DD was developed in mentally retarded children and adolescents for the purposes of diagnosis and assessment of treatment,[226] and it is a close relative of the EDRS, discussed previously. There are no data on treatment sensitivity, but it is one of few instruments to address problems of mood and emotion in this population.[115]

5. Maladaptive Behavior Scale

The Maladaptive Behavior Scale[28] was discussed under general rating instruments, above. This global index is suitable for use with developmentally disabled patients, because it can be used to assess any observable symptom or behavior and is able to be repeated.

6. Other Instruments

There are a variety of instruments that may prove to be useful for monitoring treatment effects in mentally retarded children and adolescents, though their sensitivity to pharmacological treatments is largely untested and, for other reasons, they do not seem as suitable as those discussed here. Most have been reviewed in detail elsewhere[115,227]; they include the Attention Checklist,[228] the Behaviour Disturbance Scale,[229] the Behavior Evaluation Rating Scale (BeERS),[230] the Developmental Behaviour Checklist,[231] the Diagnostic Assessment for the Severely Handicapped (DASH) Scale,[232] the Self-Injurious Behavior Questionnaire (SIB-Q),[233] and the Emotional Problems Scales (informant version) (formerly called the Strohmer–Prout Behavior Rating Scale).[234]

J. Autism

Unfortunately, in autism there are relatively few standardized measures that have been shown to be sensitive to pharmacological intervention thus far.[235]

1. The Children's Psychiatric Rating Scale (CPRS)

The CPRS[5] is a 63-item scale designed to measure a broad spectrum of psychopathology in children and adolescents, of which 28 items are rated on the basis of observation of the child's behavior, and 34 items are self-reports. All items are scored on a seven-point scale. In younger and/or nonverbal patients with autism, only the observational part of the scale is used. Of the items on this part of the scale, 14 symptoms are relevant to autistic behavior and appear to be sensitive to drug treatment in autistic youngsters.[235] Interrater reliabilities range from moderate to high, but validity is unstudied. The 14 symptoms for autism have been factor analyzed and found to contribute to four factors designated as Autism (5 items), Anger/uncooperativeness (4 items), Hyperactivity (3 items), and Speech deviance (2 items).[236] The 14-item CPRS has been shown to be sensitive to psychotropic medication[235] (see Chapter 10).

2. Aberrant Behavior Checklist

The Aberrant Behavior Checklist[222] (discussed above under mental retardation) should be relevant for assessing children with autistic disorder because problems described in three of its five subscales (II—Lethargy/Social Withdrawal, III—Stereotypic Behavior, and IV—Hyperactivity, Noncompliance) are prominent features of the disorder. It has proven to be drug-sensitive in children with autism,[210,221] and it has well-established sensitivity to treatment effects in nonautistic children with mental retardation.

3. The Nisonger Child Behavior Rating Form

The Nisonger Child Behavior Rating Form,[223,224] discussed in the section on mental retardation, is also highly relevant to autism. In particular, the subscales designated as Hyperactive, Self-isolated/ritualistic, and Self-injury/stereotypy are highly relevant to the disorder, and Conduct problem and Irritable may be relevant in individual patients.

4. The Conners Scales—Revised

In the past, Conners' Hyperactivity Index was frequently used in drug studies,[226] and, as the "offspring" of the Hyperactivity Index, it is possible that Conners' Global Index[33] will also be used. Conners' ADHD/DSM-IV Symptoms Subscale[33] may also find a niche for assessment in autism. However, hyperactivity is only one of several symptoms that are commonly found in children with autism.

5. Timed Stereotypies Rating Scale

The Timed Stereotypies Rating Scale[237] lists 22 specific stereotypies, plus an open slot for write-ins. Its purpose is to rate the frequency of stereotypies and to differentiate their reemergence upon discontinuance of drug therapy.[235]

6. Ritvo-Freeman Real Life Rating Scale for Autism

The Real Life Rating Scale (RLRS)[238] comprises 47 behaviors, rated on a four-point scale, that resolve onto five clinically derived subscales: (I) Sensory Motor, (II) Social Relationship to People, (III) Affectual Responses, (IV) Sensory Responses, and (V) Language. Reliability is low to moderate between novice observers but moderate to high between experienced observers. Test–retest reliability is unknown, but there are moderate (negative) correlations between the RLRS and the Alpern–Boll Developmental Profile, which is a scale of developmental and adaptive behavior. The RLRS was used in 8 of 27 studies of fenfluramine in autism, and one or more subscales showed significant changes in 6 studies.[239] However, the instrument is rather insensitive in other than children with autism.[219,240]

7. Conclusion

There are a number of other scales for autism described elsewhere, but most are merely diagnostic.[241] There are no psychometrically established scales for drug evaluation, although the CPRS has been used often and appears drug-sensitive. Recommendations appear in Table 2.

K. Preschool Rating Scales

1. Introduction

Most of the scales discussed thus far were developed for children of school age (usually 6 years of age and above) and adolescents. While pharmacotherapy is less indicated in preschoolers, it still may be indicated in a few disorders like autism and ADHD (see Chapter 7). Unfortunately, there is neither the diversity and the sophistication, nor the wealth of psychometric data on instruments for this age group compared with those for older children. Three of the best instruments for assessing preschoolers are discussed here. Other scales can be found elsewhere.[242]

2. Child Behavior Checklist (CBCL)

The CBCL, discussed in detail above, is normed down to age 4 years. More recently, the CBCL/2-3 was introduced for children aged 2 to 3 years.[243] Half of its 100 items were taken from the CBCL and others from scales such as the Behavioural Screening Questionnaire and the Preschool Behavior Questionnaire (see below). There are six factor-analytically derived subscales as follows: (I) Social Withdrawal (14 items), (II) Depressed (15 items), (III) Sleep Problems (8 items), (IV) Somatic Problems (12 items), (V) Aggressive (32 items), and (VI) Destructive (14 items), of which Sleep and Destructive are unique to this age group, the others being also found in the CBCL. Psychometric characteristics appear acceptable to good[243] in that 1-week test–retest reliability was high, interparent reliability was modest, and clinic children had higher scores than nonreferred children. Second-order factor analyses allow broad-band internalizing and externalizing factor scores to be calculated, and T scores are available to assess a child's clinical standing. More studies of this new scale are needed.

3. The Preschool Behavior Questionnaire (PBQ)

The PBQ[244,245] is a screening instrument for problems in preschoolers, with most of the 30 items taken from the Children's Behaviour Questionnaire[246] and with 10 additional items. There are three factor-analytically derived subscales: (I) Hostile–Aggressive, (II) Anxious–Fearful, and (III) Hyperactive–Distractible[244,245,247] and a total score as well. Interrater reliabilities range from 0.67 (Hyperactive–Distractible) to 0.81 (Hostile–Aggressive), test–retest reliabilities are adequate, and discrimination between community and clinic children is high.[244] The PBQ has been the subject of considerable psychometric research, and most is supportive, including the research on its use in children with developmental disabilities.[115,248–252]

The PBQ appears to be a convenient and useful clinical tool, which has generated much research interest. Its principal weaknesses include the fact that its Hyperactive-Distractible subscale has only four items (which tends to undermine its reliability) and that certain items seem to relate more to developmental level than emotional status (e.g., "Has wet or soiled self," "Speech difficulty"). Nevertheless, it could be valuable for monitoring treatment in some youngsters.

4. Other Preschool Instruments

a. The Behavioural Screening Questionnaire (BSQ)

The BSQ is a brief interview comprising 12 items of problem behavior scored 0–2 to provide a Behavior Score.[253] A score of 10 or above is regarded as clinically significant.[254–256] There is also a Behaviour Check List, which is a parent rating form that closely parallels the BSQ.[257] The scales are worded in a way that is highly relevant to the behavior of preschool children, but they provide only a global severity score and do not convey information about different symptom areas. They have not been used to assess drug treatment.

b. The Symptom Checklist

The Symptom Checklist[258–260] was derived by factor analysis of behavior ratings of children in preschool, kindergarten, or day-care centers and is intended to be completed by teachers or assistant teachers. It has 49 items on an Apathy–Withdrawal or an Anger–Defiance subscale; a three-point scale is used for each item.

c. Temperament Scales

Temperament scales have been discussed by Hertzig and Snow[261] and Aman.[115] The instruments are usually constructed to reflect relatively stable, constitutionally determined personality traits, and, hence, they are unlikely to be treatment-sensitive.

5. Conclusion

Scales for preschoolers are limited, and there are no data on drug sensitivity. Recommendations are, therefore, tentative. We recommend the age-appropriate version of the CBCL or the PBQ (see Table 2). Though developed for teacher ratings, the PBQ could be completed by parents so long as the teacher-based norms are not used.

IV. DIRECT OBSERVATION

Direct observation has been defined as the contemporaneous recording of spontaneously occurring, externally observable, behavioral events.[262] Given the emphasis of this book, only brief attention can be given to direct observations for assessing treatment effects, since most practitioners will not be well positioned to request formal direct observations on their patients. This should not be construed as indicating that direct observations are unimportant. In fact, direct behavioral observations comprise the second most commonly used (after rating scales) mode of assessing the effects of drugs in research and are the most objective. The use of direct observation for assessing children is detailed elsewhere.[1,2,263–265]

A. General Considerations

Although behavior may be observed in contrived settings, direct observation has traditionally taken place in the child's natural setting (e.g., home, classroom), where clinically relevant considerations are paramount. The key elements of behavioral observation[263] are: (1) a data collection system is used, (2) preset behavioral (observable) categories are recorded in specified settings and periods, (3) observation periods are sufficiently brief that they minimize reliance on memory, and (4) systematic checks on the accuracy and reliability of the data are collected. There are certain advantages and disadvantages of direct observation.[2] Advantages include the following. (1) Direct observations are highly objective and provide an accurate portrayal of clinical relevance. (2) Unlike certain instruments, like IQ tests and even rating scales, direct observations can be repeated as frequently as required without practice effects. This could be a valuable feature in determining the time of onset and offset of drug action. (3) They can be used in very disturbed, uncooperative, or nonverbal children. (4) They can be tailored to the individual clinical problems presented by a patient. Disadvantages are: (1) Direct observation usually requires extensive logistics and staff support involving high costs; (2) direct observatons can be insensitive to the overall global effects of psychoactive drugs if behavioral categories are too narrowly defined or effects in any one area are small; (3) the presence of an observer or video camera can distort the behavior of both child and eliciting agent (parent, teacher); and (4) the sampling period may be too short or otherwise atypical.

B. Types of Direct Observation Methods

There are five types of direct observation.[2] (1) Continuous records entail a real-time record of all onsets and terminations of the behavioral categories of concern. This is a labor-intensive assessment method and is rarely used in clinical drug studies. (2) Response duration measures the time during which a patient engages in a given behavior. It is most useful for long-lasting behaviors such as tantrums, application to classrooms tasks, and so forth. (3) Frequency counts entail the tallying of behaviors in a given category during a standard interval, such as a classroom period. Frequency counts are most suitable for infrequent behaviors (e.g., tantrums, fighting, property abuse) that might not be detected in briefer sessions. (4) Interval recording is used when behaviors are of moderate to high frequency, and several categories are monitored. It requires a timing device that signifies brief intervals (e.g., 15 sec) and an explicit coding scheme. The observer checks all categories of behavior that occurred in the previous interval. (5) Momentary time sampling (or point sampling) entails brief observations of behavior at fixed or random intervals and is suitable for high-rate behaviors.

Interval recording is the most usual in drug studies, but frequency counts and response duration can be used by parents or teachers, provided the number of categories is small. Momentary time sampling is attractive if the observer is in close proximity with the patient and can include it as part of the work routine (e.g., on an inpatient unit).

C. Some Illustrative Examples

As noted, direct observation is versatile and adaptable to any clinical situation. Below are a few examples from the literature. Others can be found elsewhere.[60]

1. Hyperactivity (ADHD)

An overview of observational measures that can be employed for assessing children and adolescents with ADHD is available.[266] In a popular playroom paradigm,[267] the floor is divided into sections with tape or painted squares to measure grid crossings and toy changes. More recently, a "restricted play" format has been used.[266] Typically, the child is observed in a free-play situation for part of the session, after which he or she is told to stay in one sector of the room and to play with only one toy. Grid crossings and toy changes can be assessed in the first portion, whereas number of quadrants entered and number of "forbidden toys" can be recorded during restricted play.[268]

There are several coding schemes for observing behavior relevant to hyperactivity in the classroom, of which one method[269] uses nine behavioral categories: (1) Interference with others, (2) Off-task, (3) Non-compliance, (4) Minor motor movements, (5) Gross motor movement, (6) Out-of-chair behavior, (7) Physical aggression, (8) Threat or verbal aggression, and (9) Solicitation of teacher. Another scheme[270] employs eight categories: (1) On-task, (2) Out-of-chair, (3) Movement, (4) Translocation, (5) Fidgeting, (6) Verbalization or vocalization, (7) Natural contact, and (8) Aversive physical contact. Parallel or similar procedures can be developed for use in the playground or in the home.

Gadow and colleagues[271] have developed an extensive system, called the ADHD School Observation Code (ADHD SOC), for observing behavior in the classroom and on the playground. The ADHD SOC manual contains a wealth of information on establishing and maintaining a sound observational system. As the Code includes a variety of verbal and physical aggression categories, it would likely be useful for assessing aggression as well.

2. Conduct Disorder and Aggression Problems

The Code for Observing Social Activity (COSA)[272] provides a structure for observing social interactions during class, lunch, and recess. The following behaviors are coded as present or absent in 30-sec intervals: (1) Appropriate social behavior, (2) Physical aggression, (3) Play aggression (physical force in the context of play), (4) Verbal aggression/verbal negative, (5) Symbolic aggression, (6) Overt aggression, and (7) Noncompliance.[273]

The examples thus far employ interval sampling techniques. A scan-sampling technique for social behavior, in which many brief repeated observations are made serially across several children in the playground, is similar to momentary time sampling, except that all observations are packed into one brief observational period.[274] The six categories used are as follows: (1) Participation/rule following, (2) Prosocial initiation/leadership, (3) Noncompliant/annoying, (4) Verbally or physically aggressive, (5) Social isolation/bystand, and (6) Sad/down.

3. Depression

By their very nature, internalizing conditions like major depression and anxiety disorders are more difficult to observe. One example of such an observational approach[275] used an interval-sampling procedure to record (1) crying or whimpering, (2) socially appropriate behavior, (3) inactivity, and (4) inappropriate behavior. Observational procedures were also used to gauge total hours of sleep, percentage of meals consumed, and number of screaming outbursts each day.

4. Anxiety Disorders

There are a number of procedures to assess fears and anxieties in children and adolescents.[276] One frequently used method is the Behavioral Avoidance Test[277] (also called the Behavioral Approach Test), in which a feared/phobic stimulus (e.g., an animal, darkness, heights) is brought closer to the patient (or vice versa) or the stimulus is varied in intensity (e.g., brightness to darkness). The relevant measure is the distance from the object or strength of the stimulus that the patient will tolerate. Another method is to place the child into the fear-eliciting situation, such as a social setting or public speaking, and use interval-sampling procedures to observe categories such as crying, posture, stuttering, and tremor. Ethically, this should not to be done unless the level of distress is tolerable to the youngster.

5. Conclusion

These examples are illustrative. Direct observations are highly reliable, objective tools for monitoring drug effects, and their ability to be tailored to specific clinical needs is a major strength. At the same time, they often require technical knowledge in such procedures, and, if extra staff are needed to carry out observations, they can be costly.

V. PERFORMANCE AND AUTOMATED ACTIVITY MEASURES

This section is included in case practitioners encounter performance tests in their clinical work, rather than as a guide for setting up such tests as a routine part of clinical assessment. Nevertheless, given the importance of learning in children and its disruption in psychiatric disorders, and with the increasing availability of computerized procedures, cognitive assessment may need to become a routine part of testing for drug effects.

A. Performance and Related Tests

The tests considered in this section evaluate cognitive functions by specifically *eliciting* performance. Unlike achievement and verbal parts of IQ tests, the material to be learned or processed is often novel (e.g., paired associate learning) and used for that test only, the subject is required to *perform* at that point in time, and the test is often designed to tap a specific cognitive function (e.g., sustained attention, selective attention, short-term memory). Frequently, performance tests are controlled by electronic equipment, such as personal computers. Performance tests are often used because of their ability to measure constructs of theoretical significance such as selective or sustained attention, impulsivity, or memory. However, in order to be relevant to the practitioner, such tests must also be "ecologically valid" or reflect behavior in real-world settings. Most of the numerous tests used in ADHD have only untested or modest ecological validity.[266] Only some of the more popular, used in pediatric psychopharmacology, will be discussed here, some because they could be integrated into clinical practice and others because of their historical significance. Comprehensive reviews can be found elsewhere.[278–282]

1. Continuous Performance Task (CPT)

The Continuous Performance Task (CPT) is the most frequently used test of cognitive function in pediatric psychopharmacology, perhaps because of the importance of attention span in children, perhaps because of the well-documented effects of stimulants in improving ing attention in children with ADHD, and perhaps because it is among the most sensitive indices of drug effects in children.[278] It is a vigilance task in which the child is required to make a response whenever a target stimulus appears. Two versions are often used.[283,284] In the simpler, the child presses a switch whenever the target (e.g., an X) appears; in the more difficult, the child responds to the letter X but only when preceded by the letter A. Errors of omission (failures to detect the X), errors of commission (false detections), and response time are recorded. Specific types of CPT errors, together with information regarding the speed of these errors, have been used to infer underlying problems. For example, it has been noted that an omission is suggestive of inattention, whereas some, but not all, forms of commission are suggestive of impulsivity.[285,286] Commissions that are associated with impulsivity include responses in which the child hits the response key after seeing an "A" but not waiting for an "X" to appear, whereas commissions in which the child hits the response key for other targets (e.g., a "G") are not suggestive of impulsivity.

The CPT has virtually eclipsed the classical reaction time task,[287] perhaps because it yields additional information or perhaps because it seems analogous to attention in the classroom. Indeed, error variables on the CPT have been correlated with responses on teacher behavioral ratings.[285,288] Children with ADHD make substantially more errors than children without ADHD,[289–291] thereby implicating attentional difficulties and impulsivity as part of the disorder. In recent years, simplified versions of the traditional letter- or number-based CPT stimuli have been developed that use picture-based stimuli. These simplified CPT programs have been found to discriminate children with and without ADHD in preschool populations[292] and in children with mental retardation.[293] However, as Ingersoll[294] rightly pointed out, while the CPT is a useful adjunct in the diagnosis of

ADHD, it is not a substitute for traditional diagnostic measures such as psychological testing, careful interviewing and history taking, and parent and teacher behavioral ratings. The CPT has also been found to be sensitive to methylphenidate treatment response,[295–297] as well as response to other medications, e.g., bupropion[298] and guanfacine.[299]

There are numerous versions of the CPT available, in both visual and auditory formats, from both commercial and academic sources. Two widely known commercial versions are the CPT included in the Gordon Diagnostic System[300,301] (see below) and the Conners CPT software program.[302] The Gordon system (which includes two other tests) costs about $1600 and employs dedicated equipment.* The Conners CPT is about one third the price and can be used on most PCs.† There are norms for the Conners CPT, it yields about eight scores, and the software interprets the results. For both the Gordon Diagnostic System and the Conners CPT program, once the system is purchased, there are no additional user charges. This unfortunately is not the case with a number of software products on the market.

2. Cancellation Tasks

Cancellation tasks (sometimes referred to as "checking tasks") involve marking a specified form or letter on a sheet usually interspersed with nontargets as distractors.[303] Only limited time is allowed so that the child cannot complete the task. The number of target stimuli correctly marked, the number missed, incorrect cancellations, and the total number canceled are scored.[304] Such tasks are among the most ecologically valid for assessing hyperactive children.[280] Interestingly, there is a significant improvement in the cancellation task performance of hyperactive boys when an experimenter is present, relative to when the child performs it with his mother present or when alone.[305] This finding has been noted with a variety of performance tasks, including the CPT.

3. Matching Familiar Figures Task (MFFT)

The MFFT[306] was developed as a measure of reflection–impulsivity and visual discrimination. In its most common format, the MFFT task comes as a booklet with plastic binding. The child's task is to identify which of six test stimuli is identical to one on an adjacent page. The original MFFT contains 12 sets of stimuli,[306] whereas a more recent version contains 20 sets.[307] Measures include time required for the child to make a response and the number of errors before the match is identified. The MFFT has been used extensively in research, especially with hyperactive and learning-disabled children, probably because of the characterization of response time as an index of "reflection–impulsivity."[306] Computerized versions of the MFFT were developed in recent years.[308] However, there are several serious problems with the task[309] so that this description should not be accepted at face value. Both response time and accuracy only variably discriminate between clinical and control groups,[281] and it is relatively drug-insensitive.[310] Hence, despite its clinical popularity, it would be hard to recommend this test. However, in at least one recent study, the MFFT has been shown to be sensitive to both methylphenidate and bupropion treatment in children with ADHD.[95]

---

*The Gordon Diagnostic System is available through Gordon Systems, Inc., DeWitt, NY (315-446-4849).
†The Conners CPT is available from Multihealth Systems Inc., 908 Niagara Falls Blvd., North Tonawanda, NY 14120–2060.

4. Analogue Classroom Tests

Among the most ecologically valid cognitive tests are the analogue classroom tests. These involve several sheets containing numerous arithmetic, spelling, or reading problems, well within the youngster's demonstrated ability range. Usually, the child is given a standard amount of time to solve the problems, and the measures obtained may include the number of problems attempted and the number completed correctly.[311–313] Some have suggested that increased performance reflects true gains in academic skills,[312,313] but it is more likely that they reflect changes in the child's motivation, attention span, and compliance as well as other, perhaps unrecognized, factors rather than new skills. Should worsening on such tasks occur with treatment, the value of that treatment would have to be carefully reconsidered. Like the cancellation task, this is a class of cognitive test that is almost totally free of requirements for technical equipment and is thus suited to clinical settings.

5. Paired Associate Learning (PAL)

In the PAL paradigm,[281] the subject is required to learn pairs of objects not naturally associated in any way, such as pictures of common objects or words. The first part of the pair (the stimulus) is presented and the subject is asked to name the other member before it is re-presented. Testing continues until some criterion (such as one or two perfect trials) is reached or until the completion of a predetermined number of trials. Dependent measures can include errors to criterion and trials to criterion, although the former is more sensitive. PAL appears to be largely a measure of short-term and medium-term memory, and, unlike many of the tasks previously described, PAL measures effortful performance. PAL tests have been used quite extensively to assess medication and dosage effects, and researchers have found them to be quite sensitive.[281] However, they do require technical knowledge.[281] In recent years, PAL tasks have also been used to correlate brain pathology (as assessed using magnetic resonance spectroscopy techniques) with cognitive functions.[314]

6. Delay Task

The Delay Task was devised to measure impulsivity in ADHD children, using the differential reinforcement of low (DRL) rate behavior, in which the child responds by pressing a button on a portable monitor. The Delay Task is part of the commercially available Gordon Diagnostic System,[315] which also includes a version of the CPT. The youngster is told that if he or she waits long enough between responses, a point will be forthcoming each time on a counter. The actual delay required is 6 sec, although the youngster is not told this. The Delay Task lasts 8 min and has been shown to discriminate between hyperactive and control groups of children.[300,301] Intuitively, it would seem to be a good way to assess impulsivity,[316,317] but it may be insensitive to stimulant medication.[318]

7. Short Term Recognition Memory Task

The Short Term Recognition Memory Task is discussed here more for its historical significance to the field than for its current impact, as it was used in the original studies of differential dose–response effects between behavior and cognition.[319,320] The Short Term Memory (STM) task was originally developed to assess memory in children with mental retardation[321] and involves the presentation of arrays of cartoon figures followed by a single figure. The child indicates whether the test figure was a member of the previous array by pressing a "same" or "different" response key. The STM task is quite drug-sensitive,[278] but it requires a significant amount of equipment and is not commercially available. Other short-term memory tasks, such as the Sternberg STM Task, have been found to be sensitive to drug treatment (e.g., bupropion).[298]

8. Automated Measures of Activity Level

Although they are certainly not performance tests, this is a reasonable place to discuss automated measures of activity level, given their frequent reliance on electronic equipment and their frequent pairing with performance tests. Furthermore, seat activity is often found to be inversely related to accuracy on performance tests. Automated activity measures have been discussed in greater detail elsewhere.[322,323] The wrist actometer is a self-winding wristwatch that has been modified to indicate the total amount of movement (rather than time). It is commercially available and not expensive.[322] Sprague and Toppe[324] developed a special stabilimetric seat that they used in conjunction with performance tests, and another group used pressure-sensitive mats to measure activity of autistic children.[325] The most sophisticated is a solid-state unit fastened to the trunk, which can measure free-range activity over 24 hr, but it is expensive to build.[326] Of these options, the wrist actometer is clearly of greatest interest to practitioners, but its validity has been questioned, especially when activity is sampled over brief intervals,[280] and it has other problems including resetting by the child, the need for frequent recalibration, and breakdowns during vigorous activity.[322]

B. Computer Testing

The computer revolution has yet to impinge much on clinical assessment in pediatric psychopharmacology, but, as noted in the section on diagnostic interviewing, it is likely that microcomputers will be widely used in the future for performance testing, including in the clinical situation. An example of this development is the CPT (discussed above), which is beginning to be used in a variety of clinical settings, given that standardized software packages for it can be easily installed on existing computer equipment in a clinic.

1. Advantages and Disadvantages

For the assessment of psychomotor functions in children, computers have a number of advantages and disadvantages, some of which have been previously reviewed.[327] The advantages include the following:

1. Objectivity. Practitioners and informants hold certain biases about effects of treatments, and computer assessments should provide a useful defense against this.
2. Standardization of test format. Computer tests are inherently precise and, therefore, provide an advantage over traditional manual/clinical modes of assessment.
3. Relatively culture-fair testing. Computer tests need not rely on verbal, written, or other materials taught in the educational system, since graphic presentations can be used.
4. Tests can be presented as video "games" or "puzzles," eliciting greater cooperation from children than more traditional tests.
5. Precision in recording responses.

6. Ability to handle multiple inputs. Whereas human observers can cope with only a limited amount of input, computers can cope with a multitude of responses from several channels.
7. Immediate scoring and reporting of test results.

Disadvantages include:

1. Fragility. Children with disruptive disorders are often hard on equipment, and certain components such as the keyboard are delicate.
2. Capital cost. This is becoming less and less of a problem as prices of computer hardware appear to be on the decline over time.
3. Loss of clinical flavor. Although computer tests are probably more appealing to exceptional children than traditional tests, they may also be less relevant to the real world.
4. Lack of equivalence. When traditional tests have been "translated" into a computer format, investigators have often found that their difficulty (and sometimes the precise functions tested) is altered.
5. Lack of standardization/norming procedures. Many computer tests that have been introduced have not been normed, so that comparisons are difficult.

Though computer tests have great potential and often represent a real advance in testing, we advise clinicians to be cautious in the use of such tests, as extraneous effects may be confounded with medication effects. For example, the effect of an examiner's presence has already been mentioned, and practice or boredom effects may make it difficult to interpret changes associated with adjustments in medication. They should not be used as the sole arbiter in diagnosis or evaluation of treatment.

2. Current Status and Examples

Computers have made major inroads into psychological testing in areas such as performance testing, personality assessment, interviewing, psychiatric diagnosis, test interpretation, and neuropsychological and electrophysiological assessments. There are several monographs pertinent to assessing pharmacotherapy[328–331] as well as listings of commercially available software.[331] Some examples follow.

a. Gordon Diagnostic System (GDS)

The Gordon system[315] was developed for assessing children with ADHD and comprises a continuous performance test (vigilance/sustained attention), a delay test, and a distractibility test. The first two of these tests have already been discussed in this chapter. The Gordon system uses a self-standing portable unit, rather than a microcomputer platform. In the vigilance test, similar to the original letter-based version of the CPT,[332] the child is told to press a button after seeing a particular sequence of numbers (e.g., 1 followed by 9). There is also a preschool version, in which the target is a single digit. The Distractibility task is identical to the vigilance tasks, except that distracting numbers are flashed on either side of the relevant target stimuli (which are presented in a central location). Finally, the Delay task, also included in the system, has already been described.

As of this writing, the GDS system purchase price is approximately $1600.* As noted above, one favorable feature of the GDS system is that there are no "pay as you use"

---

*The Gordon Diagnostic System is available through Gordon Systems, Inc., DeWitt, NY (315-446-4849).

costs—the purchase price includes the machine and the authorization to use it for as many administrations as desired. There is a recent "Auditory Module" that features an auditory vigilance task and an auditory interference task. The auditory vigilance task is identical to the visual vigilance task, except that the participant hears the stimuli rather than seeing them. The cost of the auditory module is approximately $400.

Finally, a compact (1 lb) GDS-compatible printer is also available. However, the output from the GDS can be obtained by attaching the unit to any standard printer. As noted previously, the ecological validity of the CPT is modest,[280] and the Gordon CPT appears to be relatively insensitive to stimulants[318] and to have mediocre diagnostic sensitivity and specificity.[333] However, it is portable and very sturdy and has become popular in some assessment centers. For instance, the vigilance and distractibility tasks have been shown to discriminate individuals with traumatic brain injury from controls.[334] The distractibility task has also been shown to differentiate children exposed either in utero or in their early childhood (environmentally) to opiates from controls.[335]

b. Test of Variables of Attention (T.O.V.A.)

The T.O.V.A.[336,337] software program controls a visual continuous performance task in which the target is a square with a small hole near the bottom and the nontarget is a square with a small hole near the top. The child's job is to hit a response key when the target stimulus appears. Dependent measures include (1) errors of omission (inattention), (2) errors of commission (impulsivity), (3) mean response time, (4) variability of response time, (5) anticipatory responses, (6) response time following commission errors, and (7) multiple responses. There is also an Auditory T.O.V.A. ("T.O.V.A.-A"), which uses two easily discriminable tones as the target and nontarget stimuli. The T.O.V.A. is now commercially available (American Guidance Service, Circle Pines, Minnesota). A strength of this program is that it is available for PCs and Macintoshes. A potential drawback is that the purchase price ($500 for Visual T.O.V.A., $500 for Auditory T.O.V.A., or $800 for the combination) does not include the additional per-use charge to clinicians for scoring and interpretive reports ($5–$25). Normative data are now available for males and females aged 6 to 19 years. The reliability between different quarters of the task of the auditory T.O.V.A. ($r = 0.63–0.93$) is somewhat higher than for the visual version ($r = 0.52–0.93$). The T.O.V.A. did not differentiate children with and without ADHD,[291] as well as adults with and without ADHD.[338] The T.O.V.A. was sensitive to neurofeedback treatment in children with ADHD[339] and effects of caffeine in school-age children without behavioral problems.[340] The developers also state that the T.O.V.A. can be used to titrate medication treatments in children with ADHD,[341] and they present means for premedication versus postmedication treatment for individual subjects, but many details are lacking, so these data are difficult to judge. We are not aware of any data on test–retest reliability. Although the T.O.V.A. appears to be a very promising and useful tool, more information regarding the present version is needed to assess its diagnostic utility and sensitivity to medication effects.

c. The Fe Psy ("Iron Psych") Test System

The Fe Psy system,[342] developed in the Netherlands for assessing antiepileptic medication, is the most sophisticated package that we have seen so far. It comprises at least 16 tests as follows: (1) auditory reaction time, (2) visual reaction time (adult version), (3) visual reaction time for children, (4) binary choice reaction time (adult version), (5) binary choice reaction time for children, (6) tapping task, (7) computerized visual searching task (adult version), (8) computerized visual searching task for children, (9) recognition of simultaneously presented words or figures, (10) recognition of serially presented words or figures, (11) vigilance task, (12) the Seashore rhythm test, (13) classification test, (14) visual half-field tasks, (15) Corsi block tapping, and (16) Binnie's blocks tapping (continuous EEG version). Most of these will not be described further, as they were discussed earlier or are available through the Fepsy website.* The visual searching task involves a grid pattern with 24 surrounding patterns, one of which is identical and must be located. The recognition memory test entails presenting arrays of words or figures, followed 2 sec later by another array, which has one element that matches the earlier group, and the child is asked to identify that element. There is also a variation of this task calling for recall of the order of the stimuli. All test results are output directly to a data base, which can then be exported to statistical programs such as SPSS, Paradox, Dbase, or Access.

This is an evolving system: a number of subtests have been added in recent years, and several more are planned for addition to later versions of the system. Normative data are available for different age levels. It has been used successfully both to compare children with epilepsy and controls and to evaluate different types of medication. It is available in 12 languages, and the software sells for NLG 3995 (or approximately U.S. $2212) at the time of this writing.†

VI. CONCLUSIONS

To sum up, a truly large variety of instruments and procedures are available for assessing the behavioral, emotional, and learning performance of children and adolescents. Whenever possible, it is wise to have any rating scale completed at least twice before instituting or changing therapy to wash out "practice" effects. Many informant, clinician, and self-rating scales are available. Some of the better instruments were identified here with an emphasis on those for assessing ADHD, conduct and oppositional problems, depression, anxiety, and problems associated with mental retardation, autism, or found in preschool-age children. However, only a few of the scales reviewed have been shown to be sensitive to drug effects.

Direct observation is also an important technique for assessing behavioral changes due to pharmacotherapy, and some procedures are suited to clinical practice. Performance tests are prominent in pediatric psychopharmacology research and some, such as the cancellation task and academic probes, are simple and promising. Wide availability of computer testing is on the horizon, and the innovative practitioner should watch this area. IQ tests are unsuitable for monitoring medication effects because they are usually insensitive to drug effects. Achievement tests may be relevant in youngsters with learning problems where medication is to be given over a period of months or years, but they are usually insensitive too.

The array of choices available may seem bewildering but, as in the case of choosing medications themselves, the practitioner should have a decision tree for choosing systematic methods for monitoring medication. Table 2 was developed to make this task easier. It is more important to have an established, well-defined set of monitoring tools rather than an elaborate but perhaps poorly understood and unwieldy system. **What is most important in monitoring drug effects is that decisions be based on systematic data, preferably from several sources, rather than solely on the practitioner's clinical impressions**. Each

---

*Homepage: http://www.euronet.nl/users/fepsy.

†More information about the Fepsy system is available through Willem Alpherts or Bert Aldenkamp (e-mail: fepsy@euronet.nl; phone: +3123 5237 555; fax: +3123 5289 412).

practitioner must determine which array of methods is most suitable for the patients seen in his or her practice. We hope that this chapter will serve both as a stimulus and as an aid to do this.

ACKNOWLEDGMENTS. Work on this chapter was supported in part by a research contract from the U.S. National Institute of Mental Health (Grant MH N01MH80011) and by a Training Initiative Project from the Administration on Developmental Disabilities (Grant 90DD0446/01) to Michael Aman. Deborah Pearson's work was supported in part by NIMH Grant MH48212.

REFERENCES

1. Werry JS: Measures in pediatric psychopharmacology, in Werry JS (ed): *Pediatric Psychopharmacology: The Use of Behavior Modifying Drugs in Children*. New York, Brunner/Mazel, 1978, pp 29–78.
2. Aman MG, White AJ: Measures of drug change in mental retardation, in Gadow KD (ed): *Advances in Learning and Behavioral Disabilities*. Greenwich, Conn, JAI Press, 1986, vol 5, pp 157–202.
3. Rutter M, Tuma H, Lann I: *Assessment and Diagnosis in Child Psychopathology*. New York, Guilford Press, 1988.
4. Sattler JM: *Assessment of Children*, ed 3. San Diego, Jerome M Sattler, Publisher, 1988.
5. *Psychopharmacology Bulletin: Rating Scales and Assessment Instruments for Use in Pediatric Psychopharmacology Research*. *Psychopharmacol Bull* 21:713–1124, 1985.
6. Hogg C, Rutter M, Richman N: *Child Psychology Portfolio: Emotional and Behavioural Problems in Children*. Windsor, UK, NFER-Nelson Publishing Company, 1997.
7. American Psychiatric Association: *Diagnostic and Statistical Manual of Mental Disorders*, ed 4. Washington, DC, American Psychiatric Association, 1994.
8. Ambrosini PJ: Structured and semi-structured diagnostic interviewing. Unpublished manuscript, Medical College of Pennsylvania/Eastern Pennsylvania Psychiatric Institute, 1992.
9. Werry JS: Child psychiatric disorders: Are they classifiable? *Br J Psychiatry*, 161:472–480, 1992.
10. Young JG, O'Brien JD, Gutterman EM, et al: Research on the clinical interview. *J Am Acad Child Adolesc Psychiatry* 26:613–620, 1987.
11. Quay HC: Classification, in Quay HC, Werry JS (eds): *Psychopathological Disorders of Childhood*, ed 3. New York, John Wiley & Sons, 1986, pp 1–34.
12. Regier DA, Myers JK, Kramer M, et al: The NIMH epidemiologic catchment area program. Historical context, major objectives, and study population characteristics. *Arch Gen Psychiatry* 41: 934–944, 1984.
13. Graham P, Rutter M: The reliability and validity of the psychiatric assessment of the child: II. Interview with the parent. *Br J Psychiatry* 114:581–592, 1968.
14. Chambers WJ, Puig-Antich J, Hirsch M, et al: The assessment of affective disorders in children and adolescents by semistructured interview. Test–retest reliability of the Schedule for Affective Disorders and Schizophrenia for School-age Children, Present Episode Version. *Arch Gen Psychiatry* 42:696–702, 1985.
15. Herjanic B, Reich W: Development of a structured interview for children: Agreement between child and parent on individual symptoms. *J Abnorm Child Psychol* 10:307–324, 1982.
16. Kovacs M: The Interview Schedule for Children (ISC): Interrater and parent–child agreement. Unpublished manuscript, University of Pittsburgh, 1983.
17. Kovacs M: The Interview Schedule for Children (ISC). *Psychopharmacol Bull* 21:991–994, 1985.
18. Gadow KD, Sprafkin J: *Manual for the Stony Brook Child Symptom Inventories. Child Symptom Inventories. Child Symptom Inventory: Parent Checklist. Child Symptom Inventory: Teacher Checklist*. Stony Brook, NY, Checkmate Plus, Limited, 1994.
19. Aman MG, Singh NN: *Manual for the Aberrant Behavior Checklist*. East Aurora, NY, Slosson Educational Publications, 1986.
20. Achenbach TM, Edelbrock C: *Manual for the Teacher's Report Form and Teacher Version of the Child Behavior Profile*. Burlington, University of Vermont, 1986.
21. Werry JS, Sprague RL: Methylphenidate in children—Effect of dosage. *Aust NZ J Psychiatry* 8:9–19, 1974.
22. Milich R, Roberts MA, Loney J, et al: Differentiating practice effects and statistical regression on the Conners Hyperkinesis Index. *J Abnorm Child Psychol* 8:549–552, 1980.

23. Klein RG: Parent–child agreement in clinical assessment of anxiety and other psychopathology: A review. *J Anxiety Disord* 5:187–198, 1991.

24. Hodges K: Depression and anxiety in children: A comparison of self-report questionnaire to clinical interview. *Psychol Assess J Consult Clin Psychol* 2:376–381, 1990.

25. Herjanic B, Reich W: Development of a structured psychiatric interview for children: Agreement between child and parent on individual symptoms. *J Abnorm Child Psychol* 25:21–31, 1997.

26. McConaughy S: Advances in empirically based assessment of children's behavioral and emotional problems. *School Psychol Rev* 22:285–307, 1993.

27. Arnold LE, Wender PH, McClosky K, et al: Levodopamine and dextroamphetamine: Comparative efficacy in hyperkinetic syndrome. *Arch Gen Psychiatry* 27:816–822, 1972.

28. Thompson TI: Maladaptive Behavior Scale. Vanderbilt University, Memphis, 1992.

29. Achenbach TM: Manual for the CBCL/4–18 and Profile. Department of Psychiatry, University of Vermont, 1991.

30. Achenbach TM: Manual for the TRF and 1991 Profile. Department of Psychiatry, University of Vermont, 1991.

31. Achenbach TM: Manual for the YSR and 1991 Profile. Department of Psychiatry, University of Vermont, 1991.

32. Werry JS: Overanxious disorder: A review of its taxonomic properties. *J Am Acad Child Adolesc Psychiatry* 30:533–544, 1991.

33. Conners CK: Conners Rating Scales—Revised. Technical Manual. North Tonawanda, NY, Multi-Health Systems Inc, 1997.

34. Quay HC, Peterson DR: Interim manual for the Revised Behavior Problem Checklist. Unpublished manuscript, 1983, available from H. C. Quay, Box 240074, University of Miami, Coral Gables, Fla 33124.

35. Quay HC, Peterson DR: Manual for the Behavior Problem Checklist. Unpublished manuscript, University of Miami, Coral Gables, Fla 1975.

36. Quay HC: A dimensional approach to behavior disorder: The Revised Behavior Problem Checklist. *School Psychol Rev* 12:244–249, 1983.

37. Aman MG, Werry JS: The Revised Behavior Problem Checklist in clinic attenders and nonattenders: Age and sex effects. *J Clin Child Psychol* 13:237–242, 1984.

38. DuPaul GJ, Power TJ, Anastopoulos AD, et al: Teacher ratings of attention deficit hyperactivity disorder symptoms: Factor structure and normative data. *Psychological Assessment*, 9:436–444, 1997.

39. DuPaul GJ, Anastopoulos AD, Power TJ, et al: Parent ratings of attention deficit/hyperactivity disorder symptoms: Factor structure and normative data. *Journal of Psychopathology and Behavioral Assessment* 20:83–102, 1997.

40. Edelbrock C: Childhood Attention Problems (CAP) Scale. Available from Dr. C Edelbrock, Pennsylvania State University, University Park, Pa, 1978.

41. Aman MG: Monitoring and measuring drug effects. II. Behavioral, emotional, and cognitive effects, in Werry JS, Aman MG (eds): *Practitioner's Guide to Psychoactive Drugs for Children and Adolescents*, New York, Plenum Medical Book Co, 1993, pp 99–159.

42. DuPaul GJ, Power TJ, McGoey KE, et al: Reliability and validity of parent and teacher ratings of attention deficit/hyperactivity disorder symptoms. *Journal of Psychoeducational Assessment* 16:55–68.

43. Barkley RA: *Attention-Deficit Hyperactivity Disorder: A Clinical Workbook.* New York: Guilford Press, 1991.

44. Barkley RA, DuPaul GJ, McMurray MB: Attention deficit disorder with and without hyperactivity: Clinical response to three dose levels of methylphenidate. *Pediatrics* 87:519–531, 1991.

45. Barkley RA, McMurray MB, Edelbrock CS, et al: The response of aggressive and nonaggressive ADHD children to two doses of methylphenidate. *J Am Acad Child Adolesc Psychiatry* 28:873–881, 1989.

46. Ullmann RK, Sleator EK, Sprague RL: Introduction to the use of ACTeRS. *Psychopharmacol Bull* 21:915–916, 1985.

47. Ullmann RK, Sleator EK, Sprague RL: *ACTeRS Teacher and Parent Forms Manual*, ed 2. Champaign, Ill, MetriTech, Inc, 1997.

48. Ullmann RK, Sleator EK: Attention deficit disorder children with or without hyperactivity. Which behaviors are helped by stimulants? *Clin Pediatr* 24:547–551, 1985.

49. Ullmann RK, Sleator EK, Sprague RL: A new rating scale for diagnosis and monitoring of ADD children. *Psychopharmacol Bull* 20:160–164, 1984.

50. Jarvinen DW, Sprague RL: Using ACTeRS to screen minority children for ADHD: An examination of item bias. *Journal of Psychological Assessment*, Special issue on ADHD, pp 172–184, 1995.

51. Loney J, Milich R: Hyperactivity, inattention, and aggression in clinical practice, in Wolraich M, Routh DK (eds): *Advances in Developmental and Behavioral Pediatrics.* Greenwich, Conn, JAI Press, 1982, pp 113–147.
52. Gadow KD, Nolan EE, Sverd J, et al: Methylphenidate in aggressive-hyperactive boys: I. Effects on peer aggression in public school settings. *J Am Acad Child Adolesc Psychiatry* 29:710–718, 1990.
53. Klorman R, Brumaghim JT, Salzman LF, et al: Effects of methylphenidate on attention-deficit hyperactivity disorder with and without aggressive/noncompliant features. *J Abnorm Psychol* 97:413–422, 1988.
54. Pelham WE, Milich R, Murphy DA, et al: Normative data on the IOWA Conners Teacher Rating Scale. *J Clin Child Psychol* 18:259–262, 1989.
55. Conners CK, Wells KC: ADD-H Adolescent Self Report Scale. *Psychopharmacol Bull* 21:921–922, 1985.
56. Werry JS: The diagnosis, etiology, and treatment of hyperactivity in children, in Hellmuth J (ed): *Learning Disorders.* Seattle, Wash, Special Child Publications, 1968, vol 3.
57. Ross DM, Ross SA: *Hyperactivity: Research, Theory, Action,* ed 2. New York, John Wiley & Sons, 1982.
58. Barkley RA, Edelbrock C: Assessing situational variations in children's problem behaviors. The Home and School Situations Questionnaire, in Prinz R (ed): *Advances in Behavioral Assessment of Children and Families.* Greenwich, Conn, JAI Press, 1987.
59. McMahon RJ, Forehand R: Conduct disorders, in Mash EJ, Terdal LG (eds): *Behavioral Assessment of Childhood Disorders,* ed 2. New York, Guilford Press, 1988, pp 105–153.
60. O'Leary KD, Johnson SB: Assessment and assessment of change, in Quay HC, Werry JS (eds): *Psychopathological Disorders of Childhood,* ed 3. New York, John Wiley & Sons, 1986, pp 423–454.
61. Hinshaw SP: Stimulant medication and the treatment of aggression in children with attention deficits. *J Clin Child Psychol* 20:301–312, 1991.
62. Miller LS, Klein RG, Piacentini J, et al: The New York Teacher Rating Scale for Disruptive and Antisocial Behavior. *J Am Acad Child Adolesc Psychiatry* 34, 359–370, 1995.
63. Brown RT, Jaffe SL, Silverstein J, et al: Methylphenidate and adolescents hospitalized with conduct disorder: Dose effects on classroom behavior, academic performance, and impulsivity. *J Clin Child Psychol* 20:282–292, 1991.
64. Werry JS, Aman MG, Lampen E: Halperidol and methylphenidate in hyperactive children. *Acta Paedopsychiatr* 42:26–40, 1975.
65. Gadow KD: Peer Conflict Scale. Unpublished instrument, State University of New York at Stony Brook, 1986.
66. Sprafkin J, Grayson P, Gadow KD: Code for Observing Social Activity. Department of Psychiatry, State University of New York at Stony Brook, 1983.
67. Nolan EE: The effects of methylphenidate on aggression in ADD boys. Doctoral dissertation completed at the State University of New York at Stony Brook, 1988.
68. Yudofsky SC, Silver JM, Jackson W, et al: The Overt Aggression Scale for the objective rating of verbal and physical aggression. *Am J Psychiatry* 143:35–39, 1986.
69. Palmstierna T, Wiestedt B: Staff Observation Aggression Scale, SOAS: Presentation and evaluation. *Acta Psychiatr Scand* 76:657–663, 1987.
70. Wiestedt B, Rasmussen A, Pedersen L, et al: The development of an observer-scale for measuring social dysfunction and aggression. *Pharmacopsychiatry* 23:249–252, 1990.
71. Finch AJ Jr, Saylor CF, Nelson WM III: Assessment of anger in children, in Prinz RJ (ed): *Advances in Behavioral Assessment of Children and Families.* Greenwich, Conn, JAI Press, 1987, vol 3, pp 235–265.
72. Whalen CK, Henker B: Social impact of stimulant treatment for hyperactive children. *J Learn Disabil* 24:231–241, 1991.
73. Kazdin AE: Childhood depression, in Mash EJ, Terdal LG (eds): *Behavioral Assessment of Childhood Disorders,* ed 2. New York, Guilford Press, 1988, pp 157–195.
74. Berstein GA, Borchardt CM: Anxiety disorders of childhood and adolescents. *J Am Acad Child Adolesc Psychiatry* 30:519–532, 1991.
75. Emslie GJ, Rush AJ, Weinberg WA, et al: A double-blind randomized placebo-controlled trial of fluoxetine in children and adolescents with depression. *Arch of Gen Psychiatry,* 54:1031–1037, 1997.
76. Cantwell DP, Carlson GA (eds): Affective disorders in children and adolescents—An update. New York, Spectrum Publications, 1983.
77. Kazdin AE: Childhood depression. *J Child Psychol Psychiatry* 31:121–160, 1990.
78. Kazdin AE, Petti TA: Self-report and interview measures of childhood and adolescent depression. *J Child Psychol Psychiatry* 23:437–457, 1982.
79. Strober M, Werry JS: The assessment of depression in children and adolescents, in Sartorius N, Ban TA (eds): *Assessment of Depression.* Berlin, Springer-Verlag, 1985, pp 324–342.

80. Nelson WM, Politano PM: Children's Depression Inventory: Stability over repeated administrations in psychiatric inpatient children. *J Clin Child Psychol* 19:254–256, 1990.
81. Petti T: Scales of potential use in the psychopharmacologic treatment of depressed children and adolescents. *Psychopharmacol Bull* 21:951–956, 1985.
82. Kovacs M: The Children's Depression Inventory (CDI). *Psychopharmacol Bull* 21:995–998, 1985.
83. Kovacs M: Children's Depression Inventory Manual. North Tonawanda, NY, Multi-Health Symptoms, 1992.
84. Beck AT: *Depression: Clinical, Experimental, and Theoretical Aspects*. New York, Harper & Row, 1967.
85. Chartier GM, Lassen MK: Adolescent depression: Children's Depression Inventory. Inventory norms, suicidal ideation, and (weak) gender effects. *Adolescence* 29:859–864, 1994.
86. DeMoss K, Milich R, DeMers S: Gender, creativity, depression, and attributional style in adolescents with high academic ability. *J Abnorm Child Psychol* 21:455–467, 1993.
87. Worchel FF, Hughes JN, Hall BM, Stanton SB, Stanton H, Little VZ: Evaluation of subclinical depression in children using self-, peer-, and teacher-report measures. *J Abnorm Child Psychol* 18:271–282, 1990.
88. Koizumi, S: The standardization of Children's Depression Inventory. *Syoni Hoken Kenkyu (The Journal of Child Health)* 50:717–721, 1991.
89. Ghareeb GA, Beshai JA: Arabic version of the Child Depression Inventory: Reliability and validity. *J Clin Child Psychol*, 18:323–326, 1989.
90. Devine D, Kemptom T, Forehand R: Adolescent depressed mood and young adult functioning: A longitudinal study. *J Abnorm Child Psychol* 22:629–640, 1994.
91. Doerfler LA, Felner RD, Rowlison RT, et al: Depression in children and adolescents: A comparative analysis of the utility and construct validity of two assessment measures. *J Consult Clin Psychol* 56:769–772, 1988.
92. Knight D, Hensley VR, Waters B: Validation of the Children's Depression Scale and The Children's Depression Inventory in a prepubertal sample. *J Child Psychol Psychiatry* 29:853–863, 1988.
93. Renouf AG, Kovacs M: Concordance between mothers' reports and children's self-reports of depressive symptoms: a longitudinal study. *J Am Acad Child Adolesc Psychiatry*. 33:208–216, 1994.
94. Barrickman LL, Perry PJ, Alle AJ, Kuperman S, Arndt SV, Hermann KJ, Schumacher E: Bupropion versus methylphenidate in the treatment of attention-deficit hyperactivity disorder. *J Am Acad Child Adolesc Psychiatry* 34:649–657, 1995.
95. Reynolds WM: Assessment of depression in children and adolescents by self-report questionnaires, in Reynolds WM, Johnston HE (eds): *Handbook of Depression in Children and Adolescents*. New York: Plenum, 1994, pp 209–234.
96. Lang M, Tisher M: Children's Depression Scale. Melbourne, Australian Council for Educational Research, 1978.
97. Tisher M, Takac E, Lang M: The Children's Depression Scale: Review of Australian and overseas experience. *Aust J Psychol* 44:27–35, 1992
98. Tisher M, Lang M: The Children's Depression Scale: Review and further developments, in Cantwell DP, Carlson GA (eds): *Affective Disorders in Childhood and Adolescence—An Update*. New York, Spectrum Publications, 1983, pp 181–203.
99. Gardiner C: An investigation of the relationships between lateral preferences and personality and emotional characteristics in children. Unpublished thesis, University of Adelaide, South Australia, 1980.
100. Patton W, Burnett PC: The Children's Depression Scale: Assessment of factor structure with data from a normal adolescent population. *Adolescence* 28:315–324, 1993.
101. Birleson P: The validity of depression in childhood and the development of a self-rating scale: A research report. *J Child Psychol Psychiatry* 22:73–88, 1981.
102. Reynolds WM: *Reynolds Child Depression Scale: Professional Manual*. Odessa, Fla, Psychological Assessment Resources, 1989.
103. Reynolds WM: *Reynolds Adolescent Depression Scale: Professional Manual*. Odessa, Fla, Psychological Assessment Resources, 1987.
104. Reynolds WM: Depression in childhood and adolescence: Diagnosis, assessment, intervention strategies and research, in Kratochwill TR (ed): *Advances in School Psychology*. Hillsdale, NJ, Lawrence Erlbaum, 1985, vol 1, pp 133–189.
105. Kobak KA, Reynolds WM, Griest JH: Computerized and clinician assessment of depression and anxiety: Respondent evaluation and satisfaction. *J Pers Assess* 63:173–180, 1994.
106. Reynolds WM, Coats KI: A comparison of cognitive-behavioral therapy and relaxation training for the treatment of depression in adolescents. *J Consult Clin Psychol* 54:653–660, 1986.
107. Reynolds WM, Miller KL: Depression and learned helplessness in mentally retarded adolescents: An initial investigation. *Appl Res Ment Retard* 6:295–306, 1985.

108. Hovey JD, King CA: Acculturative stress, depression, and suicidal ideation among immigrant and second-generation Latino adolescents. *J Am Acad Child Adolesc Psychiatry* 35:1183–1192, 1996.
109. Baron P, Campbell TL: Gender differences in the expression of depressive symptoms in middle adolescents: An extension of earlier findings. *Adolescence* 28:903–911, 1993.
110. Wierzbicki M: A parent form of the Children's Depression Inventory: Reliability and validity in nonclinical populations. *J Clin Psychol* 43:390–397, 1987.
111. Garber J: The developmental progression of depression in female children, in Achetti D, Schneider-Rosen K (eds): *Childhood Depression: New Directions for Child Development*. San Francisco, Jossey-Bass, 1984, pp 29–58.
112. Petti TA: The Bellevue Index of Depression (BID). *Psychopharmacol Bull* 21:959–968, 1985.
113. Benavidez DA, Matson JL: Assessment of depression in mentally retarded adolescents. *Res Dev Disabil* 14:179–188, 1993.
114. Kaminer Y, Feinstein C, Seifer R, et al: An observationally based scale for affective symptomatology in child psychiatry. *J Nerv Ment Dis* 178:750–754, 1990.
115. Aman MG: Assessing psychopathology and behavior problems in persons with mental retardation: A review of available instruments. DHHS publication (ADM) 91-1712. Rockville, Md, US Department of Health and Human Services, 1991.
116. Kaminer Y, Seifer R, Mastrian A: Observational measurement of symptoms responsive to treatment of major depressive disorder in children and adolescents. *J Nerv Ment Dis*, 180:639–643, 1992.
117. Lefkowitz MM, Tesiny EP, Solodow W: A rating scale for assessing dysphoria in youth. *J Abnorm Child Psychol* 17:337–347, 1989.
118. Poznanski ED, Grossman JA, Buchsbaum Y, et al: Preliminary studies of the reliability and validity of the Children's Depression Rating Scale. *J Am Acad Child Psychiatry* 23:191–197, 1984.
119. Poznanski ED, Cook SC, Carroll BJ: A depression rating scale for children. *Pediatrics* 64:442–450, 1979.
120. Kazdin AE, French NH, Unis AS, et al: Assessment of childhood depression: Correspondence of child and parent ratings. *J Am Acad Child Psychiatry* 22:157–164, 1983.
121. Weller E, Weller R: Diagnostic Interview for Depression in Children and Adolescents. Unpublished manuscript, The Ohio State University, Columbus, 1982.
122. Petti TA: School Age Depression Listed Inventory (SADLI). *Psychopharmacol Bull* 21:972–977, 1985.
123. Lefkowitz MM, Tesiny EP: Assessment of childhood depression. *J Consult Clin Psychol* 48:43–50, 1980.
124. Lefkowitz MM, Tesiny EP: Peer Nomination Index of Depression (PNID). *Psychopharmacol Bull* 21:969–971, 1985.
125. Carlson G: Childhood and adolescent mania: Diagnostic considerations. *J Child Psychol Psychiatry* 31:331–392, 1990.
126. Kovacs M: Presentation and course of major depressive disorder during childhood and later years of the life span. *J Am Acad Child Adolesc Psychiatry* 35:705–715, 1996.
127. Beigel A, Murphy DL, Bunney WE: The Manic State Rating Scale: Scale construction, reliability and validity. *Arch Gen Psychiatry* 25:256–262, 1971.
128. Goodwin FK, Jamison KR: *Manic Depressive Illness*. London, Oxford University Press, 1990, pp 321–322.
129. Weller EB, Weller RA, Fristad MA: Bipolar disorder in children: Misdiagnosis, underdiagnosis, and future directions. *J Am Acad Child Adolesc Psychiatry* 34:709–714, 1995
130. Braunig P, Shugar G, Kruger S: An investigation of the Self-Report Manic Inventory as a diagnostic and severity scale for mania. *Compr Psychiatry* 37:52–55, 1996.
131. Young RC, Biggs JT, Ziegler VE, Meyer DA: A rating scale for mania: Reliability, validity and sensitivity. *Br Psychiatry* 133:429–435, 1978.
132. Fristad MA, Weller EB, Weller RA: The Mania Rating Scale: Can it be used in children? A preliminary report. *J Am Acad Child Adolesc Psychiatry* 31:252–257, 1992.
133. Fristad MA, Weller RA, Weller EB: The Mania Rating Scale (MRS): Further reliability and validity studies with children. *Ann Clin Psychiatry* 7:127–132, 1995.
134. Fristad MA, Weller EB, Weller RA: Clinical Global Impression—Mania (CGI-M). Unpublished document. Columbus, Ohio, Ohio State University, 1988.
135. Papatheodorou G, Kutcher SP: Divalproex sodium treatment in late adolescent and young adult acute mania. *Psychopharmacol Bull* 29:213–219, 1993.
136. Werry JS, Aman MG: Anxiety in children, in Burrows GD, Davies B (eds): *Handbook of Studies on Anxiety*. Amsterdam, Elsevier North-Holland Biomedical, 1980, pp 165–192.
137. Klein RG: Parent–child agreement in clinical assessment of anxiety and other psychopathology: A review. *J Anxiety Disord* 5:187–198, 1991.

138. Barrios BA, Hartmann DP: Fears and anxieties, in Mash EJ, Terdal LG (eds): *Behavioral Assessment of Childhood Disorders*, ed 2. New York, Guilford Press, 1988, pp 196–262.

139. Miller LC, Barrett CL, Hampe E: Phobias of childhood in a prescientific era, in Davids A (ed): *Child Personality and Psychopathology: Current Topics*. New York, John Wiley & Sons, 1974, pp 89–134.

140. Klein RG: Childhood anxiety disorders, in Kestenbaum CJ, Williams DT (eds): *Clinical Assessment of Children and Adolescents—A Biopsychosocial Approach*. New York, New York University Press, 1988, pp 722–742.

141. Roberts N, Vargo B, Ferguson HB: Measurement of anxiety and depression in children and adolescents. *Pediatr Clin North Am* 12:837–860, 1989.

142. Sherer MW, Nakamura CY: A Fear Survey Schedule for Children (FSS-FC): A factor analytic comparison with manifest anxiety (CMAS). *Behav Res Ther* 24:1–8, 1968.

143. Ollendick TH: Reliability and validity of the Revised Fear Survey Schedule for Children (FSSC-R). *Behav Res Ther* 21:685–692, 1983.

144. King NJ, Gullone E, Ollendick TH: Manifest anxiety and fearfulness in children and adolescents. *J Gen Psychol* 153:63–73, 1992.

145. Spielberger CD: *State–Trait Anxiety Inventory for Children*. Palo Alto, Calif, Consulting Psychologists Press, 1973.

146. Ollendick TH, Matson JL, Helsel WJ: Fears in children and adolescents: Normative data. *Behav Res Ther* 23:465–467, 1985.

147. Spence SH, McCathie H: The stability of fears in children: A two-year prospective study: A research note. *J Child Psychol Psychiatry* 34:579–585, 1993.

148. Gullone E, King, NJ: Psychometric evaluation of a revised Fear Survey Schedule for Children and Adolescents. *J Child Psychol Psychiatry* 33:987–998, 1992.

149. Last C, Francis G, Strauss CC: Assessing fears in anxiety-disordered children with the Revised Fear Survey Schedule for Children (FSSC-R). *J Clin Child Psychol* 18:137–141, 1989.

150. Gullone E, King NJ: The fears of youth in the 1990s: Contemporary normative data. *J Genet Psychol.* 154:137–153, 1993.

151. King NJ, Josephs A, Gullone E, Madden C, Ollendick TH: Assessing the fears of children with disability using the Revised Fear Survey Schedule for Children: A comparative study. *Br J Med Psychol* 67:377–386, 1994.

152. Gullone E, Cummins RA, King NJ: Self-reported fears: A comparison study of youths with and without an intellectual disability. *J Intellect Disabil Res* 40:227–240, 1996.

153. Gullone E, King NJ, Cummins RA: Fears of youth with mental retardation: psychometric evaluation of the Fear Survey Schedule for Children-II (FSSC-II). *Res Dev Disabil.* 17:269–284, 1996.

154. Perrin S, Last CG: Do childhood anxiety measures measure anxiety? *J Abnorm Child Psychol* 20:567–578, 1992.

155. Ollendick TH, Yang B, Dong Q, Xia Y, Lin L: Perceptions of fear in other children and adolescents: The role of gender and friendship status. *J Abnorm Child Psychol* 23:439–452, 1995.

156. Erol N, Sahin N: Fears of children and the cultural context: The Turkish norms. *Eur Child Adolesc Psychiatry* 4:85–93, 1995.

157. Casteneda A, Palermo DS, McCandless BR: The children's form of the Manifest Anxiety Scale. *Child Dev* 27:317–326, 1956.

158. Taylor JA: A personality scale of manifest anxiety. *J Abnorm Soc Psychol* 48:285–290, 1953.

159. Reynolds CR, Richmond BO: What I Think and Feel: A revised measure of children's manifest anxiety. *J Abnorm Child Psychol* 6:271–280, 1978.

160. Reynolds CR, Richmond BO: *Revised Children's Manifest Anxiety Scale Manual*. Los Angeles, Western Psychological Services, 1985.

161. Reynolds CR: Concurrent validity of What I Think and Feel: The revised Children's Manifest Anxiety Scale. *J Consult Clin Psychol* 48:774–775, 1980.

162. Hodges K: Depression and anxiety in children: A comparison of self-report questionnaire to clinical interview. *Psychol Assess J Consult Clin Psychol* 2:376–381, 1990.

163. Rabian B, Peterson RA, Richters J, Jensen PS: Anxiety sensitivity among anxious children. *J Clin Child Psychol* 22:441–446, 1993.

164. Forsyth BW, Damour L, Nagler S, Adnopoz J: The psychological effects of parental human immunodeficiency virus infection on uninfected children [see comments]. *Arch Pediatr Adolesc Med.* 150:1015–1020, 1996.

165. Aman MG, Werry JS: Methylphenidate and diazepam in severe reading retardation. *J Am Acad Child Psychiatry* 21:31–37, 1982.

166. Klein RG, Koplewicz HS, Kanner A: Imipramine treatment of children with separation anxiety disorder. *J Am Acad Child Adolesc Psychiatry*, 31:21–28, 1992.

167. Nelson WM 3rd, Renzenbrink G, Kapp CJ: Sensitivity of clinically hospitalized adolescents' self-report measures to change over time. *J Clin Psychol.* 51:753–760, 1995.

168. Reynolds CR, Richmond BO: What I Think and Feel: A revised measure of the Children's Manifest Anxiety. *J Abnorm Child Psychol* 25:15–20, 1997.

169. Silverman WK, Fleisig W, Rabian B, et al: Childhood anxiety and sensitivity index. *J Clin Child Psychol* 20:162–168, 1991.

170. Reiss S, Peterson RA, Gursky DM, et al: Anxiety sensitivity, anxiety frequency, and the prediction of fearfulness. *Behav Res Ther* 24:1–8, 1986.

171. Chorpita BF, Albano AM, Barlow DH: Child Anxiety Sensitivity Index: Considerations for children with anxiety disorders. *J Clin Child Psychol* 25:77–82, 1996.

172. Montgomery LE, Finch AJ: Validity of two measures of anxiety in children. *J Abnorm Child Psychol* 2:293–295, 1974.

173. Finch AJ Jr, Nelson WM: Anxiety and locus of conflict in emotionally disturbed children. *J Abnorm Child Psychol* 2:33–37, 1974.

174. Muris P, Steerneman P, Merckelbach H, Meesters C: The role of parental fearfulness and modeling in children's fear. *Behav Res Ther* 34:265–268, 1996.

175. Canals J, Carbajo G, Fernandez J, Marti-Henneberg C, Domenech E: Biopsychopathologic risk profile of adolescents with eating disorder symptoms. *Adolescence* 31:443–450, 1996.

176. Berg CJ, Rapoport JL, Whitacker A, et al: Childhood obsessive compulsive disorder: A two year prospective follow-up of a community sample. *J Am Acad Child Adolesc Psychiatry* 28:528–533, 1989.

177. Berg CJ, Rapoport JL, Flament M: The Leyton Obsessional Inventory—Child version. *J Am Acad Child Adolesc Psychiatry* 25:84–91, 1986.

178. Berg CJ, Whitacker A, Davies M, et al: The survey form of the Leyton Obsessional Inventory—Child version: Norms from an epidemiological study. *J Am Acad Child Adolesc Psychiatry* 27:759–763, 1988.

179. Berg A, Murphy DL, Bunny WE: The Manic State Rating Scale: Scale construction, reliability, and validity. *Arch Gen Psychiatry* 25:256–262, 1971.

180. King NJ, Myerson NN, Inglis S, Jenkins M, Ollendick TH: Obsessive-compulsive behaviour in children and adolescents: A cross-sectional Australian study. *J Paediatr Child Health* 31:527–531, 1995.

181. King N, Inglis S, Jenkins M, Myerson N, Ollendick T: Test-retest reliability of the survey form of the Leyton Obsessional Inventory—Child Version. *Percept Mot Skills* 80:1200–1202, 1995.

182. Goodman WK, Price LH, Rasmussen SA, et al.: The Yale-Brown Obsessive Compulsive Scale I. Development, use, and reliability. *Arch Gen Psychiatry* 46:1006–1011, 1989.

183. Goodman WK, Price LH, Rasmussen SA, et al.: The Yale-Brown Obsessive Compulsive Scale II. Validity. *Arch Gen Psychiatry* 46:1012–1016, 1989.

184. Steketee G, Frost R, Bogart K: The Yale-Brown Obsessive Compulsive Scale: Interview versus self-report. *Behav Res Ther* 34:675–684, 1996.

185. Woody SR, Steketee G, Chambless DL: Reliability and validity of the Yale-Brown Obsessive-Compulsive Scale. *Behav Res Therapy* 33:597–605, 1995.

186. Lombroso PJ, Scahill L, King RA, et al.: Risperidone treatment of children and adolescents with chronic tic disorders: A preliminary report. *J Am Acad Child Adolesc Psychiatry* 34:1147–1152, 1995.

187. March JS, Mulle K, Herbal B: Behavioral psychotherapy for children and adolescents with obsessive–compulsive disorder: An open trial of a new protocol-driven treatment package. *J Am Acad Child Adolesc Psychiatry* 33:333–341, 1994.

188. Vitiello B, Behar D, Wolfson S, et al: Diagnosis of panic disorder in prepubertal children. *J Am Acad Child Adolesc Psychiatry* 29:782–784, 1989.

189. King NJ, Gullone E, Tonge BJ, Ollendick TH: Self-reports of panic attacks and manifest anxiety in adolescents. *Behav Res Ther.* 31:111–116, 1993.

190. Schwab-Stone M, Fallon T, Briggs M, Crowther B: Reliability of diagnostic reporting for children aged 6-11 years: a test-retest study of the Diagnostic Interview Schedule for Children-Revised. *Am J Psychiatry.* 151:1048–1054, 1994.

191. Ollendick TH, Mattis SG, King NJ: Panic in children and adolescents: A review. *J Child Psychol Psychiatry Allied Discip.* 35:113–134, 1994.

192. Milne JM, Garrison CZ, Addy CL, McKeown RE, Jackson KL, Cuffe SP, Waller JL: Frequency of phobic disorder in a community sample of young adolescents. *J Am Acad Child Adolesc Psychiatry.* 34:1202–1211, 1995

193. Stuber MC, Nader K, Yasuda P, et al: Stress responses after pediatric bone marrow transplantation. *J Am Acad Child Adolesc Psychiatry* 30:952–957, 1991.

194. Lonigan CJ, Shannon MP, Taylor CM, Finch AJ Jr., Sallee FR: Children exposed to disaster: II. Risk factors for the development of post-traumatic symptomatology. *J Am Acad Child Adolesc Psychiatry*. 33:94–105, 1994

195. Shannon MP, Lonigan CJ, Finch AJ Jr., Taylor CM: Children exposed to disaster: I. Epidemiology of post-traumatic symptoms and symptom profiles. *J Am Acad Child Adolesc Psychiatry* 33:80–93, 1994.

196. Sack WH, Seeley JR, Clarke GN: Does PTSD transcend cultural barriers? A study from the Khmer Adolescent Refugee Project. *J Am Acad Child Adolesc Psychiatry* 36:49–54, 1997

197. Wirt RD, Lachar D, Klinedinst JK, Seat PD: *Multidimensional Description of Child Personality: A Manual for the Personality Inventory for Children (Revised)*. Los Angeles: Western Psychological Institute, 1984.

198. Miller LC, Barrett CL, Hampe E, et al: Revised anxiety scales for the Louisville Behavior Check List. *Psychol Rep* 29:503–511, 1971.

199. Miller LC, Barrett CL, Hampe E, et al: Factor structure of childhood fears. *J Consult Clin Psychol* 39:264–268, 1972.

200. Silverman WK, Nelles WB: The Anxiety Disorders Interview Schedule for Children. *J Am Acad Child Adolesc Psychiatry* 27:772–778, 1988.

201. Russell AT: Schizophrenia, in Hooper SR, Hynd GW, Mattison RE (eds): *Child Psychopathology: Diagnostic Criteria and Clinical Assessment*. Hillsdale, NJ, Lawrence Erlbaum, 1992, pp 23–63.

202. Werry JS: Schizophrenia and allied disorders, in Rutter M, Hersov L, Taylor E (eds): *Child and Adolescent Psychiatry: Modern Approaches*, ed 3. Oxford, Blackwell, 1994, pp 594–615.

203. Leckman JF, Towbin JF, Ort SI, et al: Clinical assessment of tic severity, in Cohen DJ, Bruun RD, Leckman JF (eds): *Tourette's Syndrome and Tic Disorders: Clinical Understanding and Treatment*. New York, John Wiley & Sons, 1988, pp 56–78.

204. Shapiro AK, Shapiro ES, Young JG, et al: Measurement in tic disorders, in Shapiro AK, Shapiro, ES, Young JG, et al (eds): *Gilles de la Tourette Syndrome*, ed 2. New York, Raven Press, 1998, pp 451–480.

205. Leckman JF, Riddle MA, Hardin MT, et al: Yale Global Tic Scale. Initial testing of a clinician-rated scale of tic severity. *J Am Acad Child Adolesc Psychiatry* 28:566–573, 1989.

206. Harcherik DF, Leckman JF, Detlor J, et al: A new instrument for clinical studies of Tourette's Syndrome. *J Am Acad Child Psychiatry* 23:153–160, 1984.

207. Shapiro AK, Shapiro E: Controlled study of pimozide vs. placebo in Tourette's syndrome. *J Am Acad Child Psychiatry* 23:161–173, 1984.

208. Gaffney GR, Sieg K, Hellings J: The MOVES: A self-rating scale for Tourette's Syndrome. *J Child Adolesc Psychopharmacol* 4:269–280, 1994.

209. Aman MG, Singh NN, Stewart AW, et al: The Aberrant Behavior Checklist: A behavior rating scale for the assessment of treatment effects. *Am J Ment Defic* 89:485–491, 1985.

210. Aman MG: Annotated bibliography on the Aberrant Behavior Checklist (ABC). Unpublished manuscript, The Nisonger Center UAP, Ohio State University, Columbus, Ohio, 1997.

211. Aman MG, Singh NN, Turbott SH: Reliability of the Aberrant Behavior Checklist and the effects of variations in instructions. *Am J Ment Defic* 92:237–240, 1987.

212. Aman MG, Singh NN, Stewart AW, et al: Psychometric characteristics of the Aberrant Behavior Checklist. *Am J Ment Defic* 89:492–502, 1985.

213. Aman MG, Richmond G, Stewart AW, et al: The Aberrant Behavior Checklist: Factor structure and the effect of subject variables in American and New Zealand facilities. *Am J Ment Defic* 91:570–578, 1987.

214. Bihm E, Poindexter AR: Cross-validation of the Aberrant Behavior Checklist. *Am J Ment Retard* 96:209–211, 1991.

215. Newton JT, Sturmey P: The Aberrant Behavior Checklist: A British replication and extension of its psychometric properties. *J Ment Defic Res* 32:87–92, 1988.

216. Freund LS, Reiss AL: Rating problem behaviors in outpatients with mental retardation: Use of the Aberrant Behavior Checklist. *Res Dev Disabil* 12:435–451, 1991.

217. Marshburn EC, Aman MG: Factor validity and norms for the Aberrant Behavior Checklist in a community sample of children with mental retardation. *J Autism Dev Disord* 22:357–373, 1992.

218. Rojahn J, Helsel WJ: The Aberrant Behavior Checklist in children and adolescents with dual diagnosis. *J Autism Dev Disord* 21:17–28, 1991.

219. Aman MG, Kern RA, McGhee D, et al: Fenfluramine and methylphenidate in children with mental retardation and ADHD: Clinical and side effects. *J Am Acad Child Adolesc Psychiatry* 32:851–859, 1993.

220. Gadow KD, Pomeroy JC: A controlled case study of methylphenidate and fenfluramine in a young mentally retarded hyperactive child. *Aust NZ J Dev Disabil* 16:323–334, 1990.

221. Realmuto GM, August GJ, Garfinkel BD: Clinical effect of buspirone in autistic children. *J Clin Psycho-pharmacol* 9:122–125, 1989.
222. Aman MG, Singh NN: *Aberrant Behavior Checklist—Community. Supplementary Manual.* East Aurora, NY, Slosson Educational Publications, 1994.
223. Aman MG, Tassé MJ, Rojahn J, et al: The Nisonger CBRF: A child behavior rating form for children with developmental disabilities. *Res Dev Disabil* 17:41–57, 1996.
224. Tassé MJ, Aman MG, Hammer D, et al: The Nisonger Child Behavior Rating Form: Age and gender effects and norms. *Res Dev Disabil* 17:59–75, 1996.
225. Rojahn J, Polster LM, Mulick JA, et al: Reliability of the Behavior Problems Inventory. *J Multihandicapped Person* 2:283–293, 1989.
226. Feinstein C, Kaminer Y, Barrett RP, et al: The assessment of mood and affect in developmentally disabled children and adolescents: The Emotional Disorders Rating Scale. *Res Dev Disabil* 9:109–121, 1988.
227. Aman, MG: Instruments for assessing treatment effects in developmentally disabled populations. *Assessment in Rehabilitation and Exceptionality* 1:1–20, 1994.
228. Das JP, Melnyk L: Attention Checklist: A scale for mildly mentally handicapped adolescents. *Psychol Rep* 64:1267–1274, 1989.
229. Leudar I, Fraser WI, Jeeves MA: Behaviour disturbance and mental handicap: Typology and longitudinal trends. *Psychol Med* 14:923–935, 1984.
230. Sprague RL: BeERS (Behavior Evaluation Rating Scale). Unpublished scale, University of Illinois, Champaign, 1982.
231. Einfeld S, Tonge BJ: *Manual for the Developmental Behaviour Checklist.* University of New South Wales, Sydney, Australia, 1994.
232. Matson JL, Gardner WI, Coe DA, et al: Diagnostic Assessment for the Severely Handicapped (DASH). Unpublished manuscript, Louisiana State University, Baton Rouge, 1990.
233. Gualtieri CT, Schroeder SR: Pharmacotherapy for self-injurious behavior: Preliminary tests of the D_1 hypothesis. *Psychopharmacol Bull* 25:364–371, 1989.
234. Strohmer DC, Prout HT: Strohmer—Prout Behavior Rating Scale Manual. Schenectady, NY, Genium Publishing Corporation, 1989.
235. Campbell M, Palij M: Behavioral and cognitive measures used in psychopharmacological studies of infantile autism. *Psychopharmacol Bull* 21:1047–1052, 1985.
236. Overall JE, Campbell M: Behavioral assessment of psychopathology in children: Infantile autism. *J Clin Psychol* 44:708–716, 1988.
237. Campbell M: Timed Stereotypies Rating Scale. *Psychopharmacol Bull* 21:1082, 1985.
238. Freeman BJ, Ritvo ER, Yokota A, et al: A scale for rating symptoms of patients with syndrome of autism in real life settings. *J Am Acad Child Psychiatry* 25:130–136, 1986.
239. Aman MG, Kern RA: Review of fenfluramine in the treatment of the developmental disabilities. *J Am Acad Child Adolesc Psychiatry* 28:549–565, 1989.
240. Aman MG, Marks RE, Turbott SH, et al: The clinical effects of methylphenidate and thioridazine in intellectually subaverage children. *J Am Acad Child Adolesc Psychiatry* 30:246–256, 1991.
241. Schopler E, Mesibov GB: *Diagnosis and Assessment of Autism.* New York, Plenum Press, 1988, pp 123–165.
242. Martin RP: Assessment of the social and emotional functioning of preschool children. *School Psychol Rev* 15:216–232, 1986.
243. Achenbach TM, Edelbrock C, Howell CT: Empirically based assessment of the behavioral/emotional problems of 2- and 3-year-old children. *J Abnorm Child Psychol* 15:629–650, 1987.
244. Behar LB, Stringfield SA: *Manual for the Preschool Behavior Questionnaire.* Durham, NC, Learning Institute of North Carolina, 1974.
245. Behar LB, Stringfield SA: A behavior rating scale for the preschool child. *Dev Psychol* 10:601–610, 1974.
246. Rutter M: Children's behaviour questionnaire for completion by teachers. Preliminary findings. *J Child Psychol Psychiatry* 8:1–11, 1967.
247. Behar LB: The Preschool Behavior Questionnaire. *J Abnorm Child Psychol* 5:265–275, 1977.
248. Rubin KH, Moller L, Emptage A: The Preschool Behavior Questionnaire: A useful index of behavior problems in elementary school-age children? *Can J Behav Sci/Rev Can Sci Comp* 19:86–100, 1987.
249. Rheinscheld TL: A factor analytic study of the Preschool Behavior Questionnaire with developmentally delayed children ages 3–6. Unpublished master's thesis, The Ohio State University, Columbus, 1989.
250. Aman MG, Rojahn J: The psychometric characteristics of the Behavior Questionnaire in preschoolers with developmental handicaps. *J Dev Phys Disabil* 6:311–325, 1994.

251. Rubin KH, Clark ML: Preschool teachers' rating of behavior problems: Observational, sociometric, and social-cognitive correlates. *J Abnorm Child Psychol* 11:273–286, 1983.
252. Hoge RD, Meginbir L, Kahn Y, et al: A multitrait-multimethod analysis of the Preschool Behavior Questionnaire. *J Abnorm Child Psychol* 13:119–127, 1985.
253. Richman N, Graham PJ: A behavioural screening questionnaire for use with three-year-old children: Preliminary findings. *J Child Psychol Psychiatry* 12:5–33, 1971.
254. Earls F, Richman N: Behaviour problems in pre-school children of West Indian-born parents: A re-examination of family and social factors. *J Child Psychol Psychiatry* 21:107–117, 1980.
255. Richman N: Behaviour problems in pre-school children: Family and social factors. *Br J Psychiatry* 131:523–527, 1977.
256. Richman N, Stevenson JE, Graham, PJ: Prevalence of behaviour problems in three-year-old children: An epidemiological study in a London borough. *J Child Psychol Psychiatry* 16:277–287, 1975.
257. Richman N, Stevenson J, Graham PJ: Pre-school to school: A behavioural study, in Schaffer R (ed): *Behavioural Development: A Series of Monographs.* New York, Academic Press, 1982.
258. Kohn M, Rosman BL: A social competence scale and symptom checklist for the preschool child: Factor dimensions, their cross-instrument generality, and longitudinal persistence. *Dev Psychol* 6:430–444, 1972.
259. Kohn M, Rosman BL: Relationship of preschool social–emotional functioning to later intellectual achievement. *Dev Psychol* 6:445–452, 1972.
260. Kohn M, Rosman BL: A two-factor model of emotional disturbance in the young child: Validity and screening efficiency. *J Child Psychol Psychiatry* 14:31–56, 1973.
261. Hertzig ME, Snow ME: The assessment of temperament, in Kestenbaum CJ, Williams DT (eds): *Handbook of Clinical Assessment of Children and Adolescents.* New York, New York University Press, 1988, vol 1, pp 133–153.
262. Werry JS: Behavior observations and activity measures for use in pediatric psychopharmacology, in Guidelines for the Clinical Evaluation of Psychoactive Drugs in Infants and Children. FDA publication HEW 79-3055. Rockville, Md, Food and Drug Administration, 1979.
263. Reid JB, Patterson GR, Baldwin DV, et al: Observations in the assessment of childhood disorders, in Rutter M, Tuma H, Lann I (eds): *Assessment and Diagnosis in Child Psychopathology.* New York, Guilford Press, 1988, pp 156–195.
264. Rojahn J, Schroeder SR: Behavioral assessment, in Matson JL, Mulick JA (eds): *Handbook of Mental Retardation,* ed 2. New York, Pergamon Press, 1991, pp 240–259.
265. Singh NN, Beale IL: Behavioural assessment of pharmacotherapy. *Behav Change* 3:34–40, 1986.
266. Barkley RA: *Attention Deficit Hyperactivity Disorder: A Handbook for Diagnosis and Treatment.* New York, Guilford Press, 1990.
267. Rapoport J, Abramson A, Alexander D, et al: Playroom observations of hyperactive children on medication. *J Am Acad Child Psychiatry* 10:524–534, 1971.
268. Routh DK, Schroeder CS: Standardized playroom measures as indices of hyperactivity. *J Abnorm Child Psychol* 4:144–207, 1976.
269. Abikoff H, Gittelman R: Classroom Observation Code: A modification of the Stony Brook Code. *Psychopharmacol Bull* 21:901–909, 1985.
270. Whalen CK, Henker B, Collins BE, et al: A social ecology of hyperactive boys: Medication effects in structured classroom environments. *J Appl Behav Anal* 12:65–81, 1979.
271. Gadow KD, Sprafkin J, Nolan EE: *ADHD School Observation Code.* Stony Brook, NY, Checkmate Plus, Ltd, 1996.
272. Sprafkin J, Gadow KD: An observational study of emotionally disturbed and learning-disabled children in school settings. *J Abnorm Child Psychol* 15:393–408, 1987.
273. Sprafkin J, Grayson P, Gadow KD, et al: Code for Observing Social Activity (COSA). Unpublished document, Department of Psychiatry and Behavioral Science, State University of New York at Stony Brook, 1986.
274. Hinshaw SP, Henker B, Whalen CK, et al: Aggressive, prosocial, and nonsocial behavior in hyperactive boys: Dose effects of methylphenidate in naturalistic settings. *J Consult Clin Psychol* 57:636–643, 1989.
275. Field CJ, Aman MG, White AJ, et al: A single-subject study of imipramine in a mentally retarded woman with depressive symptoms. *J Ment Defic Res* 30:191–198, 1986.
276. Cohen NJ, Douglas VI, Morgenstern G: The effect of methylphenidate on attentive behavior and autonomic activity in hyperactive children. *Psychopharmacologia* 22:282–294, 1971.
277. Lang PJ, Lazovik AD: Experimental desensitization of a phobia. *J Abnorm Soc Psychol* 66:519–525, 1963.
278. Aman MG: Drugs, learning and psychotherapies, in Werry JS (ed): *Pediatric Psychopharmacology: The Use of Behavior Modifying Drugs in Children.* New York, Brunner/Mazel, 1978, pp 79–108.

279. Aman MG: Drugs and learning in mentally retarded persons, in Burrows GD, Werry JS (eds): *Advances in Human Psychopharmacology.* Greenwich, Conn, JAI Press, 1984, vol 4, pp 121–163.
280. Barkley RA: The ecological validity of laboratory and analogue assessment methods of ADHD symptoms. *J Abnorm Child Psychol* 19:149–178, 1991.
281. Swanson JM: Measures of cognitive functioning appropriate for use in pediatric psychopharmacology research studies. *Psychopharmacol Bull* 21:887–892, 1985.
282. Werry JS: Drugs, learning, and cognitive function in children—An update. *J Child Psychol Psychiatry* 28:129–144, 1988.
283. Sykes DH, Douglas VI, Weiss G, et al: Attention in hyperactive children and the effect of methylphenidate (Ritalin). *J Child Psychol Psychiatry* 12:129–139, 1971.
284. Sykes DH, Douglas VI, Morgenstern G: The effect of methylphenidate (Ritalin) on sustained attention in hyperactive children. *Psychopharmacologia* 25:262–274, 1972.
285. Halperin JM, Wolf LE, Pascualvaca DM, Newcorn JH, Healey JM, O'Brien JD, Morganstein A, Young JG: Differential assessment of attention and impulsivity in children. *J Am Acad Child Adolesc Psychiatry* 27: 326–329, 1988.
286. Halperin JM, Wolf L, Greenblatt ER, Young G: Subtype analysis of commission errors on the Continuous Performance Test in children. *Dev Neuropsychol* 7:207–217, 1991.
287. Cohen NJ, Douglas VI, Morgenstern G: The effect of methylphenidate on attentive behavior and autonomic activity in hyperactive children. *Psychopharmacologia* 22:282–294, 1971.
288. Fischer M, Newby RF, Gordon M: Who are the false negatives on Continuous Performance Tests? *J Clin Child Psychol* 24:427–433, 1995.
289. Halperin JM, Newcorn JH, Matier K, Sharma V, McKay KE, Schwartz S: Discriminant validity of attention-deficit hyperactivity disorder. *J Am Acad Child Adolesc Psychiatry* 32:1038–1043, 1993.
290. Halperin JM, Newcorn JH, Matier K, Bedi G, Hall S, Sharma V: Impulsivity and the initiation of fights in children with disruptive behavior disorders. *J Child Psychol Psychiatry* 36:1199–1211, 1995.
291. Teicher MH, Ito Y, Glod CA, Barber NI: Objective measurement of hyperactivity and attentional problems in ADHD. *J Am Acad Child Adolesc Psychiatry* 35:334–342, 1996
292. Harper, GW, Ottinger DR: The performance of hyperactive and control preschoolers on a new computerized measure of visual vigilance: The Preschool Vigilance Task. *J Child Psychol Psychiatry* 33:1365–1372, 1992.
293. Pearson DA, Yaffee LS, Loveland KA, Lewis KR: A comparison of sustained and selective attention in children who have mental retardation with and without attention deficit hyperactivity disorder. *Am J Ment Retard* 100:592–607, 1996.
294. Ingersoll BD: Computerized Continuous Performance Tests: A clinician's perspective. *Behav Ther* 19: 20–22, 1996.
295. Gross-Tsur V, Manor O, van der Meere J, Joseph A, Shalev RS: Epilepsy and attention deficit hyperactivity disorder: Is methylphenidate safe and effective? *J Pediatr* 130:40–44, 1997.
296. Matier K, Halperin JM, Sharma V, Newcorn JH, Sathaye N: Methylphenidate response in aggressive and nonaggressive ADHD children: Distinctions on laboratory measures of symptoms. *J Am Acad Child Adolesc Psychiatry* 31:219–225, 1992.
297. Nigg JT, Hinshaw SP, Halperin JM: Continuous Performance Test in boys with attention deficit hyperactivity disorder: Methylphenidate dose response and relations with observed behaviors. *J Clin Child Psychol* 25:330–340, 1996.
298. Conners CK, Casat CD, Gualtieri CT, Weller E, Reader M, Reiss A, Weller RA, Khayrallah M, Ascher J: Bupropion hydrochloride in attention deficit disorder with hyperactivity. *J Am Acad Child Adolesc Psychiatry* 35:1314–1321, 1996
299. Chappell PB, Riddle MA, Scahill L, et al: Guanfacine treatment of comorbid attention-deficit hyperactivity disorder and Tourette's syndrome: Preliminary clinical experience. *J Am Acad Child Adolesc Psychiatry* 34: 1140–1146, 1995
300. Gordon M: The assessment of impulsivity and mediating behavior in hyperactive and non-hyperactive children. *J Abnorm Child Psychol* 7:317–326, 1979.
301. McClure FD, Gordon M: Performance of disturbed hyperactive and nonhyperactive children on an objective measure of hyperactivity. *J Abnorm Child Psychol* 12:561–572, 1984.
302. Conners CK: *Continuous Performance Test: Users Guide.* North Tonawanda, NY, Multi-Health Systems, Inc., 1994.
303. Charles L, Schain RJ, Zelniker T, et al: Effects of methylphenidate on hyperactive children's ability to sustain attention. *Pediatrics* 64:412–418, 1979.
304. Aman MG, Turbott SH: Incidental learning, distraction, and sustained attention in hyperactive and control subjects. *J Abnorm Child Psychol* 14:441–456, 1986.

305. Gomez R, Sanson AV: Effects of experimenter and mother presence on the attentional performance and activity of hyperactive boys. *J Abnorm Child Psychol* 22:517–529, 1994.
306. Kagan J: Reflection-impulsivity and reading ability in primary grade children. *Child Dev* 36:609–628, 1965.
307. Cairns E, Cammock T: Development of a more reliable version of the Matching Familiar Figures Test. *Dev Psychol* 11:244–248, 1978.
308. Sonuga-Barke EJ, Houlberg K, Hall M: When is "impulsiveness" not impulsive? The case of hyperactive children's cognitive style. *J Child Psychol Psychiatry Allied Discipl* 35:1247–1253, 1994.
309. Milich R, Kramer J: Reflections on impulsivity: An empirical investigation of impulsivity as a construct, in Gadow K (ed): *Advances in Learning and Behavior Disabilities.* Greenwich, Conn, JAI Press, 1984, vol 3, pp 57–94.
310. Aman MG: Applications of computerized cognitive–motor measures to the assessment of psychoactive drugs, in Dodson WE, Kinsbourne M (eds): *Assessing Cognitive Function in Patients with Epilepsy.* New York, Demos Press, 1982, pp 69–96.
311. Handen BL, Breaux AM, Gosling A, et al: Efficacy of Ritalin among mentally retarded children with ADHD. *Pediatrics* 86:922–930, 1990.
312. Douglas VI, Barr RG, O'Neill ME, et al: Short term effects of methylphenidate on the cognition, learning and academic performance of children with attention deficit disorder in the laboratory and the classroom. *J Child Psychol Psychiatry* 27:191–211, 1986.
313. Pelham WE, Bender ME, Caddell J, et al: Methylphenidate and children with attention deficit disorder. *Arch Gen Psychiatry* 42:941–952, 1985.
314. Gadian DG, Isaacs EB, Cross JH, Connelly A, Jackson GD, King MD, Neville BG, Vargha-Khadem, F: Lateralization of brain function in childhood revealed by magnetic resonance spectroscopy. *Neurology* 46: 974–977, 1996.
315. Gordon M: The Gordon Diagnostic System. DeWitt, NY, Gordon Systems, 1983.
316. Bjorklund DF, Kipp K: Parental investment theory and gender differences in the evolution of inhibition mechanisms. *Psychol Bull* 120:163–188, 1996.
317. Krueger RF, Caspi A, Moffitt TE, White J, Stouthamer-Loeber M: Delay of gratification, psychopathology, and personality: Is low self-control specific to externalizing problems? *J Pers* 64:107–129, 1996.
318. Barkley RA, Fischer M, Newby R, et al: Development of a multi-method clinical protocol for assessing stimulant drug responses in ADHD children. *J Clin Child Psychol* 17:14–24, 1988.
319. Sprague RL, Sleator EK: Effects of psychopharmacologic agents on learning disorders. *Pediatr Clin North Am* 20:719–735, 1973.
320. Sprague RL, Sleator EK: Methylphenidate in hyperkinetic children: Differences in dose effects on learning and social behavior. *Science* 198:1274–1276, 1977.
321. Scott KG: Recognition memory: A research strategy and summary of initial findings. *Int Rev Res Men Retard* 5:83–111, 1971.
322. Conners CK, Kronsberg S: Measuring activity level in children. *Psychopharmacol Bull* 21:893–897, 1985.
323. Pfadt A, Tyron WW: Issues in the selection and use of mechanical transducers to directly measure motor activity in clinical settings. *Appl Res Ment Retard* 4:251–270, 1983.
324. Sprague RL, Toppe LK: Relationship between activity level and delay of reinforcement. *J Exp Psychol* 3:390–397, 1966.
325. Anderson LT, Campbell M, Grega DM, et al: Haloperidol in infantile autism: Effects on learning and behavioral symptoms. *Am J Psychiatry* 141:1195–1202, 1984.
326. Rapoport JL, Buchsbaum MS, Weingartner H, et al: Dextroamphetamine—its cognitive and behavioral effects in normal and hyperactive boys and normal men. *Arch Gen Psychiatry* 37:933–943, 1980.
327. Cull, CA, Trimble MR: Automated testing and psychopharmacology, in Hineman I, Hansen KE (eds): *Human Psychopharmacology.* New York, John Wiley & Sons, 1987, pp 113–153.
328. Butcher JN (ed): *Computerized Psychological Assessment.* New York, Basic Books, 1987.
329. Dodson WE, Kinsbourne M (eds): *Assessing Cognitive Function in Patients with Epilepsy.* New York, Demos Press, 1992.
330. Maarse FJ, Mulder LJM, Sjouw WPB, et al: *Computers in Psychology: Methods, Instrumentation, and Psychodiagnostics.* Amsterdam, Smets & Zeitlinger, 1988.
331. Butcher JN: Appendix A: Commercially available computerized psychological software and services, in Butcher JN (ed): *Computerized Psychological Assessment.* New York, Basic Books, 1987, pp 367–412.
332. Rosvold HE, Mirsky AF, Sarason I, Bransome SD Jr., Beck, LH: A continuous performance test of brain damage. *J Consult Psychol* 20:343–350, 1956.
333. Trommer BL, Hoeppner JB, Lorber R, et al: Pitfalls in the use of a continuous performance test as a diagnostic tool in attention deficit disorder. *J Dev Behav Pediatr* 9:339–345, 1988.

334. Burg JS, Burright RG, Donovick PJ: Performance data for traumatic brain-injured subjects on the Gordon Diagnostic System (GDS) tests of attention. *Brain Inj* 9:395–403, 1995.
335. Hickey JE, Suess PE, Newlin DB, Spurgeon L, Porges SW: Vagal tone regulation during sustained attention in boys exposed to opiates in utero. *Addict Behav* 20:43–59, 1995.
336. Leark RA, Dupuy TR, Greenberg LM, Corman CL, Kindschi CL: *T.O.V.A.: Test of Variables of Attention Professional Manual*. Los Alamitos, Calif, Universal Attention Disorders, Inc., 1996.
337. Greenberg LM, Waldman ID: Developmental normative data on the Test of Variables of Attention (T.O.V.A.®). *J Child Adolesc Psychiatry* 34:1019–1030, 1993.
338. Downey KK, Stelson FW, Pomerleau OF, Giordani B: Adult attention deficit hyperactivity disorder: Psychological test profiles in a clinical population. *J Nervous Ment Dis* 185:32–38, 1997.
339. Lubar JF, Swartwood MO, Swartwood JN, O'Donnell PH: Evaluation of the effectiveness of EEG neurofeedback training for ADHD in a clinical setting as measured by changes in T.O.V.A. scores, behavioral ratings, and WISC-R performance. *Biofeedback Self-Regul* 20:83–99, 1995.
340. Bernstein GA, Carroll ME, Crosby RD, Perwien AR, Go FS, Benowitz NL: Caffeine effects on learning, performance, and anxiety in normal school-age children. *J Am Acad Child Adolesc Psychiatry* 33:407–415, 1994
341. Greenberg, LM, Kindschi, CL: *T.O.V.A.: Test of Variables of Attention Clinical Guide*. Los Alamitos, Calif, Universal Attention Disorders, Inc., 1996.
342. Alpherts WCJ, Aldenkamp AP: Computerized neuropsychological assessment of cognitive functioning in children with epilepsy. *Epilepsia* 31(suppl 4):S35–S40, 1990.

6

Medicolegal and Ethical Issues in the Pharmacologic Treatment of Children

RONALD SCHOUTEN, M.D., J.D., and KENNETH S. DUCKWORTH, M.D.

I. INTRODUCTION

Physicians who prescribe psychotropic medications to children face unique legal and ethical challenges. The issues of competency, consent to treatment, patient autonomy, and confidentiality are important in this work, just as they are in adult medicine. The child and adolescent psychopharmacologist must also deal with the complex influences of family dynamics, child development, divorce, and custody as well as the involvement of parents, school personnel, and social service agencies in the treatment process. The fact that much remains to be understood in child psychiatry, the probabilistic rather than certain outcomes of medication trials, and the uncertain effects of new treatments on developing nervous systems all add additional layers of complexity.

This chapter focuses on selected legal and ethical issues surrounding the use of psychopharmacological agents with children. The issues of informed consent, competency to accept and refuse treatment, confidentiality, malpractice, and off-label use of medications will be highlighted.

Throughout this chapter, we will use two terms frequently: law and jurisdiction. The word law refers to a wide range of requirements and proscriptions that society applies to individual and group behavior. The law can be found in constitutions, statutes enacted by legislation, in the decisions of the courts (common or case law), and regulations promulgated by administrative bodies.

RONALD SCHOUTEN, M.D., J.D. • Law and Psychiatry Service, Massachusetts General Hospital, Boston, Massachusetts 02114–2517. **KENNETH S. DUCKWORTH, M.D.** • Massachusetts Mental Health Center, Boston, Massachusetts 02114.

Practitioner's Guide to Psychoactive Drugs for Children and Adolescents (Second Edition), Werry and Aman, eds. Plenum Publishing Corporation, New York, 1999.

Jurisdiction refers to a place or subject matter over which a particular court has authority. A jurisdiction is usually defined on the basis of either governmental entity or geography. For example, in the United States each state has its own courts that rule on matters arising under state law. In addition, the federal government has courts in each of the states to handle matters that arise under federal law. The state systems may have courts that handle specific topics (e.g., guardianship and family law matters, criminal cases, civil cases, land disputes). Each of these courts is then said to have jurisdiction over its assigned subject matter.

II. OBTAINING CONSENT FOR TREATMENT

A. The Doctrine of Informed Consent

Informed consent is the embodiment of ethical and clinical principles that protect patient autonomy by ensuring that patients are informed of the diagnosis, treatment options, and risks and benefits of those options. The establishment of informed consent as a legal as well as an ethical principle is one of the most significant developments in modern medicine.

Informed consent traces its origins to the tort of battery: the intentional touching of another person without permission or legal privilege.[1] Traditionally, a physician could avoid charges of battery by obtaining the patient's agreement to be treated; the consent process required only that permission be requested and a simple "yes" received in reply. It was enough if a patient consented to the basic type of treatment proposed or acted in a manner consistent with consent; the details or risks of the treatment did not need to be explained. For example, the physician's explanation that medication was needed and the patient's agreement to take it were adequate for consent, without a discussion of the risks and side effects.

This model of consent, known as simple consent, prevailed in the United States until the late 1950s and early 1960s, when a series of cases gave rise to the modern principles of informed consent.[2-4] These cases, and others, led to the following definition of informed consent: "The willing and uncoerced acceptance of a medical intervention by a patient after adequate disclosure by the physician of the nature of the intervention, its risks and benefits, as well as the alternatives with their risks and benefits."[5] In the United Kingdom, the obligation to obtain informed consent has been defined as follows: "... if a patient is fit to receive information and wishes to receive it, the doctor must 'brief' the patient so that he can make a free and informed choice."[6] The English model remains closer to the concept of simple consent and allows a physician to withhold information if he or she feels it is clinically appropriate. The reader is advised to note the variations in the definition of informed consent among jurisdictions as well as countries. Every physician should learn the standard that applies where he or she practices.

B. Elements of Informed Consent

Informed consent differs from simple consent by requiring that the physician disclose relevant information to the consenting party. In addition, the consent must be given voluntarily and by an individual competent to do so.

1. Information

The amount and type of information disclosed to the patient, patient's parents, or other decision maker is mandated by standards that vary according to legal jurisdiction. Under the professional standard, the physician must provide the patient or decision maker that information that the average physician in the community would convey under similar circumstances. This standard applies in a small majority of jurisdictions in the United States as well as in the United Kingdom.[7] The reasonable-person standard requires that the physician convey that amount of knowledge that the average patient or decision maker would require in order to make a decision under similar circumstances. A third approach looks to the professional standard first but focuses on what this parent or patient would require in order to make an informed decision.[8] Thus, the first standard is physician-oriented, the second standard is patient-oriented, and the third standard combines features of both.

In most jurisdictions in the United States and Canada, the information requirement of informed consent can be satisfied if the physician has discussed those details of the treatment that the average patient would require to make a decision. Specific items of information to be covered are listed in Table 1.[9]

Physicians in the United Kingdom traditionally have been given more latitude in determining the amount of information disclosed to the patient. The American model of informed consent has been specifically rejected in England and Wales. In 1990, however, the National Health Service issued guidelines for consent to treatment that attempt to move England closer to the American and Canadian models.[10]

It is important for the physician to explain what is not known as well as what is known. For example, when a new treatment is being offered, the patient should be informed of the novelty of the treatment and the possibility of unknown side effects. The limited amount of data on the long-term effects and side effects of psychotropics in children underscores the importance of the informed consent process. Popper[11] has suggested that the physician prescribing for children and adolescents should state explicitly that the medication in question may pose risks that are currently unknown. Recent experience with newly discovered adverse side effects of pemoline (hepatotoxicity) and fenfluramine (cardiac effects and neurotoxicity) lends new weight to this recommendation.

When prescribing antipsychotic medication, the physician must discuss the risk of tar-

TABLE 1. Informational Requirements for Informed Consent[a]

1. The condition to be treated
2. Nature of the proposed treatment
3. Nature and probability of the material risks of the treatment
4. The benefits that may be expected from treatment
5. The physician's inability to predict results
6. The irreversibility of the procedure (if applicable)
7. Likely results of no treatment
8. Likely results, risks, and benefits of alternative treatments

[a]From *Harnish vs Children's Hospital Medical Center*, 387 Mass 152, 439 NE 2d 240, 1982.

dive dyskinesia with the decision maker. The appearance of tardive dyskinesia in children appears to be positively related to dose and length of exposure.[12,13] Estimates of the risk of tardive dyskinesia vary, but the significance of this side effect warrants a clear and open discussion with emphasis on the likelihood of occurrence, the potential irreversibility, available alternatives, and the risk–benefit analysis supporting the use of antipsychotic medication. Tardive dyskinesia and antipsychotic medications have received considerable attention from the legal community, and every physician should be aware of the risks in this area.[14] In the event that abnormal movements develop, the parents or guardian must be informed of this fact and the responses available. These should include a careful assessment for all causes of involuntary movements, such as other neurologic disorders and medications.[15]

2. Voluntariness

The law of informed consent requires that the patient's decision to accept treatment be free of coercion from the proponent of the treatment. When the patient is a child, it is the parent's or guardian's decision that must be free of coercion. Coercion refers to any situation in which the patient's refusal to cooperate with the proposed treatment results in a threat or imposition of some negative consequence. The physician who coerces consent from the patient is open to a charge of battery. Physicians and patients do have disagreements over treatment, and patient nonadherence (once called "noncompliance") is a major clinical problem. How does the physician obtain adherence from the resistant patient without coercion and invalidation of the consent? There is a fine line between a physician's legitimate expectations and coercive threats. In the United States, it is considered acceptable for a physician to refuse to treat a patient who is noncompliant, so long as adequate notice and opportunity to arrange alternative care are provided. Sudden termination of treatment and failure to provide an opportunity for alternative care leaves the physician open to a charge of abandonment and potential liability for any harm that results from the lack of care.

Parents and guardians may attempt to coerce the child patient to accept treatment. From ethical and legal standpoints, coercion by family members may be permissible while coercion from the treating physician is not.[16] When the patient's agreement is extracted under duress by his or her parent, the primary concern is clinical rather than legal. If frustrated parents make an explicit threat in an effort to coerce compliance, the resulting compliance usually will be temporary and partial at best. In addition, the psychiatrist may be seen as just another adult who is party to the coercion. The physician must be aware of the possibility of real or perceived parental duress and the potential harm it poses to the alliance between physician and patient.

3. Competency

Competency in the context of informed consent refers to a person's legal ability to make binding decisions about his or her life. The formal declaration of incompetence is a legal, not a clinical, matter; only a judge can declare an individual incompetent. A judicial declaration of incompetence strips the individual of status as a "legal person," depriving him or her of the power to make treatment decisions, make contracts, vote, hold licenses, and engage in a wide range of normal adult activities. Clinicians are called upon to assess the capacity of individuals to engage in certain activities. These clinical assessments are then used by judges to make a legal determination of either global or specific competency (competency to engage in a single activity). The assessments are routinely referred to as "competency evaluations." While technically inaccurate, this use is widely accepted, and we will use the terms competency and capacity interchangeably.

There are many different types of capacities or competencies, but the capacity to give informed consent is our focus. As a rule, adults are presumed to possess the capacity to give informed consent and children under the age of majority (18 years) are presumed to lack this capacity. The age of majority varies by country and according to the issue in question. In New Zealand, individuals aged 16 and older are presumed competent to make medical treatment decisions, but for abortion there is no minimum age. In the United Kingdom, the age of majority is 18. Generally, capacity to give informed consent exists if the patient:

1. can attain a factual understanding of the situation, including the relevant needs and alternatives involved;
2. has an appreciation of the seriousness of the condition and the consequences of accepting or rejecting treatment;
3. is able to express a preference; and
4. is capable of manipulating the information provided in a rational fashion.[17]

In the United Kingdom, valid consent to treatment may be given by children aged 16 and older, as well as children under 16 if "they have the intelligence and maturity to make up their own minds and have achieved a sufficient understanding and intelligence to understand fully what is proposed."[18] The Children's Act of 1989 required that the ascertainable wishes of any child be incorporated into the decision making. However, since the Act came into force in 1991, the Court of Appeal has held that while children may consent to treatment, they may not refuse treatment. Treatment refusal, even by a competent child, can be overridden by parental or judicial authority.[19,20]

C. Exceptions to the Requirement of Informed Consent

There are four basic exceptions to the requirement of informed consent. Informed consent need not be obtained:

1. In an emergency, where delaying treatment to obtain full informed consent would result in serious deterioration of the patient's condition. Consent must be obtained in the usual fashion once the patient is stabilized, however.
2. Where the patient has waived informed consent.
3. Where the patient is incompetent and the treating person is unable to identify or locate the patient's parent or guardian.
4. Under the principle of therapeutic privilege, where the process of obtaining consent itself could lead to worsening of the physical or emotional condition.[8]

In the United States, therapeutic privilege is invoked infrequently. For therapeutic privilege to be applicable, the disclosure of information must itself have the potential to cause deterioration, such as when a patient is suffering an unstable arrhythmia and the anxiety associated with this knowledge might cause cardiac arrest. The fact that a patient might refuse treatment if full information is provided is not sufficient basis for invoking therapeutic privilege in the United States. In the United Kingdom, the potential for treatment refusal would provide justification for withholding information.[18]

D. Special Consent Issues with Children and Adolescents

There are a number of special issues relevant to informed consent and competency in the treatment of children.

1. Parental Authority

The relationship between parent and child has special status under the law. Under the common law, children were deemed to be chattel—property of their parents. While parents are generally held to have a duty to provide housing, food, and medical care to their children, they in turn have a right to custody of and control over their children.[21] All decisions concerning the child, including decisions about medical treatment, are deemed to fall within the province of the parent, although there is variability among jurisdictions as to when the child may assume responsibility. The law presumes that a parent will act in the best interests of the child.[22,23]

However, parental authority has limits. Parents may not waive a child's common law or constitutionally protected due process rights to a civil commitment hearing[24] or maintain control over the child where such control is contrary to the child's best interests.[25] The parameters of this authority are often inconsistent, even within a single jurisdiction. In Connecticut, parents have been held to have the authority to consent to nontherapeutic surgery for the sole benefit of a sibling[26] (transplant of kidney from one sibling to another) but to lack authority to admit a child to a psychiatric school where the court deemed it unnecessary for the child's welfare.[27] In a series of cases involving conflicts between the religious beliefs of parents and proposed medical treatment for their children, courts have balanced the parents' right to control the religious training of their children against the best interests of the child. Where the interests of the child are served by the proposed treatment, the state may intervene even where treatment is in direct opposition to the religious beliefs of the parents.[28-30] In some jurisdictions, statutes require that the welfare of the child serve as the controlling factor in all treatment decisions (e.g., the New Zealand Children and Young Persons Act). Two Canadian provinces, British Columbia and New Brunswick, have passed legislation allowing children to consent to health care. Under the former statute, the physician must be convinced that the child understands the foreseeable risks and benefits. Under the latter statute, two qualified medical practitioners must conclude that the child has the capacity to give consent. In both cases, the physician must conclude that the treatment is in the child's best interests. Once this capacity threshold is reached, consent need not be obtained from the child's parent or guardian.[31]

2. The Authority of Children

While there is a presumption that children lack the capacity to make competent treatment decisions, there has been growing recognition that children of all ages have some capacity to evaluate treatment options.[32] This ability has been demonstrated to be more dependent on developmental stage than chronological age.[32,33]

The point at which a child becomes competent to make his or her own treatment decisions has been debated for centuries. One indicator of a child's capacity to take on the rights and responsibilities of adulthood has been the degree of emancipation from parental control.[34] Tests of competency have included the ability to join the armed forces or bear children. The law recognizes that while children are presumed to be incompetent, many children are forced to take full responsibility for themselves. Under the emancipated minor rule, a child who lives separately and apart from his or her parents, manages his or her own financial affairs, and has either the explicit or implied consent of his or her parents to undertake these activities is considered an emancipated minor and an adult in the eyes of the law.[35] In Massachusetts, for example, a minor who has been married, has had a child, is in the military, is pregnant or believes herself to be pregnant, or lives apart from his or her parents and manages his or her own finances is considered emancipated and capable of making treatment decisions.[36] Emancipation usually relieves parents of their obligations to the child and confers full responsibility on the child.[37] Other minors who do not meet the statutory requirements for emancipation may still be considered capable of giving informed consent under the mature minor rule.[34–38] A child is considered a mature minor if he or she is near the age of majority and is able to comprehend clearly the nature and potential impact of the treatment decision in question.

In the United Kingdom, children over 16 and those under 16 who possess a necessary degree of understanding and intelligence may consent to treatment. However, if these individuals refuse treatment while subject to wardship, contrary to the wishes of parents or guardians, their refusal may be overridden.[18–20] In the United States, the competent child patient's decision would be definitive.[34]

A number of jurisdictions have enacted specific measures to allow minors to consent to certain types of treatment with or without their parents' consent.[34] Many states have statutes that allow minors to consent to treatment for substance abuse,[39] treatment for sexually transmitted diseases,[40] abortion, and psychotherapy.[41] Every physician should consult with his or her medical or psychiatric association and become familiar with the law on these issues in his or her jurisdiction.

3. Developmental Aspects of Competency

One of the key issues related to competency is whether or not the minor child actually has the cognitive and emotional capacity to make treatment decisions. A study by Weithorn and Campbell[42] showed that 14-year-olds have the same capacities for making complicated treatment decisions as 18- and 21-year-olds. Nine-year-olds who were part of the study seemed to have less capacity to work with hypothetical situations but did demonstrate a capacity to understand situations and manipulate the information placed before them. It is noteworthy that the development of these abilities coincides with theories of development and the capacity for formal operations.[33] Dorn et al.[43] concluded that, in the research setting, decreased anxiety and increased sense of control were more strongly correlated with understanding of research participation than age. Cauffman and Steinberg[44] urge caution before assuming that cognitive capacity equates with capacity to make mature judgments. They note that important psychosocial differences exist between early adolescents and adults and that these differences may have considerable implications for judgment.

4. Assent

Where the child is not capable of giving informed consent to treatment, he or she is usually still capable of assent—general agreement to treatment, similar to the notion of simple consent. By seeking the patient's assent, the physician fosters the child's sense of autonomy and responsibility.

The American Academy of Pediatrics has suggested that assent include at least the following elements[45]:

1. Helping the patient achieve a developmentally appropriate awareness of the nature of his or her condition.
2. Telling the patient what to expect from the tests or treatment.
3. Making a clinical assessment of the patient's understanding of the situation and what factors are influencing his or her response.
4. Soliciting a statement of the patient's willingness to accept the proposed tests or treatment.

Assent is no panacea for conflicts over autonomy, however, as it may mask important underlying clinical concerns. For example, Mike, an 8-year-old boy with attention-deficit hyperactivity disorder (ADHD) and a learning disability, was compliant with his prescription for methylphenidate, 10 mg, b.i.d. When asked why he took the medicine, he said it was because "I am hyper and stupid and bad." In this case, Mike technically assented to treatment, but his assent was grounded in his own low self-esteem and misconceptions of how others viewed him. The physician should consider the basis of the child's assent and be prepared to address those issues that foster compliance but risk causing other types of harm.

E. Consent Procedures in Practice

The child psychopharmacologist should view informed consent as a set of guidelines for proposing and carrying out the treatment of the patient. These guidelines should be followed both with the patient and with the patient's parents or guardian. Although the physician's primary obligation is to the patient, the parents or guardians must be included in a discussion of the risks and benefits of treatment. Unless treatment of the child without parental consent is specifically allowed by statute, the physician is well advised to obtain the formal consent of the parent or guardian. Failure to do so leaves the physician open to allegations of battery or malpractice and sets the stage for conflicts between parents, patient, and physician.[34]

In some situations, the clinician may have doubts about the family's competence to manage the child's medication. This can be addressed initially by direct discussion with the family. If a question remains, the family may agree to voluntary assistance, such as a visiting nurse or social worker.

In extreme circumstances, a family may be totally incapable of providing adequate care for the patient, and it may be necessary to file a neglect petition with the appropriate social service agency. While often a necessity, the entry of the social service agency into the process can have negative effects, as when the involved parties have conflicting attitudes about medication. For example, if a child is in the custody of a social service agency during the week but stays with his mother on weekends, the mother's beliefs about the medication may lead her to withhold it. This sends a mixed message to the child and can undermine the likelihood of successful treatment if left unaddressed.

When an adolescent refuses treatment, the explanation may be found in the patient's dynamics or developmental stage. Adolescents are preoccupied with their bodies and with increasing autonomy from their parents through identification with a peer group. The decision to introduce a medication may strike at the core developmental tasks of becoming comfortable with bodily changes and forming an identity separate from parents. If the patient views the medication as a means of parental control, there is little hope of successful treatment. This is a delicate clinical matter, requiring a balance between respect for the patient's autonomy and the role of the parents. Especially in older children and adolescents, the doctor should endeavor to emphasize the patient's control over the treatment and information imparted to facilitate this sense of autonomy. These situations require patience, listening, explanations, reassurance, and the highest of professional skill on the part of the physician.

F. Documenting Informed Consent

Formal consent forms, signed by the patient, are required by many treatment facilities. In many jurisdictions, they are required by law for certain types of treatment. Too often, these forms are legalistic, impersonal, and ill suited to conveying information. The purpose of documentation is to provide evidence that informed consent was obtained. The signing of the form does not constitute informed consent; it merely memorializes it. While such forms obviously should be used where required, they should be used in conjunction with a note in the patient's record. The note should document the following in summary form: (1) the topic under discussion, (2) parties present, (3) discussion of risks and benefits, (4) questions asked, (5) subsequent consent, and (6) the opportunity to ask further questions. Documentation is especially important for child psychiatrists because as yet unknown adverse effects of treatment may not manifest themselves until many years after treatment has ended. Careful documentation of the consent process and assessment of the competence of the decision maker are essential. A sample note documenting informed consent is provided in Fig. 1. If the physician chooses to withhold some or all of the relevant information, the justification for doing so should be documented in the patient's record.

III. THE RIGHT TO REFUSE TREATMENT

The doctrine of informed consent establishes that patients, and not their physicians, are to be the primary decision makers with regard to medical care. The question of who makes treatment decisions on behalf of incompetent patients has received different answers in different jurisdictions. In a growing number of jurisdictions in the United States, the decision to treat an incompetent adult patient with antipsychotic medication (which is regarded as intrusive and extraordinary treatment) can only be made by a judge after a full adversarial hearing.[46,47] In Massachusetts, the state's highest court held that family members, guardians, and physicians are too biased by their relationships with the patient to reach appropriate decisions for the incompetent adult, even where the patient assents to the treatment, and such decisions require a full adversarial hearing.[48] In some countries, civil commitment of a patient automatically confers authority to treat, even over a patient's objections. Independent reviewing committees consisting of physicians and other caretakers may serve as the decision makers in some jurisdictions, or the matter may be left to the patient and his or her family or within the confines of the treatment relationship.[43]

Even in states that require full adversarial proceedings before an incompetent patient

October 17, 1997 Meeting with JM's parents

I have reviewed JM's diagnosis of ADHD, his treatment course, available

treatments, and prognosis with Mr. & Mrs. M.

(1)   The available pharmacological treatment options were reviewed, including the

        option of no treatment with medication. Specifically, we discussed

        methylphenidate and desipramine.

(2)   Possible behavioral treatments were reviewed at length.

(3)   The risks and benefits of each medication, behavioral treatment, and no treatment

        were reviewed in the usual fashion. These included, but were not limited to,

        worsening of behavior, growth inhibition, and the risks of motor tics for

        methylphenidate. We discussed reports of sudden death in children taking

        desipramine, as well as other more common side effects. Mr. & Mrs. M could

        recall no family history of sudden death or cardiac problems.

(4)   Mr. & Mrs. M indicated a clear understanding of JM's illness, treatment options,

        and prognosis.

(5)   Mr. & Mrs. M are aware that research in this area is ongoing, and additional side

        effects from these medications may be discovered in the future.

(6)   Following a review of this information and their other questions, Mr. & Mrs. M

        consented to a trial of methylphenidate for JM.

FIGURE 1.   Sample note documenting informed consent.

can be treated with antipsychotic medication, the situation with regard to children and adolescents is unclear. In the United States, most states that have established a right to refuse treatment with antipsychotic medication have extended this right to adolescents at least down to the age of 16. In other words, a 16-year-old may refuse the treatment and cannot be treated involuntarily without judicial approval. However, a child of 13, deemed incompetent to make treatment decisions because of his age, may be treated with antipsychotics with the consent of his parents, even over his objections. The ability of parents to consent to treatment of their minor children with antipsychotics reflects a tacit decision that parental rights of control outweigh the child's interests in being spared treatment that would be considered intrusive for adults.[26,27] It is something of a paradox that the same courts that consider antipsychotics harmful and intrusive allow minor children to be treated at their parents' requests, while incompetent adults who live independently have multiple layers of procedural protections from their parents and treaters.

Some states, either by statute or by administrative regulation, provide guidelines for judicial involvement in these decisions.[49,50] Generally speaking, in the absence of such regulations or statutes, parents are presumed to act in the child's best interests. Therefore, the physician need not seek judicial approval unless there are doubts as to the parents' competence to make the decision for the child. When parents refuse treatment for a child, physicians generally are successful in obtaining judicial authorization to override the parent's refusal as long as the risk–benefit analysis favors treatment. Courts are less inclined to override parental authority when the risks of treatment are substantial and the benefits are less clear-cut.[34]

IV. CONSENT TO TREATMENT AND THE CUSTODY PROBLEM

With the divorce rate rising in most countries and approaching 50% in the United States, it is not unusual for the child psychiatrist to be treating the child of a divorced couple. The same difficulties that led to the dissolution of the marriage often lead to conflicts over custody of the children. Concepts such as joint custody, legal custody, and physical custody are poorly defined in most jurisdictions and give physicians little guidance as to which parent has authority to consent to treatment of the child. This can lead to significant problems when treating a child with mental illness. The following example points up some of these problems.

> Billy was an 11-year-old only child referred for psychiatric evaluation because of worsening grades and isolative behavior. After a careful evaluation, he was diagnosed as having obsessive–compulsive disorder, and a trial of clomipramine was recommended. Billy's parents had been divorced three years prior to his evaluation. Under the joint custody agreement, Billy lived with his mother during the school year and spent alternating weekends and vacations with his father. The parents shared authority for medical treatment decisions. Billy's mother brought him to the appointment with the child psychiatrist and agreed to treatment with clomipramine. One week after starting the medication, Billy visited his father and brought his medication with him. Over the course of the weekend, Billy's father took the medication from him and refused to return it, telling Billy he was opposed to treatment with drugs. Billy's mother returned to the child psychiatrist, who refused to treat Billy until the legal issue was resolved because Billy's father had recently threatened a lawsuit if the psychiatrist prescribed medication for Billy again.

While the child psychiatrist in this situation was in something of a bind, her problems were not nearly as great as Billy's. In joint custody situations, both parents have an equal say in determining such matters as the religious training and medical treatment of the child. Day-to-day authority rests with the parent who has physical and legal custody. For example, in a joint custody situation, the parent with physical custody has the authority to control religious instruction. If the other parent has objections, he or she may intervene by turning to the court and showing that the child is at risk of substantial harm.[51] Where divorced parents disagree over proposed medical treatment, the noncustodial parent has the right to suggest a physician for another opinion.[52]

Conflicts between parents like the one outlined above can cause tremendous harm to the treatment. The psychiatrist in this example resorted to a legalistic approach that did very little for Billy but may have let the psychiatrist feel less vulnerable to a malpractice complaint. In fact, there was no basis for a lawsuit against her; the psychiatrist was prescribing the medication with the agreement of an appropriate decision maker. Neverthe-less, the psychiatrist must acknowledge the concerns of Billy's father and address them. The approach with the highest likelihood of success in such cases is to invite the objecting parent into the office to discuss his or her opposition. The opposition often has more to do with interpersonal conflict between the accepting and the refusing parent than actual objection to the medication. The noncustodial parent often feels left out of significant portions of the child's life. By soliciting the opinion and concerns of the objecting parent, the physician may be able to move him or her out of the adversarial position. If this ap-proach is unsuccessful, the physician must consider the risk of poor compliance when treatment is pursued in the face of parental conflict. Involvement of the court may be the only means of resolving this problem.

Bernet[53] notes the differing opinions about the rights of noncustodial parents to authorize different types of treatment: emergency treatment, nonemergent medical care, psychiatric evaluation, and psychiatric care. He advocates resolution of these decisions at the time of the custody decision, as well as limiting the right of the noncustodial parent to consent to psychiatric evaluation and treatment.

V. CONFIDENTIALITY

Confidentiality is the responsibility of physicians and other professionals to keep those matters revealed in confidence from the ears of third parties. For example, if an adult patient confides that he had an extramarital affair, the psychiatrist is obliged not to disclose this information to the community or to the patient's family. Exceptions to the rule of absolute confidentiality are numerous and include incompetence. In most jurisdictions, confiden-tiality can be broken where the patient poses a danger to himself, in an emergency, or where the patient poses a risk of harm to third parties.[54]

Confidentiality is limited for young children because they are presumed to be incom-petent; information must be shared with the child's parents in order for the parents to make treatment decisions. The duty of confidentiality owed to the child patient increases as the child approaches the age of majority or emancipation.

The traditional psychotherapy model relies on complete confidentiality as the basis for a trusting relationship between physician and patient. Actual or potential breaches of confidentiality can weaken the therapeutic alliance and impair the ability of the therapist and patient to work together. Although confidentiality is valued in psychopharmacology as well, adequate pharmacotherapy often requires communication with the patient's family. Many child psychiatrists are both psychotherapists and psychopharmacologists, giving rise to some difficult situations, as exemplified by the following case.

> Maryanne was a 16-year-old girl referred for treatment because of behavioral problems at school. During her weekly psychotherapy visits, she discussed a number of problems related to the divorce of her parents. At one visit, Maryanne told her doctor that she had missed her last menses and was concerned that she might be pregnant. She confirmed her pregnancy at the next visit, and they discussed a number of issues, including the need to inform her parents. She adamantly refused to tell her parents and refused to allow her psychiatrist to contact them.

Rules and regulations regarding pregnancy counseling, especially with minors, vary among countries and jurisdictions within countries. Barring any absolute statutory require-ment in his jurisdiction that would compel him to inform the parents over the objections of

Maryanne, her psychiatrist has both a legal and an ethical obligation to maintain her confidence. However, he also has an obligation to help her reach a decision that will best serve her needs. This may include assisting her to tell her parents that she is pregnant and helping her to obtain appropriate emotional support from them.

It is important to clarify the limits on confidentiality for children and adolescents in anticipation of any breach. For instance, if a child who requires medication is a student at a boarding school, on-site after-hours assistance may be needed. If the school nurse leaves at 5 p.m., the clinician may need to include the dormitory parent in the treatment team by asking the dormitory parent to dispense medications and offer observations. The clinician should assess the patient's relationship with the dormitory parent and document the reasons for involving him or her in the treatment. The patient should be alerted to the new role of the dormitory parent, so the inclusion of this adult will be seen as a necessary expansion of the treatment team rather than as a breach of confidentiality.

VI. RISK MANAGEMENT IN THE TREATMENT OF CHILDREN AND ADOLESCENTS

While not all countries share the penchant for litigation seen in the United States, the risk of a malpractice suit or complaint is an ongoing concern for all physicians.[55–57] Psychiatrists seem to be sued less often than other medical specialists, but psychiatry does have its share of malpractice litigation and complaints. A study by the Risk Management Foundation of the Harvard Medical Institutions showed that suicide and harm to others headed the list of events leading to psychiatric malpractice claims, with medication-related claims accounting for approximately 11% of all claims at the Harvard facilities.[58]

Medical malpractice is one of the subdivisions of the general category of law known as tort or personal-injury law. In order to prove a claim of medical malpractice, four elements must be established.

1. The psychiatrist owed a duty of due care to the patient. The physician's duty is usually defined as a duty to possess and use that degree of skill and knowledge that are commonly possessed and applied by reasonable physicians in the community practicing the same specialty.[1] This is referred to as the standard of care. The physician's duty is to the patient; however, the physician may be held to have a duty of care to third parties, such as where a patient poses a risk of violence to another person.[59]

2. The psychiatrist was derelict in his or her duty to the patient. Dereliction of a duty implies a negligent departure from the standard of care, either through failure to follow standard practice or through improper application of the standard of care.[1] For example, failure to monitor white blood cell counts in a patient on clozapine constitutes a departure from the standard of care. Obtaining white blood cell counts on patients taking clozapine but then failing either to review the results or to act appropriately in response to the results constitutes a negligent application of the standard of care. In either case, there has been an unjustified departure from the standard of care.

3. The negligent behavior was the proximate cause of some injury. Proximate cause is a legal concept that attempts to determine whether an event, A, caused a subsequent event, B. Proximate cause will not be found where the consequences of an act were not foreseeable by a reasonable person. The "But for" test is used to determine proximate cause: "But for" the dereliction of the duty in question the injury would not have occurred.[1]

4. The negligent behavior caused damages that can be proved. Unless actual damages can be shown, the malpractice action cannot be successful. For example, let us imagine that a psychiatrist prescribes lithium carbonate to an 18-year-old patient but then does not check lithium levels in subsequent months. At the 6-month follow-up visit, the patient complains of unsteadiness and increased tremors as well as nausea and vomiting. A blood sample is drawn and shows a lithium level of 3.0 mEq/liter, i.e., a concentration clearly falling in the toxic range. Instead of hospitalizing the patient for treatment, the psychiatrist sends him home with instructions to take no lithium for 3 days and then to take a reduced daily dose. The patient remains mildly ataxic for the next several days but loses no time from school or work. On subsequent testing, his lithium level has returned to 0.6 mEq/liter and he is asymptomatic. The psychiatrist's behavior in this case demonstrates a departure from the standard of care resulting in significant symptoms. Nevertheless, if no actual financial, physical, or emotional damages are shown in this case, the legal elements of malpractice would not be established.

In some areas of the United States, the frequency of malpractice suits has begun to decline in recent years, perhaps because of improved teaching of risk-management techniques and continuing-education programs. One of the aspects of medical practice that has received the most attention in risk-management seminars is the notion of informed consent and sharing uncertainty, both as clinical and as risk-management tools.[60] As Gutheil and colleagues[61] point out, sharing the uncertainty inherent in medical practice serves to strengthen the physician–patient relationship, which in turn decreases the likelihood that a patient will bring suit should an adverse event occur.

While good relations with patient and family members are likely to reduce the risk of malpractice litigation and complaints to medical disciplinary bodies, listed below are concrete risk-management tools that improve the defensibility of a malpractice complaint, should one be filed.

1. Documentation of the history, mental status examination, current symptoms, diagnosis, plan, risk–benefit analysis, and informed consent during the treatment process is essential. A complete physical examination and the existence of any preexisting or concurrent illnesses should be documented as well.

2. Consultation with one's colleagues or an independent consultant can serve several purposes. (a) From a clinical perspective, it provides the clinician with some additional insight from either another colleague or one with more experience in the field. (b) It may be used to establish the standard of care in the community. (c) It may help show the physician to be an open-minded practitioner who is willing to ask for advice from others.[62]

3. Avoid making promises. When a physician guarantees a certain outcome, the dispute is removed from the area of tort law and placed in the area of contract law. Thus, even though negligence may not be established, a disgruntled patient could bring an action based on breach of contract.[63]

4. Apologize to patients for adverse events. In general, a well-intentioned and sincere apology regarding the occurrence of an event humanizes the medical treatment experience, greatly reducing the bad feelings that increase the risk of malpractice litigation.[64] The physician must take care to avoid accepting or laying blame. The point of the apology is to express ongoing concern for the patient and regret that an event occurred. Too often, conscientious physicians place the fault on themselves when no objective party would find them blameworthy. In such cases, an admission of fault serves the physician poorly in any subsequent legal proceedings.

Off-Label Use of Medication

Pediatric and adolescent psychopharmacologists frequently find themselves prescribing medications to their patients which have either not been approved for use in children or have not yet been approved by the US Food and Drug Administration (FDA) for that specific purpose. This common practice is totally within the bounds of the law and is consistent with the policy of the FDA. The FDA limits what can be stated in the promotional materials for a product, based upon the established research on efficacy and safety. It was not Congress's intent to interfere with the practice of medicine when the act creating the FDA was passed. The decision as to how a specific medication is to be used, once approved for a purpose, is left to the physician and the patient.[65] The fact that it is legal to prescribe medications for purposes other than those formally approved by the FDA (off-label use) does not insulate the prescribing physician from a possible malpractice action in the event of an adverse event with the medication. A plaintiff may use the absence of FDA approval for a certain use to establish departure from the standard of care, but the lack of approval is not dispositive of the issue. Evidence of established use of the medication for that purpose in the community or the presence of studies showing efficacy and safety of the medication for that use serve to establish that the practice comports with the standard of care.[66–69]

The lack of FDA approval has been held not to constitute a material risk factor which must be revealed to a patient as part of the informed consent process, although the decision to prescribe medications for an off-label use is a matter of medical judgment and does leave the physician open to a claim for malpractice.[70] The physician prescribing medication for off-label uses is well advised to discuss this fact with the decision maker, however. This discussion should include information related to the risks and side effects associated with the medication, the reasons for using the medication as planned, and the support for using the medication in this way.

VII. CONCLUSIONS

Child psychopharmacology, like the rest of medicine, has more than its share of legal risks and ethical dilemmas, but they are not insurmountable. The law requires that physicians practice with a reasonable degree of care; it does not require perfection. Our ethical responsibilities as physicians compel us to act in the best interests of the patient. Often this can lead to real and perceived conflicts between our ethical responsibilities and the legal rights of parent and child. The means of negotiating this difficult passage are to be found in the conscientious practice of good medicine, not in legalistic posturing. The child psychiatrist encounters the special challenges of working with one patient but multiple decision makers. Sensitivity to these issues and respect for the rights of others, along with a solid knowledge of his or her field, will allow the physician to minimize legal risks and provide the greatest benefits for patients.

REFERENCES

1. Keeton WP, Dobbs DB, Keeton RE, et al: *Prosser & Keeton on Torts*, ed 5. St. Paul, Minn, West Publishing Co, 1984.

2. *Salgo vs Leland Stanford Jr. Univ. Board of Trustees*, 317 P 2d 170 (Calif Ct App), 1957.
3. *Natanson vs Kline*, 186 Kans 393, 350 P 2d 1093, 1960.
4. *Canterbury vs Spence*, 464 F 2d 772 (DC Cir), 1972.
5. Jansen AR, Siegler M, Winslade WJ: *Clinical Ethics*, ed 2. New York, Macmillan, 1986.
6. Scarman L, quoted in Marsh BT: Informed consent: Help or hindrance? *J R Soc Med* 83:603–606, 1990.
7. Havard JDJ: The responsibility of the doctor. *Br Med J* 299:503–508, 1989.
8. Appelbaum PS, Lidz CW, Meisel A: *Informed Consent*. London, Oxford University Press, 1987.
9. *Harnish vs Children's Hospital Medical Center*, 387 Mass 152, 439 NE 2d 240, 1982.
10. Heneghan C: Consent to medical treatment. *Lancet* 337:421, 1991.
11. Popper C: Medical unknowns and ethical consent: Prescribing psychotropic medications for children in the face of uncertainty, in Popper C (ed): *Psychiatric Pharmacosciences of Children and Adolescents*. Washington DC, American Psychiatric Press, 1987, pp 127–161.
12. Campbell M, Grega DM, Green WH, et al: Neuroleptic-induced dyskinesias in children. *Clin Neuropharmacol* 6:207–222, 1983.
13. Gualtieri CT, Barnhill J, McGimsey J, et al: Tardive dyskinesia and other movement disorder in children treated with psychotropic drugs. *J Am Acad Child Psychiatry* 19:491–510, 1980.
14. Beyer HA: Litigation and use of psychoactive drugs in developmental disabilities, in Aman MG, Singh NN (eds): *Psychopharmacology of the Developmental Disabilities*. Berlin, Springer-Verlag, 29–57, 1988.
15. Golden GS: Tardive dyskinesia and developmental disabilities, in Aman MG, Singh NN (eds): *Psychopharmacology of the Developmental Disabilities*. Berlin, Springer-Verlag, 197–215, 1988.
16. Mallary SD, Gert B, Culver CM: Family coercion and valid consent. *Theor Med* 7:123–126, 1986.
17. Appelbaum PS, Grisso T: Assessing patients' capacities to consent to treatment. *N Engl J Med* 319:1635–1638, 1988.
18. Brahams D: Consent for treatment of minors in wardship. *Lancet 1* 338:564–565, 1991.
19. Kessel R: In the U.K., children can't just say no. *Hastings Center Report* 23(2):20–21, 1993.
20. Dickinson D: Children's informed consent to treatment: Is the law an ass? *J Med Ethics* 20:205–206, 222, 1994.
21. *Schleiffer vs Meyers*, 644 F 2d 656 (7th Cir), 1981, cert den 454 US 823, 102 S Ct 110.
22. *Parham vs J.R.*, 442 US 584, 1979.
23. *R.J.D. vs Vaughan Clinic, P.C.*, 572 So 2d 1225 (Ala Sup Ct), 1990.
24. *In re Roger S.*, 141 Calif Rptr 298, 569 P 2d 1286 (Calif S Ct), 1977.
25. *Corpus Juris Secundum*, Parent and Child Sec 16.
26. *Hart vs Brown*, 29 Conn Sup 368, 289 A 2d 386 (Conn Sup), 1972.
27. *Melville vs Sabbatino*, 30 Conn Sup 320, 313 A 2d 886 (Conn Sup), 1973.
28. *In re Sampson*, 65 Misc 2d 658, 317 NYS 2d 641, 1970, aff'd 29 NY 2d 900, 278 NE 2d 918, 1972.
29. *In re Green*, 448 Pa 338, 292 A 2d 387, 1972.
30. *Custody of a Minor*, 375 Mass 733, 375 NE 2d 373, 1978.
31. Kluge EH: Informed consent by children: The new reality. *Can Med Assoc J* 152:1495–1497, 1995.
32. Redding RE: Children's competence to provide informed consent for mental health treatment. *Washington & Lee Law Review* 50:695–753, 1993.
33. Koocher GP: Children under the law: The paradigm of consent, in Melton GB (ed): *Reforming the Law*. New York, Guilford Press, 1987.
34. Holder AR: Disclosure and consent problems in pediatrics. *Law Med Health Care* 16:219–228, 1988.
35. *Corpus Juris Secundum*, Parent and Child Sec 5–9.
36. Massachusetts General Laws, Ch 112 Sec 12F.
37. Code of Virginia, Art 15 Sec 16.1-334, 1990.
38. *Baird vs Attorney General*, 371 Mass 741, 360 NE 2d 288, 1971.
39. Arizona Laws of 1962, Title 44 Sec 44-133.01.
40. Arizona Laws of 1971, Title 44 Sec 44-132.01.
41. Code of Virginia, Art 6 Sec 54.1-2969.
42. Weithorn LA, Campbell SB: The competency of children and adolescents to make informed treatment decisions. *Child Dev* 53:1589–1598, 1982.
43. Dorn LD, Susman EJ, Fletcher JC: Informed consent in children and adolescents: Age, motivation and psychological state. *J Adolesc Health* 16:185–190, 1995.
44. Cauffman E, Steinberg L: The cognitive and affective influences on adolescent decision making. *Temple Law Review* 68:1763–1789, 1995.
45. American Academy of Pediatrics Committee on Broethics: Informed consent, parental permission, and assent in pediatric practice. *Pediatrics* 95(2):314–317, 1995.
46. *Rogers vs Commissioner of the Department of Mental Health*, 390 Mass 489, 458 NE 2d 308, 1983.

47. Appelbaum PS: The right to refuse treatment with antipsychotic medication: Retrospect and prospect. *Am J Psychiatry* 145:413–419, 1988.
48. *Guardianship of Roe*, 383 Mass 415, 421 NE 2d 40, 1981.
49. 110 Code of Massachusetts Regulations 11.00.
50. Barnum R: Decision making for children: The regulation of psychopharmacological treatment for children in public custody in Massachusetts. *Mass Family Law J* 7:21–31, 1989.
51. *Zummo vs Zummo*, 394 Pa S 30, 574 A 2d 1130 (Pa Super), 1990.
52. *Durfee vs Durfee*, 194 Misc 594, 87 NYS 2d 275 (NY S Ct), 1949.
53. Bernet W: The noncustodial parent and medical treatment. *Bull Am Acad Psychiatry Law* 21(3):357–364, 1993.
54. Weinstock R, Leong GB, Silva JA: Confidentiality and privilege, in Simon RI (ed): *Review of Clinical Psychiatry and the Law*. Washington DC, American Psychiatric Association Press, 1990, vol 1, pp 90–98.
55. Coyte PC, Dewees DN, Trebilcock MJ: Medical malpractice—The Canadian experience. *N Engl J Med* 324:89–93, 1991.
56. Danzon PM: The "crisis" in medical malpractice: A comparison of trends in the United States, Canada, the United Kingdom, and Australia. *Law Med Health Care* 18:48–58, 1990.
57. Quam L, Fenn P, Dingwale R: Medical malpractice in perspective II—The implications for Britain. *Br Med J* 294:1597–1600, 1987.
58. Tan MW, McDonough VJ: Risk management in psychiatry. *Psychiatric Clin North Am* 13:135–147, 1990.
59. *Tarasoff vs Regents of University of California*, 17 Calif 3d 425, 551 P 2d 334, 1976.
60. Schouten R: Informed consent: Resistance and reappraisal. *Crit Care Med* 17:1359–1361, 1989.
61. Gutheil TG, Bursztajn H, Brodsky A: Liability prevention through the sharing of uncertainty: Informed consent and the therapeutic alliance. *N Engl J Med* 311:49–51, 1984.
62. Appelbaum PS, Gutheil TG: *Clinical Handbook of Psychiatry and the Law*. Baltimore, Williams & Wilkins, 1991.
63. *Woods vs Brumlop*, 377 P 2d 520 (NM), 1962.
64. Gutheil TG: On apologizing to patients. *Risk Manage Found Forum* 8:3–4, 1987.
65. *Weaver vs. Reagen*, 886 F. 2d 194 (C.A. 8, 1989).
66. Rayburn WF: A physician's preogative to prescibe drugs for off-label uses during pregnancy. *Obstet Gynecol* 81:1052–1055, 1993.
67. Stoffelmayr KJ: Products liability and "off-label" uses of prescription drugs. *University of Chicago Law Review* 63:275–306, 1996.
68. American Academy of Pediatrics Committee on Drugs: Unapproved uses of approved drugs: The physician, the package insert, and the Food and Drug Administration: Subject review. *Pediatrics* 98(1):143–145, 1996.
69. Torres A: The use of Food and Drug Administration-approved medications for unlabelled (off-label) uses. *Arch Dermatol* 130:32–36, 1994.
70. *Klein vs. Biscup*, 109 Ohio App.3d 855, 673 N.E.2d 225 (Ohio App. 8 Dist.).

7

Disorders, Symptoms, and Their Pharmacotherapy

KELLY BOTTERON, M.D., and BARBARA GELLER, M.D.

I. INTRODUCTION

In this chapter, the issue of the relationship of diagnoses and dimensions to potential pharmacotherapeutic agents will be examined. The scope of this chapter does not include differential diagnoses, nor does it claim to cover the clinical aspects of any disorder in detail. For more in-depth diagnostic considerations, the reader should consult more comprehensive diagnostic texts in child and adolescent psychiatry.[1-3]

When the pioneering child psychopharmacology text[4] was published, the third edition of the *Diagnostic and Statistical Manual of Mental Disorders* (DSM-lll)[5] had been developed but not yet published. Psychiatry was just beginning to evolve the concept of empirically based criteria for psychiatric diagnostic classification. In the above-cited text,[4] Gittelman-Klein et al.[6] provided extensive discussion of and justification for the usefulness and benefits of specific categorical diagnoses. Currently, it is generally accepted in child psychiatry that categorical diagnoses may be relevant to pharmacotherapy and nondrug treatments. They improve treatment planning by providing a framework for the assessment of long-term prognosis and the consideration of typical comorbid conditions and by allowing a more critical assessment of the risk/benefit ratio for treatments. Operationally defined diagnostic classification has also enabled the study of more homogeneous populations of children; the latter has facilitated comparison of results between different institutions and across age groups.

KELLY BOTTERON, M.D. • Mallinckrodt Institute of Radiology, Washington University School of Medicine, St. Louis, Missouri 63110. BARBARA GELLER, M.D. • Department of Psychiatry, Washington University School of Medicine, St. Louis, Missouri 63110.

Practitioner's Guide to Psychoactive Drugs for Children and Adolescents (Second Edition), Werry and Aman, eds. Plenum Publishing Corporation, New York, 1999.

This chapter serves as a guide or map to the remainder of the book. It will provide a general discussion of both established and investigational medications for diagnostic categories applicable to child psychiatry. In addition, the pharmacotherapy of psychopathological dimensions (e.g., aggression, attention) will be outlined. The reader will then be referred to the appropriate chapter (and to recent review articles) for more specific discussions of each medication's potential benefits, side effects, pharmacokinetics, dosing, and so forth.

The diagnostic categorization and specific criteria discussed are in accordance with DSM-IV guidelines.[7] A brief review of important changes in criteria from DSM-III-R to DSM-IV is included in the description of each disorder. This is no reflection on other diagnostic systems such as RDC or ICD-10; however, most of the work on pharmacotherapy in children and adolescents during the past decade has been based on DSM criteria.

Before pharmacotherapy is instituted, a thorough psychiatric evaluation is necessary in order to establish the diagnoses and develop a comprehensive treatment plan. Guidelines for considering and prescribing medications are discussed in depth in Chapter 1. Pharmacotherapy should be evaluated on an individual case-by-case basis as a potential component of comprehensive management. The benefits and risks of pharmacotherapy must be thoughtfully weighed in the decision to initiate a trial of medication. **Additionally, it should be emphasized that this chapter only discusses pharmacotherapeutic indications for each disorder and does not cover psychotherapeutic, psychosocial, or other treatments which may be indicated.**

The importance of diagnostic categorization was dramatically illustrated by the early experience with lithium salts in the 1950s. Bipolar manic–depressive patients showed significant improvement and stabilization in contrast to minimal response in schizophrenic patients. Although diagnostic categorization is important, few medications are diagnosis-specific. For example, neuroleptics are potentially useful in multiple diagnostic disorders including schizophrenic or affective psychoses, tic disorders, pervasive developmental disorders, and aggressive conduct disorder.[8] Children and adolescents who present for treatment with psychiatric disorders often also demonstrate comorbid psychiatric disorders.[9,10] Thus, it is important to assess and consider comorbidity when formulating pharmacotherapeutic treatment plans. For example, attention-deficit hyperactivity disorder may be comorbid with an affective disorder,[11] and one could expect altered or attenuated treatment response if the pharmacotherapy only addresses one disorder. Treatment decisions may also be based on dimensional or symptomological considerations, as is often the case with the problems of aggression and hyperactivity. Thus, the choice of medication can be influenced not only by primary and comorbid diagnoses but also by certain individual symptoms.

Under each diagnostic category and dimensional heading where relevant data are available, the subsection of "potential pharmacotherapeutic mechanisms" will provide a discussion in broad terms of the neurochemical systems that are currently hypothesized to be related to the pharmacotherapeutic response in relation to the pathogenesis of the disorder. It should be emphasized that in all cases these hypotheses remain generally speculative and have undergone significant change over the past decade as knowledge continues to evolve. Thus, it is anticipated that these hypotheses will continue to be modified.

II. DISRUPTIVE BEHAVIOR DISORDERS

A. Attention-Deficit Hyperactivity Disorder

1. Diagnostic Features and Pharmacotherapy

Attention-deficit hyperactivity disorder (ADHD) has been historically described by a variety of clinical terms (e.g., minimal brain dysfunction, hyperactivity disorder, attention-deficit disorder, hyperkinetic reaction, etc.) and is characterized by inattention, motoric hyperactivity, and impulsive behaviors which significantly interfere with a child's social and academic functioning and which frequently persist into adolescence and adulthood. DSM-IV specifies three as yet unproven diagnostic types: ADHD, Predominantly Hyperactive–Impulsive Type; ADHD, Predominantly Inattentive Type; and ADHD, Combined Type. DSM-III-R only specified a combined type of ADHD; thus, many systematic investigations have been done only on the combined type of ADHD. The pharmacotherapeutic agents that are potentially useful in ADHD are summarized in Table 1.

a. Stimulants

Amphetamines were the first drugs studied for behavioral disorders in children. In 1937, Bradley[12] reported that amphetamine improved hyperactivity and impulsivity in children with conduct and emotional problems. Since that time, stimulants have been widely and successfully used for the treatment of inattention, hyperactivity, and impulsivity (see Chapter 8). The most commonly used stimulants are methylphenidate, dextroamphetamine, and magnesium pemoline. These agents are generally the first choice over tricyclic (TCAs) or heterocyclic antidepressants because of superiority in clinical improvement and fewer side effects. They may be effective for the cognitive and behavioral symptoms of ADHD throughout the life span[13–15](see Chapter 8). Stimulants have a more variable response

TABLE 1. Pharmacotherapy of Disruptive Disorders

Disorder	Potential drugs	Clinical priority[a]	Chapter
ADHD	Stimulants (methylphenidate, dextroamphetamine, pemoline)	1st	8
	Tricyclic antidepressants	2nd or 3rd	9
	Bupropion	2nd or 3rd	9
	α-agonists (clonidine, guanfacine)	Uncertain	15
	Neuroleptics	Uncertain	10
	MAOIs	Uncertain	9
Conduct disorder	Stimulants	1st	8
	Neuroleptics	2nd or 3rd	10
	Lithium	2nd or 3rd	9
	Carbamazepine	Uncertain	12
Oppositional defiant disorder	None		

[a]Refers to established efficacy in controlled studies. The numerical ordering (1st, 2nd, etc.) refers to suggested use based on a balance of efficacy and adverse effects. "Uncertain" means that the drug has not been established as effective via double-blind, placebo-controlled studies in children and adolescents.

in preschoolers, with the potential for increased side effects and the need for a lower dose. ADHD, predominantly inattentive type, may also be responsive to stimulants[16].

b. Antidepressants

Although tricyclic antidepressants have been demonstrated to be an alternative that can be useful in some cases (see Chapter 9), this must be tempered by occasional reports of sudden, unexplained deaths[17] and by high lethality from overdose. Several factors can influence the decision to use TCAs, such as patients who are poorly responsive or intolerant to stimulants or who have a significant component of anxiety or affective symptoms a strong family history of mood disorder, a personal or family history of tic disorder, or a family member who is at risk for abusing or selling stimulants. Desipramine, imipramine, and clomipramine have been investigated.[18–20]

Bupropion, a novel antidepressant, has also shown some promise in open and double-blind studies for the treatment of ADHD.[21,22]

c. Neuroleptics (Antipsychotics)

Neuroleptic medications have also been shown to reduce symptoms and improve hyperactive and impulsive behavior (see Chapter 10). However, serious concerns about potential tardive dyskinesia may limit their use to difficult and refractory cases.[20]

d. Other Drugs

Several other drugs have had limited investigation and may be useful for certain subgroups. These include clonidine[23] and guanfacine[24,25] (see Chapter 15), monoamine oxidase inhibitor antidepressants (MAOIs)[26] (see Chapter 9) and, lithium (see Chapter 9).

Several medications that were thought to have potential usefulness have yet to be proven effective in the treatment of ADHD. These include caffeine and several dopamine agonists: piribedil, amantadine, and L-DOPA.[15]

2. Potential Pharmacotherapeutic Mechanisms

Neurotransmitter hypotheses of ADHD have focused on the noradrenergic and dopaminergic systems.[15,27,28] Dopaminergic dysfunction is supported based on dopamine agonist poperties of all three commonly used stimulants. In support of noradrenergic dysfunction, there is evidence for altered autonomic (noradrenergic) function in ADHD children, and most of the clinically effective medications have some noradrenergic effects.[15] It has been hypothesized that medications which are effective in the treatment of ADHD have two common properties. First, they increase dopamine release, which results in enhanced autoreceptor-mediated inhibition of ascending dopamine neurons. Second, they increase inhibition of the noradrenergic locus coeruleus via increased adrenergic-mediated inhibition.[28] The proposed mechanism of action of several effective medications is outlined in further detail to illustrate the support for this hypothesis. Dextroamphetamine and methylphenidate increase dopamine and norepinephrine neurotransmission by increasing dopamine release, blocking presynaptic uptake, and inhibiting monoamine oxidase activity. Dextroamphetamine has an additional effect of increasing serotonin transmission, and methylphenidate has additional direct postsynaptic agonist activity.[29] Magnesium pemoline primarily affects dopamine transmission, with little sympathomimetic effects.[30] The effects of bupropion are unclear; however, it is reported to have indirect dopamine agonist effects.[31] MAOIs affect dopamine, serotonin, and norepinephrine. TCAs are primarily catecholamine reuptake inhibitors and thus enhance central noradrenergic tone.

B. Conduct Disorders

1. Diagnostic Features and Pharmacotherapy

Children with conduct disorder are characterized by a variety of persistent behavioral problems which violate the basic rights of others and which violate major age-appropriate societal norms and rules. Aggressive behavior, including fights, use of weapons, destruction of property, and cruelty to animals, is common. Other problem behaviors include stealing, lying, and running away.

The pharmacotherapy of conduct disorder (see Table 1) has been poorly studied. However, there is reason to believe that, because of the high degree of comorbidity in conduct disorder with ADHD,[32] at least some of the pharmacologic findings in ADHD may be applicable to conduct disorder. This awaits definitive confirmation. In fact, many of the early studies of ADHD included children with conduct disorder in addition to their ADHD, and there are repeated reports of improvement in symptoms like "aggression" and "noncompliance."[33,34]

Haloperidol and lithium are currently the best studied pharmacotherapeutic agents for conduct disorder. These drugs may reduce certain types of aggressive behavior, more typically impulsive aggression.[8,33,34] There are two types of aggression: impulsive, which is not part of a planned crime and is accompanied by guilt, versus predatory, which is part of a planned crime and is guiltless. Medications that help predatory aggression are not yet available (see Chapters 9 and 10). Older studies identified carbamazepine as potentially useful for impulsive aggression.[35] Although this was further supported in an open trial,[36] a recent double-blind trial with aggressive inpatient children did not find carbamazepine superior to placebo during a 6-week trial.[37] Other recent studies suggest that stimulants improve behavior in children with conduct disorder, and this evidence is discussed in Chapter 8.[33,34] There may be some role for the use of buspirone or trazodone.[38]

2. Potential Pharmacotherapeutic Mechanisms

Aggressive behavior, especially impulsive aggression, has been linked to alterations in central serotonergic (5-HT) function, which is seen as mediating inhibitory mechanisms. This hypothesis has been supported by the demonstration of decreased levels of 5-hydroxyindoleacetic acid (5-HIAA) in cerebrospinal fluid (CSF) in several adult investigations[39] and in children and adolescents.[40,41] Lithium, carbamazepine, β-blockers, buspirone, and trazodone all function in part as 5-HT blockers. This mechanism may be important to their antiaggressive properties.

C. Oppositional Defiant Disorder

Diagnostic Features and Pharmacotherapy

Children with oppositional defiant disorder (ODD) are characterized by chronic negativistic, hostile, and defiant behavior. They do not demonstrate the pattern of behavior that violates the rights of others which is seen in conduct disorder. There are no specific psychotropic medications currently used in the treatment of ODD; however, ODD is frequently a comorbid diagnosis in children with other psychiatric disorders such as ADHD or affective disorders. Treatment of the primary disorder often does improve the ODD behavior.

III. MOOD DISORDERS

A. Major Depressive Disorder

1. Diagnostic Features and Pharmacotherapy

Major depressive disorder (MDD) in children is phenomenologically similar to MDD in adults.[42,43] Childhood MDD in DSM-IV is characterized by dysphoric or irritable mood and at least four additional symptoms from the following eight: decreased interest; feelings of worthlessness or excessive guilt; impairment in concentration; decreased energy; sleep disturbance; change in appetite; psychomotor retardation or agitation; and morbid or suicidal ideation (DSM-lll-R). MDD may also be delusional.[42,44]

TABLE 2. Pharmacotherapy of Mood, Schizophrenic, and Developmental Disorders

Disorder	Potential drugs	Clinical priority[a]	Chapter
Major depressive disorder	Fluoxetine	1st	9
(MDD)	Tricyclic antidepressants	Uncertain	9
	MAOIs	Uncertain	9
	Lithium	Uncertain	9
Delusional MDD	Neuroleptics	Uncertain	10
Mania	Lithium	Uncertain	9
	Neuroleptics	Uncertain	10
	Carbamazepine	Uncertain	12
	Valproic acid	Uncertain	12
	Benzodiazepines	Uncertain	15
	Levothyroxine	Uncertain	
Comorbid: Bipolar, substance dependency	Lithium	1st	9
Schizophrenia	Typical neuroleptics	1st	10
	Atypical neuroleptics (clozapine)	1st or 2nd	10
	Lithium	Uncertain	9
	Carbamazepine	Uncertain	9
Dyslexia	Piracetam	Uncertain	14
Pervasive developmental	SSRIs (fluoxetine)	1st	9
disorders (autism)	Clomipramine	2nd	9
	Neuroleptics	3rd	10
	Naltrexone	Uncertain	15
	Buspirone	Uncertain	15
	Methylphenidate	Uncertain	8

[a]Refers to established efficacy in controlled studies. The numerical ordering (1st, 2nd, etc.) refers to suggested use based on a balance of efficacy and adverse effects. "Uncertain" means that the drug has not been established as effective via double-blind, placebo-controlled studies in children and adolescents.

The pharmacotherapeutics that are potentially useful in MDD are summarized in Table 2. TCAs have established efficacy in the treatment of adults with MDD. There were initially promising findings of response to TCAs in prepubertal children and adolescents in case reports and open study designs. Systematic investigations, however, have failed to demonstrate significant efficacy for TCAs over placebo[18,45–47] (see Chapter 9). Recently, fluoxetine has been demonstrated to be superior to placebo for children and adolescents with major depression,[48] though caution is needed since this is a single study. There are a number of case reports and small case series suggesting a possible role for other specific serotonin reuptake inhibitors (SSRIs) such as sertraline, fluvoxamine, or paroxeitine.[49,50] Other medications which are of potential use in depressed children include MAOIs or bupropion[18] (see Chapter 9). A double-blind controlled study of lithium for depressed prepubertal children with bipolar family histories was negative.[51]

2. Potential Pharmacotherapeutic Mechanisms

The neurotransmitter pathogenesis of MDD is generally hypothesized to be secondary to dysregulation of the noradrenergic, cholinergic, or serotonergic systems[52–54] Noradrenergic and serotonergic hypotheses are supported by characteristics of sleep disturbance, neuroendocrine changes, and pharmacotherapeutic response. For example, decreased norepinephrine correlates with decreased REM sleep latency (a common feature in adult MDD), and potentiating serotonin increases REM sleep latency.[53] In addition, postmortem studies of suicide victims generally show decreased levels of serotonin metabolites. TCAs affect noradrenergic and serotonergic systems to differential degrees but generally all work as catecholamine reuptake inhibitors.[18] MAOIs and lithium affect serotonergic and, to a lesser degree, noradrenergic mechanisms. Numerous findings in adults suggest that the therapeutic response to antidepressants is related to the upregulation of both serotonergic and noradrenergic systems.[18] Conversely, also consistently, downregulation (e.g., by antihypertensive agents) can provoke depression.

B. Bipolar Disorder

1. Diagnostic Features and Pharmacotherapy

In some instances, bipolar disorder may have its onset in prepubertal children and in adolescents.[55,56] Typical adult manic episodes are characterized by a distinct period of abnormally elevated, expansive, or irritable mood which causes marked functional impairment and is present along with at least three additional symptoms. These include grandiosity; decreased need for sleep; hypertalkativeness; racing thoughts; distractibility; increased goal-directed activity or agitation; and poor judgment with excessive involvement in pleasurable activities with potentially painful consequences. Prepubertal onset in children and adolescents may have mixed manic, nonepisodic, rapid-cycling features and comorbidity with ADHD.[55–57]

Lithium is the mainstay of treatment of bipolar disorder in adults (see Table 2). It may be useful in children and adolescents with the disorder, but no systematic study is yet available[45,56,58,59] (see Chapter 9). A recently completed double-blind, placebo-controlled study of adolescents with comorbid bipolar and secondary substance dependency disorders showed a positive outcome by both completer and intent-to-treat analyses for both the bipolar and substance dependency disorders.[60]

Other mood stabilizers which have been shown to be efficacious in adults have received only limited investigation in children, including carbamazepine[61] and valproic acid[59] (see Chapters 9 and 12), and benzodiazepines (e.g., clonazepam) (see Chapters 12 and 15). Similarly, calcium-channel blockers have received minimal attention in children and adolescents. Neuroleptics are also often used when psychotic symptoms are present and may be useful in prophylaxis (see Chapter 10). High-dose levothyroxine may have some benefit in rapid-cycling treatment-refractory cases.[62,63]

2. Potential Pharmacotherapeutic Mechanisms

Dysfunction in dopaminergic, noradrenergic, serotonergic, and/or GABAergic neurotransmitter systems has been reasonably implicated in the pathogenesis of bipolar affective disorder. Medication effects support these hypotheses. Neuroleptics clearly affect dopaminergic transmission. Carbamazepine has been demonstrated to reduce amygdaloid firing and stabilize the limbic system, probably through changes in all four above-mentioned neurotransmitter systems. Valproic acid may exert its effect secondary to its potentiation of GABAergic systems. The therapeutic mechanism of action of lithium in treating bipolar disorder is unknown. There are several theories, including reduction in catecholamine transmission through an effect on Na^+ and K^+-activated adenosine triphosphatase (Na^+-K^+ pump) with resulting reduced cAMP concentrations or on other second messenger systems.[64,65]

IV. SCHIZOPHRENIC DISORDERS

A. Diagnostic Features and Pharmacotherapy

Schizophrenia is a fluctuating but chronic disorder marked by characteristic psychotic symptoms such as hallucinations and delusions, disturbances in affect and form of thought, and markedly impaired function. Although it is recognized that schizophrenia frequently begins in adolescence and may in rare cases develop in childhood, there is a paucity of studies regarding the treatment of schizophrenia in this age group.

Antipsychotics have been shown clearly to be effective in the treatment of adult patients in more than 100 double-blind controlled studies.[66] There have recently been a few rigorous studies with DSM-III-R (or DSM-IV) criteria of neuroleptics in schizophrenic children.[67,68] There are reports that standard neuroleptics may be effective in adolescents[69] and children (see Chapter 10). Some investigators speculate that because of the increased evidence of negative symptoms in early-onset schizophrenia, newer atypical antipsychotics such as clozapine, risperidone, or olanzapine[8] may prove more useful (see Chapter 10). Clozapine has been demonstrated to decrease psychoses and improve function when compared to placebo.[68,70] Prepubertal-onset schizophrenia is understudied and rare.[68] Although antipsychotics, which are a standard and important part of treatment of adults, had previously been thought to be less effective in prepubertal schizophrenia,[71] recent investigation indicates that children respond favorably to haloperidol, the response being similar to that of adults[67,72] (see Chapter 10). Drugs (e.g., lithium or carbamazepine) more recently used in adults have not yet been studied in younger populations[61,73] (see Table 2).

B. Potential Pharmacotherapeutic Mechanisms

Complex abnormalities in the dopaminergic system, including differential areas of excessive and deficient dopaminergic function, are hypothesized to be related to schizophrenia.[66] More recent hypotheses implicate GABAergic systems interacting with dopaminergic systems.[74] In support of these hypotheses, all neuroleptic medications are dopamine reuptake blockers and alter dopaminergic systems. Newer atypical neuroleptics such as clozapine are less potent dopaminergic antagonists but have serotonergic properties and are reportedly more clinically effective. Additional support for this hypothesis comes from post-mortem, clinical, animal-model, and position-emission tomography (PET) studies which have found some supporting evidence for increased basal ganglia and decreased frontal cortex dopaminergic function.

V. DEVELOPMENTAL DISORDERS

A. Mental Retardation

1. Diagnostic Features and Pharmacotherapy

Mental retardation is defined by significantly subaverage intelligence (IQ < 70) and significant impairments in adaptive functioning with an onset before age 18. There are no specific treatments for the primary cognitive deficits of mental retardation. However, individuals with mental retardation are known to have the potential to develop the entire spectrum of other psychiatric disorders. They are reported to have a four- to- sixfold increased frequency of psychiatric disorders compared to the general population.[75,76] There is no reason *a priori* that a developmentally disabled individual may not suffer from any specific disorder and thus, when diagnosed, that pharmacotherapy should differ. However, most attention has been focused not on disorder but on troublesome behaviors.

In general, the reports of medication trials in the mentally retarded population have had methodologic limitations.[77] The pharmacotherapy of individuals with mental retardation has often focused on aggressive and self-injurious behaviors rather than diagnostic disorders. Various drugs may be clinically useful for aggression in this population including neuroleptics[78] (see Chapter 10), lithium[79] (see Chapter 9), carbamazepine[61,80] (see Chapter 12), β blockers[81–83] (see Chapter 15), and opiate agonists and antagonists (e.g., naloxone and naltrexone)[81] (see Chapter 15).

Earlier, it had been hypothesized that attentional difficulties were a part of the syndrome of mental retardation that were not amenable to pharmacotherapy. Recent studies have, however, supported the usefulness and efficacy of treating attention-deficit symptoms in the mildly mentally retarded with stimulant medications[16,84] (see Chapter 8). Stimulants may not improve attention and may exacerbate stereotypies or behavioral problems in some mentally retarded patients; generally, this is more likely in the more severe or profoundly retarded subgroup[84,85] (see Chapter 8). Fenfluramine has been demonstrated to be beneficial for attentional difficulties and hyperactivity in some of these children[86,87] but has recently been pulled off the market in the United States secondary to an association with valvular heart disease and pulmonary hypertension in adults taking fenfluramine for weight loss.

2. Potential Pharmacotherapeutic Mechanisms

Mental retardation is a heterogeneous diagnosis encompassing multiple etiologies, including a wide variety of chromosomal, metabolic, structural, and perinatal disorders which have a variety of associated neurochemical changes. As noted, more attention needs to be given to making specific disorder diagnoses, with less overinclusive thinking using "mental retardation."

B. Specific Developmental Disorders

Diagnostic Features and Pharmacotherapy (see Table II)

There are eight specific developmental disorders currently classified in DSM-IV: reading disorder, mathematics disorder, disorder of written expression, phonological disorder, expressive language disorder, mixed receptive–expressive language disorder, stuttering, and developmental coordination disorder. Currently, medications are not clinically available for the treatment of specific developmental disorders. There have been several investigations of dyslexic reading disorder children treated with piracetam[88-90] (see Chapter 14); however, piracetam is not currently clincally available in the United States. These disorders may benefit from treatment of comorbid ADHD.

C. Pervasive Developmental Disorder

1. Diagnostic Features and Pharmacotherapy

The pervasive developmental disorders (PDD) are a heterogeneous group of disorders which have undergone several changes in their classification during the evolution of DSM criteria. DSM-IV currently specifies five related PDD diagnoses: autistic disorder, Rett's disorder, childhood disintegrative disorder, Asperger's disorder, and PDD not otherwise specified. There is reason to suspect that all of these, except Rett's disorder, are variants of autism (except the rare cases of disintegrative disorder). The subgroup of infantile autism has been the focus of the majority of drug studies in this category. Children with infantile autism are characterized by impairments in social relatedness, language, cognition, communicative behaviors, and sensory modulation. They also are characteristically resistant to change and often exhibit stereotypic movements and behaviors.

Recently, several serotonin reuptake inhibitors (SSRIs), including clomipramine, fluoxetine, and fluvoxamine (see Chapter 9), have been shown to have significant effects in reducing aggressive and stereotypic behaviors along with demonstrated improvement in cognitive flexibility and social relatedness.[91-93]

Haloperidol, a dopamine antagonist, has been shown to be superior to placebo in producing clinical improvement in stereotypies, hyperactivity, aggression, and discriminant learning in autistic children[71,94] (see Chapter 10). The use of haloperidol in this population is associated with a significant rate (approximately 30%) of drug-related dyskinesias.[71] Lower-potency neuroleptics have been reported to be associated with more side effects, including impairment in cognitive functioning in this population. Pimozide, a high-potency neuroleptic, may prove useful (see Chapter 10). Haloperidol may also be effective for the control of hyperactivity and aggression in childhood-onset and atypical pervasive development disorder.[95] Newer atypical neuroleptics, such as risperidone and olanzapine, may offer significant benefits with improved side-effect profiles.[96]

Because problems with attention, distractibility, and hyperactivity are highly prevalent features in children with PDD, DSM-IV criteria exclude a separate diagnosis of ADHD if a child is diagnosed with PDD. However, significant difficulties with hyperactivity, distractibility, and impulsivity may respond to stimulant medications in some children with PDD or autism[84,97,98] (see Chapter 8). Drugs that may be useful for some patients with hyperactivity, withdrawal, or stereotypies include fenfluramine (now withdrawn from the U.S. market), naltrexone, clonidine (see Chapter 15), or buspirone[94] (see Chapter 15).

Pharmacotherapy in autism (see Table 2) can decrease aggressivity and hyperactivity and can facilitate the child's responsiveness and ability to participate in other treatment modalities, including behavioral and educational interventions.[99]

2. Potential Pharmacotherapeutic Mechanisms (see Table II)

Neurobiochemical studies in autism suggest that there may be several subgroups of patients who show either increased serotonergic or dopaminergic function and noradrenergic or endogenous opioid dysfunction.[100–102] These subgroups have not yet been clearly identified, and it is not currently possible to distinguish them clinically. Antidopaminergic drugs such as haloperidol and other neuroleptics may be useful in lessening some symptoms. Additionally, a subgroup of patients show increased CSF levels of homovanillic acid (HVA; a major dopamine metabolite) which correlate with some symptoms. In support of serotonergic dysfunction, there is a subgroup of children with autism with increased serum serotonin and altered CSF serotonin metabolites.[102] There are several serotonergic medications which are potentially useful, including flenfluramine (see Chapter 15), clomipramine, and fluoxetine (see Chapter 9). In support of opioid dysfunction, some autistic children have elevated CSF endorphin levels. This finding is hypothesized to be related to self-injurious behavior in some patients with autism.[101,103] Additionally, opiate antagonists such as naltrexone have shown some promise (see Chapter 15).

VI. EATING DISORDERS

A. Anorexia Nervosa

Diagnostic Features and Pharmacotherapy

Anorexia nervosa is an eating disorder which is characterized by marked weight loss or failure to make expected weight gain during a period of growth that leads to a maintenance body weight at least 15% below an ideal weight. Additionally, anorectics exhibit distortions in body image and profound fear of becoming fat. Significant medical and psychiatric sequelae are also present (DSM-IV).

Numerous pharmacotherapies have been investigated in the treatment of anorexia, including TCAs, neuroleptics, lithium, and cyproheptadine. However, none has yet been shown to be efficacious in the treatment of primary anorexia nervosa.[104–105] Clomipramine, fluoxetine, and cyproheptadine may be useful (Table 3) (see Chapters 9, 10, and 15).

**TABLE 3. Pharmacotherapy of Eating,
Anxiety, Tic, and Sleep Disorders**

Disorder	Potential drugs	Clinical priority[a]	Chapter
Anorexia nervosa	Fluoxetine	Uncertain	9
	Cyproheptadine	Uncertain	15
Bulimia nervosa	Tricyclic antidepressants	1st or 2nd	9
	Fluoxetine/SSRIs	1st or 2nd	9
	MAOIs	Uncertain	9
	Lithium	Uncertain	9
	Carbamazepine	Uncertain	12
Pica	None		
Rumination disorder of infancy	None		
Generalized anxiety disorder	Unknown		
Separation anxiety disorder	Imipramine	Uncertain	9
Posttraumatic stress disorder	Imipramine	Uncertain	9
	Benzodiazepines	Uncertain	15
	β-Blockers	Uncertain	15
Obsessive–compulsive disorder	SSRIs	1st	9
	Clomipramine	2nd	9
Tourette's disorder	Pimozide	1st	10
	Haloperidol	2nd	10
	Clonidine	Uncertain	15
	SSRIs	Uncertain	9
	Clonazepam	Uncertain	15
	Nifedipine	Uncertain	15
	Verapamil	Uncertain	15
Night terrors and	Imipramine	Uncertain	9
somnambulism	Benzodiazepines	Uncertain	15
Enuresis	Imipramine	1st	9
	Desmopressin	1st	
Encopresis	None		

[a]Refers to established efficacy in controlled studies. The numerical ordering (1st, 2nd, etc.) refers to suggested use based on a balance of efficacy and adverse effects. "Uncertain" means that the drug has not been established as effective via double-blind, placebo-controlled studies in children and adolescents.

B. Bulimia Nervosa

1. Diagnostic Features and Pharmacotherapy

There can be substantial comorbidity between anorexia and bulimia nervosa. By DSM-IV criteria, bulimia is characterized by recurrent episodes of binge eating along with efforts to counteract the binge by purging, vigorous exercise, use of laxatives, or strict dieting. There is a preoccupation with shape and weight. Several antidepressant medications have shown promise for the reduction of binging behavior in those with bulimia. These include imipramine, desipramine, amitriptyline, fluoxetine, and MAOIs[104–106] (see Chapter 9). Several other drugs have received some preliminary attention including lithium, carbamazepine, and fenfluramine[106] (Table 3) (see Chapters 9, 12, and 15).

2. Potential Pharmacotherapeutic Mechanisms

There is evidence of neurochemical dysfunction for both patients with anorexia nervosa and those with bulimia. There is support for noradrenergic, serotonergic, dopaminergic, and opioid dysregulation.[107] The exact alterations and their potential relationship to loss of weight rather than disease factors are not yet clearly defined.[107]

C. Pica

Diagnostic Features and Pharmacotherapy

Children with pica persistently eat non-nutritive substances such as paint, plaster, string, and dirt. The disorder tends to occur in toddlers and rarely persists past early childhood. Sometimes it is coexistent with mental retardation or other developmental disorders.[1] The presence of pica may be associated with a nutritional, generally mineral, deficiency and may respond to appropriate replacement therapy (see Chapter 14). Behavioral management techniques are used to decrease the frequency of the behavior. There are no specific medications that are currently recommended unless the pica is of lead-based substances (e.g., older interior wall paint). Chelating agents would then be indicated.

D. Rumination Disorder of Infancy

Diagnostic Features and Pharmacotherapy

Rumination disorder is a rare disorder wherein an infant with previously normal development experiences repeated regurgitation of food with subsequent weight loss and malnutrition (DSM-IV). There can be life-threatening complications. Current treatment focuses on hospitalization with refeeding and copious attention. No psychotropics are currently recommended.

VII. SEXUAL DISORDERS

DSM-IV specifies two main categories of sexual disorders: (1) sexual dysfunction disorders (desire, arousal, orgasmic, and pain disorders) and (2) paraphilias. There is little psychiatric literature in general on adolescent sexual dysfunction disorders or paraphilias. Psychopharmacology studies with adolescents with sexual disorders are virtually nonexistent. However, given the potentially serious nature of sexually aggressive behavior associated with some paraphilic disorders or within the context of other Axis I psychiatric disorders, it is worth noting some treatment strategies studied for adults with these disorders. In adults, there is substantial experience with the use of antiandrogen therapies.[108] High-dose intramuscular medroxyprogesterone acetate (MPA), oral medroxyprogesterone,[109] or cyproterone[110] have been reported to decrease paraphilic obsessions and behaviors. Early experience suggests there may also be a role for SSRIs in the treatment of paraphilias.[111]

VIII. GENDER IDENTITY DISORDERS

Gender identity disorder is characterized by an intense chronic distress over the biological gender and expressed strong desire to be the opposite sex. Currently, there are no pharmacologic treatments.[112]

IX. ANXIETY DISORDERS

Childhood anxiety disorders are characterized by pervasive, functionally impairing, nonpsychotic anxiety. Classification of childhood anxiety disorders was revised and reorganized in the transition from DSM-III-R to DSM-IV. DSM-IV shifts toward maintaining continuity between anxiety disorders in children and adults. However, these changes influence the generalizability of earlier pharmacologic (and other) studies in childhood anxiety disorders, which have largely been completed using DSM-III or DSM-III-R criteria. Despite the frequency of anxiety disorders, there have been relatively few well-designed medication trials reported.[113] The major changes from DSM-III-R to DSM-IV are the inclusion of overanxious disorder of childhood under generalized anxiety disorder, the elimination of school phobia, which appears now to be more generally subsumed under separation anxiety disorder, and the elimination of childhood avoidant disorder. Many children with avoidant disorder would now be classified under the diagnosis of social phobia.

A. Generalized Anxiety Disorder

Diagnostic Features and Pharmacotherapy

DSM-IV eliminated the previous category in DSM-III-R of overanxious disorder of childhood and included it under the more general adult category of generalized anxiety disorder. By DSM-III-R criteria, children with overanxious disorder are characterized by excessive anxiety and doubts which persist over long periods and are functionally impairing. These children often worry about future and past events and about self-competence and performance; they may have coexisting somatic complaints and other anxiety or depressive disorders. Generalized anxiety disorder is characterized by excessive anxiety and worry associated with at least one of the following symptoms: restlessness, fatigue, difficulty concentrating, irritability, muscle tension, and sleep disturbance. At present, little is known about the role of pharmacotherapy for either children previously described as having overanxious disorder or children currently defined as having generalized anxiety disorder.[113] Anectodal case reports suggest a possible role for buspirone (Chapter 15) and SSRIs.[114]

B. Separation Anxiety Disorder

Diagnostic Features and Pharmacotherapy

Separation anxiety disorder is characterized by excessive anxiety about separation from parents or major attachment figures that is more pronounced than would be expected for the child's developmental level. When separation does occur, the child's anxiety may escalate to the point of panic. The patients are generally preoccupied with worries about the safety of their parents or themselves. A majority of children with separation anxiety disorder also manifest school phobia or school refusal. School phobia is no longer listed as a separate disorder in DSM-IV. Separation anxiety and school phobia are often related to later panic disorder and agoraphobia in adulthood, where antidepressants and benzodiazepines have been shown to be helpful.

Earlier investigations had demonstrated imipramine to be effective in the treatment of school phobia in children;[18,115] however, recent studies with imipramine and other tricyclic antidepressants have not replicated these positive results.[116] Small doses of short-acting benzodiazepines may have a role in the treatment of anticipatory anxiety in children with school phobia and separation anxiety disorder[82] (see Chapter 15). Recent studies have also begun to examine the potential role of serotonin reuptake inhibitors[114] and clonazepam[117] (see Chapter 15).

C. Panic Disorder

Diagnostic Features and Pharmacotherapy

Panic disorder is characterized by recurrent unexpected panic attacks (a discrete period of intense fear or discomfort with associated symptoms such as elevated heart rate, sweating, trembling, feeling short of breath, and dizziness). Panic disorder is frequently comorbid with other anxiety disorders and may respond to treatment for these anxiety disorders. Panic has not been well studied in children or adolescents. A few studies suggest possible usefulness of clonazepam[118] though serotonergic antidepressants such as imipramine or clomipramine are the mainstay in adult treatment and are not potential drugs of dependence like benzodiazepines (see Chapters 11 and 15).

D. Selective Mutism

Diagnostic Features and Pharmacotherapy

Children with selective mutism do not speak in certain situations. Generally, they do not speak with people outside their immediate family and thus are impaired at school and in social situations. Selective mutism may be related to social phobia. There has recently been some support for the role of fluoxetine in the treatment for this disorder.[119]

E. Social Phobia

Diagnostic Features and Pharmacotherapy

Social phobia in DSM-IV replaces what was previously termed childhood avoidant disorder in DSM-III-R. Children with avoidant disorder are generally characterized by their avoidance of contact with strangers or new situations although they interact warmly and comfortably with close family and familiar people. Their avoidance significantly interferes with social functioning and peer relationships and is of long-standing duration. Children with avoidant disorder often have other comorbid anxiety disorders. Along with other features of this disorder, pharmacotherapy has not been well studied. There is some support for the usefulness of SSRIs in reducing social anxiety.[113]

F. Posttraumatic Stress Disorder

Diagnostic Features and Pharmacotherapy

Posttraumatic stress disorder (PTSD) can develop in children and adolescents follow-ing a severe stressor that is outside the realm of usual human expcrience. The general symptoms include greater than one month of intrusive recurrent recollection of the event, avoidance of associated stimuli, numbing of general responsiveness, and persistent in-creased arousal. Currently, little is known about pharmacotherapy of this disorder in children and adolescents. Propranolol may improve affective, cognitive, and physiologic symptoms of PTSD.[120] Other medications which may be useful as adjuvants to treatment include clonidine (see Chapter 15), TCAs (see Chapter 9), and benzodiazepines[121] (see Chapters 12 and 15).

G. Reactive Attachment Disorder of Infancy or Early Childhood

Diagnostic Features and Pharmacotherapy

Children with reactive attachment disorder show significant disturbance and develop-mentally inappropriate social relatedness in multiple contexts beginning before the age of 5 years. Associated with this behavior DSM-IV specifies that there be evidence of patho-genic care, such as persistent disregard of the child's basic emotional or physical needs and/ or repeated changes of a primary caregiver. Any role of pharmacotherapy in this disorder is not defined at this time.

H. Obsessive—Compulsive Disorder

1. Diagnostic Features and Pharmacotherapy

Obsessive–compulsive disorder (OCD) can be a particularly disabling disorder which begins in one-half to one-third of cases in childhood or adolescence.[122,123] Children with OCD have intrusive repetitive thoughts and repetitive compulsive behaviors which disrupt their functioning. Significant advances in the treatment of OCD have been made over the past several years. Although in the past there was little effective pharmacotherapy avail-able, several of the SSRIs have now been demonstrated to be effective in decreasing obsessive and compulsive symptoms in children and adolescents with OCD. Clomipra-mine, fluvoxamine, and fluoxetine have been demonstrated in double-blind trials to be efficacious in the treatment of childhood and adolescent OCD[49,124,125] (see Chapter 9). Anectodal evidence supports the potential utility of newer SSRIs, such as paroxetine, sertraline, or nefazodone.[113]

2. Potential Pharmacotherapeutic Mechanisms

There are several neurotransmitter systems which are hypothesized to be involved in the expression of fear and anxiety.[126,127] Current thinking emphasizes the importance of serotonergic dysfunction in conjunction with alterations in noradrenergic and GABAergic systems. γ-Aminobutyric acid (GABA) is recognized as the most important and pervasive inhibitory neurotransmitter in the CNS. Benzodiazepines interact directly with GABA receptors to facilitate GABA release. Changes in plasma serotonin precursor levels are associated with stress and anxiety, and SSRIs have been demonstrated to be effective treatments in adults. Additionally, TCAs have been shown to decrease measures of noradrenergic function[126,127] and may be an effective treatment.

The serotonergic system is hypothesized to be the major neurotransmitter system involved in the pathophysiology of OCD, along with possible dopaminergic dysfunction.[128] Clomipramine and fluoxetine exert their main pharmacologic effects via selective serotonin reuptake inhibition. Additionally, decreases in CSF serotonin metabolites during clomipramine treatment have been shown to correlate with clinical response.[128]

X. TIC DISORDERS

A. Simple Tics

Diagnostic Features and Pharmacotherapy

Tics are repetitive, stereotyped, rapid involuntary movements usually in the head and neck region. They are common in children aged 7–12 years and are seldom a problem except when severe, chronic, or multiple. Most of the pharmacotherapy studies have therefore focused on Tourette syndrome, especially since the pharmacotherapy of tic disorders is not without hazards.

B. Tourette's Disorder

1. Diagnostic Features and Pharmacotherapy

Tourette syndrome is a debilitating disorder of childhood onset which is characterized by motor and phonic tics and by behavioral and psychological problems. The most effective drugs for reducing motor and verbal tics are neuroleptics, notably haloperidol, pimozide, and fluphenazine.[8,129,130] There is some evidence for differential relative efficacy, with pimozide being superior to haloperidol in treatment efficacy and side-effect profile[131] (see Chapter 10). Clonidine may have potential for treating behavioral and attentional problems in Tourette syndrome along with less efficacious reduction of tics, either when used alone or in combination with a neuroleptic[23,81,130] (see Chapter 15). Newer atypical neuroleptics, such as risperidone, which have fewer of the extrapyramidal side effects that limit the usefulness of other neuroleptics may have some role in reducing tics and comorbid OCD symptoms.[132]

A portion of Tourette syndrome patients also meet criteria for obsessive–compulsive disorder, which, though perhaps integral to the disorder, can be conveniently represented as a comorbid disorder. Preliminary reports suggest, as would be expected, that these symptoms may benefit from medications efficacious in OCD alone, including clomipramine and fluoxetine[134] (see Chapter 9).

Other potentially useful medications for Tourette's disorder include clonazepam (see Chapter 12), nifedipine and verapamil (see Chapter 15), and naloxone and tetrabenazine[129] (see Chapter 15).

A significant percentage of patients with Tourette's disorder also may have problems with hyperactivity, concentration, impulsivity, and distractibility. It was previously believed that stimulant medications were contraindicated in these children because of the possibility of precipitating or exacerbating the tic disorder. Current family history and drug study data suggest that stimulants may be safe to use in many of these patients[135,136] (see Chapter 8) or that these patients may benefit from TCAs.[133]

2. Potential Pharmacotherapeutic Mechanisms

There are hypotheses implicating several neurochemical systems in the pathophysiology of Tourette syndrome, specifically dopaminergic, noradrenergic, and serotonergic dysfunction in basal ganglia–frontal cortex circuits.[138]

XI. PSYCHOACTIVE SUBSTANCE ABUSE AND DEPENDENCE DISORDERS

Alcohol and illicit substance abuse can begin in late childhood and early adolescence and cause significant impairment and morbidity. Children and adolescents with substance disorders often have coexisting additional psychiatric diagnoses, including bipolar disorder.[139,140] Recently, there has been interest in the investigation of the potential pharmacotherapy of substance abuse in adolescents [National Institute of Drug Abuse (NIDA)].[141] There are three distinct potential aims of pharmacotherapy for substance abuse and dependence in adolescents: (1) treatment of the abuse and dependence itself, (2) treatment of withdrawal effects, and (3) treatment of comorbid or underlying psychiatric disorders. The pharmacotherapy of substance abuse has largely been studied in adults but has potential application to adolescents. Examples of treatment aimed at the primary abuse and dependence include disulfiram (Antabuse®) for alcohol dependence and methadone for opiate dependence (see Chapter 11). Withdrawal syndromes can be distressing and potentially life-threatening. Alcohol and other sedative withdrawal is potentially dangerous and is treated by substituting a cross-tolerant drug, such as a benzodiazepine (see Chapter 11), which is gradually tapered. Opiate withdrawal can be treated with methadone or clonidine (see Chapter 11). Substance abuse in adolescents with comorbid or psychiatric disorders may improve with treatment of the underlying psychiatric disorder. A double-blind controlled trial of lithium for comorbid bipolar disorder and substance dependency in adolescents showed a positive outcome for both disorders[60,141] (see Chapter 9). Substance abuse is covered in more detail in Chapter 11.

XII. SLEEP DISORDERS

Night terrors and somnambulism are the most important sleep disorders in children. Somnambulism, or sleepwalking, is characterized by sudden apparent arousal wherein the child walks about clumsily and may utter words and have stereotyped movements. Night terrors are characterized by sudden arousal with terrified screaming, difficulty in being consoled, and signs of intense autonomic discharge. As is true with somnambulism, the child is amnestic for the experience. Both disorders have been shown to be phenomena of disturbed stage 3 and stage 4 sleep.[142,143]

Generally, these disorders are short-lived with only sporadic episodes and do not warrant pharmacotherapy. However, benzodiazepines (such as clonazepam) or imipramine may be useful when these disorders are severe enough to warrant pharmacotherapy.[82,142,143]

XIII. ELIMINATION DISORDERS

A. Enuresis

1. Diagnostic Features and Pharmacotherapy

Children with enuresis are characterized by repeated involuntary elimination of urine at inappropriate times after the age of 3 or 4. This disorder can be primary, meaning that bladder control was never fully achieved, or secondary. Behavioral therapies are the treatment of choice in enuresis; however, pharmacotherapy with imipramine has been shown to be helpful in lessening the symptoms[18,144] (see Chapter 9). Treatment with imipramine, however, carries risks, and many relapses occur during and after medication withdrawal. Desmopressin has been demonstrated to be an effective treatment option.[145] Several other drugs have been less well studied but may be useful, including clomipramine (see Chapter 9).

2. Potential Pharmacotherapeutic Mechanisms

The mechanism of therapeutic action of the TCAs in enuresis is hypothesized to be secondary to changes in norepinephrine metabolism. Other strictly anticholinergic drugs are not effective, and antidepressants with stronger noradrenergic and weaker serotonergic effects have been found to be most efficacious.[18]

B. Encopresis

Diagnostic Features and Pharmacotherapy

A child can be classified as encopretic if the child has repeated passage of feces in inappropriate places at least once a month for six months. Encopresis can be primary or secondary, based on the absence or presence of a prior period of at least one year of fecal continence. The treatment and evaluation of encopresis involves a thorough medical exam, and drug treatment consists of stool softeners and laxatives.[146] There are no known effective psychotropic medications.

XIV. PERSONALITY DISORDERS (AXIS II DISORDERS)

Personality disorders are generally defined by long-standing, enduring patterns of behavior and inner experience that have their onset in childhood or adolescence and deviate markedly from the expectation of the individual's culture. DSM-IV defines that problem behavior or inner experience is manifested in at least two of the following areas: (1) cognitive perceptions of the self and others, (2) affective responsiveness, (3) interpersonal functioning, and (4) impulse control. The pattern of behavior is inflexible and generalized across different environments and social situations and leads to clinically significant impairment and distress. Finally, the symptoms and enduring pattern cannot be Nbetter accounted for as a manifestation or consequence of another disorder.[7]

The 10 personality disorders specified in DSM-IV are clustered into three different subtypes. Cluster A includes paranoid, schizoid, and schizotypal personality disorders. Cluster B includes antisocial, borderline, and histrionic personality disorders. Cluster C includes avoidant, dependent, and obsessive–compulsive personality disorders. A full description of their symptoms and classification is beyond the scope of this chapter. There is no empirical support in child or adolescent populations for pharmacotherapeutic treatment of a primary personality disorder diagnosis. Individuals with a clear comorbid Axis I disorder may benefit from treatment of the Axis I disorder; however, their response is often less robust than that of individuals without comorbid personality disorders. This is an area in need of much further research to clarify the indication or efficacy of pharmacotherapeutic agents.

XV. DIMENSIONAL CONSIDERATIONS

A. Aggression

1. Clinical Features and Pharmacotherapy

Aggression can be subclassified into two different types: impulsive–reactive and proactive. In the former, the aggression is impulsive and often reactive, and in the latter it is more premeditated and calculated (e.g., intimidation for theft). Pharmacotherapy appears to have more potential for helping to diminish or prevent reactive–impulsive aggression.[147] Aggression and violent behavior directed toward self or others can be features of several diagnoses. Treatment may be difficult. Many different medications, and medication classes, have been tried and reported to be modestly helpful in the treatment of impulsive aggression,[33,148] including neuroleptics (see Chapter 10), lithium (see Chapter 9), anticonvulsants (see Chapter 12), benzodiazepines (see Chapters 12 and 15), stimulants (see Chapter 8), and β-blockers, clonidine, buspirone, trazodone, naloxone, and naltrexone (see Chapter 15).

2. Potential Pharmacotherapeutic Mechanisms

Changes in serotonin metabolism associated with suicidal behavior have been reported in many, but not all, studies.[149,150] Postmortem brain studies of suicide victims and CSF studies in suicide attempters have demonstrated decreased levels of 5-HIAA, a serotonin metabolite. These changes are felt to reflect reduced CNS serotonin tone and have been reported across diagnostic categories including affective disorders, alcoholism, schizophrenia, and personality disorders. Additionally, irritability and nonpremeditated aggression have been associated with decreased CSF levels of 5-HIAA.[39] It is hypothesized that 5-HT may play a role in inhibitory behavioral systems mitigating against impulsive or affect-driven acts.

Self-injurious or self-mutilatory behavior may have different underlying mechanisms from suicidal or outwardly directed impulsive aggressive behavior. There are two main theories of neurotransmitter abnormalities related to self-injurious behavior: dysregulation of dopaminergic systems or dysregulation of endogenous opiate systems.[151] The dopamine model, which posits a link to endogenous reward systems, is based on animal lesion studies and neuropathic findings in select self-mutilating patients. Neuroleptics and dopamine receptor antagonists may be useful in the treatment of self-injurious behavior,[152,153] although not all neuroleptics appear to be equally effective: those with higher D_1 antagonist activity may be more effective[152] (See Chapter 10). Dysregulation in the endogenous opiate system has been demonstrated in some patients with self-injurious behavior, as well as subgroups of autistic children.[100,101,153,154] The opiate antagonists naltrexone and naloxone have both been investigated for their role in decreasing self-injurious behavior[81,152] (see Chapter 15). This endogenous opiate model differs from the pleasure-seeking dopamine model by positing a decreased pain threshhold and self-reinforcing effect of injurious behavior related to increased levels of endogenous opioids in these individuals.

B. Attention

Clinical Features and Pharmacotherapy

Problems with attention and concentration are present as a feature of many diagnostic categories other than ADHD, including mental retardation, pervasive developmental disorders, major depressive disorder, mania, Tourette's disorder, and psychotic disorders. The same mechanisms may not underlie the attentional disturbances in all of these disorders, and thus they are observed to respond differently to pharmacotherapy. Attentional deficits in affective and psychotic disorders are best remediated by treatment of the primary disorder (see Chapters 9 and 10). However, in children with Tourette's disorder, attentional problems and impulsivity may persist or be partially remediated by treatment with neuroleptics or clonidine (see Chapter 10). There has been debate about, and recent support for, the potential usefulness of stimulant medication (as in traditional ADHD treatment) despite its potential to exacerbate tics[135,136](see Chapter 8). Children and adolescents with mental retardation in the milder ranges appear to respond to stimulant medications similarly to ADHD children; however, response is more variable for individuals with more profound retardation.[87]

Aman[84,87,155] has proposed a model to explain this phenomenon, noting that stimulant medications constrict and focus attention in anyone who takes them; this is true in normal adults and children, subjects with attention-deficit disorder, and mentally retarded subjects. Attentional difficulties in many individuals with mental retardation can be characterized as being narrow and overselective, and this in general intensifies with increasingly severe intellectual impairment. Thus, this subgroup is thought to be less likely to respond and may develop increased problems with stimulant medications. However, there is variability in response, and some children and adults with moderate to severe mental retardation have a positive response to stimulants. Additional work is needed to assess levels of restricted attention in order to better predict treatment responses.[84] Similarly, some, but not all, children with autism may have a poor response to stimulants, related to the mechanism discussed above.

XVI. SUMMARY

This overview shows that pharmacotherapy has a solid and growing role in the treatment of children and adolescents. The specific indications and usefulness of psychotropic medications have often been discovered serendipitously; however, increasingly over the past several decades the development of useful psychotropic agents has been based on neurochemical rationales. Some of these rationales have been briefly outlined here to high-light how pharmacotherapy research is moving from an exclusively empirically driven approach to theoretically driven pharmacotherapies which are then empirically tested. This is likely to lead to escalating progress in pediatric psychopharmacology. Similarly, there is an increasingly rational approach to prescribing psychotropics in children, and their use presupposes good diagnostic ability and procedures. Additionally, no child or adolescent should receive pharmacotherapy without simultaneous attention to other facets of their presenting problems within the supportive relationship which every prescribing physician should provide for the child and his or her family.

It is our expressed hope that this chapter provides practitioners with a useful "algo-rithm" to pharmacologic treatment for children with psychiatric disorders and serves as a guide to the remaining chapters of the book.

ACKNOWLEDGMENT. This work was supported in part by National Institute of Mental Health grants MH01292, (Dr. Botteron) and R01MH40273 and R01MH53063 (Dr. Geller).

REFERENCES

1. Lewis M: *Child and Adolescent Psychiatry: A Comprehensive Textbook.* Baltimore: Williams & Wilkins, 1996.
2. Rutter M, Hersov L, and Taylor E: *Child and Adolescent Psychiatry: Modern Approaches* ed 3. Oxford, England, Blackwell Scientific Publications, 1993.
3. Weiner JM: *Textbook of Child and Adolescent Psychiatry.* Washington, DC, American Psychiatric Press, 1997.
4. Werry JS *Pediatric Psychopharmacology: The Use of Behavior Modifying Drugs in Children.* New York, Brunner/Mazel, 1978.
5. American Psychiatric Association: *Diagnostic and Statistical Manual of Mental Disorders,* 3rd ed revised (DSM-III-R). Washington, DC, American Psychiatric Association Press, 1987.
6. Gittelman-Klein R, Spitzer RL, Cantwell DP: Diagnostic classifications and psychopharmacological indica-tions, In Werry JS, (ed): *Pediatric Psychopharmacology: The Use of Behavior Modifying Drugs in Children.* New York, Brunner/Mazel, 1978.
7. American Psychiatric Association: *Diagnostic and Statistical Manual of Mental Disorders,* ed 4. (DSM-IV). Washington, DC, American Psychiatric Association Press, 1994.
8. Teicher MH, Glod CA: Neuroleptic drugs: Indications and guidelines for their rational use in children and adolescents. *J Child Adolesc Psychopharmacol,* 1:33–56, 1990.
9. Bird HR, Gould MS, Staghezza BM: Patterns of diagnostic comorbidity in a community sample of children aged 9 through 16 years. *J Am Acad Child Adolesc Psychiatry,* 32:361–368, 1993.
10. Fergusson DM, Horwood J, Lynskey MT: Prevalence and comorbidity of DSM-III-R diagnoses in a birth cohort of 15 year olds. *J Am Acad Child Adolesc Psychiatry* 32:1127–1134, 1993.
11. Biederman J, et al: Child behavior checklist findings further support comorbidity between ADHD and major depression in a referred sample. *J Am Acad Child Adolesc Psychiatry* 35:734–42, 1996.
12. Bradley C: The behavior of children receiving Benzedrine. *Am J Orthopsychiatry* 94:577–585, 1937.
13. Schachar R, Tannock R: Childhood hyperactivity and psychostimulants: A review of extended treatment studies. *J Child and Adolesc Psychopharmacol.* 3:81-97, 1993.
14. Klein RG: The role of methylphenidate in psychiatry. *Arch Gen Psychiatry* 52:429–433, 1995.
15. Zametkin AJ, Rapoport JL: Neurobiology of attention deficit disorder with hyperactivity: Where have we come in 50 years? *J Am Acad Child Adolesc Psychiatry* 26:676–886, 1987.
16. Dulcan MK: Using psychostimulants to treat behavioral disorders of children and adolescents. *J Child Adolesc Psychopharmacol* 1:7–20, 1990.
17. Riddle MA, Geller B, Ryan N: Another sudden death in a child treated with desipramine. *J Am Acad Child Adolesc Psychiatry* 32:792–797, 1993.

18. Ryan ND: Heterocyclic antidepressants in children and adolescents. *J Child Adolesc Psychopharmacol* 1: 21–31, 1990.
19. Plizka SR: Tricyclic antidepressants in the treatment of children with attention deficit disorder. *J Am Acad Child Adolesc Psychiatry* 26:127–132, 1987.
20. Biederman J, Baldessarini RJ, Wright VD: A double-blind placebo controlled study of desipramine in the treatment of ADD: I. Efficacy. *J Am Acad Child Adolesc Psychiatry* 28:777–784, 1989.
21. Barrickman LL, et al: Bupropion versus methylphenidate in the treatment of attention-deficit hyperactivity disorder. *J Am Acad Child Adolesc Psychiatry* 34:649–657, 1995.
22. Casat CD, Pleasants DZ, Fleet JVS: A double-blind trial of bupropion in children with attention deficit disorder. *Psychopharmacol Bull* 23:120–122, 1987.
23. Hunt RD, Capper L, O'Connell P: Clonidine in child and adolescent psychiatry. *J Child Adolesc Psychopharmacol* 1:87–102, 1990.
24. Hunt RD, Arnsten AFT, Asbell MD: An open trial of guanfacine in the treatment of attention-deficit hyperactivity disorder. *J Am Acad Child Adolesc Psychiatry* 34:50–54, 1995.
25. Horrigan JP, Barnhill, LJ: Guanfacine for treatment of attention-deficit hyperactivity disorder in boys. *J Child Adolesc Psychopharmacol* 5:215–223, 1995.
26. Zametkin A, et al.: Treatment of hyperactive children with monoamine oxidase inhibitors. *Arch Gen Psychiatry.* 42:962–966, 1985.
27. Weizman R, Weizman A, Deutsch S: Biological studies of attention-deficit disorder, in Deutsch S, Weizman A, Weizman R (eds): *Application of Basic Neuroscience to Child Psychiatry.* New York, Plenum Press, 1990.
28. McCracken JT: A two-part model of stimulant action on attention-deficit hyperactivity disorder in children. *J Neuropsychiatry Clin Neurosci* 3:201–209, 1991.
29. Kuczenski R: Biochemical actions of amphetamine and other stimulants, in Creese I (ed): *Stimulants: Neurochemical, Behavioral and Clinical Perspectives.* New York, Raven Press, 1983.
30. Fuller RW, Perry KW, Bymaster FP: Comparative effects of pemoline, amfonelic acid and amphetamine on dopamine uptake and release in vitro and on brain 3,4-dihydroxyphenylacetic acid concentration in spiperone-treated rats. *J Pharm Pharmacol* 30:197–198, 1978.
31. Preskorn SH, Othmer, SC: Evaluation of bupropion hydrochloride: The first of a new class of atypical antidepressants. *Pharmacotherapy* 4:20–34, 1984.
32. Klein RG, Mannuzza S: Long-term outcome of hyperactive children: A review. *J Am Acad Child Adolesc Psychiatry* 30:383–387, 1992.
33. Campbell M, Gonzalez N, Silva R: The pharmacological treatment of conduct disorders and rage outbursts. *Psychiatr Clin North Am* 15:69–85, 1992.
34. Kaplan S, Busner J, Kupietz S: Effects of methylphenidate on adolescents with aggressive conduct disorder and ADHD. *J Am Acad Child Adolesc Psychiatry* 29:719–724, 1990.
35. Remschmidt H: The psychotropic effect of carbamazepine in non-epileptic patients, with particular reference to problems posed by clinical studies in children with behavioural disorders, in Birkmayer W (ed): *Epileptic Seizures: Behavior-Pain.* London, University Park Press, pp. 253–258, 1976.
36. Kafantaris V, et al: Carbamazepine in hospitalized aggressive conduct disorder children: An open pilot study. *Psychopharmacol Bull* 28:193–199, 1992.
37. Cueva JE, et al: Carbamazepine in aggressive children with conduct disorder: A double-blind and placebo-controlled study. *J Am Acad Child Adolesc Psychiatry* 35:480–490, 1996.
38. Ghaziuddin N, Alessi NE: An open clinical trial of trazodone in aggressive children. *J Child Adolesc Psychopharmacol* 2:291–297, 1992.
39. Linnoila M, Virkkunen M, Scheinin M: Low cerebrospinal fluid 5-hydroyindolacetic acid concentration differentiates impulsive from nonimpulsive violent behavior. *Life Sd* 33:2609–2614, 1983.
40. Kruesi MJP, et al: Cerebrospinal fluid monamine metabolites, aggression, and impulsivity in disruptive behavior disorders of children and adolescents. *Arch Gen Psychiatry* 47:419–426, 1990.
41. Kruesi MJP, et al: A 2-year prospective follow-up study of children and adolescents with disruptive behavior disorders. *Arch Gen Psychiatry.* 49:429–435, 1992.
42. Puig-Antich J: Affective disorders in childhood: A review and perspective. *Psychiatr Clin North Am* 3:403–424, 1980.
43. Ryan ND, et al: The clinical picture of major depression in children and adolescents. *Arch Gen Psychiatry* 44:854–861, 1987.
44. Geller B, et al: Dose and plasma levels of nortriptyline and chlorpromazine in delusionally depressed adolescents and of nortriptyline in nondelusionally depressed adolescents. *Am J Psychiatry* 142:336–338, 1985.

45. Fetner HH, Geller B: Lithium and tricyclic antidepressants. *Psychiatr Clin North Am* 15:223–224, 1992.
46. Birmaher R, et al: Childhood and adolescent depression: A review of the past 10 years. Part II. *J Am Acad Child Adolesc Psychiatry* 35:1575–1583, 1996.
47. Geller B, et al: Treatment-resistant depression in children and adolescents. *Psychiatr Clin North Am* 19:253–267, 1996.
48. Emslie G, Rush AJ, Weinberg AW: A double-blind, randomized placebo-controlled trial of fluoxetine in depressed children and adolescents with depression. *Arch Gen Psychiatry* 54:1030–1037, 1997.
49. Apter A, Ratzoni G, King RA, et al: Fluvoxamine open-label treatment of adolescent inpatients with obsessive-compulsive disorder or depression. *J Am Acad Child Adolesc Psychiatry* 33:342–348, 1994.
50. McConville BJ, et al: An open study of the effects of sertraline on adolescent major depression. *J Child and Adolesc Psychopharmacol* 6:41–51, 1996.
51. Geller B, et al: Lithium for prepubertal depressed children with family history predictors of future bipolarity: A double-blind, placebo controlled study. *J Affect Disord*, in press.
52. Dahl RE, Ryan ND, Williamson DE: The regulation of sleep and growth hormone in adolescent depression. *J Am Acad Child Adolesc Psychiatry* 31:615–621, 1992.
53. Puig-Antich J: Sleep and neuroendocrine correlates of affective illness in childhood and adolescence. *J Adolesc Health Care* 8:505–529, 1987.
54. Yaylayan SA, Weller EB, Weller RA: Biology of depression in children and adolescents. *J Child Adolesc Psychopharmacol.* 1:215–227, 1991.
55. Geller B, et al: Complex and rapid-cycling in bipolar children and adolescents: A preliminary study. *J Affect Disord* 34:259–268, 1995.
56. Geller B, Luby J: Child and adolescent bipolar disorder: A review of the past 10 years. *J Am Acad Child Adolesc Psychiatry*, 36:1168–1176, 1997.
57. Wozniak J, et al: Mania-like symptoms suggestive of childhood-onset bipolar disorder in clinically referred children. *J Am Acad Child Adolesc Psychiatry* 34:867–876, 1995.
58. Varanka TM, et al: Lithium treatment of manic episodes with psychotic features in prepubertal children. *Am J Psychiatry* 145:1557–1559, 1988.
59. Botteron K, Geller B, Cooper TB, Sun K, et al: Pharmacologic treatment of childhood and adolescent mania. *Child Adolesc Psychiatr Clin North Am* 4:283–304, 1995.
60. Geller B, Cooper TB, Sun K, et al: Double-blind and placebo controlled study of lithium for adolescent bipolar disorders with secondary substance dependency. *J Am Acad Child Adolesc Psychiatry*, 37:171–178, 1998.
61. Evans RW, Clay TH, Gualtieri CT: Carbamazepine in pediatric psychiatry. *J Am Acad Child Adolesc Psychiatry* 26:2–8, 1987.
62. Weeston TF, Constantino J: High-dose T4 for rapid-cycling bipolar disorder. *J Am Acad Child Adolesc Psychiatry* 35:131–132, 1996.
63. Bauer MS, Whybrow PC: Rapid cycling bipolar affective disorder. *Arch Gen Psychiatry.* 47:435–440, 1990.
64. Baraban JM, Worley R, Snyder SH: Second messenger systems and psychoactive drug action: Focus on the phosphoinositide system and lithium. *Am J Psychiatry* 146:1251–1260, 1989.
65. El-Mallakh RS, Barrett JL, Wyatt RJ: The Na,K-ATPase hypothesis for bipolar disorder: Implications of normal development. *J Child Adolesc Psychopharmacol* 3:37–52, 1993.
66. Davis KL, Kahn RS, Ko G: Dopamine in schizophrenia: A review and reconceptualization. *Am J Psychiatry* 148:1474–1486, 1991.
67. Spencer EK, Campbell M: Children with schizophrenia: Diagnosis, phenomenology, and pharmacotherapy. *Schizophren Bull* 20:713–725, 1994.
68. Gordon CT, et al: Childhood-onset schizophrenia: An NIMH study in progress. *Schizophren Bull* 20:697–712, 1994.
69. McClellan J, Werry J: Practice parameters for the assessment and treatment of children and adolescents with schizophrenia. *J Am Acad Child Adolesc Psychiatry* 33:616–635, 1994.
70. Kumra S, et al: Childhood-onset schizophrenia. *Arch Gen Psychiatry* 53:1090–1097, 1996.
71. Campbell M, Spencer KM: Psychopharmacology in child and adolescent psychiatry: A review of the past five years. *J Am Acad Child Adolesc Psychiatry* 3:269–279, 1988.
72. Spencer E, et al: Haloperidol in schizophrenic children: Early findings from a study in progress. *Psychopharmacol Bull* 28:183–186, 1992.
73. Trimble MR: Anticonvulsants in children and adolescents. *J Child Adolesc Psychopharmacol* 1:107–124, 1990.
74. Olney JW, Farber NB: Glutamate receptor dysfunction and schizophrenia. *Arch Gen Psychiatry* 52:998–1007, 1995.

75. Jacobsen JW: Problem behavior and psychiatric impairment within a developmentally disabled population I: Behavior frequency. *Appl Res Ment Retard* 3:212–239, 1982.

76. Rutter M, Tizard J, Yule W: Isle of Wight studies. *Psychol Med* 6:313–332, 1976.

77. Aman MG: Psychoactive drugs in mental retardation, In Matson JL(ed): *Treatment Issues and Innovation in Mental Retardation.* New York, Plenum, 1985, pp. 455–513.

78. Schroeder SR: Neuroleptic Medications for persons with developmental disabilities, in Aman MG, (ed): *Psychopharmacology of the Developmental Disabilities.* New York, Springer-Verlag, 1988.

79. Gualtieri CT: Mental retardation: Antidepressant drugs and lithium, in Karosu TB (ed): *Treatment of Psychiatric Disorders,* Vol 1. Washington, DC, APA Press, 1989.

80. Stores G: Antiepileptic drugs. In Aman MG, (ed): *Psychopharmacology of the Developmental Disabilities.* New York, Springer-Verlag, 1988.

81. Sokol MS, Campbell M: Novel psychoactive agents in the treatment of developmental disorders, In Aman MG, (ed): *Psychopharmacology of the Developmental Disabilities.* New York, Springer-Verlag, 1988.

82. Coffey BJ: Anxiolytics for children and adolescents: Traditional and new drugs. *J Child Adolesc Psychopharmacol* 1:57–83, 1990.

83. Arnold LE, Aman MG: Beta blockers in mental retardation and developmental disorders. *J Child and Adolesc Psychopharmacol* 1:361–374, 1991.

84. Aman MG: Stimulant drugs in the developmental disabilities revisited. *J Dev Phys Disabil* 8:347–365, 1996.

85. Chandler M, Gualtieri CT, Fahs J: Other psychotropic drugs: Stimulants, antidepressants, anxiolytics and lithium carbonate. In Aman MG, Singh NN, eds: *Psychopharmacology of the Developmental Disabilities.* New York, Springer-Verlag, 1988.

86. Aman MG, et al: Fenfluramine and methylphenidate in children with mental retardation and ADHD: Clinical and side effects. *J Am Acad Child Adolesc Psychiatry* 32:851–859, 1992.

87. Aman MG, et al: Fenfluramine and methylphenidate in children with mental retardation and borderline IQ: Clinical effects. *Am J Men Retard* 101:521–534, 1997.

88. Conners CK, Bloum AG, Winglee M: Piracetam and event-related potentials in dyslexic children. *Psychopharmacol Bull* 20:667–673, 1984.

89. Aman MG, Rojahn J: Pharmacological intervention. In Singh NN, (ed): *Current Perspectives in Learning Disabilities.* New York, 1992, pp. 478–525.

90. Helfgott E, Rudel RG, Kneger J: Effect of piracetam on the single word and prose reading of dyslexic children. *Psychopharmacol Bull* 20:688–696, 1984.

91. Gordon CT, et al: A double-blind comparison of clomipramine, desipramine and placebo in the treatment of autistic disorder. *Arch Gen Psychiatry* 50:441–447, 1993.

92. Cook EH, et al: Fluoxetine treatment of children and adults with autistic disorder and mental retardation. *J Am Acad Child Adolesc Psychiatry* 31:739–745, 1992.

93. McDougle CJ, et al: A double-blind, placebo-controlled study of fluvoxamine in adults with autistic disorder. *Arch Gen Psychiatry* 53:1001–1008, 1996.

94. Campbell M, et al: Treatment of autistic disorder. *J Am Acad Child Adolesc Psychiatry* 35:134–143, 1996.

95. Joshi PT, Capozzoli JA, Coyle JT: Low dose neuroleptic therapy for children with childhood-onset pervasive developmental disorder. *Am J Psychiatry* 145:335–338, 1988.

96. McDougle CJ, et al: Risperidone in adults with autism or pervasive developmental disorder. *J Child Adolesc Psychopharmacol* 5:273–282, 1995.

97. Geller B, Guttmacher L, Bleeg M: The coexistence of childhood onset pervasive developmental disorder and attention deficit disorder with hyperactivity. *Am J Psychiatry* 38:338–339, 1981.

98. Birmaher B, Quintana H, Greenhill LL: Methylphenidate treatment of hyperactive autistic children. *J Am Acad Child Adoles Psychiatry* 27:248–251, 1988.

99. Campbell M, Anderson LT, Mejer M: A comparison of haloperidol and behavior therapy and their interaction in autistic children. *J Am Acad Child Adolesc Psychiatry* 23:640–645, 1984.

100. Deutsch SI: Rationale for the administration of opiate antagonists in treating infantile autism. *Am J Ment Defic* 90:631–635, 1986.

101. Sandman C: The opiate hypothesis in autism and self-injury. *J Child Adolesc Psychopharmacol* 1:237–250, 1990.

102. Young JG, Leven LI, Newcorn JH: Genetic and neurobiological approaches to the pathophysiology of autism and the pervasive developmental disorders, in Meltzer HY (ed): *Psychopharmacology: The Third Generation of Progress.* New York, Raven Press, 1987.

103. Ernst M, et al: Plasma beta-endorphin levels, naltrexone, and haloperidol in autistic children. *Psychopharm Bull* 29:221–227, 1993.

104. Walsh BT, Devlin MJ: The pharmacologic treatment of eating disorders (review). *Psychiatr Clin North Am* 15:149–160, 1992.
105. Agras WS: Treatment of eating disorders, in Nemeroff CB (ed): *The American Psychiatric Press Textbook of Psychopharmacology.* Washington, DC, APA Press, pp. 725–734, 1995.
106. Walsh TB: Long-term outcome of antidepressant treatment for bulimia nervosa. *Am J Psychiatry* 148:1206–1212, 1991.
107. Halmi KA, Ackerman S, Gibbs J, et al: Basic biological overview of the eating disorders, in Meltzer HY (ed): *Psychopharmacology: The Third Generation of Progress.* New York, Raven Press, pp. 1255–1266, 1987.
108. Hall GCN: Sexual offender recidivism revisited: A meta-analysis of recent treatment studies. *J Consult Clin Psychol* 63:802–809, 1995.
109. Gottesman HG, Schubert DSP: Low-dose oral medroxyprogesterone acetate in the management of the paraphilias. *J Clin Psychiatry* 54:182–188, 1993.
110. Bradford JMW, Pawlak A: Double-blind placebo crossover study of cyproterone acetate in the treatment of the paraphilias. *Arch Sex Behav* 22:383–402, 1993.
111. Kafka MP: Sertraline pharmacotherapy for paraphilias and paraphilia-related disorders: An open trial. *Ann Clin Psychiatry* 6:189–195, 1994.
112. Meyer-Bahlburg HFL: Can homosexuality in adolescents be treated by sex hormones? *J Child Adolesc Psychopharmacol* 1:231–236, 1990/1991.
113. Allen AJ, Leonard H, Swedo SE: Current knowledge of medications for the treatment of childhood anxiety disorders. *J Am Acad Child Adolesc Psychiatry* 34:976–986, 1995.
114. Birmaher B, et al: Fluoxetine for childhood anxiety disorders. *J Am Acad Child Adolesc Psychiatry* 33:993–999, 1994.
115. Bernstein GA, Garfinkel BD, Borchardt CM: Comparative studies of pharmacotherapy for school refusal. *J Am Acad Child Adolesc Psychiatry* 29:773–781, 1990.
116. Bernstein GA, Perwien AR: Anxiety disorders. *Child Adolesc Psychiatr Clin* 4:305–322, 1995.
117. Graae F, et al: Clonazepam in childhood anxiety disorders. *J Am Acad Child Adolesc Psychiatry* 33:372–376, 1994.
118. Kutcher SP, et al: The pharmacotherapy of anxiety disorders in children and adolescents. *Psychiatr Clin North Am* 15:41–67, 1992.
119. Black B, Uhde TW: Treatment of elective mutism with fluoxetine: A double-blind, placebo-controlled study. *J Am Acad Child Adolesc Psychiatry* 33:1000–1006, 1994.
120. Famularo R, Kinscherff R, Fenton T: Propranolol treatment for childhood posttraumatic stress disorder, acute type. A pilot study. *Am J Dis Child* 142:1244–1247, 1988.
121. Tern LC: Acute response to external events and post traumatic stress disorder, in Lewis M, (ed): *Child and Adolescent Psychiatry: A Comprehensive Textbook.* Baltimore, Williams & Wilkins; 1991.
122. Rapaport JL: *Obsessive Compulsive Disorder in Children and Adolescents.* Washington, DC, American Psychiatric Press, 1988.
123. March JS, Leonard HL: Obsessive–compulsive disorder in children and adolescents: A review of the past 10 years. *J Am Acad Child Adolesc Psychiatry* 34:1265–1273, 1996.
124. Leonard H, Swedo S, Rapoport JL: Treatment of childhood obsessive compulsive, disorder with clomipramine and desmethylimipramine: A double-blind crossover comparison. *Psychopharmacol Bull* 24:93–95, 1988.
125. DeVeaugh-Geiss J, et al: Clomipramine hydrochloride in childhood and adolescent obsessive–compulsive disorder—a multicenter trial. *J Am Acad Child Adolesc Psychiatry* 31:45–49, 1992.
126. Hoehn-Saric R: Neurotransmitters in anxiety. *Arch Gen Psychiatry* 39:735–742, 1982.
127. Charney DS, Redmond DE: Neurobiological mechanisms in human anxiety. *Neuropharmacology* 22:1531–1536, 1983.
128. Swedo SE, JL Rapoport: Neurochemical and neuroendocrine considerations of obsessive–compulsive disorders in childhood. In Deutcsh SI, Weizman A, Weizman R (eds): *Application of Basic Neuroscience to Child Psychiatry.* Plenum, New York, pp. 275–284, 1990.
129. Robertson MM: The Gilles de La Tourette syndrome: The current status. *Br J Psychiatry* 154:147–169, 1989.
130. Cohen DJ, Leckman JF, Shaywitz BA: The Tourette syndrome and other tics, in Shaffer D, (ed): *The Clinical Guide to Child Psychiatry.* New York, Free Press, 1985.
131. Sallee FR, et al: Relative efficacy of haloperidol and pimozide in children and adolescents with Tourette's disorder. *Am J Psychiatry* 154:1057–1062, 1997.
132. Lombroso PJ, et al: Risperidone treatment of children and adolescents with chronic tic disorders: A preliminary report. *J Am Acad Child Adolesc Psychiatry* 34:1147–1152, 1995.

133. Riddle MA, Hardin MT, Churl S: Desipramine treatment of boys with attention deficit hyperactivity disorder and tics: Preliminary clinical experience. *J Am Acad Child Adolesc Psychiatry* 27:811–814, 1988.

134. Riddle MA, Hardin MT, King R: Fluoxetine treatment of children and adolescents with Tourette's and obsessive compulsive disorders: Preliminary clinical experience. *J Am Acad Child Adolesc Psychiatry* 29:45–48, 1990.

135. Cohen DJ, Riddle MA, Leckman JF: Pharmacotherapy of Tourette's syndrome and associated disorders. *Psychiatr Clin North Am* 15:109–129, 1992.

136. Gadow KD, Nolan EE, Sverd J: Methylphenidate in hyperactive boys with comorbid tic disorder II: Behavioral effects in school settings. *J Am Acad Child Adolesc Psychiatry* 31:462–471, 1992.

137. Spencer T, Biederman J, Wilens T: Tricyclic antidepressant treatment of children with ADHD and tic disorders. *J Am Acad Child Adolesc Psychiatry* 33:1203–1204, 1994.

138. Chappell PB, et al: Biochemical and genetic studies of Tourette's syndrome, in Deutsch SI, (ed): *Application of Basic Neuroscience to Child Psychiatry*. New York, Plenum Medical Book Company, pp. 241–260, 1990.

139. Geller B: Pharmacotherapy of concomitant psychiatric disorders in adolescent substance abusers, in Rahdert ER (ed): *Adolescent Drug Abuse: Analyses of Treatment Research*. Washington, DC, DHHS Publications, National Institute on Drug Abuse Monograph Series, pp. 85–1523, 1988.

140. Rahdert ER: Adolescent Drug Abuse: Analysis of Treatment Research. *NIDA Resarch Monograph*, 77:1–3, 1988.

141. Geller B, et al: Early findings from a pharmacokinetically designed double-blind and placebo-controlled study of lithium for adolescents comorbid with bipolar and substance dependency disorders. *Prog Neuropsychopharmacol Biol Psychiatry* 16:281–299, 1992.

142. Nino-Murcia G, Dement WC: Psychophysiological and pharmacological aspects of somnambulism and night terrors in children, in Meltzer HY (ed): *Psychopharmacology: The Third Generation of Progress*. New York, Raven Press, 1987.

143. Dahl RE: Child and adolescent sleep disorders. *Pediatr Psychopharmacol* 4:323–341, 1995.

144. Houts AC, Berman JS, Abramson H: Effectiveness of psychological and pharmacological treatments for nocturnal enuresis. *J Consul Clin Psychol* 62:737–745, 1994.

145. Thompson S, Rey JM: Functional enuresis: Is desmopressin the answer? *J Am Acad Child Adolesc Psychiatry* 34:266–271, 1995.

146. Kirschner B: Constipation, in Kelly VC, (ed): *Practice of Pediatrics*. Philadelphia, Harper & Row, 1987.

147. Dodge KA: Social-cognitive mechanisms in the development of conduct disorder and depression. *Annu Rev Psychol* 44:559–584, 1993.

148. Stewart JT, Myers WC, Burket MD: A review of pharmacotherapy of aggression in children and adolescents. *J Am Acad Child Adolesc Psychiatry* 29:269–277, 1990.

149. Winchel RM, Stanley M: Self-injurious behavior: A review of the behavior and biology of self-mutilation. *Am J Psychiatry* 148:308–317, 1991.

150. Birmaher B, Greenhill LL, Stanley M: Biochemical studies of suicide, in Deutsch SI, (ed): *Application of Basic Neuroscience to Child Psychiatry*. New York, Plenum, 1990.

151. Gualitieri CT: Self-injurious behavior, in Gualtieri CT, (ed): *Neuropsychiatry and Behavioral Pharmacology*. New York, Springer-Verlag, 1991.

152. Aman MG: Efficacy of psychotropic drugs for reducing self-injurious behavior in the developmental disabilities. *Ann Clin Psychiatry* 5:171–188, 1993.

153. Cold J, Allolio B, Rees LH: Raised plasma metenkephalin in patients who habitually mutilate themselves. *Lancet* ii:545–546, 1983.

154. Gillberg C, Terenius L, Lonnerholm G: Endorphin activity in childhood psychoses: Spinal fluid levels in 24 cases. *Arch Gen Psychiatry* 42:780–783, 1985.

155. Aman MG: Stimulant drug effects in developmental disorders and hyperactivity—toward a resolution of disparate findings. *J Autism Dev Disord* 12:385–398, 1982.

II

Specific Drugs

8

Stimulants

RUSSELL A. BARKLEY, Ph.D.,
GEORGE J. DuPAUL, Ph.D.,
and DANIEL F. CONNOR, M.D.

The stimulant medications are the most commonly used psychotropic drugs employed with children, especially where inattentive, hyperactive, and/or impulsive behavior is sufficiently severe to impact adversely on school functioning or social adjustment. It has been estimated that 1.5 million children annually, 2.8% of the school-age population, may be using stimulants for behavior management.[1] Historically, most of the individuals for whom stimulants were prescribed were children between 5 and 12 years of age. But, more recently, there has been a significant increase in the prescription of these medications for adolescents, particularly for those diagnosed as having attention-deficit hyperactivity disorder (ADHD).[2]

Substantial research has been conducted on the effects of stimulant medications on children. This has clearly demonstrated the efficacy of the stimulants in improving behavioral, academic, and social functioning in about 50–95% of children treated, depending on the presence of other, comorbid child psychiatric and developmental disorders. Despite the plethora of studies on their efficacy, the stimulants are no panacea for treating children with behavioral problems or even ADHD nor should they ordinarily be the sole form of therapy for most such children. Having said this, however, *we also recognize that the stimulants are the only treatment modality to date to demonstrate the normalization of inattentive, impulsive, and restless behavior in children.* There are some cases, in fact, for which medication alone may be adequate or the only practical way to address the concerns of parents and teachers about the child's performance. For most cases, though, one of the greatest benefits of stimulant therapy seems to be the *theoretical* possibility of maximizing the effects of concurrently applied psychosocial and educational treatments (e.g., behavior modification, academic tutoring).

Despite this tremendous body of scientific research, the use of stimulants with children continues to be controversial, both publicly and professionally. The inaccurate, and, regrettably, successful media propaganda campaign conducted in the late 1980s by certain religious groups and pseudo-civil-libertarian groups against the use of stimulants, partic-

RUSSELL A. BARKLEY, Ph.D., and DANIEL F. CONNOR, M.D. • Department of Psychiatry, University of Massachusetts Medical Center, Worcester, Massachusetts 01655.   GEORGE J. DuPAUL, Ph.D. • Department of School Psychology, Lehigh University, Bethlehem, Pennsylvania 18015.

Practitioner's Guide to Psychoactive Drugs for Children and Adolescents (Second Edition), Werry and Aman, eds. Plenum Publishing Corporation, New York, 1999.

ularly Ritalin® (methylphenidate), with children[3] may have been the basis for the dramatic decline in the prescribing of this medication that occurred between 1988 and 1990 (D.J. Safer, personal communication, September 1991). Recent television reports of cases of stimulant abuse by adolescents, rare as they apparently turned out to be, may have another chilling effect on the prescribing of stimulants, particularly Ritalin, for ADHD. This latest wave of media attention to Ritalin, much of it sensationalized, may have been fueled in part by a dispute between the Drug Enforcement Agency and CHADD, the national organization for children and adults with ADHD, surrounding the efforts of CHADD to have Ritalin reclassified into the Schedule III category from its current placement with Schedule II drugs. Though that petition was eventually unsuccessful, the whirlwind of media stories concerning increasing rates of prescribing of Ritalin and potential abuse contributed once again to a public atmosphere of concern and even alarm about this otherwise safe and effective form of treatment for children and adults with ADHD.

In this chapter, we summarize knowledge about the stimulant medications, particularly as used in treating ADHD, and to suggest guidelines for their clinical use.

I. PHARMACOLOGICAL ASPECTS OF STIMULANT MEDICATION: DEFINITION AND NOMENCLATURE

The stimulants are referred to as such because of their ability to activate the level of activity, arousal, or alertness of the central nervous system (CNS). They are structurally similar to brain catecholamines (dopamine and norepinephrine) and are called sympathomimetic compounds because they may mimic the actions of these brain neurotransmitters. The three most commonly employed stimulants are dextroamphetamine (Dexedrine®), methylphenidate (Ritalin®), and magnesium pemoline (Cylert®). A new stimulant, Adderall®, comprising a combination of amphetamine and dextroamphetamine, has recently been approved for use in children and adults with ADHD. Methamphetamine (Desoxyn®) has also been used in a small percentage of cases of ADHD; however, in view of its higher abuse potential, the dearth of controlled research on its efficacy, and limited availability in some geographic regions, it will not be discussed here as a treatment option for children with ADHD. Other (noncatecholaminergic) stimulant compounds (e.g., caffeine, deanol) are not discussed here since they have not been found to be nearly as effective as the CNS stimulants and cannot be recommended for clinical use.

A. Pharmacology

The primary mode of action of dextroamphetamine is believed to be that of enhancing catecholamine activity in the CNS, probably by increasing the availability of norepinephrine and/or dopamine at the synaptic cleft. The precise mechanism is still poorly understood, and the increasing availability of molecular probes to investigate receptor sites, as well as other new investigational techniques, makes this an area in which knowledge is likely to change rapidly in the next few years. Methylphenidate is a piperidine derivative structurally similar to dextroamphetamine. Its specific mode of action is even less clearly understood. It may be that methylphenidate has a greater effect on dopamine activity than on other neurotransmitters, but this remains speculative at this time. Investigation of the pharmacology of Adderall® is only now being completed, but its mode of action is highly likely to prove similar, if not identical, to that of the amphetamines, given its composition of various amphetamines. Pemoline is similar in function to the other CNS stimulants, though it has minimal sympathomimetic effects and is structurally dissimilar. The specific mechanism of action of pemoline is poorly understood.

Catecholaminergic (especially noradrenergic) receptors are widely distributed throughout the brain. However, catecholaminergic neurons are few and localized to the brainstem. Partly because of this wide receptor distribution, the actual site of action of the stimulants within the CNS also remains speculative. Early investigators conjectured that brainstem activation was the primary locus, but lately the midbrain or frontal cortex has been favored. Recent studies of cerebral blood flow have shown that activity in the area of the striatum and the connections between the orbital-frontal and limbic regions are enhanced during stimulant medication treatment.[4,5] Moreover, Zametkin and colleagues,[6] using position-emission tomography (PET), have demonstrated increased brain metabolic activity in the bilateral orbital-frontal area and in the left sensorimotor and parietal areas following a single dose of methylphenidate in seven adults with ADHD. Surprisingly, a *suppression* of activity was noted in the left temporal region following stimulant administration, but the brain is an exceedingly complex organ, and changes in one area of the brain may be consequences of those in other areas.

Gualtieri, Hicks, and Mayo[7] have hypothesized that the stimulants act to "canalize" or decrease fluctuation and variability in arousal, attention, and CNS reactivity, thereby enhancing the persistence of responding and increasing cortical inhibition. Others[8] have proposed that the stimulants decrease the threshold for reinforcement through enhancement of the arousal of the CNS behavioral activation (reward) system, thereby creating a persistence of responding to tasks or activities; that is, activities in which the organism engages are now more reinforcing, resulting in prolonged responding to them.

B. Pharmacokinetics

Stimulants are almost always given orally, are swiftly absorbed from the gastrointestinal tract, cross the blood–brain barrier quickly and easily, and are rapidly eliminated from the body within 24 hr.[9] Dextroamphetamine achieves peak plasma levels in children within 2–3 hr and has a plasma half-life of between 4 and 6 hr (but with substantial *interindividual* variability). The breakdown of dextroamphetamine occurs mainly in the liver, where deamination and *p*-hydroxylation transform it mainly to benzoic acid. A significant proportion is excreted in the urine, ranging from 2% in very alkaline urine to as much as 80% in very acidic urine, so that high gastric activity (which produces alkaline urine) and some treatments for urinary infections may affect concentration substantially.[10] Behavioral effects are noticeable within 30–60 min, appear to peak between 1 and 2 hr post ingestion, and usually dissipate within 4–6 hr.[11] Although data on Adderall® have not yet been published, its pharmacokinetics are likely to be similar to those for dextroamphetamine and amphetamine given that these two drugs make up this hybrid stimulant compound.

Methylphenidate reaches peak plasma levels somewhat more quickly, within 1.5–2.5 hr after ingestion. The plasma half-life is usually shorter as well, between 2 and 3 hr, and the drug is entirely metabolized within 12–24 hr, with almost none of the drug appearing in the urine.[9,12] The metabolic pathway for its decomposition and elimination seems to be via deesterification to ritalinic acid and, to a lesser degree, via hydroxylation to *p*-hydroxymethylphenidate, with the remainder transformed to oxoritalinic acid and oxomethylpheni-

date; all of these metabolites are pharmacologically inactive.[13] As with dextroamphetamine, behavioral effects occur within 30–60 min, peak within 1–3 hr and are dissipated
within 3–6 hr after oral ingestion, creating an effective span of clinical improvement
ranging from about 4 to 6 hr in most children. The plasma half-life of so-called "sustained-
release" methylphenidate has been found to be nearly twice as long as that of the standard
preparation.[14] Behavioral effects of this preparation appear to occur within 1–2 hr, peak
within 3–5 hr, and slowly diminish until approximately 8 hr post ingestion.[15,16] These
effects are equivalent to those produced by the standard preparation.[17] It is important to note
that considerable interindividual variability exists with respect to these parameters, however, with clinical implications for the frequency of dosage. The plasma level does appear
to be dose-related.[18]

Pemoline appears to have a longer half-life than the other stimulants. Even so, this
half-life seems to be shorter with children (i.e., 7–8 hr) than with adults (i.e., 11–13 hr) and
peak plasma levels are reached 2–4 hr postingestion.[19] Within 24 hr, 50–75% of the dose
seems to be excreted in the urine. The time-course and response characteristics of its
behavioral effects have not been well documented. More recently, behavioral effects have
been noted to develop by 2 hr after ingestion and last through the 7th hour postingestion.[20]
The half-life of this compound possibly increases with chronic use, which may lead to a
buildup in plasma levels thereby explaining the considerably delayed behavioral effects (up
to 3–4 weeks) of the medication.[11]

Behavioral effects for the stimulants do not appear to be well predicted from peak or
absolute blood levels compared to knowledge of dose alone.[21,22] Peak behavioral changes
often seem to lag behind peak blood levels by as much as an hour. However, changes in
learning on laboratory learning tasks may correspond more closely to blood levels,[21,23]
though there is insufficient data to be sure. Consequently, where *behavioral change* is the
goal of treatment, blood levels play little role in establishing the therapeutic range or
response for any individual case beyond knowledge of the oral dose itself. Where changes
in *learning performance* are more important, blood levels may eventually provide more
promising information about establishing a therapeutic range, although here, again, inter-
and intraindividual variability is quite high.[21] Despite such promise, drawing blood to
establish drug levels for guiding therapeutic adjustments to children's stimulant medication
is not recommended[22,24] except possibly in resistant cases.

Tolerance to these drugs has not been established in research, but clinical anecdotes
suggest decreased efficacy of the drugs in some cases over prolonged administration.
Dulcan[11] conjectures that this may stem from hepatic autoinduction, behavioral noncompliance with the prescribed regimen, weight gain, or contextual factors such as an intercurrent stress event (e.g., moves, divorce, change in school classroom) or altered caregiver
expectations. It is also possible, given the inherent complexity of dopamine receptors, that
compensatory changes in the number of receptor sites may occur.

II. CLINICAL EFFECTS: SHORT-TERM

A vast number of studies exist on the effects of the stimulants on children's behavior
and learning, most of which have studied children with hyperactivity, attention-deficit
disorder (ADD), or, more recently, ADHD. Space does not permit reviewing these studies
in any detail. Instead, this chapter will focus on extracting from this rich vein of research
those findings that are most substantiated or most applicable to clinical practice. Most of

these studies have been conducted with methylphenidate, and considerably less with dextroamphetamine. Only a few have employed pemoline, but these suggest similar effects on learning and behavior as with the other two stimulants.[20] No controlled studies of clinical effects using Adderall® have yet been published, but those recently completed by Swanson at the University of California Medical School at Irvine and by Greenhill at Columbia University in New York suggest that these effects may be similar to those of the other stimulants.

A. General Clinical Effects

Barkley's[25] initial review of more than 120 studies up to 1977 indicated that between 73% and 77% of children treated with stimulants were seen as improved in their "behavior," variously measured. In contrast, the proportion responding to placebo was 39%. More recent studies[26-28] and reviews of this literature, including meta–analyses, have reached similar conclusions concerning the response rates to the stimulants, although some have found lower response rates to placebo than Barkley originally reported.[29-31] The stimulants, therefore, have substantial documentation for their efficacy relative to other types of child therapy. Nevertheless, as many as 20–30% of children tried on stimulants may display no positive response to these medications or are made worse by them in their behavioral adjustment. Thus, it should not be assumed that all ADHD children respond positively or in the same manner to these medications. Further complicating the clinical picture is the finding that children may respond well on one or a few measures of behavior and learning while showing no response or an adverse reaction on other types of measures. Moreover, when some children respond poorly to one type of stimulant, such as methylphenidate, it is possible that they might respond to a different one, such as dextroamphetamine,[32] though this remains to be well established. All of this suggests that the response of children to stimulants can be quite idiosyncratic and individualization clinically is essential.

B. Physical Effects

Both methylphenidate and dextroamphetamine produce acute growth hormone release in both children and adults, which could lead to alterations in prolactin, cortisol, and β-endorphins.[33] However, as Reeve and Garfinkel noted,[33] long-term effects on the hypothalamic–pituitary–growth hormone axis have not been demonstrated. Despite some evidence of initial growth inhibition by these drugs, effects on eventual adult height or skeletal stature are often clinically insignificant.[34] Effects on weight are also frequently minimal, resulting in a loss of 0.5–1.0 kg during the initial year of treatment and often showing a rebound in growth by the second or later years of treatment.[11,33,35] The effects on weight are likely to be the same for Adderall®, although there is a report of a single case involving severe weight loss associated with this drug.[36] All of the stimulants seem to reduce appetite to some degree, although this is temporary and mainly limited to the time of peak effects.[13]

A large, albeit inconclusive literature exists on the psychophysiological effects of the stimulants.[37-39] Heart rate, as well as systolic and diastolic blood pressure, may be increased by these medications; however, these effects appear to be small and moderated by a number of factors. For instance, higher dosages of stimulants are linearly related to increasing levels of heart rate, and these effects are dependent upon both the initial (i.e., premedication) heart rate and the time course of the medication.[40] What changes in cardiovascular functioning that do occur are often mild (about 6–15 bpm, mean = 11 bpm), are clearly dose dependent, and are often outweighed by other normal daily physiologic stresses (e.g., digestion).[37,41,42] The effect on heart rate may attenuate somewhat with continued use of the medication.[42] No electrocardiogram irregularities for any of the stimulants have been identified in the few studies examining this issue.[42] Dextroamphetamine and pemoline may be less likely to produce these effects on heart rate and blood pressure.[42,43] Heart rate variability is reduced by methylphenidate, as is heart rate deceleration to a reaction time task. The latter result is consistent with changes in cognitive functions such as attention span and concentration. In all studies, cardiovascular effects of stimulants are subject to tremendous intra- and interindividual variability. Effects on blood pressure from all three stimulants are quite modest, when noted, and are not consistently found across studies.[42] However, the possibility exists that African-American adolescents may have a greater risk for developing an increase in diastolic blood pressure.[44]

Stimulant effects on autonomic nervous system functioning have been noted in the literature for several decades. Skin conductance is often increased, primarily at doses of methylphenidate over 15 mg/day,[37] while effects on both nonspecific and specific galvanic skin responses are equivocal.[45,46]

Background electrical activity of the CNS is sometimes increased by the stimulants, usually noted in reduced alpha or slow-wave activity, and CNS sensitivity to stimulation may also be heightened as measured by electroencephalograms (EEGs) and audio- and visual-evoked potentials.[37,47,48] Consequently, cerebral blood flow and brain metabolic activity may be increased. These effects seem to be selective, however, being concentrated primarily in the anterior frontal regions bilaterally as documented in recent studies using cerebral blood flow and PET.[5,6,49] Effects on the reticular activating system may also be noted, probably leading to the increases in heart rate, blood pressure, and in a few cases, respiration. Effects on various aspects of sleep seem insignificant other than a mild delay to sleep onset, or insomnia, experienced by the majority of children on stimulants, noted below. Some evidence points to a temporary reduction in REM sleep, which often returns to normal within several months.[37]

In summary, the stimulants appear to have minor effects on physical systems. What effects are seen involve increased aspects of both autonomic and central nervous system activity, but these are typically small and relatively insignificant clinically.

C. Effects on Behavior and Emotion

Unquestionably, the stimulants produce positive effects on sustained attention and persistence of effort to assigned tasks while reducing task-irrelevant restlessness and motor activity.[25,50–54] In significant numbers of cases, attention to assigned classwork is improved to the extent that the child's behavior appears highly similar to that of his or her non-ADHD classmates.[55–57] Attention while playing sports may also improve in response to stimulant use.[58] Problems with aggression, impulsive behavior, noisiness, noncompliance, and disruptiveness have also been shown to improve with these medications.[59–64] More recently, some research using an open-trial format has suggested that using stimulants with conduct disordered youth who also have ADHD may reduce the symptoms of conduct disorder as well.[65] This report is consistent with a study in a laboratory setting showing that stimulants reduced covert antisocial behavior, such as stealing and property destruction, in boys with ADHD.[66] This suggests that ADHD may amplify or increase conduct problem behaviors in some children and so the reduction in ADHD symptoms achieved by the stimulants may be the basis for these reductions in antisocial behavior.

Despite the finding that adults generally report elevations in mood and euphoria when taking stimulant medications, these effects are rarely reported in children.[25,67] Some children do describe feeling "funny," "different," or dizzy. It may be that actual developmental differences in response to stimulant medication make adults more likely to experience temporary elevations in mood. It is also possible, however, that children are not as adept at labeling their feelings and thus under–report euphoria (e.g., referring to it as feeling "funny").

Some children may evidence various mild negative moods or emotions in reaction to the stimulants,[25] described in Section V below. These mood changes occur later in the time course of the dose response, typically as the drugs are "washing out" of the body in late morning or late afternoon. Such reactions are frequently mild and are dose-related, being more prevalent among children treated with higher dosages.

D. Effects on Cognition, Learning, and Academic Performance

Numerous studies have been conducted on the effects of stimulants on measures of intellect, memory, vigilance, attention, concentration, and learning. A plethora of studies have found that these drugs enhance performance on measures of vigilance, impulse control, fine motor coordination, and reaction time.[43,62] Further, positive though inconsistent drug effects have been obtained on measures of short-term memory and learning of paired verbal or nonverbal material.[50,52,68] Performance on both simple and complex learning paradigms appears to be enhanced[69–71] but not always consistently.[68] In addition, stimulant-related improvements are noted, albeit again not reliably, in perceptual efficiency and speed of symbolic or verbal retrieval (both short- and long-term).[25,72,73] Changes in functioning on more traditional measures of cognitive abilities (e.g., intelligence tests) have not been found.[25] In general, drug effects seem particularly salient in situations that require children to restrict their behavior and concentrate on assigned tasks. As Werry[74] has noted previously, the stimulant drugs allow children to show what they know but are unlikely to alter children's knowledge of what needs to be done.

Concern has arisen over whether CNS stimulants result in state-dependent learning,[70] that is, whether information children learn while on the medication may not be as easily recalled when they are off the medication, or vice versa. The findings are contradictory, however, and, where such effects have been found, they are of such a small magnitude when they do occur as to be clinically insignificant. In general, the weight of the evidence is against such effects occurring with the stimulants.[75,76]

Stimulant medication treatment is associated with minimal improvement in academic achievement, as defined by the grade level of difficulty of the material children are asked to perform.[25,77,78] Stimulant-induced improvements in academic productivity and, to a less reliable degree, accuracy have been found in many studies.[57,62] Although the evidence so far is largely negative, it remains to be seen whether these short-term improvements in academic *performance* lead to greater scholastic *success* in the long run.[77,79]

E. Effects on Social Systems

Treatment with stimulant medication has been found to reduce the intensity and improve the quality of social interactions between children with ADHD and their parents, teachers, and peers. Stimulants increase children's compliance with parental commands and enhance their responsiveness to the interactions of others.[51,80,81] Negative and off-task behaviors are also reduced in compliance situations. In turn, parents and teachers reduce their rate of commands and degree of supervision over these children, while increasing their praise and positive responsiveness to the children's behavior. These effects on social behavior do not differ as a function of sex of the ADHD child.[82,83] Positive medication effects have also been noted on the interactions of ADHD children with their teachers[84] and peers across a variety of situations, with concomitant improvements in the degree to which such children are accepted by their peers.[60,85,86] These medications do not appreciably decrease the frequency of initiations of appropriate interactions in most children but may do so in a minority of cases, particularly at high doses,[87] possibly leading some children to be judged as passive or socially inhibited.[88] Stimulant medications not only directly alter the behavior of children with ADHD but also indirectly affect the behaviors of important adults and peers toward those children. When the latter changes are obtained, they may contribute further to a positive drug response in the child.

Some concern has been raised that taking stimulant medication may undermine children's perceptions of their self-efficacy, leading them to attribute the source of their success while on medication to external rather than internal factors.[89] Recent studies of the attributions of ADHD children about their task performance and successes, however, have not been able to document any deleterious effects of stimulants on their attributions.[90-92]

F. Dose Effects on Behavior and Learning

Early research seemed to demonstrate that different doses of the stimulants had effects on different domains of behavior and learning in hyperactive children.[93,94] Specifically, it was believed that lower doses (0.3 mg/kg) produced maximum improvement in learning while higher doses were more beneficial for social behavior while being detrimental to learning. Further, these results implied that, to the extent that physicians rely on parent and teacher reports to titrate dosage, they may be unnecessarily overdosing ADHD children if the true goal of treatment is improved classroom learning. Several other interpretations of these results are possible (e.g., teacher ratings are less sensitive to medication effects than are laboratory tasks), but the above conclusions have been the most popular ones. More recently, studies show that functioning on a large number of learning and behavioral measures is enhanced in a stepwise fashion across doses, reaching a peak at 20 mg, or 1 mg/kg.[15,59,61,68] No constriction of flexible thinking has been found at doses of methylphenidate up to 0.9 mg/kg.[95] Alternatively, dose–response effects at the individual level can be characterized by significant intersubject variability. The response of individual children to methylphenidate could be categorized as: (a) improvement related to stepwise increases in dose; (b) subject to a "threshold" effect at a moderate or high dose; (c) reaching a peak at a moderate dose with a decrement in performance at higher doses; or (d) inconsistent across doses.[61] These patterns were found to be independent of a child's body weight and to vary across specific measures.

Research to date suggests that several factors moderate the dosage effects of the stimulants on the functioning of children: (1) results are highly variable across individual children and must be assessed at the latter level to be clinically useful; (2) dosage effects may vary across areas of functioning, but not necessarily in the systematic fashion suggested by Sprague and Sleator's study[94]; (3) this task specificity of dosage effects also appears to be subject to individual differences; (4) dosages between 0.3 mg/kg and 1.0 mg/kg have been found to optimize cognitive, academic, *and* behavioral performance at the group level, thus casting doubt on the notion of low doses being exclusively related to enhancement of learning; and (5) poor compliance to the prescribed regimen of taking the stimulant medication may also contribute to the apparent intraindividual variability of drug response.[96] To this list might be added the tendency of some caregivers, or even clinicians, to expect far too much clinical improvement from the stimulants and thus to report somewhat disappointing medication responses when perfection in the eyes of the caregiver or clinician is not achieved.

To summarize, substantial evidence exists to show that the stimulants produce positive effects in many behavioral domains of children which translate into increased social acceptability. Effects on learning and academic performance are less clear-cut and are primarily limited to increases in work productivity and, less consistently, work accuracy. However, an improved ability to master increasingly difficult or higher level academic material, such as that assessed in achievement tests, has not been demonstrated. These effects are highly variable across children and doses, again, mandating that individualization of drug, dosage, and titration occur in clinical practice.

III. CLINICAL EFFECTS: LONG-TERM

Few studies employing rigorous methodology have evaluated the long-term efficacy of stimulant medications. Those that have examined the issue have generally found little advantage.[79,97] Children with ADHD who had been on medication but were off at the time of follow-up were not found to differ in any important respect from those who had never received pharmacotherapy. Hence, no enduring effects of up to 5 years of medication treatment were observed in these studies. Many important shortcomings of long-term outcome investigations have been identified and will not be specifically reviewed here.[98] Suffice it to say that there is abundant evidence of short-term benefit in studies of up to 7 months' duration which, if continued, would be posited to produce ongoing symptomatic relief from ADHD.[98] Enduring effects of these medications after treatment termination seem unlikely, yet this issue must await more rigorous examination than has been possible to date. Further, the chronic and pervasive difficulties associated with more serious ADHD (most likely to be treated with medication) are probably not going to be permanently eradicated by any single treatment, even one with demonstrated short-term efficacy like stimulant medication.[99]

IV. PREDICTING THE CLINICAL RESPONSE TO STIMULANTS

Predicting the response to psychostimulant treatment is an important clinical issue, and a variety of factors have been proposed to distinguish children with ADHD who would respond favorably to stimulant medications (responders) from those who would not (nonresponders), including psychophysiological factors, neurological variables, familial characteristics, demographic/sociological factors, diagnostic categories, rating scale scores, psychological profiles, and behavioral characteristics.[100–102] Those behavioral and psychophysiological measures related to *attention span* are typically the most reliable predictors of improvement during stimulant drug treatment. This is hardly surprising given that stimulants have their primary mode of action on attention span. This conclusion is in keeping with related research which has indicated that the behavioral effects of stimulants may be dependent upon the drug-free rate of the behavior in question (i.e., rate-dependent). In other words, the greater the inattention of children, the better is their reaction to medication (i.e., the more pronounced the effect on attention span). Note, however, that the statistical magnitude of such rate-dependent effects has been found to exceed what would be predicted simply on the basis of regression to the mean.[103]

Some studies have also found that the quality of the relationship between parent and child was a good predictor of drug response: the better the mother–child relationship, the greater the response to medication. This is related to the findings reported earlier that for many children the medication produces positive changes in the behavior of both the children and their mothers. It may be that mothers who are more appreciative and rewarding of these initial positive changes in their children's behavior while on stimulants produce further gains associated with treatment. This is supported by results obtained by Cunningham and Barkley[104] indicating that children whose mothers were more interactive with them and more rewarding of child compliance prior to pharmacotherapy exhibited greater positive changes in behavior as a result of treatment with medication.

Taylor[39] found that higher levels of restless behavior (e.g., hyperactivity), poor motor coordination, younger age, and the absence of symptoms of overt emotional disorder predicted better stimulant response among a large sample of children with ADHD. Similar reports[105,106] suggest that children who are more anxious or depressed according to parent and/or teacher ratings (e.g., Conners' Rating Scales) have a poorer response to stimulant medications and are less likely to exhibit "normalized" behavior as a result of treatment.[107]

Less research exists on the response to stimulants of developmentally delayed children who may also have ADHD.[108] What research exists suggests that the percentage of delayed children responding to these medications may be somewhat less than the corresponding percentage for normal-IQ children, particularly at IQ levels below 50.[108–111]

For clinical purposes, the current evidence would suggest that the younger (but still school-age), more inattentive, less coordinated, more hyperactive, less anxious, and less intellectually delayed a child may be, and the better the parental management and involvement in the care of the child, the better is the response to psychostimulant treatment.

Some clinicians have attempted to use neurometric tests as a means of predicting children's probable drug responses to the stimulants and even to monitor such responses during their drug trial. To date, the authors are aware of no consistent body of research that would support this rather expensive and inconvenient practice.

V. SIDE EFFECTS AND TOXICITY

A. Lethal Dose

No data could be located on deaths that could be directly attributable to the use of acute toxic doses of stimulants in humans. Deaths and the need for liver transplants are noted below as a secondary consequence of the hepatic dysfunction that can occur in some cases from prolonged use of pemoline. In rats, evidence suggests that doses over 100 mg/kg are lethal within 12 hr after ingestion. This dose in dogs did not produce mortality but did produce convulsions. While simple extrapolation to humans is hazardous, the margin of safety, therefore, would seem likely to be at least 100:1 between a single dose representing the high end of the human clinical dose range (1.0 mg/kg) and lethal doses in small mammals.[9]

B. Short-Term Side Effects

1. Usual Side Effects

The results of a study of prevalence of parent- and teacher-reported side effects to two doses (i.e., 0.3 mg/kg and 0.5 mg/kg) of methylphenidate, given twice daily, in a sample of 82 children with ADHD[112] are shown in Table 1. Over half of the sample exhibited decreased appetite, insomnia, anxiousness, irritability, or proneness to crying with both doses of methylphenidate. However, it should be noted that *many of these apparent side effects (especially those associated with mood) were present during the placebo condition* and may represent characteristics associated with the disorder rather than its treatment.[113] In most cases, the severity of these side effects has been shown to be quite mild. Stomachaches and headaches were reported in about a third of the subjects, but these were usually of mild severity as well. Thus, clinicians can expect some mild side effects such as insomnia or diminished appetite; however, care should be taken to assess the presence of these during nonmedication conditions to determine their "true" relation to stimulant use. A similar profile of side effects has been obtained in two more recent studies using a much larger sample.[113,114] These studies have also found that some teacher-reported side effects on this same rating scale actually *declined* significantly during the drug trial,[114] further supporting the notion that some "side effects" may actually be preexisting behavioral/emotional problems of ADHD children. These studies also suggest that more side effects are associated with the "wash out" phase of the time course rather than the peak phase. Others[115] have reported similar results.

2. Tics

One side effect that should receive serious attention from clinicians is the possible increase in nervous tics produced by stimulant medications. A number of cases of irreversible Tourette's disorder have also been reported as secondary to stimulant treatment, although these findings are somewhat controversial.[116–123] It has been estimated that fewer than 1% of ADHD children treated with stimulants will develop a tic disorder and that in 13% of the cases in which there is a preexisting tic disorder, it may exacerbate preexisting tics.[124] Thus, while it is not clear whether stimulant medications cause Tourette's disorder in previously unafflicted individuals, these compounds certainly may exacerbate symptoms in patients who already exhibit this disorder.[125–128] Although the vast majority of such reactions subside once pharmacotherapy is discontinued, there are a few cases reported in the literature where the tics apparently did not diminish in frequency and severity following termination of treatment.[116] More recent studies have suggested that the effects of stimulants on tics are less than was originally believed, with the use of stimulants resulting in minor increases in some motor tics but possible decreases in vocal tics.[129,130] *It still seems*

TABLE 1. Percentage of 82 Subjects (Rated by Parents) Displaying Each of 17 Side Effects of Methylphenidate during Each Drug Condition[a,b]

Side effect	Placebo	Methylphenidate Low dose (0.3 mg/kg)	Medium dose (0.5 mg/kg)
Decreased appetite			
Percent	15	52	56
Percent severe	1	7	13
Insomnia			
Percent	40	62	68
Percent severe	7	18	18
Stomachaches			
Percent	18	39	35
Percent severe	0	1	6
Headaches			
Percent	11	26	21
Percent severe	0	1	4
Prone to crying			
Percent	49	59	54
Percent severe	10	16	10
Tics/nervous movements			
Percent	18	18	28
Percent severe	4	7	5
Dizziness			
Percent	4	10	7
Percent severe	0	0	1
Drowsiness			
Percent	18	23	20
Percent severe	1	2	1
Nail biting			
Percent	22	26	29
Percent severe	7	4	9
Talks less			
Percent	16	20	22
Percent severe	1	1	2
Anxiousness			
Percent	58	58	52
Percent severe	12	9	7
Disinterested in others			
Percent	18	18	15
Percent severe	0	1	2
Euphoria			
Percent	41	34	43
Percent severe	9	4	7
Irritable			
Percent	72	65	66
Percent severe	18	15	13
Nightmares			
Percent	20	20	21
Percent severe	0	0	3
Sadness			
Percent	43	48	41
Percent severe	5	6	8
Staring			
Percent	40	38	38
Percent severe	2	4	1

[a]From Barkley RA, McMurray MB, Edelbrock CS, Robbins K: Side effects of methylphenidate in children with attention deficit hyperactivity disorder: A systematic, placebo-controlled evaluation. *Pediatrics* 86:184–192, 1990. Copyright by the American Academy of Pediatrics. Reprinted with permission.

[b]Percent refers to the number of subjects rated a 1 or higher on the scale of severity (1 to 9) whereas percent severe refers to the number of subjects whose severity rating was 7 or higher.

prudent to adequately screen children with ADHD for a personal or family history of tics or Tourette's syndrome prior to initiating stimulant therapy and to proceed cautiously with such treatment in those with positive histories. When these medications are used in children without these risk factors and tics develop, the dose can be lowered to see if the tics subside or be discontinued if the tics are proving to be significantly impairing. The tics will usually subside within 7–10 days. Treatment can then be resumed at a lower dose if the child's behavioral adjustment has dramatically deteriorated, to determine if a lower dose can be tolerated without production of tics. If not, then trying an alternative stimulant medication or an antidepressant may prove successful. Failing this, the parents should be warned not to have their children treated with stimulants in the future without alerting the treating physician to this history of stimulant-induced tic reactions.

3. "Behavioral Rebound"

Typically, "behavioral rebound" is described as a deterioration in behavior (exceeding that which occurs during baseline or placebo conditions) that occurs in the late afternoon and evening following daytime administrations of medication. Johnston and colleagues[131] conducted a rigorous, placebo-controlled study of this in a sample of 21 children with ADHD treated with two doses of methylphenidate and found that about a third of their sample exhibited rebound effects. The magnitude of these effects varied considerably across days for individual children. Thus this phenomenon is not as widespread as believed (once certain biases are controlled for), and even when it does occur, its magnitude across days is highly variable. When observed, several options can be pursued which may diminish the severity of the rebound. Giving the child a lower dosage of medication in the late afternoon (provided that this does not lead to insomnia or loss of appetite at dinnertime) may help. The noontime dosage may also be reduced. In any case, one rarely has to resort to discontinuing the medication entirely because of rebound effects. Even so, it is a good idea to warn the parents about the possibility of a rebound effect; otherwise, they may misinterpret this phenomenon as the drug making their child permanently worse.

4. Cognitive Toxicity

As noted earlier, the possibility exists that high doses of stimulants may produce an adverse impact on learning or other higher mental functions. High doses of stimulants conceivably may produce an overfocusing or constriction of attention[42,68,70,73] and, perhaps, even a mental equivalent of motor stereotypies, such as perseverative responding or diminished flexibility in problem solving. Such findings have been demonstrated in only a few studies of small numbers of subjects[132] or in subgroups of larger samples to date[133] (K. Voeller, personal communication, October 1991) but not in the overall samples under study. These results imply that some children may have cognitively toxic effects on high doses of stimulants (above 0.6 mg/kg). However, a more recent study of the issue was unable to document any constriction of cognitive flexibility at doses of methylphenidate up to 0.9 mg/kg.[95] Equally important, doses within the therapeutic range recommended here have typically not produced such effects nor have they decreased mental creativity.[134]

5. Behavioral Toxicity

There is some debate about whether higher dosages of these drugs can reduce not only negative, aggressive interactions but prosocial behavior as well. Research indicates that low and moderate doses of methylphenidate do reduce the frequency of aggression and noncompliance in groups of ADHD children but have no appreciable effect, in either direction, on prosocial or nonsocial behavior.[135] Nevertheless, isolated cases may arise where parents note that a child is no longer "spontaneous" or childlike in his or her behavior and appears too controlled or socially aloof. In such cases, the dosage may need to be reduced or the medication discontinued.

6. Idiosyncratic Side Effects

Each stimulant medication may produce unique side effects. A few children may develop allergic skin rashes after a few weeks or more of treatment with pemoline. Ceasing the drug seems to eliminate the rash, and the practitioner may be able to put the child back on the medication with no recurrence of the rash.[136] In animals, stimulants at higher doses can produce stereotyped behavior, and this effect is occasionally seen in children. All may also tend to increase choreiform movements[137] and self-directed behavior, such as lip licking, lip biting, and light picking of the fingertips (not the nails). Dose reduction seems to eliminate the problem. Pemoline has also been associated with chemical hepatitis (which may not always be reversible) in up to 3% of children taking this drug.[11] As a consequence of 10 reports of acute liver failure in children in the United States, and additional reports of liver failure in children and adults in foreign countries, the company manufacturing this drug recently changed its package labeling to indicate that "Cylert should not ordinarily be considered as first line drug therapy for Attention Deficit Hyperactivity Disorder (ADHD)" (Letter from Abbott Pharmaceutical Products Division, December 1996, Ref. 03-4735-R18). The earliest reported onset of hepatic abnormalities occurred six months after initiation of pemoline. The company recommends that the drug be discontinued at the first signs of clinically significant hepatic dysfunction during its use.

All of the medications can produce temporary symptoms of psychosis (thought disorganization, press of speech, tactile hallucinations, extreme anxiety, hyperacusis, etc.) at very high doses, or even at smaller doses in a rare child. *Such reactions are quite uncommon.*[11,25] There may also occur rare cases of bone marrow suppression and neutropenia, thrombocytopenia, and anemia associated with stimulant use, leading some physicians to monitor complete blood counts (CBC) in all children during their initial drug trial. Yet the rarity of these cases may not justify the expense involved in screening all children for this side effect.

7. Summary of Short-Term Side Effects

Most of the short-term side effects of stimulants are clearly dose-related and subject to individual differences. Many of them diminish within 1–2 weeks of beginning medication, and all, except possibly the occasional tic, disappear upon ceasing pharmacotherapy. Where side effects persist beyond 1–2 weeks of treatment initiation, they can be made more tolerable by a slight lowering of the dose. Alternatively, a trial of a different stimulant medication can be initiated, as some side effects may be unique to the specific stimulant employed. It has been estimated that 1–3% of children with ADHD cannot tolerate any dose of stimulant medication.[25]

C. Long-Term Side Effects

For obvious practical reasons, the deleterious effects of using stimulant medications over several years with children has not been well studied. Nevertheless, there are now a number of follow-up studies, some of quite substantial duration,[79] which have not found any significant disadvantages associated with long-term stimulant treatment.

1. Drug Dependence and Abuse

Parents are often quite concerned about their children's possible addiction to stimulants or increased risk of abusing other drugs as teenagers. There are no reported individual cases of addiction or serious drug dependence to date with these medications. Several studies[79] have examined the question of whether children on these drugs are more likely to abuse other substances as teenagers than those not taking them. The results suggest that they are not, although more research is needed to rule this out conclusively.

2. Height and Weight Suppression

As noted earlier, one long-term side effect that has been of concern to many clinicians and scientists, though unlikely, is the suppression of height and weight gain. Early reports[138,139] indicated that both methylphenidate and dextroamphetamine produced this effect. Later studies have found this to be a dose-related phenomenon, more prevalent with dextroamphetamine, and to occur primarily within the first year of treatment. The loss in weight is typically minimal (1 kg or less). A rebound in growth or habituation to this effect seems to occur thereafter, and there is no appreciable effect on eventual adult height or weight.[140–142] Effects on growth are thought to be secondary to appetite suppression produced by these drugs, although several studies have indicated that stimulants may have some direct effects on growth hormone levels in the blood.[33] Thus, it seems reasonable to conclude that any suppression in growth is typically minor, is a relatively transient side effect of the first year or so of treatment, and has no significant effect on eventual adult height or weight. Recent evidence[141] indicates that children with ADHD may be somewhat smaller than normal prior to puberty and catch up with normal peers during adolescence, yet such growth delay is associated with the disorder and not with stimulant treatment. However, as always with group studies, a few individuals within the group may experience more serious weight loss as a function of stimulant treatment but, being so few in number, may be averaged out of the resulting mean statistics. Consequently, it still behooves the clinician to monitor weight and height periodically in children receiving stimulant medications and to alter dosage scheduling should clinically significant changes in these growth parameters occur as a function of stimulant treatment.

3. Cardiovascular Effects

While there is no evidence available on either side of the issue, some parents may express concern as to the effects of chronic stimulant drug use on the development of the cardiovascular system in children. All of the medications reviewed here have some effects on heart rate and blood pressure, albeit relatively mild. Even these effects appear to diminish or even dissipate with extended use of medication (measured up to 1.75 years).[142] The concern, however, is that children taking stimulants over a number of years might be at an increased risk for cardiovascular problems in middle-to-late life. At present, other than the single report of acutely increased blood pressure in African-American males, studies have not specifically addressed this important issue, but there is no reason from the extant data to suggest that such long-term cardiovascular problems might arise.

VI. CLINICAL INDICATIONS AND USAGE

A. Standard Indications

The stimulants are routinely indicated where children have significant problems with inattention, hyperactivity, impulsivity, and other symptoms associated with ADHD Combined Type (e.g., academic underproductivity, poor peer relations, aggression, etc.). The drugs are also useful in children with the Inattentive Type of ADHD, but the percentage of such children responding to medication may be somewhat lower (55–65%) than that seen in children with the Combined Type (70–90%), and the doses needed to achieve a therapeutic response may also be lower.[143,144] No studies have specifically examined children having the newest subtype of ADHD, that being the Predominantly Hyperactive–Impulsive Type, but this type is likely a preschool developmental precursor to the Combined Type and so these children may be just as likely to respond well to the medication as are children with the Combined Type, their young age notwithstanding.

Where ADHD symptoms are associated with *mental retardation*, the stimulants may also be useful in the management of those symptoms. However, clinical response may vary with the intellectual level of the child. One writer has argued that stimulants generally cause a focusing of attention and that some children who are mentally retarded (especially those with severe mental retardation) may already have overfocused attention.[145] In one study, children with mental ages greater than 4.5 years or IQs above 45 often had positive clinical responses whereas those with lower mental ages or IQs generally responded poorly.[146] It also appears that the closer the clinical picture of the patient with mental retardation approximates that of classical ADHD, the better may be the response to stimulant treatment.[146] However, one research group observed what appears to be a higher rate of unacceptable side effects due to methylphenidate in children with mental retardation than is typically the case in children of normal IQ.[147] In general, however, it appears that stimulants are useful in the management of ADHD symptoms in children with mental retardation.[108,109]

ADHD has become increasingly recognized as likely to persist into the adult years in at least 8–66% of all diagnosed childhood cases, with more recent studies using more contemporary diagnostic criteria tending to favor the higher figure. The recognition of adult ADHD has led to several studies involving stimulant medication trials with adults having ADHD. The most recent of these using current diagnostic criteria has shown that approximately 80% of adults respond well to methylphenidate.[148] These results indicate that as children with ADHD become adults, stimulant medication treatment can be a relatively successful means of continuing to manage their symptoms should this continue to be necessary.

B. Probable Indications

In the past it was commonly believed that stimulants lowered seizure thresholds, thereby ruling against their use in children with epilepsy or seizure disorders who also had ADHD. More recent studies have not found this to be the case[149,150] and so the drugs may be used safely with this population as well. However, one study (M. Fischer, personal communication, 1990) found more behavioral side effects among ADHD children with epilepsy when placed on stimulants than in a control group of ADHD children with epilepsy.

Similarly, the use of stimulants with ADHD children having tics or Tourette's syndrome has also been controversial (and potentially litigious). As noted above, the stimulants may exacerbate an existing tic disorder or Tourette's syndrome. While this is unlikely to be permanent and the tics return to their pretreatment frequency within 1–2 weeks, cases do exist in which exacerbation of tics or Tourette syndrome persists after cessation of medication. Current evidence implies that where Tourette's syndrome emerges in association with stimulant treatment, it may simply be coincidental in that the children were likely to have developed the disorder independent of their stimulant treatment.[151] Nevertheless, this area continues to be highly controversial, and clinicians are advised to proceed with caution in giving stimulants to children with tic disorders.

The role of stimulants in the treatment of children with pervasive developmental disorders is unclear owing to conflicting evidence. Single case reports have suggested positive responses while other studies of larger groups found evidence suggesting that such children were more likely to have an adverse response to medication than children without PDD who had mental retardation.[145,152]

Some children with traumatic brain injuries may develop symptoms of ADHD to a degree that warrants consideration of a stimulant drug trial. Gualtieri[153] reports that adults with ADHD symptoms, anergia/apathy, or disinhibition secondary to such brain injuries show a positive response to the stimulants. However, we are aware of no data available on this subject dealing with children with such brain injuries.

Recently, Fernandez[154] noted that the stimulants may also be beneficial in the management of HIV-related dementia and other concomitant organic mental disorders secondary to the HIV disease in adults. Of 97 HIV patients, 91% showed at least mild improvement and 72% were markedly improved. Among the patients with major depression or an organic mental disorder, 67–85% experienced a marked improvement. No controlled studies exist to show whether HIV-related mental disorders in children would respond this favorably, so this must await future confirmation.

Over 35 years ago, several reports noted the beneficial effects of stimulants on inpatients with drowsiness and lethargy associated with other medications, especially reserpine and anticonvulsants.[152] Little research has been conducted recently to follow up on these earlier positive reports.

The reduction of oppositional–defiant behavior and social aggressiveness by the stimulants in ADHD children has recently led to trials of the stimulants with adolescents diagnosed primarily as having conduct disorder. The response of inpatient conduct disordered teens has generally been positive, even in patients with no comorbid ADHD.[155] Not all studies agree on this issue, however. Thus, these positive findings should not automatically indicate widespread use of stimulants for conduct disordered youth, but they do imply that consideration of such medication be raised where ADHD may be comorbid with conduct disorder and be resulting in significant impairment.

C. Usage

Suggestions for ways in which to medicate and monitor stimulant use for children vary widely. We offer here an amalgamation of suggestions from our clinical practice and research and the advice of other respected scientist-practitioners in this area.[11,13,24,156,157]

1. When to Use Medication

The decision to use stimulant medications with children should not be undertaken lightly, despite the efficacy of these medications and their relative safety with children. As we have noted elsewhere,[99,104] *the diagnosis of ADHD should not constitute automatic drug treatment.* We suggest following several rules as aids in making the decision to use medication. They are intended only as rules of thumb. Clinicians should clearly remain flexible to the unique needs and circumstances of each case.

1. *Has the child had adequate physical and psychological evaluations?* Medications should never be prescribed if the child has not been directly examined in a thorough manner or if there is no other good evidence of physical health (e.g., pediatric or family physician assessment).

2. *How old is the child?* Pharmacotherapy is often less effective or leads to more severe side effects among children below the age of 4 years and is therefore not usually recommended in this age group.

3. *Have other therapies been used?* If this is the family's initial contact with the professional, prescription of medication might be postponed until other interventions (e.g., parent training in child management skills) have been attempted. Alternatively, when the child's behavior presents a severe problem and the family cannot participate in child management training, medication may be the most viable initial treatment.

4. *How severe are the child's current symptoms?* In some cases, the child's behavior is so unmanageable or distressing to the family that medication may prove the fastest and most effective manner of dealing with the crisis until other forms of treatment can commence. Once progress is obtained with other therapies, some effort can be made to reduce or terminate the medication, although this is not always possible.

5. *Can the family afford the medication and associated costs (e.g., follow-up visits)?* Long-term compliance rates are typically poor and may be especially problematic among families of low socioeconomic status. Of course, the family's ability to afford, and its compliance with, alternative treatments would also be suspect.

6. *Are the parents sufficiently able to adequately supervise the use of the medications and guard against their abuse?*

7. *What is (are) the parents' attitude(s) toward pharmacotherapy?* Some parents are simply "antidrug" and should not be coerced into agreeing to this treatment as they will probably sabotage its efficacy.

8. *Is there a substance-abusing sibling or drug-abusing parent in the household?* In this case, psychostimulant medication should not be prescribed since there is a high risk of its illicit use or sale. One might consider the use of pemoline, which seems to have little or no street value or potential for abuse, or alternative medications such as the tricyclic antidepressants or bupropion.

9. *Does the child have any history of psychosis, or thought disorder?* If so, the stimulants are contraindicated as they may exacerbate such difficulties.

10. *Is the child highly anxious, fearful, or more likely to complain of psychosomatic disturbances?* Such children are less likely to respond positively to stimulant medications and may exhibit a better response to antidepressant medications.

11. *Does the physician have the time to monitor medication effects properly?* In addition to an initial assessment of drug efficacy and establishing the optimal dosage, periodic reassessment of drug response and effects on height and weight should be conducted throughout the year.

12. *How does the child feel about medication and its alternatives?* With older children and adolescents, it is important that the use of medication be discussed with them and its rationale fully explained. In cases where children are "antidrug" or oppositional, they may resist efforts to use medication (e.g., refuse to swallow the pill).

13. *Is this child or adolescent involved in competitive sports in which urine screens for illicit drug use are routine?* If so, the clinician should discuss this issue with the parents as some children may be disqualified from participation in competitive sports as a result of taking methylphenidate immediately prior to or during such competitive events.

14. *Is the older adolescent being considered for medication treatment planning on entering the military?* A number of instances have been reported in the United States where teenagers planning to enlist in the military have been denied admission because of a history of having ADHD and, in particular, of having been treated with stimulant medication within the past few years. Again, clinicians should discuss this issue with parents and the adolescent before initiating stimulant medication treatment.

2. Initial Medical Workup

Although the monitoring of physical, behavioral, cognitive, emotional, and social parameters in children undergoing medication trials has been dealt with earlier in this text (see Chapters 4 and 5), a few recommendations seem in order here. Height and weight should always be recorded and, if possible, earlier measurements obtained so that the child's position and former trajectory on a growth velocity curve can be estimated. This makes it easier to evaluate any subsequent change in growth rate. Possible cardiological abnormality should be excluded, and blood pressures and pulse should be taken. Before giving stimulants, it is important to establish the child's previous eating and sleeping patterns. The pretreatment levels of potential behavioral side effects of stimulants should also be obtained by giving the Side-Effects Questionnaire (see below) at this time as many clinic-referred children show such behavioral/emotional problems before even beginning medication. Without such monitoring, these preexisting conditions might easily be confused with "side effects" during the subsequent trial. Finally, a careful history should be taken for evidence of possible seizure disorders and tics, and follow-up investigation done if indicated. Other laboratory tests (CBC, liver function tests) are only needed as baseline data or as part of a routine physical evaluation and have no routine specific application in preparation for prescribing stimulants, unless pemoline is to be used. In view of the extraordinary rarity of reports of bone marrow suppression on stimulants, it is not clear that screening of all stimulant-treated ADHD children with CBC tests would be sufficiently cost-effective to be recommended as standard care.

3. Prescribing and Titrating

Very young children (i.e., under the age of 4 years old) should not be given stimulant medications as a treatment of first choice, given the lower probability of a positive response ($<65\%$) and a higher incidence of side effects.[158] In general, however, very few well-controlled investigations of stimulant effects have been conducted with this age group, warranting the exercise of prudence when a child in this age group presents with significant symptoms of ADHD and no contraindications to pharmacotherapy. Similarly, the percentage of clinic-referred adolescents with ADHD who respond to stimulant medication may be somewhat lower (approximately 50%) than the response rate seen in 5- to 12-year-olds with

ADHD (70–95%).[159] Whether this has to do with true developmental changes in the response of children to the stimulants or to differences in the extent of comorbid conditions associated with poorer drug response (or poorer compliance!) that may be likely to be seen in clinic-referred adolescents relative to children is unclear. The risk of drug abuse of stimulants is clearly higher in adolescents, especially those with comorbid conduct disorder and abuse of other substances.

The first choice of medication is usually methylphenidate because of its greater documentation in research, proven efficacy across a wide age range, and the greater amount of dose–response information available. Since a child's failure to respond to one stimulant may not preclude a positive response to an alternate drug in the same class,[32] we recommend a trial of dextroamphetamine as the next step. Some clinicians, however, may still prefer to abandon stimulant medication treatment at this point until more evidence is available from research that response to one stimulant may not be predictive of response to the others. But failing a good response to dextroamphetamine, a trial of Adderall® could be considered, as clinical reports suggest that some patients may tolerate this combination better than dextroamphetamine, at least according to its manufacturer. If these medications are not effective, then a trial of pemoline could be considered, though the risk of hepatic toxicity of this medication requires closer monitoring and periodic assessment of liver functioning, making it a less benign medication than the other stimulants. Alternatively, we suggest switching to a tricyclic antidepressant (e.g., desipramine or imipramine), discussed in Chapter 9, fluoxetine or buproprion. If these, too, fail, then pharmacotherapy may need to be discontinued for at least one year, if not altogether eliminated from consideration. Children younger than the age of 6 years who evidence a poor response to stimulants may well respond positively in later years (i.e., after the age of 6). (The authors are aware that not all of these medications may be available outside of the United States, and so the availability of these or related medications will certainly dictate the stepwise sequence of medications to be tried in a particular clinical practice.)

The stimulant medications, their available tablet sizes, and typical dose ranges are displayed in Table 2. Although body weight has not been shown to be related to drug response, using it as a rough guideline for determining a starting dose continues to have some merit, in our opinion. Even so, idiosyncratic response is typically found among children of similar body weights and so the clinician must be prepared to titrate the dose to the individual responding of each case (which presumes careful monitoring). With methylphenidate, the usual practice is to start a child at a low dose such as 2.5–5 mg given twice daily; children below the age of 5 years can be started on 2.5 mg given once daily to lessen the likelihood of an immediate adverse response. We recommend beginning with a twice-daily dose (morning and noon) for school age children to assess dose response and then progressing to a third dose for some children, as needed. Other practitioners with whom we are familiar prefer to start with a single morning dose only as a few children may require only this scheduling of medication to achieve a therapeutic response. Third dosing may be beneficial to some children and not result in detrimental effects on sleep onset or duration for most taking such a t.i.d. schedule.[160,161] The dose is increased by 2.5- to 5-mg increments on a weekly basis until therapeutic effects are reported or a dose of 1 mg/kg is reached. Even then, a few children may require doses slightly higher than this recommended threshold. Children who rise early or who have a more rapid elimination of the drug may require doses three times per day. The daily dose needed to achieve optimum behavior change typically does not need to exceed 20 mg per dose given two to three times daily. However, once again, some children may benefit from somewhat higher doses than this traditional level,

TABLE 2. Stimulant Drugs, Available Doses, and Costs

Drug	Trade name	Manufacturer	Doses	Costs[a]
Dextroamphetamine	Dexedrine®	Smith, Kline, & French	5, 10, and 15 mg	
			Tablets (5 mg)	$0.13
			Spansule (5, 10, and 15 mg)	$0.29–0.46
			Elixir (5 mg/5 mL)	
	Generic		5- and 10-mg tablets	$0.03–0.04
			Recommended range: 2.5–20 mg	
Methylphenidate	Ritalin®	CIBA	5, 10, and 20 mg	$0.23–0.47
			20 mg SR	$0.71
	Generic		5, 10, and 20 mg	$0.17–0.36
			Recommended range: 2.5–60 mg	
Amphetamine/ dextroamphetamine	Adderall®	Shire	10- and 20-mg tablets	$0.46–0.67
			Recommended range: 2.5–40 mg	
Pemoline	Cylert®	Abbott	18.75-, 37.5-, and 75-mg tablets	$0.36–0.97
			Chewable tablets (37.5 mg)	
			Recommended range: 18.75–112.5 mg	

[a]Sources: Dulcan M: Using psychostimulants to treat behavioral disorders of children and adolescents. *J Child Adolesc Psychopharmacol* 1:7–20, 1990, and Adderall® product information sheet, Richwood Pharmaceuticals.

although there is a possible increase in the severity of side effects. We rarely go beyond 40–60 mg per day in our clinic. Other clinicians have reported to us an average dose range of 5–15 mg per dose in the morning, tapering down to a half dose at noon, and then a third of the morning dose in the afternoon.

Giving the doses with or after meals may lessen the anorexia or stomachaches sometimes associated with these drugs. Where such side effects are not problematic, it has been traditionally suggested that the medications be given 30 min before mealtimes to minimize excretion rates. A very small study[162] suggests that the effect of meals is not statistically significant, but the trend of the data supported administration prior to meals. So, while this may not typically be significant in individual cases, it may be worth adhering to this traditional advice in a child who is responding only marginally to medication despite adequate dosage.

As noted earlier, it is a matter of some controversy whether behavioral tolerance develops with chronic administration of stimulants. Extant research indicates that failure to maintain clinical response at a given dose is more likely to occur with higher dosages (i.e., 15 mg or 20 mg b.i.d.) after a period of six months or more of chronic use. This is, by no means, a universal phenomenon, and each case must be evaluated individually. A reevaluation of a child's maintenance dose on an annual basis, as discussed below, to determine the necessity of a dosage change is strongly recommended.

As Table 2 indicates, dextroamphetamine is typically given in doses about half those of methylphenidate due to its greater potency. However, since the potency equivalence of these medications has not been properly established, a dose of dextroamphetamine that is one-fourth that of methylphenidate can be used. Pemoline is prescribed and titrated quite differently, given that it is a "steady-state" medication (i.e., requiring several days to develop a pharmacodynamic equilibrium). It is generally given only once a day, in the morning. The initial dose is usually 37.5 mg and is titrated upward in 18.75-mg increments every 3–5 days until a therapeutic effect is reported, up to a maximum of 112.5 mg or 2.2 mg/kg for adolescents.[11] On occasion, a second dose, often half that of the morning dose, may be given in mid-afternoon if the morning dose is proving ineffective during the afternoon. This, however, may increase the chances of insomnia occurring. Several investigations have indicated that pemoline is slower in achieving its peak effects and in "washing out" of the body than the other stimulants. Thus, its effects may last 2–3 days following its discontinuation.

Both methylphenidate and dextroamphetamine are available in short-acting and sustained-release forms. The sustained-release forms have several benefits such as making noontime medication administration at school unnecessary and affording greater confidentiality of treatment. At the peak of their time course, the sustained-release forms of these medications appear to be as effective as their standard preparations. However, there is both research and clinical evidence that sustained-release methylphenidate may be less effective than the standard preparation during the first several hours post ingestion.[15] In our experience, some patients may demonstrate a diminished efficacy, particularly during the morning hours, when switching from standard methylphenidate to the sustained-release compound. For these reasons, the use of the shorter-acting forms of these medications may be more ideal except in situations where in-school administration of the drugs is significantly problematic (e.g., no school nurse to dispense the medication or for teenagers who may be more sensitive to teasing or censure by peers).

Generic forms of the stimulants are now available and provide a less expensive alternative to their brand-name counterparts. Although no empirical investigations of differences in their efficacy have been reported, brands may possibly vary in quality, leading to complaints from parents or teachers of greater variability in the behavioral control achieved with the generic as compared to the brand-name medication.

Methylphenidate and dextroamphetamine can be dispensed according to various schedules depending upon the severity of the child's ADHD and associated difficulties. In a minority of cases, the medication may be used primarily for classroom management. If so, it is usually suggested that it be discontinued on weekends, holidays, and summer vacations. When reinitiation of the medication each Monday produces a renewal of side effects exhibited only at the start of each week, keeping the child on one-half or less of the regular dose during the weekend may maintain habituation to side effects. Most ADHD children, however, exhibit significant behavioral control difficulties at home and in the community as well as during school. Indeed, this might be considered almost a requirement of diagnosis if DSM-IV criteria for ADHD are to be strictly adhered to in clinical practice (i.e., the requirement of impairing symptoms in at least two settings). In these cases, it is recommended that the child receive medication 7 days a week with an attempt to discontinue pharmacotherapy during school vacations, when possible or feasible. As noted above, it may be necessary to recommend the use of a twice-daily or even three-times-a-day dose schedule with methylphenidate, primarily because effects may last 3–4 hr or less with some children. This problem is often discovered in contacts with the child's teachers, who may observe that the morning dose has essentially worn off by mid-morning. In such cases, the following schedule may be employed: a breakfast dose at 7:00–8:00 A.M., a second dose at 10:30–11:00 A.M., and a final dose at 2:00–3:00 P.M.

In general, the dose should always be the lowest possible and should be given only as many times per day as necessary to achieve adequate management of the child's behavior. In many cases, pharmacotherapy need not be discontinued on holidays or summer vacations because of the benefits that accrue to increased self-control, social conduct, and task persistence from stimulants in settings other than school. Should a significant change in the child's growth trajectory be evident from such medication use, then returning to the traditional drug holidays on weekends and school vacations may be necessary for some children.

Titration should be based on a wide range and objective assessment whenever possible (as described below) and should start with the lowest possible increments. Sufficient time (e.g., 5–7 days) should be allowed to evaluate the efficacy of each dosage.

Parents should never be given permission to adjust the dosage of medication without consultation with the physician. Otherwise, parents may overmedicate the child, as they may increase the dose every time the child is temperamental, noncompliant, or obstinant. Such occurrences are usually better treated by the altering of parent management styles.

D. Monitoring Response to Medication

The methods used by practicing clinicians to monitor medication response vary widely in content and quality. Unfortunately, all too frequently, titration of dosage and long-term assessment of efficacy are based solely on the subjective reports of parents, thereby increasing the chances of erroneous decisions. Indeed, the most appropriate clinical dosage for a child cannot be adequately established without school-based information, which can be obtained directly or via the parent and through standardized rating scales. Monitoring procedures are discussed in more detail in Chapter 5.

1. Assessing Initial Response to Medication

Objective data regarding changes in an ADHD child's behavior should always be collected across several doses, given the frequently unique and idiosyncratic reactions of children to these drugs. Under ideal circumstances, a child's optimal dose should be established in the context of a double-blind, placebo-controlled assessment paradigm which includes multiple measures collected across several settings (i.e., home, school, and clinic). This type of evaluation not only involves the aggregation of objective, quantitative data regarding a child's treatment response but also the use of a placebo control wherein teachers, parents, and children do not know the dosage being administered.[59,162] In addition, it is often helpful for the parents and teachers to complete a weekly Side-Effects Questionnaire.[99]

There is a high likelihood of apparent "practice effects" on these rating scales between their first and second, and possibly later, administrations. Many parent and teacher rating scales show significant declines in scores between their first and second administrations even when there has been no intervening treatment. Clinicians who give the scales once, begin drug treatment, and then give them again a week or two later are likely to confuse the drug effects with these practice effects, concluding that the medication or that dose of it was helpful when it may not have been. Clinicians using these scales should give them twice before using them in drug trials and to use the *second* administration as the baseline against which to measure changes due to medication trials.

2. Maintenance on Medication

a. Assessing Progress

Once a child's optimal dosage is established, then some, or preferably all, of the above measures should be collected periodically throughout the school year to evaluate the need for dosage adjustments or the onset of side effects. The vast majority of the questionnaires need only be readministered every several months or so. However, it is usually a good idea to review items from the Side-Effects Questionnaire each month when the parents call to obtain another prescription. In addition, at each monthly contact (usually by telephone), a checklist of questions is reviewed with parents to assess continued drug efficacy.[99]

b. When the Effect Appears to Diminish

Parents may call to complain about ineffective doses that were formerly effective. Physicians should employ caution before deciding to increase the level of medication. If no family turmoil or precipitating stressful events are occurring, then it may indeed be true that the current dosage has become less effective. Careful questioning of the parent as to the ways in which the child's behavior is different or worse can be useful in making the decision. In addition, the child's teacher should be contacted to ascertain whether similar deterioration in functioning has occurred in the school setting. The parent and teacher questionnaires discussed above should be administered and compared to previously collected data in an effort to specify which behaviors have actually worsened and to quantify the amount of behavioral change. After this is done, if there are no side effects, a cautious increment in dosage may be tried, providing the dosage has not yet exceeded 1 mg/kg/per dose.

c. Side Effects

Side effects should be asked about at every monthly contact, and the parents should be informed in advance about the presenting symptoms of any serious side effects, for example, depression, weight loss, induction of tics, or, with pemoline, hepatic damage. For children receiving pemoline, at 6-month intervals, or whenever suspicions are prompted by symptoms, blood should be drawn for liver function tests, given the findings that this drug may rarely and idiosyncratically adversely affect liver functions. This is no substitute for a review of possible presenting symptoms of such dysfunction at each monthly contact.

d. Reassessment

Approximately every 3–4 months that a child is on medication, it is advisable to administer a more thorough follow-up clinic examination. At this time, height, weight, blood pressure, and heart rate can be recorded to determine potential side effects and any blood tests can be done. Parent and teacher ratings should be collected concurrently with this visit as well. Difficulties that continue to plague the child or family can be discussed, and referrals to appropriate professionals can be made as necessary. When parents are called for the appointment, they should be encouraged to write down in advance any concerns or questions they might have, so that the visit can be as useful as possible.

E. Discontinuing Medication

There are no firm guidelines regarding when to discontinue treatment, other than a determination that medication no longer seems to be necessary. Up to 20% of children may be able to have medication stopped after a year or so. These drugs do not need to be discontinued at onset of puberty, as their efficacy with adolescents has been established.[47,148] Further, chronic administration of these drugs does not appear to increase the probability of substance abuse and may, in fact, decrease it.[79]

Treatment can be discontinued annually for a short time (e.g., a few days to 2 weeks) usually a month or so after the beginning of the new academic year, and standardized measures, such as rating scales, can be collected during both medication and nonmedication periods. We recommend that children who have been on medication the previous school year begin a new academic year on that medication so as not to have the child fail at the beginning of a new school year, thereby establishing for himself or herself a reputation that may be difficult to overcome thereafter. The reassessment of drug responding should not take place right at the beginning of the school year to ensure that the child has acclimated to the new classroom and to prevent erroneous decisions being made on the basis of a "honeymoon" effect with a new teacher, which may occur during the initial stages of the academic year. If there is no significant difference in the child's behavior when he or she is on or off medication, then treatment may be discontinued for a longer period. If there is no appreciable difference with treatment and the child continues to display behavioral control difficulties, it may be time to reevaluate the dosage or switch to a different medication.

VII. CONTRAINDICATIONS AND DRUG INTERACTIONS

As stated earlier, children with a history of tics, Tourette's disorder, psychosis, autism, or pervasive developmental disorder should be given stimulant medications with great caution, for the latter often exacerbate the symptoms of such disorders. Children with high levels of anxiety (e.g., generalized anxiety disorder) are also likely to respond poorly to these medications. Furthermore, children under 4 years of age tend to be poor responders to stimulant compounds, and there are few research studies investigating drug effects and side effects in this age group. There is some controversy over whether stimulants should be given to children with seizures or epilepsy; doubts about the practice are based on the possibility that these drugs may lower seizure thresholds. Studies[148,149] showed that this does not often occur. This phenomenon is rarely, if ever, seen clinically, and it can be avoided by a slight increase in the level of anticonvulsants. High blood pressure, cardiac, or cardiovascular problems in children may also be contraindications for the stimulants, given their mild but significant cardiac pressor effects, but a pediatric cardiologist should be consulted in these cases.

The stimulants can alter the actions of other medications. Though such interactions are unusual, some are potentially serious. The sedating effects of antihistamines and benzodiazepines may be inhibited by stimulants, and stimulants can potentiate the effect of all sympathomimetic drugs, including street drugs and cocaine. The effect of combining heterocyclic antidepressants with stimulants may be beneficial, and in small doses this combination may give better and more even control of ADHD symptoms. However, cardiac arrhythmias and hypertensive crises have been reported, as have unusual cognitive and mood disturbances.[163] Stimulant and antidepressant drugs also may accentuate the effects of one another. The combination of monoamine oxidase inhibitors (MAOIs), sometimes used as antidepressants, with stimulants is dangerous and may lead to a fatal hypertensive crisis. If an MAOI has been used, a minimum two-week washout interval should be allowed before beginning stimulants. Lithium inhibits the stimulatory effects of amphetamines, and probably those of other stimulants. Though the manufacturers suggest that the seizure threshold may be lowered by methylphenidate, in practice concomitant administration of methylphenidate and anticonvulsants for children with documented seizure disorder appears safe,[149,150] It has been suggested that amphetamines may act synergistically with phenytoin and phenobarbital to increase anticonvulsant activity. Other interactions have been documented with medications unlikely to be used in pediatric practice.

VIII. DRUG COMBINATIONS*

In rare cases, it may be necessary to combine the stimulants with other medications in order to achieve greater therapeutic management of the child with ADHD. This is likely to be so where comorbid disorders exist that may not respond satisfactorily to stimulants. Such disorders may include major depressive disorder, generalized anxiety disorder, juvenile-onset bipolar disorder, Tourette syndrome, or enuresis. In recent years, two types of drug combinations have increased in frequency in the clinical management of ADHD children, these being combined stimulant/antidepressant therapy and combined stimulant/clonidine therapy. Although these other medications are discussed in detail in their respective chapters in this text, some special considerations involved in these drug combinations are briefly discussed below.

A. Combined Stimulant/Antidepressant Therapy

Combinations of stimulant with tricyclic antidepressants can be considered when ADHD presents with comorbid, socially serious enuresis that remains refractory to behavioral treatment or with comorbid affective (mood and anxiety) disorders. In a series of studies, the separate and combined effects of methylphenidate and desipramine on ADHD and comorbid affective disorders have been investigated.[164–166] Although both medications alone produced reductions in ADHD symptoms, the combination produced positive effects on learning over and above the efficacy of each single agent. The combination was associated with more side effects than either drug alone, yet there was no evidence that combined use was associated with any unique or serious side effects. Stimulants have also been successfully combined with fluoxetine (a specific serotonin reuptake inhibitor antidepressant) in the management of ADHD and depression.[167] Again, such a combination has not been found to produce unique or serious side effects apart from those side effects associated with either drug used individually. Data are sparse on the issue, however, and continued vigilance in such cases seems prudent.

B. Combined Stimulant/Clonidine Therapy

Clonidine is a presynaptic α-adrenergic receptor agonist that downregulates norepinephrine outflow from the CNS (see Chapter 15). It has been combined with stimulants when ADHD children present with comorbid conduct disorder, extreme hyperactivity/impulsivity, and aggression. Clonidine does not improve attention span or academic productivity significantly but may be helpful in decreasing overarousal that contributes to behavior problems in these children.[168] Because of its acute sedative properties, clonidine may also be used with stimulants for sleep disorders which commonly present as part of ADHD in children.[30] Clonidine decreases blood pressure and pulse. Children with preexist-

---

*See also Chapter 1.

ing syncope, bradycardic arrhythmias, or cardiac conditions are not candidates for clonidine therapy. Recently, three cases of sudden death were reported in children taking combined methylphenidate/clonidine therapy.[169] Although the hazard may have been merely coincidental, prudence suggests that practitioners be cautious in prescribing the combination and in monitoring any physical effects.[170] In addition, abrupt clonidine withdrawal (e.g., from noncompliance) can result in adrenergic rebound and associated treatment-emergent symptoms of hypertension, diaphoresis, tachycardia, diarrhea, and anxiety. A baseline child and family cardiac history, recent physical examination, and baseline and on drug electrocardiogram, pulse, and blood pressure monitoring are recommended when clonidine is combined with stimulants. Clonidine is discussed in detail in Chapter 15.

IX. MANAGEMENT OF STIMULANT OVERDOSE

Stimulant overdose is rarely, if ever, fatal on its own. In fact, we are aware of no cases of fatalities from oral administration. Signs and symptoms of acute overdose result from overstimulation of the central nervous system and from excessive sympathomimetic effects. These may include symptoms such as vomiting, agitation, tremor, convulsions, confusion, hallucinations, hyperpyrexia, tachycardia, arrhythmias, hypertension, and delirium. Treatment consists of prompt medical referral and appropriate supportive measures. The patient must be protected from self-injury and from environmental overstimulation that would aggravate heightened sympathomimetic arousal. Chlorpromazine has been reported in the literature to be useful in decreasing CNS stimulation and sympathomimetic effects. Sedation with a barbiturate may also be helpful. If the patient is alert and conscious, gastric contents may be evacuated by induction of emesis or gastric lavage. For amphetamine intoxication, acidification of the urine will increase excretion. For more severe overdose, intensive care must be provided to maintain adequate cardiopulmonary function and treat hyperpyrexia. The efficacy of peritoneal dialysis or extracorporeal hemodialysis for stimulant overdosage has not been established.

X. SUMMARY

This survey of the clinical effects and side effects of stimulant medications suggests the following conclusions about their use in the treatment of children, particularly those with ADHD.[99]

1. Up to 70–80% of children with carefully diagnosed ADHD appear to exhibit a positive response to CNS stimulants. Primary effects are the improvement of attention span and the reduction of disruptive, inappropriate, and impulsive behavior. Compliance with authority-figure commands is increased, and children's peer relations may also improve, primarily through reductions in aggression. If the medication is titrated according to changes in academic performance, improvements may also be seen in productivity and accuracy, at least in the short term. Dosages and regimens should be individualized and adjusted slowly to suit each child and never given according to some formula. Many of the problems attributed to stimulants may be the result of excessive dose levels and schedules for a particular child, as well as to overly ambitious clinical objectives in inadequately assessed and monitored children.

2. While these medications are certainly helpful in the day-to-day management of ADHD, they have not been demonstrated to lead to enduring positive changes after their cessation. Thus, this treatment is not a quick solution to ADHD but rather an intervention that must often be employed on a chronic basis to maintain positive effects.

3. The side effects, both short- and long-term, are generally mild, often transient, and diminish with reduction or discontinuance of pharmacotherapy. Children with ADHD who also have a personal or family history of tics or Tourette syndrome may be prescribed stimulants, but closer monitoring of such children and the use of lower doses during initial titration may be in order. Tics may be induced or exacerbated by the stimulants in some children even though recent studies have not documented such reactions to be as likely as early reports indicated initially. Whether such tics may prove irreversible seems unlikely but is not yet known.

4. Despite the lack of established long-term success of these medications, they are useful in managing the behavior of children with symptoms of ADHD. While the issue of controlling the behavior of children with drugs is highly controversial, the difficulties these youngsters present to others who must live, work, or attend school with them must not be overlooked. Not only do such children frustrate parents and teachers, but the effects of their disruptive behavior on the ability of their classmates to receive adequate instruction is at times considerable. If medications can temporarily ameliorate these difficulties, while reducing the level of ostracism, censure, and punishment that children with ADHD receive, then they seem certainly worthwhile.

5. Stimulant medications are not a panacea for ADHD or its symptoms and should not be the sole treatment employed in most cases. Other therapies focusing on the myriad of social, psychological, educational, and physical problems these children often display will be necessary.[3] Medications do not teach the child anything; they merely alter the likelihood of occurrence of behaviors already in the child's repertoire. The numerous skill deficits that these children may present with will still require attention. Thus, the medication may enhance the efficacy of other interventions by aiding the child to attend and respond to the environment in a more successful fashion. Nevertheless, parents will require child management training and other forms of counseling to cope with the child during periods when the medication can not be used. Each professional must, therefore, be knowledgeable about the resources within the community that will be necessary to treat the "total child."

XI. CONCLUSION

The stimulant medications are effective and safe treatments for the symptomatic management of children with symptoms of ADHD. Indeed, they are the best studied treatment applied to this disorder and are among the safest and most effective symptomatic treatments in medicine. Most children who receive stimulants will show improvements in their attention, impulse control, task-irrelevant activity, academic productivity and accuracy, handwriting, play, social conduct, and/or compliance to commands and rules. These result in a diminution of the supervision, reprimands, punishment, and censure from those adults and peers who must frequently interact with them. Changes in the long-term outcome of children on stimulants have not been reliably obtained to date. Even though the stimulants are quite useful in the day-to-day management of symptoms of ADHD, other treatments are usually required to maximize the chances for better short- and long-term adjustment. This is because the stimulants do not teach appropriate or prosocial behavior but increase the probabilities of a child displaying "good" behavior that is already in the child's repertoire. Such displays of behavior require that the right environment be present to reinforce and maintain their occurrence. While the absence of such positive environments or adjunctive treatments cannot be a sole reason to give medication to children, neither is it a reason to withhold it.

REFERENCES

1. Safer DJ, Zito JM, Fine EM: Increased methylphenidate usage for attention deficit disorder in the 1990s. *Pediatrics* 98:1084–1088, 1996.
2. American Psychiatric Association: *Diagnostic and Statistical Manual of Mental Disorders,* 3 ed, revised. Washington DC, American Psychiatric Association, 1987.
3. Barkley RA: *Attention Deficit Hyperactivity Disorder: A Handbook for Diagnosis and Treatment.* New York, Guilford, 1990.
4. Lou HC, Henriksen L, Bruhn P: Focal cerebral hypoperfusion in children with dysphasia and/or attention deficit disorder. *Arch Neurol* 41:825–829, 1984.
5. Lou HC, Henriksen L, Bruhn P, et al: Striatal dysfunction in attention deficit and hyperkinetic disorder. *Arch Neurol* 46:48–52, 1989.
6. Redman CA, Zametkin AJ: Ritalin and brain metabolism, in Greenhill LL, Osmon BB (eds): *Ritalin: Theory and Patient Management.* New York, Mary Ann Liebert, 1991, pp 301–309.
7. Gualtieri CT, Hicks RE, Mayo JP: Hyperactivity and homeostasis. *J Am Acad Child Adolesc Psychiatry* 22:382–384, 1983.
8. Haenlein M, Caul WF: Attention deficit disorder with hyperactivity: A specific hypothesis of reward dysfunction. *J Am Acad Child Adolesc Psychiatry* 26:356–362, 1987.
9. Diener RM: Toxicology of Ritalin, in Greenhill LL, Osmon BB (eds): Ritalin: *Theory and Patient Management.* New York, Mary Ann Liebert, 1991, pp 34–43.
10. Brown GL, Hunt RD, Ebert MH, et al: Plasma levels of d- amphetamine in hyperactive children. *Psychopharmacology* 62:133–140, 1979.
11. Dulcan MK: Using psychostimulants to treat behavioral disorders of children and adolescents. *J Child Adolesc Psychopharmacol* 1:7–20, 1990.
12. Wargin W, Patrick K, Kilts C, et al: Pharmacokinetics of methylphenidate in man, rat, and monkey. *J Pharmacol Exp Ther* 226:382–386, 1983.
13. Cantwell D, Carlson G: Stimulants, in Werry J (ed): *Pediatric Psychopharmacology.* New York, Brunner/Mazel, 1978, pp 171–207.
14. Birmaher B, Greenhill LL, Cooper TB, Fried J, Maminski B: Sustained release methylphenidate: Pharmacokinetic studies in ADDH males. *J Am Acad Child Adolesc Psychiatry* 28:768–772, 1989.
15. Pelham WE, Sturges J, Hoza J, et al: Sustained release and standard methylphenidate effects on cognitive and social behavior in children with attention deficit disorder. *Pediatrics* 4:491–501, 1987.
16. Pelham WE, Greenslade KE, Vodde-Hamilton M, et al: Relative efficacy of long-acting stimulants on children with attention deficit-hyperactivity disorder: A comparison of standard methylphenidate, sustained-release methylphenidate, sustained-release dextroamphetamine, and pemoline. *Pediatrics* 86:226–237, 1990.
17. Fitzpatrick PA, Klorman R, Brumaghim JT, Borgstedt AD: Effects of sustained-release and standard preparations of methylphenidate on attention deficit disorder. *J Am Acad Child Adolesc Psychiatry* 31:226–234, 1992.
18. Patrick KS, Mueller RA, Gualtieri CT, et al: Pharmacokinetics and actions of methylphenidate, in Meltzer HY (ed): *Psychopharmacology: The Third Generation of Progress.* New York, Raven Press, 1987.
19. Sallee F, Stiller R, Perel J, et al: Oral pemoline kinetics in hyperactive children. *Clin Pharmacol Ther* 37:606–609, 1985.
20. Pelham WE, Swanson JM, Furman MB, Schwindt H: Pemoline effects on children with ADHD: A time-response by dose-response analysis on classroom measures. *J Am Acad Child Adolesc Psychiatry* 34:1504–1513, 1995.
21. Kupietz SS: Ritalin blood levels and their correlations with measures of learning, in Greenhill LL, Osmon BB (eds): *Ritalin: Theory and Patient Management.* New York, Mary Ann Liebert, 1991, pp 247–256.

22. Swanson JM: Measurement of serum concentrations and behavioral response in ADDH children to acute doses of methylphenidate, in LB Bloomingdale (ed): *Attention Deficit Disorder: New Research in Attention, Treatment, and Psychopharmacology*. New York, Pergamon Press, 1988.
23. Swanson J, Kinsbourne M, Roberts W, et al: Time-response analysis of the effect of medication on the learning ability of children referred for hyperactivity. *Pediatrics* 61:21–29, 1978.
24. Shaywitz SE, Shaywitz BA: Attention deficit disorder: Diagnosis and role of Ritalin in management, in Greenhill LL, Osmon BB (eds): *Ritalin: Theory and Patient Management*. New York, Mary Ann Liebert, 1991, pp 45–68.
25. Barkley RA: A review of stimulant drug research with hyperactive children. *J Child Psychol Psychiatry* 18:137–165, 1977.
26. DuPaul GJ, Rapport MD: Does methylphenidate normalize the classroom performance of children with attention deficit disorder? *J Am Acad Child Adolesc Psychiatry* 32:190–198, 1993.
27. Rapport MD, Denny C, DuPaul GJ, Gardner MJ: Attention deficit disorder and methylphenidate: Normalization rates, clinical effectiveness, and response prediction in 76 children. *J Am Acad Child Adolesc Psychiatry* 33:882–893, 1994.
28. DuPaul GJ, Barkley RA, McMurray MD: Response of children with ADHD to methylphenidate: Interaction with internalizing symptoms. *J Am Acad Child Adolesc Psychiatry* 33:894–903, 1994.
29. Pelham WE: Pharmacotherapy for children with attention-deficit hyperactivity disorder. *School Psychol Rev* 22:199–227, 1993.
30. Spencer T, Biederman J, Wilens T, Harding M, O'Donnell D, Griffin S: Pharmacotherapy of attention-deficit hyperactivity disorder across the life cycle. *J Am Acad Child Adolesc Psychiatry* 35:409–432, 1996.
31. Swanson JM, McBurnett K, Christian DL, Wigal T: Stimulant medications and the treatment of children with ADHD, in Ollendick TH, Prinz RJ (eds): *Advances in Clinical Child Psychology*, New York, Plenum, 1995, vol 17, pp 265–322.
32. Elia J, Rapoport JL: Ritalin versus dextroamphetamine in ADHD: Both should be tried, in Greenhill LL, Osmon BB (eds): *Ritalin: Theory and Patient Management*. New York, Mary Ann Liebert, 1991, pp 69–74.
33. Reeve E, Garfinkel B: Neuroendocrine and growth regulation: The role of sympathomimetic medication, in Greenhill LL, Osmon BB (eds): *Ritalin: Theory and Patient Management*. New York, Mary Ann Liebert, 1991, pp 289–300.
34. Klein RG, Mannuzza S: Hyperactive boys almost grown up: III. Methylphenidate effects on ultimate height. *Arch Gen Psychiatry* 45:1131–1134, 1988.
35. Gittelman R, Landa B, Mattes JA, et al: Methylphenidate and growth in hyperactive children. *Arch Gen Psychiatry* 45:1127–1130, 1988.
36. Kalikow KT, Blumencranz H: Severe weight loss induced by Adderall in a child with ADHD. *J Child Adolesc Psychopharmacol* 6:81–82.
37. Hastings JE, Barkley RA: A review of psychophysiological research with hyperactive children. *J Abnorm Child Psychol* 7:413–447, 1978.
38. Rosenthal RH, Allen TW: An examination of attention, arousal, and learning dysfunctions of hyperkinetic children. *Psychol Bull* 85:689–715, 1978.
39. Taylor EA: *The Overactive Child*. Philadelphia, LP Lippincott, 1986.
40. Kelly KL, Rapport MD, DuPaul GJ: Attention deficit disorder and methylphenidate: A multi-step analysis of dose response effects on children's cardiovascular functioning. *Int Clin Psychopharmacol* 3:167–181, 1988.
41. Aman MG, Werry JS: The effects of methylphenidate and haloperidol on the heart rate and blood pressure of hyperactive children with special reference to time of action. *Psychopharmacology* 43:163–168, 1975.
42. Safer DJ: Relative cardiovascular safety of psychostimulants used to treat attention-deficit hyperactivity disorder. *J Child Adolesc Psychopharmacol* 2:279–290, 1992.
43. Knights RM, Viets A: Effects of pemoline on hyperactive boys. *Pharmacol Biochem Behav* 3:1107–1114, 1975.
44. Brown RT, Sexson SB: Effects of methylphenidate on cardiovascular responses in attention deficit hyperactivity disordered adolescents. *J Adolesc Health Care* 10:179–183, 1989.
45. Barkley RA, Jackson T Jr: Hyperkinesis, autonomic nervous system activity, and stimulant drug effects. *J Child Psychol Psychiatry* 18:347–357, 1977.
46. Satterfield JH, Dawson ME: Electrodermal correlates of hyperactivity in children. *Psychophysiology* 8:191–197, 1971.
47. Coons HW, Klorman R, Borgstedt AD: Effects of methylphenidate on adolescents with a childhood history of attention deficit disorder: II. Information processing. *J. Am Acad Child Adolesc Psychiatry* 26:368–374, 1987.
48. Peloquin LJ, Klorman R: Effects of methylphenidate on normal children's mood, event-related potentials, and performance in memory scanning and vigilance. *J Abnorm Psychol* 95:88–98, 1986.

49. Zametkin A, Nordahl T, Gross M, et al: Brain metabolism in hyperactive adults with childhood onset. *N Engl J Med* 323:1361–1366, 1990.

50. Bergman A, Winters L, Cornblatt B: Methylphenidate: Effects on sustained attention, in Greenhill LL, Osmon BB (eds): *Ritalin: Theory and Patient Management*. New York, Mary Ann Liebert, 1991, pp 223–232.

51. Barkley RA, Cunningham CE: The effects of methylphenidate on the mother-child interactions of hyperactive children. *Arch Gen Psychiatry* 36:201–208, 1979.

52. Swanson J, Kinsbourne M: The cognitive effects of stimulant drugs on hyperactive children, in Hale GA, Lewis M (eds): *Attention and Cognitive Development*. New York, Plenum, 1978, pp 249–274.

53. Elia J, Borcherding BG, Rapoport JL, Keysor CS: Methylphenidate and dextroamphetamine treatments of hyperactivity: Are there true nonresponders? *Psychiatry Res* 36:141–155, 1991.

54. Milich R, Carlson CL, Pelham WE, Licht BG: Effects of methylphenidate on the persistence of ADHD boys following failure experiences. *J Abnorm Child Psychol* 19:519–536, 1991.

55. Abikoff H, Gittelman R: Does behavior therapy normalize the classroom behavior of hyperactive children? *Arch Gen Psychiatry* 41:449–454, 1984.

56. DuPaul GJ, Rapport M: Attention deficit disorder: Does methylphenidate normalize classroom functioning? Paper presented at the American Psychological Association, August, San Francisco, Calif, 1991.

57. Pelham WE, Milich R: Individual differences in response to Ritalin in classwork and social behavior, in Greenhill LL, Osmon BB (eds): *Ritalin: Theory and Patient Management*. New York, Mary Ann Liebert, 1991, pp 203–221.

58. Pelham WE, McBurnet K, Harper GW, Milich R, et al: Methylphenidate and baseball playing in ADHD children: Who's on first? *J Consult Clin Psychol* 58:130–133, 1990.

59. Barkley RA, Fischer M, Newby R, et al: Development of a multi-method clinical protocol for assessing stimulant drug responses in ADHD children. *J Clin Child Psychol* 17:14–24, 1988.

60. Hinshaw SP: Stimulant medication and the treatment of aggression in children with attentional deficits. *J Clin Child Psychol* 20:301–312, 1991.

61. Rapport MD, DuPaul GJ, Stoner G, et al: Comparing classroom and clinic measures of attention deficit disorder: Differential, idiosyncratic, and dose-response effects of methylphenidate. *J Consult Clin Psychol* 54:334–341, 1986.

62. Rapport MD, Kelly KL: Psychostimulant effects on learning and cognitive function in children with attention deficit hyperactivity disorder: Findings and implications, in Matson JL (ed): *Hyperactivity in Children: A Handbook*. New York, Pergamon, 1991.

63. Hinshaw SP, Henker B, Whalen CK, Erhardt D, Dunnington RE: Aggressive, prosocial, and nonsocial behavior in hyperactive boys: Dose effects of methylphenidate in naturalistic settings. *J Consult Clin Psychol* 57:636–643, 1989.

64. Murphy DA, Pelham WE, Lang AR: Aggression in boys with attention deficit-hyperactivity disorder: Methylphenidate effects on naturalistically observed aggression, response to provocation, and social information processing. *J Abnorm Child Psychol* 20:451–465, 1992.

65. Shah MR, Seese LM, Abikoff H, Klein RG: Pemoline for children and adolescents with conduct disorder: A pilot investigation. *J Child Adolesc Psychopharmacol* 4:255–261, 1994.

66. Hinshaw SP, Heller T, McHale JP: Covert antisocial behavior in boys with attention-deficit hyperactivity disorder: External validation and effects of methylphenidate. *J Consult Clin Psychol* 60:274–281, 1992.

67. Rapoport JL, Buchsbaum MS, Zahn TP, et al: Dextroamphetamine: Cognitive and behavioral effects in normal prepubertal boys. *Science* 199:560–563, 1978.

68. Solanto MV: Dosage effects of Ritalin on cognition, in Greenhill LL, Osmon BB (eds): *Ritalin: Theory and Patient Management*. New York, Mary Ann Liebert, 1991, pp 233–246.

69. Douglas VI, Barr RG, O'Neill ME, et al: Dosage effects and individual responsivity to methylphenidate in attention deficit disorder. *J Child Psychol Psychiatry* 29:453–475, 1988.

70. Swanson JM: Paired-associate learning in the assessment of ADD-H children, in Bloomingdale LM, Swanson J (eds): *Attention Deficit Disorder: Current Concepts and Emerging Trends in Attentional and Behavioral Disorders of Childhood*. New York, Pergamon Press, 1989, pp 87–123.

71. Vyse SA, Rapport MD: The effects of methylphenidate on learning in children with ADDH: The stimulus-equivalence paradigm. *J Consult Clin Psychol* 57:425–435, 1989.

72. Sergeant J, van der Meere JJ: Ritalin effects and information processing in hyperactivity, in Greenhill LL, Osmon BB (eds): *Ritalin: Theory and Patient Management*. New York, Mary Ann Liebert, 1991, pp 1–13.

73. Swanson JM: What do psychopharmacological studies tell us about information processing deficits in ADDH?, in Bloomingdale LM, Sergeant J (eds): *Attention Deficit Disorder: Criteria, Cognition, Intervention*. New York, Pergamon Press, 1988, pp 97–116.

74. Werry J: *Pediatric Psychopharmacology*. New York, Brunner/Mazel, 1978.
75. Becker-Mattes A, Mattes JA, Abikoff H, et al: State-dependent learning in hyperactive children receiving methylphenidate. *Am J Psychiatry* 142:455–459, 1985.
76. Stephens RS, Pelham WE, Skinner R: State-dependent and main effects of methylphenidate and pemoline on paired-associate learning and spelling in hyperactive children. *J Consult Clin Psychol* 52:104–113, 1984.
77. Barkley RA, Cunningham CE: Do stimulant drugs improve the academic performance of hyperkinetic children? A review of outcome research. *Clin Pediatrics* 17:85–92, 1978.
78. Gittelman R, Klein DF, Feingold I: Children with reading disorders - II: Effects of methylphenidate in combination with reading remediation. *J Child Psychol Psychiatry* 24:193–212, 1983.
79. Weiss G, Hechtman L: *Hyperactive Children Grown Up*. New York, Guilford Press, 1986.
80. Barkley RA, Karlsson J, Pollard S, et al: Developmental changes in the mother-child interactions of hyperactive boys: Effects of two doses of Ritalin. *J Child Psychol Psychiatry* 26:705–715, 1985.
81. Humphries T, Kinsbourne M, Swanson J: Stimulant effects on cooperation and social interaction between hyperactive children and their mothers. *J Child Psychol Psychiatry* 19:13–22, 1978.
82. Barkley RA: Hyperactive girls and boys: Stimulant drug effects on mother–child interactions. *J Child Psychol Psychiatry Allied Discip* 30:379–390, 1989.
83. Pelham WE, Walker JL, Sturges J, Hoza J: Comparative effects of methylphenidate on ADD girls and ADD boys. *J Am Acad Child Adolesc Psychiatry* 28:773–776, 1989.
84. Whalen CK, Henker D, Dotemoto S: Methylphenidate and hyperactivity: Effects on teacher behaviors. *Science* 208:1280–1282, 1980.
85. Cunningham CE, Siegel LS, Offord DR: A developmental dose response analysis of the effects of methylphenidate on the peer interactions of attention deficit disordered boys. *J Child Psychol Psychiatry* 26:955–971, 1985.
86. Whalen CK, Henker B, Collins BE, et al: Peer interaction in structured communication task: Comparisons of normal and hyperactive boys and of methylphenidate (Ritalin) and placebo effects. *Child Dev* 50:388–401, 1979.
87. Mino Y, Ohara H: Methylphenidate and interpersonal relationships of children with attention deficit hyperactivity disorder. *Jpn J Psychiatry Neurol* 45:45–51, 1991.
88. Granger DA, Whalen CK, Henker B: Perceptions of methylphenidate effects on hyperactive children's peer interactions. *J Abnorm Child Psychol* 21:535–549, 1993.
89. Whalen CK, Henker B, Hinshaw SP, et al: Messages of medication: Effects of actual versus informed medication status on hyperactive boys' expectancies and self-evaluations. *J Consult Clin Psychol* 59:602–606, 1991.
90. Iaolongo NS, Lopez, M, Horn WF, et al: Effects of psychostimulant medication on self-perceptions of competence, control, and mood in children with attention deficit hyperactivity disorder. *J Clin Child Psychol* 23:161–173, 1994.
91. Pelham WE, Murphy DA, Vannatta K, Milich R, et al: Methylphenidate and attributions in boys with attention-deficit hyperactivity disorder. *J Consult Clin Psychol* 60:282–292, 1992.
92. Carlson CL, Pelham WE, Milich R, Hoza B: ADHD boys' performance and attributions following success and failure: Drug effects and individual differences. *Cognit Ther Res* 17:269–287, 1993.
93. Sprague R, Sleator E: Drugs and dosages: Implications for learning disabilities, in Knights RM, Bakker DJ (eds): *The Neuropsychology of Learning Disorders*, Baltimore, Md, University Park Press, 1976, pp 351–366.
94. Sprague R, Sleator E: Methylphenidate in hyperkinetic children: Differences in dose effects on learning and social behavior. *Science* 198:1274–1276, 1977.
95. Douglas VI, Barr RD, Desilets J, Sherman E: Do high doses of stimulants impair flexible thinking in attention-deficit hyperactivity disorder? *J Am Acad Child Adolesc Psychiatry* 34:877–885, 1995.
96. Kaufman RE, Smith-Wright D, Reese CA, Simpson R, Jones F: Medication compliance in hyperactive children. *Pediatr Pharmacol* 1:231–237, 1981.
97. Pelham WE: The effects of stimulant drugs on learning and achievement in hyperactive and learning disabled children, in Torgesen JK, Wong B (eds): *Psychological and Educational Perspectives on Learning Disabilities*. New York, Academic Press, 1985, pp 259–295.
98. Schachar R, Tannock R: Childhood hyperactivity and psychostimulants: A review of extended treatment studies. *J Child Adolesc Psychopharmacol* 3:81–97, 1993.
99. DuPaul GJ, Barkley RA: Medication therapy, in Barkley RA (ed): *Attention Deficit Hyperactivity Disorder: A Handbook for Diagnosis and Treatment*. New York, Guilford Press, 1990, pp 573–612.
100. Aman MG, Turbott SH: Prediction of clinical response in children taking methylphenidate. *J Autism Dev Disord* 21:211–227, 1991.

101. Barkley RA: Predicting the response of hyperactive children to stimulant drugs: A review. *J Abnorm Child Psychol* 4:327–348, 1976.
102. Taylor EA: Drug response and diagnostic validation, in Rutter M (ed): *Developmental Neuropsychiatry.* New York, Guilford Press, 1983, pp 348–368.
103. Rapport MD, DuPaul GJ, Smith NF: Rate-dependency and hyperactivity: Methylphenidate effects on operant responding. *Pharmacol Biochem Behav* 23:77–83, 1985.
104. Barkley RA: *Hyperactive Children: A Handbook for Diagnosis and Treatment.* New York, Guilford Press, 1981.
105. Pliszka SR: Effect of anxiety on cognition, behavior, and stimulant response in ADHD. *J. Am Acad Child Adolesc Psychiatry* 28:882–887, 1989.
106. Voelker S, Lachar D, Gdowski C: The Personality Inventory for Children and response to methylphenidate: Preliminary evidence for predictive validity. *J Pediatr Psychol* 8:161–169, 1983.
107. Barkley RA, DuPaul JG: Psychostimulant response of children with ADHD: Interaction with internalizing symptoms. Paper presented at the American Psychological Association, August, San Francisco, Calif, 1991.
108. Aman MG: Stimulant drugs in developmental disabilities revisited. *J Dev Phys Disabil,* 8:347–365, 1996.
109. Aman MG, Kern RA, Osborne P, et al: Fenfluramine and methylphenidate in children with mental retardation and borderline IQ: Clinical effects. *Am J Ment Retard,* in press.
110. Handen BL, Breaux AM, Janosky J, et al: Effects and noneffects of methylphenidate in children with mental retardation and ADHD. *J Am Acad Child Adolesc Psychiatry* 31:455–461, 1992.
111. Handen BL, Janosky J, McAuliffe S, et al: Prediction of response to methylphenidate among children with ADHD and mental retardation. *J Am Acad Child Adolesc Psychiatry* 33:1185–1193, 1994.
112. Barkley RA, McMurray MB, Edelbrock CS, et al: The side effects of Ritalin: A systematic placebo controlled evaluation of two doses. *Pediatrics* 86:184–192, 1990.
113. Fine S, Johnston C: Drug and placebo side effects in methylphenidate–placebo trial for attention deficit hyperactivity disorder. *Child Psychiatry Hum Dev* 24:25–30, 1993.
114. Ahmann PA, Waltonen SJ, Olson KA, et al: Placebo-controlled evaluation of Ritalin side effects. *Pediatrics* 91:1101–1106, 1993.
115. Werry J, Sprague R: Methylphenidate in children: Effect of dosage. *Aust N Z J Psychiatry* 8:9–19, 1974.
116. Barkley RA: Tic disorders and Gilles de la Tourette syndrome, in Mash E, Terdal L (eds): *Behavioral Assessment of Childhood Disorders.* ed 2, New York, Guilford Press, 1988.
117. Bremness AB, Sverd J: Methylphenidate-induced Tourette syndrome: Case report. *Am J Psychiatry* 136:1334–1335, 1979.
118. Case ED, McAndrew JB: Dexedrine dyskinesia: An unusual iatrogenic tic. *Clin Pediatr* 13:69–70, 1974.
119. Golden GS: Gilles de la Tourette's syndrome following methylphenidate administration. *Dev Med Child Neurol* 16:76–78, 1974.
120. Lowe TL, Cohen DJ, Detlor J, et al: Stimulant medications precipitate Tourette's syndrome. *JAMA* 247:1729–1731, 1982.
121. Mitchel E, Matthews KL: Gilles de la Tourette's disorder associated with pemoline. *Am J Psychiat* 137:1618–1619, 1980.
122. Pollack MA, Cohen NL, Friedhoff AJ: Gilles de la Tourette's syndrome: Familial occurrence and precipitation by methylphenidate therapy. *Arch Neurol* 34:630–632, 1977.
123. Weiner WJ, Nausieda PA, Klawans HL: Methylphenidate-induced chorea: Case report and pharmacologic implications. *Neurology* 28:1041–1044, 1978.
124. Caine ED, Ludlow CL, Polinsky RJ, et al: Provocative drug testing in Tourette's syndrome: d- and l-amphetamine and haloperidol. *J Am Acad Child Psychiatry* 23:147–152, 1984.
125. Erenberg G, Cruse RP, Rothner AD: The effect of stimulant drugs on Tourette syndrome. *Neurology* 34:84, 1984.
126. Fras I, Karlavage J: The use of methylphenidate and imipramine in Gilles de la Tourette's disease in children. *Am J Psychiatry* 134:195–197, 1977.
127. Denckla MB, Bemporad JR, MacKay MC: Tics following methylphenidate administration. *JAMA* 235:1349–1351, 1976.
128. Golden GS: The use of stimulants in the treatment of Tourette's syndrome, in Cohen DJ, Bruun RD, Leckman JF (eds): *Tourette's Syndrome & Tic Disorders: Clinical Understanding and Treatment.* New York, John Wiley & Sons, 1988.
129. Gadow KD, Nolan EE, Sverd J: Methylphenidate in hyperactive boys with comorbid tic disorder: II. Short-term behavioral effects in school settings. *J Am Acad Child Adolesc Psychiatry* 31:462–471, 1992.
130. Gadow KD, Sverd J, Sprafkin J, Nolan EE, Ezor SN: Efficacy of methylphenidate for attention-deficit hyperactivity disorder in children with tic disorder. *Arch Gen Psychiatry* 52:444–455, 1995.

131. Johnston C, Pelham WE, Hoza J, et al: Psychostimulant rebound in attention deficit disordered boys. *J Am Acad Child Adolesc Psychiatry* 27:806–810, 1988.
132. Dyme IZ, Sahakian BJ, Golinko B, et al: Perseveration induced by methylphenidate in children: Preliminary findings. *Prog Neuro-psychopharmacol Biol Psychiatry* 6:269–273, 1982.
133. Solanto MV, Wender EK: Does methylphenidate constrict cognitive functioning? *J. Am Acad Child Adolesc Psychiatry* 28:897–902, 1989.
134. Fiedler N, Ullman DG: The effects of stimulant drugs on curiousity behaviors of hyperactive boys. *J Abnorm Child Psychol* 11:193–206, 1983.
135. Hinshaw SP, Buhrmester D, Heller T: Anger control in response to verbal provocation: Effects of stimulant medication for boys with ADHD. *J Abnorm Child Psychol* 17:393–407, 1989.
136. Conners CK, Taylor E: Pemoline, methylphenidate, and placebo in children with minimal brain dysfunction. *Arch Gen Psychiatry* 37:922–932, 1980.
137. Sallee FR, Stiller RL, Perel JM, et al: Pemoline-induced abnormal involuntary movements. *J Clin Psychopharmacol* 9:125–129, 1989.
138. Safer DJ, Allen RP, Barr E: Depression of growth in hyperactive children on stimulant drugs. *N Engl J Med* 287:217–220, 1972.
139. Safer RP, Allen DJ: Factors influencing the suppressant effects of two stimulant drugs on the growth of hyperactive children. *Pediatrics* 51:660–667, 1973.
140. Mattes JA, Gittelman R: Growth of hyperactive children on maintenance regimen of methylphenidate. *Arch Gen Psychiatry* 40:317–321, 1983.
141. Spencer TJ, Biederman J, Harding M, O'Donnell D, Faraone SV, Wilens TE: Growth deficits in ADHD children revisited: Evidence for disorder-associated growth delays? J Am Acad Child Adolesc Psychiatry 35:1460–1469, 1996.
142. Zeiner P: Body growth and cardiovascular function after extended (1.75 years) treatment with methylphenidate in boys with attention-deficit hyperactivity disorder. *J Child Adolesc Psychopharmacol* 5:129–138, 1995.
143. Barkley RA, DuPaul GJ, McMurray MB: Attention deficit disorder with and without hyperactivity: Clinical response to three dose levels of methylphenidate. *Pediatrics* 87:519–531, 1991.
144. McBurnett K, Lahey BB, Swanson JM: Ritalin treatment in attention deficit disorder without hyperactivity, in Greenhill LL, Osmon BB (eds): *Ritalin: Theory and Patient Management*. New York, Mary Ann Liebert, 1991, pp 257–265.
145. Aman MG: Stimulant drug effects in developmental disorders and hyperactivity: Toward a resolution of disparate findings. *J Autism Dev Disord* 12:385–398, 1982.
146. Aman MG, Marks RE, Turbott SH, et al: Clinical effects of methylphenidate and thioridazine in intellectually subaverage children. *J. Am Acad Child Adolesc Psychiatry* 30:246–256, 1991.
147. Handen BL, Feldman H, Gosling A, et al: Adverse side effects of methylphenidate among mentally retarded children with ADHD. *J. Am Acad Child Adolesc Psychiatry* 30:241–245, 1991.
148. Spencer T, Wilens T, Biederman J, Faraone SV, Ablon S, Lapey K: A double-blind, crossover comparison of methylphenidate and placebo in adults with childhood-onset attention deficit hyperactivity disorder. *Arch Gen Psychiatry* 52:434–443.
149. Crumrine PK, Feldman HM, Teodori J, et al: The use of methylphenidate in children with seizures and attention deficit disorder. Paper presented at the Child Neurology Society, October 1987.
150. McBridge MC, Wang DD, Torres CF: Methylphenidate in therapeutic doses does not lower seizure threshold. *Ann Neurol* 20;428, 1986.
151. Cohen D, Bruun RD, Leckman JF: *Tourette Syndrome and Tic Disorders*. New York, John Wiley & Sons, 1987.
152. Demb HB: Use of Ritalin in the treatment of children with mental retardation, in Greenhill LL, Osmon BB (eds): *Ritalin: Theory and Patient Management*. New York, Mary Ann Liebert, 1991, pp 155–170.
153. Gualtieri CT: Psychostimulants in traumatic brain injury, in Greenhill LL, Osmon BB (eds): *Ritalin: Theory and Patient Management*. New York, Mary Ann Liebert, 1991, pp 171–176.
154. Fernandez F: Ritalin in HIV dementia, in Greenhill LL, Osmon BB (eds): *Ritalin: Theory and Patient Management*. New York, Mary Ann Liebert, 1991, pp 177–186.
155. Brown RT, Jaffe SL, Silverstein J, et al: Methylphenidate and adolescents hospitalized with conduct disorder: Dose effects on classroom behavior, academic performance, and impulsivity. *J Clin Child Psychol* 20: 282–292, 1991.
156. Donnelly M, Rapoport JL: Attention deficit disorders, in Wiener JM (ed): *Diagnosis and Psychopharmacology of Childhood and Adolescent Disorders*. New York, John Wiley & Sons, 1985, pp 178–198.
157. Greenhill LL: Methylphenidate in the clinical office practice of child psychiatry, in Greenhill LL, Osmon BB (eds): *Ritalin: Theory and Patient Management*. New York, Mary Ann Liebert, 1991, pp 97–118.

158. Barkley RA: The effects of methylphenidate on the interactions of preschool ADHD children with their mothers. *J. Am Acad Child Adolesc Psychiatry* 27:336–341, 1988.
159. Pelham WE, Vodde-Hamilton M, Murphy DA, et al: The effects of methylphenidate on ADHD adolescents in recreational, peer group, and classroom settings. *J Clin Child Psychol* 20:293–300, 1990.
160. Stein MA, Blondis TA, Schnitzler ER, et al: Methylphenidate dosing: b.i.d. versus t.i.d. *Pediatrics*, 98:748–756, 1996.
161. Kent JD, Blader JC, Koplewicz HS, et al: Effects of late-afternoon methylphenidate administration on behavior and sleep in attention-deficit hyperactivity disorder. *Pediatrics* 96:320–325, 1995.
162. Chan YM, Swanson JM, Soldin SS, et al: Methylphenidate hydrochloride given with or before breakfast: II. Effects on plasma concentrations of methylphenidate and ritalinic acid. *Pediatrics* 72:56–59, 1983
163. Gadow KD, Nolan EE, Paolicelli LM, et al: A procedure for assessing the effects of methylphenidate on hyperactive children in public school settings. *J Clin Child Psychol* 20:268–276, 1991.
164. Grob CS, Coyle JT: Suspected adverse methylphenidate- imipramine interactions in children. *J Dev Behav Pediatr* 7:265, 1986.
165. Rapport MD, Carlson GA, Kelly KL, Pataki C: Methylphenidate and desipramine in hospitalized children: I. Separate and combined effects on cognitive function. *J Am Acad Child Adolesc Psychiatry* 32:333–342, 1993.
166. Pataki C, Carlson G, Kelly K, Rapport M, Biancaniello T: Side effects of methylphenidate and desipramine alone and in combination in children. *Am J Psychiatry* 32: 1065–1072, 1993.
167. Gammon BD, Brown TE: Fluoxetine and methylphenidate in combination for treatment of attention deficit disorder and comorbid depressive disorder. *J Child Adolesc Psychopharmacol* 3:1–10, 1993.
168. Gunning B: A controlled trial of clonidine in hyperkinetic children. Thesis, Department of Child and Adolescent Psychiatry, Academic Hospital Rotterdam, Sophia Children's Hospital Rotterdam, The Netherlands, 1992.
169. Popper C: Combining methylphenidate and clonidine: Pharmacologic questions and new reports about sudden death. *J Child Adolesc Psychopharmacol* 5:157–166, 1995.
170. Swanson JM, Flockhart D, Udrea D, Cantwell D, Connor D, Williams L: Clonidine in the treatment of ADHD: Questions about safety and efficacy. *J Child Adolesc Psychopharmacol* 5:301–304, 1996.

9

Antidepressant and Antimanic Drugs

JOHN O. VIESSELMAN, M.D.

I. INTRODUCTION

This chapter summarizes the use of antidepressants and antimanic medications in children and adolescents. Antimanic medications that are also antiepileptics, such as carbamazepine, valproate, and clonazepam, are discussed here, but their pharmacological details are found in Chapter 12. The discussion on the use of antidepressants will focus on their use in mood disorders (for which they were originally introduced) and on their use in anxiety disorders, attention-deficit disorders, and enuresis.[1–7] Since the first edition of this guide, more data concerning the use of selective or specific serotonin reuptake inhibitors (SSRIs) has become available, and treatment with more than one medication has become more common. This chapter will discuss the uses of SSRIs as well as combinations of medications in children and adolescents. Toxicity and treatment for toxicity will also be discussed.

II. DIAGNOSIS AND EPIDEMIOLOGY OF DEPRESSION IN CHILDREN AND ADOLESCENTS

The diagnosis and epidemiology of depression in children and adolescents has been discussed in Chapter 7. However, although depression is often used loosely to describe any unhappiness, in child psychiatry it has a very precise meaning as detailed in the DSM-IV and ICD-10. Anyone not thoroughly familiar with these diagnostic criteria and how to apply them should not be prescribing psychotropic medication for children and adolescents (see Chapter 1).

According to DSM-IV, mood disorders such as depression occur in children and adolescents.[8] In DSM-IV, the criteria for a major depressive episode are the same for children, adolescents, and adults. These criteria require that a depressed mood or loss of

JOHN O. VIESSELMAN, M.D. • Children's Services, Ventura County Behavioral Health, and private practice, Ventura, California 93003; Consulting Child Psychiatrist, Casa Pacifica Residential Facility and Shelter Care, Camarillo, California 93012.

Practitioner's Guide to Psychoactive Drugs for Children and Adolescents (Second Edition), Werry and Aman, eds. Plenum Publishing Corporation, New York, 1999.

interest or pleasure be present for at least 2 weeks with at least four key symptoms, including weight changes, sleep disturbance, agitation or retardation, fatigue, worthlessness, diminished ability to think, and recurrent thoughts of death or suicide.[8]

In children and adolescents an irritable and cranky mood, failure to meet expected weight gains, and decline in school grades may be substituted for depressed mood, weight changes, and diminished ability to think. While ICD-10 has diagnostic criteria that differ somewhat from those of DSM-IV, in the remainder of this chapter we will refer to DSM-IV terminology when discussing mood disorders because it is the most widely used classification system in most countries and in research. In a series of epidemiological studies, the prevalence of depression was reported to be 0.8% in preschoolers, 2% in school-aged children, and 4.5% in adolescents.[9]

III. ANTIDEPRESSANTS

A. Types

There are several types of antidepressants. The oldest types are monoamine oxidase inhibitors (MAOIs) and tricyclic antidepressants (TCAs). Some of the newer antidepressants almost exclusively inhibit the reuptake of serotonin and are frequently referred to as selective or specific serotonin reuptake inhibitors (SSRIs). A number of other antidepressants have various nontricyclic configurations,[10] and where relevant they will be discussed under the TCAs as "others." Table 1 lists antidepressants that are available for clinical use in children and adolescents,[11-15] together with suggested ranges and starting doses for pediatric use. Venlafaxine and mirtazapine are newer antidepressants which have both serotonergic and noradrenergic effects. Other antidepressants such as citalopram and moclobemide are not yet available in the United States but have been used in other countries.

B. Tricyclic (TCAs) and Heterocyclic Antidepressants

1. Definition and Classes

All TCAs have a three-ring nucleus in their chemical structure. Amitriptyline, doxepin, imipramine, and clomipramine are classified as *tertiary amines* because they have two methyl groups attached to the nitrogen atom of the side chain. Desipramine, nortriptyline, protriptyline, and trimipramine are *secondary amines* because there is one methyl group attached to the nitrogen atom of the side chain.[16] *Heterocyclic antidepressants* refers to other cyclic antidepressants with pharmacologic properties similar to TCAs but which do not have a typical tricyclic nucleus.

2. Cellular Actions

The primary cellular actions of antidepressants are on the neurotransmitter system. Some of the neurotransmitters primarily affected by antidepressants include norepinephrine, serotonin, dopamine, and acetylcholine. Generally, antidepressants act by influencing the metabolism and/or reuptake of neurotransmitters, which results in functionally increased

TABLE 1. Antidepressants[a]

Generic name	Trade name	Pediatric dosing		
		Usual range (mg/day)	mg/kg range	Starting dose (mg/day)
Tricyclics				
Tertiary amines				
Amitriptyline	Elavil®, Endep®, Amitril®	25–300	1–5	10–25
Clomipramine	Anafranil®	50–200 div[b]	2–3	25
Doxepin	Sinequan®, Adapin®	50–300	2–5	25
Imipramine	Tofranil®, Janimine®, Dumex®	20–450 div	1–5	10–25
Secondary amines				
Desipramine	Norpramin®, Pertofrane®	25–300 div	1–5	10–25
Nortriptyline	Pamelor®, Aventyl®, Allegron®	25–200 div	1–3	10–25
Protriptyline	Vivactil®, Concordin®	10–60 div	—	5
Trimipramine	Surmontil®	25–300	2–5	25
Dibenzoxazepine				
Amoxapine	Asendin®	25–300	—	25
Tetracyclic				
Maprotiline	Ludiomil®	50–225	—	25
Propiophenone				
Bupropion	Wellbutrin®	75–450 div	3–6	75
Benzenepropanamine (SSRIs)				
Fluoxetine	Prozac®	2.5–60	0.25–1	10
Fluvoxamine	Luvox®	50–200	1.5–4.5	50
Paroxetine	Paxil®	5–60	0.25–1	10
Sertraline	Zoloft®	25–200	1.5–3	25
Phenylethylamine				
Venlafaxine	Effexor®	75–200 div	1–3	37.5
Phenylpiperazine				
Nefazodone	Serzone®	50–400 div	—	25
Triazolopyridine				
Trazodone	Desyrel®	25–300	2–5	50
MAOIs				
Isocarboxazid	Marplan®	10–30 div	—	5
Moclobemide	Aurorix®	100–600 div	2.3–5	100
Phenelzine	Nardil®	15–45 div	0.5–1.0	15
Selegiline	Deprenyl®	5–15 div	0.07–0.20	5
Tranylcypromine	Parnate®	10–30 div	0.5–1.0	10
Other				
Mirtazapine	Remeron®	15–45	—	5

[a]Refs. 11–15.
[b]div, Usually given in divided doses.

levels of available neurotransmitters. Table 2 shows the estimated potency of the noradrenergic (NE), serotonergic (5-HT), dopaminergic (DA), and anticholinergic (Ach) effects of the various antidepressants at equivalent dosages. The data are based predominately on in vitro studies.[17]

Though most of the currently available antidepressants used in children have broad-spectrum effects, some drugs influence specific brain neurotransmitter systems: desipramine mainly affects norepinephrine reuptake, the SSRIs affect serotonin, and bupropion affects dopamine. The others affect reuptake in several of the neurotransmitter

**TABLE 2. Relative Potency of Antidepressants
in Producing Neurotransmitter Effects[a]**

Antidepressant	Relative potency[b,c]				Antidepressant	Relative potency[b,c]			
	NE	5-HT	DA	Ach		NE	5-HT	DA	Ach
Tertiary amines					Triazolopyridine				
Imipramine	8	2	0	1	Trazodone	0	0.5	0	0
Amitriptyline	4	2	0	6	Phenylpiperazine				
Clomipramine	4	18	0	3	Nefazodone	0.2	0.7	0	0
Doxepin	5	0.4	0	1	Benzenepropanamine				
Trimiprimine	0.2	0	0	2	(SSRIs)				
Secondary					Fluoxetine	0.4	8	0	0
amines					Fluvoxamine	0.2	14	0	0
Desipramine	110	0.3	0	0.5	Paroxetine	3	136	0	1
Nortriptyline	25	0.4	0	0.7	Sertraline	0.5	29	0.4	0.2
Protriptyline	100	0.4	0	4	Phenylethylamine				
Dibenzoxazepine					Venlafaxine	3	3	0	0
Amoxapine	23	0.2	0	0.1	Propiophenone				
Tetracyclic					Bupropion	0	0	0.2	0
Maprotiline	13	0	0	0.2					

[a]Ref. 17.
[b]Abbreviations: Ach, anticholinergic effect; NE, norepinephrine effect; 5-HT, 5-hydroxytryptamine (serotonin) effect; DA, dopamine effect.
[c]Numbers refers to the in vitro potency of the antidepressants in equimolar amounts in rat brain synaptosomes, so, for example, imipramine has more potent effects on NE than amitriptyline, about the same effect on 5-HT and DA as amitriptyline, and is less anticholinergic.

systems. Desipramine, nortriptyline, maprotiline, amoxapine, trazodone, nefazodone, most SSRIs, and bupropion have minimal anticholinergic effects.

3. Pharmacokinetics

Developmental factors are important in the pharmacokinetics of antidepressants. As described in Chapter 2, children and adolescents display a more rapid metabolism of drugs.[18,19] Children and adolescents may need larger doses of psychotropic drugs relative to adults.[20] Other factors such as gastrointestinal absorption, body adipose stores, and rate of drug biotransformation may result in different serum drug concentrations in children than in adults (Chapter 2).

The half-lives of antidepressants vary widely. The data presented in Table 3 are based on adult laboratory values.[12,13–15,21] Half-lives generally are shorter in children; for example, the half-life of nortriptyline ranges from 11 to 42 hr in 5- to 12-year-olds, from 14 to 77 hr in 13- to 16-year-olds,[22] and from 15 to 93 hr in adults. For clomipramine, the half-life ranges from 5 to 17 hr in 5- to 19-year-olds and from 19 to 37 hr in adults. Based on these data for nortriptyline and clomipramine, the half-life of antidepressants in children under 12 may be assumed to be from one-third to two-thirds of the adult level. The pharmacokinetics of most of the other antidepressants in Table 3 have not been adequately studied in children.

Plasma levels of antidepressants usually should be obtained only when the antidepressant has reached pharmacological steady state, for which imipramine is about 5 days. Plasma levels of imipramine should be measured about 12 hr after the last dose so as to detect the steady-state level. However, the time to reach steady state varies depending on

TABLE 3. Half-lives of Antidepressants[a]

Antidepressant	Half-life range (hr)	Average half-life (hr)	Steady state (days)
Tertiary amines			
Amitriptyline	10–50	24	4–10
Clomipramine	19–37	32	7–14
Doxepin	8–36	8	2–8
Trimipramine	7–30	9	2–6
Imipramine	6–24	16	2–5
Secondary amines			
Desipramine	12–76	22	2–11
Nortriptyline	15–93	24	4–19
Protriptyline	54–198	126	10
Dibenzoxazepine			
Amoxapine	—	8	2–7
SSRIs			
Fluoxetine	24–216	72	28–35
Fluvoxamine	—	20	7
Paroxetine	7–37	20[b]	7–14
Sertraline	26	26	7–12
Others			
Venlafaxine	4	4	16
Nefazodone	2–4	—[c]	—
Trazodone	4–9	5	3–7
Maprotiline	27–58	51	6–10
Buproprion	8–24	14	2–5
Nomifensine	2–10	—	2–5
Mirtazapine	20–40	22	5

[a]Refs. 13–15, 21, and 22.
[b]Highly variable.
[c]Dose dependent.

the antidepressant used. A rule of thumb for roughly estimating steady state is that it is achieved after five half-life time periods have elapsed (e.g., for imipramine the half-life range is 6–24 hr, so steady state would conservatively be achieved in 5 × 24 hr = 120 hr, or 5 days).

Therapeutic levels of a number of antidepressants that have been studied in children and adolescents are shown in Table 4.[23–28] Those for enuresis and major depression are tentative and are representative of what the studies cited have found to be therapeutic. The level for attention-deficit hyperactivity disorder (ADHD) is listed as less than 300 ng/mL since studies do not show an association between plasma level and therapeutic response.[27,29] However, one study found that children whose ADHD symptoms were rated as "markedly improved" were more likely to have blood levels in the therapeutic range established for depression.[29]

The steady-state plasma level of antidepressant varies 6- to 27-fold for imipramine in different children at the same mg/kg or fixed (75 mg) dosage[25,26,30] and 40-fold for desipramine.[31] Although the variability of plasma levels of most antidepressants has not been systematically studied in children and adolescents, it is reasonable to assume that the same findings would hold. The variability in plasma level means that *the actual plasma level could vary from subtherapeutic to toxic* with the same dose, depending on the

TABLE 4. Therapeutic Antidepressant Plasma Levels

Diagnosis	Medication	Plasma level (ng/mL)	Reference
Enuresis	Clomipramine	20–60	23
	Imipramine	80–225[a]	24
Major depression	Imipramine	125–250	25
	Nortriptyline	60–100	26
Attention deficit	Desipramine	<300[b]	27
	Nortriptyline	50–150	28

[a]Combined imipramine and desipramine level.
[b]No lower bound for the therapeutic level has been established for improvement of ADHD symptoms.

individual. Therefore, initial daily doses should be low (e.g., the equivalent of 25 mg of imipramine) to prevent toxicity until response to the initial dosage can be evaluated either clinically or on the basis of blood levels. Other conditions that can cause plasma-level variability are fever, minor intercurrent illnesses, and concurrent administration of medications such as aspirin, acetaminophen, SSRIs, grapefruit juice, erythromycin, ketoconazole, and cimetidine.[26,32]

Although not all centers have access to plasma-level estimations, a number of rationales exist for monitoring blood levels of antidepressants.[22] Blood levels are helpful in determining patient compliance with medication, determining "therapeutic" blood levels when they exist, determining and treating possible toxic levels, and documenting "adequate" blood levels prior to changing treatments or for medicolegal purposes. In children, serious toxic effects such as electrocardiogram (ECG) changes and reversible organic brain syndromes occur at higher plasma levels.[25] Plasma levels should be drawn at steady state, and the dosage adjusted based on the plasma level. If the initial plasma level is undetectable, then the daily dosage may be increased, the plasma level redetermined, and the dosage adjusted if necessary.

The pharmacokinetics of cyclic antidepressants are linear within the usual therapeutic range.[21] Therefore, it is possible to predict the approximate blood level of a TCA by multiplying the proposed dosage by a **clearance index**.[31] The clearance index is calculated by dividing the current blood level by the current dosage in mg/kg. For example, if the current level of desipramine is 99 ng/mL and the current dose if 4.1 mg/kg, the clearance index is 99/4.1 = 24.1. With a decrease of the dosage to 3.2 mg/kg, the predicted blood level is 24.1 times 3.2 or 77 ng/mL. In actual practice, the level after the dosage change was 51 ng/mL.[31]

4. Behavioral and Emotional Effects

Sedation is a common effect of many of the antidepressants (see Table 5). This can be advantageous when treating children and adolescents with insomnia but may be deleterious in children attending school if it impairs learning. Amitriptyline, trazodone, and doxepin are among the most sedating, and desipramine, protriptyline, bupropion, and fluoxetine among the least sedating.[33] Sedation is related to a combination of the anticholinergic, antihistaminic, and serotonergic potency of the medications.[34]

Other possible favorable behavioral effects noted are decreased hyperactivity, inattentiveness, impulsiveness,[1,2] and anxiety[35,36]; improved cooperativeness; and decreased seat

TABLE 5. Sedative Potencies of Antidepressants[a]

Antidepressant	Sedative effect	Antidepressant	Sedative effect
Amitriptyline	+ + + + +	Amoxapine	+ +
Trazodone	+ + + + +	Nortriptyline	+ +
Nefazodone	+ + + +	Fluvoxamine	+ +
Doxepin	+ + + +	Sertraline	+ +
Trimipramine	+ + + +	Venlafaxine	+ +
Clomipramine	+ + + +	Protriptyline	+
Maprotiline	+ + + +	Desipramine	+
Imipramine	+ + +	Fluoxetine	+
Paroxetine	+ + +	Bupropion	+

[a]Refs. 10, 14, 33, and 34.

movement[3] in both psychiatric and normal children.[6] These effects might be mediated through the noradrenergic or "simulantlike" effects of the medication,[37] although recent studies of attention-deficit disorder show similar effects with bupropion, which has dopaminergic effects and minimal noradrenergic effects.[38–40]

5. Cognitive and Learning Effects

There is little information on the cognitive and learning effects of antidepressants in children and adolescents. A review of this issue concluded that TCAs neither impair nor significantly improve functioning on tests of short-term memory or cognitive functions.[41] Low-dose imipramine may have stimulantlike effects in children and increase vigilance, decrease impulsivity, and have no apparent effect on IQ.[2,6]

6. Physiological Side Effects

Dry mouth, drowsiness, dizziness, lethargy, tremors, sleep problems, nausea, constipation, palpitations, chest pain, blurred vision, stomachache, and perspiration can occur with imipramine.[35,36] There was no marked change in side-effect scores between 3 and 6 weeks in one study,[35] and severity of side effects was not related to plasma level of imipramine, its active metabolite desipramine, or total TCA.

Physiological side effects will depend on the relative effects on cholinergic, noradrenergic, serotonergic, histaminic, and dopaminergic systems (see Table 2). In general, the side effects will vary depending on the profile of these individual effects. Adverse side effects of TCAs will be discussed below.

7. Adverse Effects

a. Cardiovascular

Cardiovascular effects include slowing of cardiac conduction, elevation of systolic and diastolic blood pressure, and tachycardia (an increase of 5–13 bpm).[42] Combined imipramine and desipramine (imipramine's active metabolite) levels above 225 ng/mL caused slowing of intracardiac conduction, a greater elevation of diastolic blood pressure, and a greater increase in heart rate than did lower levels. There also have been reports of elevated blood pressures in hospitalized adolescents receiving imipramine.[43] The definition of hypertension in children varies with age. Table 6 shows recommended upper blood pressure parameters for children and adolescents.[44]

There have been eight reports of **sudden death** that may be related to the cardiovascular effects of TCAs.[45-50] Six unexplained deaths are reported as specifically associated with desipramine.[45-49] and two with imipramine.[48,50] It is difficult to form definite conclusions about the cause of these deaths. A number of factors might be involved with sudden death.[48]

Most speculation about the mechanism of sudden death concerns the effect of desipramine on cardiac functioning, particularly the defects in cardiac conduction. TCAs affect the PR, QRS, and QT_c intervals. The increase in the QT_c (which takes heart rate into account) is one of the best predictors of dysrhythmias and arrhythmias. Desipramine can increase the QT_c in children to >440 msec.[51] Desipramine increases the PR interval and the QRS interval more than does clomipramine.[52] The percentage of children who develop incomplete intraventricular conduction defect (IVCD) is higher among those taking desipramine (23%) than among those taking clomipramine (4%). Clomipramine also increases the QT_c more than desipramine, but they both increase the QT_c. Dosages and plasma levels do not correlate with the ECG changes. Increases in the PR, QRS, and QT_c intervals are associated with ventricular dysrhythmias and arrhythmias. Because dysrhythmias and arrhythmias can potentially lead to syncope and sudden death,[51] if desipramine or clomipramine is used in children, they need to be monitored extremely carefully.

There is little justification for using a drug with even a small degree of lethality in nonlife-threatening conditions in children. There are a large number of safer antidepressants on the market such as trazodone, bupropion, fluoxetine, sertraline, and paroxetine, with minimal lethality (even in overdose).[14] If medications that have less risk have been tried and failed and the distress, disability, and durability of the disorder are significant, then it may be justifiable to switch to a medication with a greater risk of lethality. In such cases it is important to get informed consents from the parents and child, specifically mentioning the possibility of death. In addition, medicolegally it is probably unwise to use desipramine considering the number of "sudden deaths" reported in the literature.

Clinicians should proceed very carefully in using TCAs in healthy children and adolescents in higher doses (>4 mg/kg of imipramine) and in those with cardiac conduction problems. Clinically insignificant changes occur in the ECG when serum imipramine levels are kept in the therapeutic range (125–250 ng/mL).[53]

In adults it is recommended that patients with bundle branch block be (1) hospitalized, (2) assessed with ECGs and 24-hr continuous ECG recordings prior to starting TCAs, and (3) closely monitored regarding their cardiac status until steady-state plasma concentra-

TABLE 6. Blood Pressure Parameters in Children and Adolescents[a]

Age group	Significant hypertension	Severe hypertension
Less than 2	Over 112/74	Over 118/82
3–5	Over 116/76	Over 124/84
6–9	Over 122/78	Over 130/86
10–12	Over 126/82	Over 134/90
13–15	Over 136/86	Over 144/92
16–18	Over 142/92	Over 150/96

[a]Ref. 44.

TABLE 7. ECG Parameters to Be Observed When Prescribing Antidepressants[a]

Acceptable baseline ECG parameters
  Do not start a tricyclic or tricyclic-like antidepressant if ECG indicates any of the following:
  1. PR interval **greater than or equal to** 210 millisec
  2. QRS interval **greater than or equal to** 120 millisec
  3. QTC interval **greater than or equal to** 425 millisec

Parameters during treatment
  Consider decreasing or discontinuing a tricyclic or tricyclic-like antidepressant if ECG indicates any of the following:
  1. PR interval **greater than** 210 millisec
  2. QRS interval **greater than** 30% over baseline value
  3. Heart rate **greater than** 130 bpm
  4. Blood pressure **greater than** 130 mm Hg systolic or 85 mm Hg diastolic

[a]Refs. 10, 55, and 56.

tions are achieved.[54] In children with bundle branch block, TCAs should be avoided since there are other safer alternatives. Suggested ECG parameters to follow clinically are set out in Table 7.[10,55,56]

b. Hematologic

Transient eosinophilia has been reported to occur in some adults receiving antidepressants during the first few weeks of treatment. Agranulocytosis is also a rare complication reported in adults.[57]

c. Hepatic

Jaundice has been reported with TCA use in adults. Elevation of alkaline phosphatase and/or the transaminases is common but is considered benign.[57]

d. Autonomic

Common anticholinergic side effects include burred vision, urinary retention, dry mouth, and constipation.[34]

e. Endocrine/Metabolic

Excessive weight gain has been reported. Also galactorrhea and amenorrhea can occur in women. The galactorrhea and amenorrhea can usually be managed by dose reduction.[57]

f. Neuropsychiatric

Delirium of the atropinic type characterized by disorientation, loss of memory, ataxia, flushed and dry skin, and psychosis can be treated by physostigmine, though conservative treatment may be safer. A child with a total TCA plasma level of 481 ng/mL developed a delirium with moderate electroencephalogram (EEG) abnormalities. The delirium was dose-related and resolved when the dose was reduced.[42] Tremors of the tongue and upper extremities are common.[58] Antidepressants also lower seizure threshold and may increase the likelihood of seizures in subjects who have epilepsy. Sedation can occur with most antidepressants (see Table 5). With the more sedating antidepressants, sedation can be severe enough to impair concentration and the ability to function in school. Irritability occurred in 45% of children receiving imipramine for anxiety disorders,[36] so TCAs may exacerbate symptoms in some clinical populations.

g. Withdrawal

Withdrawal effects from antidepressants are characterized by a flulike syndrome with the following symptoms: nausea, vomiting, headache, lethargy, and irritability.[59] These are due to tolerance and resulting rebound cholinergic and adrenergic effects. It has been reported that children seldom show withdrawal symptoms if TCAs are given once daily,[10] possibly because of the long half-life; however, if withdrawal symptoms occur, giving the medication in two or three smaller divided doses can prevent them. Withdrawal effects can be alleviated by restarting the patient on lower doses of the same drug and tapering it.[10]

8. Clinical Indications

a. Mood Disorders

i. Effectiveness of TCAs in Child Mood Disorders. The effectiveness of TCAs in children with mood disorders was reviewed in studies where accepted diagnostic criteria, adequate dosages, and systematic follow-up were used.[60] There were three controlled studies[61–63] and five uncontrolled studies.[22,61,64–66] All used structured methods for diagnosis and assessment of efficacy, and plasma levels were used to assess adequacy of antidepressant dosage. Imipramine was studied in two of the controlled studies,[61,62] and nortriptyline in one.[63] Medications studied in the five uncontrolled studies were imipramine,[61,64,65] amitriptyline,[66] and nortriptyline.[22] The controlled studies showed no difference in the rate of response to antidepressant treatment compared with placebo, but one study[61] demonstrated that response was greater in those patients who had positive (nonsuppressed) dexamethasone suppression tests (DSTs). As ever, response rate in the uncontrolled studies (46–70%) were higher than in the controlled studies (38–56%). Higher plasma levels were associated with a somewhat better clinical response for imipramine[61,62,64] but not for nortriptyline.[22,63,75] A metaanalysis of the placebo-controlled studies using TCAs in children and adolescents also concluded that there was no appreciable difference between TCAs and placebo.[67]

ii. Effectiveness of TCAs in Adolescent Mood Disorders. There have been eight systematic studies in adolescents, five controlled[68–72] and three open trials.[73–75] Medications studied were imipramine,[70,74] nortriptyline,[69,75] amitriptyline,[68,71] desipramine,[72] and a variety of antidepressants.[73] The results of the studies in adolescents are similar to those in children. That is, a placebo response of 30–50% was observed, no difference in response between placebo and active medication was found, and higher response rates were noted in the uncontrolled studies. There was no correlation between plasma levels and clinical outcome when assessed by decrease in severity of symptoms.[69,70,74] However, when subjects were divided into responder and nonresponder categories, the responders tended to have higher plasma levels.[74]

iii. Summary. The effectiveness of TCAs in child and adolescent depression has yet to be demonstrated. However, while there is no difference in the percentages of patients classified as responding well to TCAs compared with placebo, TCAs may decrease the severity of depressive symptoms more than placebo.[61] Blood levels may influence the results, although the results are inconsistent. Some of the problem may be a diagnostic one relating to the persistent difficulty of separating depression from comorbid disorders.[63] While all of this indicates a need for more clinical research, it does not support widespread use of TCAs in depressed children and adolescents. Alternatives such as SSRIs and others may be better choices. SSRIs will be discussed below.

b. Attention-Deficit Hyperactivity Disorder (ADHD)

Although TCAs are less effective in ADHD than are stimulants, they have consistently been found to be more effective than placebo in reducing restlessness and hyperactivity.[1-5] They may also help inattentiveness, but the evidence for this is less conclusive.[5] The most commonly studied antidepressant has been imipramine; others such as nortriptyline, desipramine, and bupropion have also been shown to be effective.[10,27,28,38–40] In ADHD, imipramine can be started at a low dosage to minimize anticholinergic side effects (see Section III.B.7), such as constipation, dry mouth, sedation, and tachycardia.[3] There does not seem to be any consistent relationship between dosage and therapeutic effect in ADHD.[3,5] The usual starting dosage is as found in Table 1, and the usual dosage range is up to 5 mg/kg per day for imipramine, desipramine, and nortriptyline and up to 3.0 mg/kg per day for clomipramine.[76] If anxiety is present, most studies also show that it can be alleviated or reduced. However, aggressiveness and conduct symptoms do not seem to respond.[5]

As previously mentioned, it is necessary to be cautious when prescribing these medications. Medicolegally, it is prudent not to choose desipramine as the first antidepressant to be tried in ADHD. If a cyclic antidepressant is to be used, it would be generally better to start with imipramine although sudden death has been reported to be associated with imipramine as well.[49,50] Too little is known about antidepressants in children, and more research is needed.[45]

Although antidepressants are generally less effective than stimulants for treating ADHD, they are clearly superior to placebo and are a sound second-choice drug when stimulants have failed or cannot be used (e.g., in Tourette syndrome). Parents should be told that antidepressants are less effective than stimulants and that anxiety, restlessness, and attention can be expected to improve the most. They should be told that conduct symptoms and aggressiveness will probably not improve. Because imipramine is the most frequently studied drug, it should be considered first. If it fails or cannot be used, bupropion or another antidepressant might be tried, although there is no evidence to suggest clearly any superiority among antidepressants. There is very little data to support the use of SSRIs as a treatment for ADHD, and this will be mentioned when SSRIs are discussed below.

Bupropion has been demonstrated to be effective in ADHD in dosages from 3 to 6 mg/kg per day.[38–40] In addition to the standard 75-mg and 100-mg tablets, a sustained-released preparation is available in 100- and 150-mg dosages. It has the advantages that it can be taken twice a day, enhancing compliance, and results in peak blood levels that are 15% lower than those for the standard preparation. Theoretically, the lower peak levels could reduce the risk of seizures, although no evidence exists yet to show that this is true.[77]

c. Enuresis

Antidepressants of all types (except possibly trimipramine) are effective in enuresis[6,7] and at relatively low dosages (25–75 mg/day). Therapeutic effect does not seem to be correlated with dosage, which must be individualized. Although the immediate success rate for antidepressants is high while the child is taking the medication, enuresis usually resumes when medication is stopped, and development of tolerance requiring increased dosage is common. Among children treated for enuresis with antidepressants, 10–40% stay dry at night and continue to remain dry when followed up 6–16 months later. These figures approximate spontaneous remission rates and are considerably less than the 50–100% recovery rates found with conditioning or "bell and pad" treatment.[7,78]

Antidepressants may be indicated in treating enuresis in situations where the "bell and pad" cannot or will not be used, where it has failed, or in social emergencies (e.g., camp). Antidepressants may be tried to augment improvement obtained with the "bell and pad." However, it is important to realize the enuresis is a self-limiting disorder, and antidepressants are not without risks and discomforts. Desmopressin (DDAVP®) is effective in suppressing enuresis and perhaps is a better alternative for symptomatic treatment.

d. Anxiety Disorders

As in adults, antidepressants have been used to treat anxiety disorders in children, including school phobia, separation anxiety disorder, panic disorder, obsessive compulsive disorder (OCD), and an allied disorder, trichotillomania. In separation anxiety and school phobia, imipramine was helpful.[35,36] Recent attempted replications[35,79–81] including the use of clomipramine did not show a clear advantage even though blood levels were within the therapeutic range (125–250 ng/mL).[80] From the evidence, it is not yet clear if antidepressants are effective in separation anxiety or phobic disorders. It may be that imipramine is helpful at lower dosages and no help at higher dosages. There is a higher incidence of irritability in children treated with imipramine for anxiety disorders (45%) than in those treated for affective disorders.[81] Children with anxiety disorders may respond differently to imipramine at the therapeutic levels used for affective disorders.

In children with OCD, clomipramine was helpful by the 5th week[82] and superior to desipramine by the 10th week.[83] Dosages of clomipramine were adjusted not to exceed 5 mg/kg. These results have now been replicated in large multicenter study,[84] which also found that therapeutic effects persisted for at least 1 year. Sedative, atropinic, and adrenergic side effects (anorexia, tremor) were common. The finding that the greater the change in serotonin concentration at 4 weeks, the greater the improvement in obsessive–compulsive symptoms at 8 weeks[85] supports the idea that OCD improvement is mediated by serotonin. Fluoxetine, which has minimal effect on neurotransmitters other than serotonin, has been shown in recent trials to be effective in OCD. Thus, it would appear that as in adults, serotonergic antidepressants are the medications of choice in childhood OCD although minor side effects are to be expected.

Trichotillomania, which has features of both an anxiety and a compulsive disorder, has been treated in adults with clomipramine and desipramine.[86] In adults, clomipramine significantly decreased the severity of hair pulling, whereas desipramine did not. However, in children, only case studies are available. A case study of clomipramine in two children showed mixed results[87]: one child showed resolution of hair pulling and decreased anxiety, and the other child showed no benefit. Dosages were modest, 75 mg qhs and 100 mg qhs. A case study using imipramine showed it to be effective in a prepubertal child,[88] and another showed fluoxetine to be effective.[89] These findings suggest that antidepressants may be helpful; however, controlled studies are needed.

e. Aggressiveness

Two-thirds of children with disruptive behavior disorders treated in an open trial with trazodone at 5.0 mg/kg per day (100–800 mg daily) showed improvement in impulsivity, hyperactivity, cruelty, fighting, arguing, losing their temper, easy excitability, being easily frustrated, and "outward aggression."[90] Follow-up 8–14 months later showed sustained improvement. A case series treated with lower doses [0.35 mg/kg (75 mg daily)] showed decreases in aggression after one week.[91] Trazodone might be helpful in decreasing aggressiveness in children and adolescents; however, these findings are only suggestive.

f. Autism and Developmental Disabilities

Because of clomipramine's effectiveness in OCD, two studies examined its effectiveness in treating the repetitive self-injurious and stereotypic behaviors seen in children and adolescents with autism and mental retardation.[92,93] An open study with adolescents[92] noted a 50–90% reduction in target behaviors on dosages of clomipramine ranging from 50 to 125 mg daily (average 75 mg daily). A double-blind, placebo-controlled study with children[93] in which clomipramine was compared with desipramine and with placebo showed clomipramine to be significantly more effective than desipramine or placebo in reducing target behaviors. Dosages of clomipramine averaged 150 mg daily, and doses of desipramine averaged 125 mg daily. There was no correlation between improvement and blood levels. Target repetitive behaviors and rituals in the studies included head banging, head/face slapping, hand/arm biting, hair pulling, eye gouging, hand wringing/flapping, nose/ear/finger flicking, rocking, weaving, spinning, questioning/vocalizations, grimacing, shrugging, pacing, touching/tapping, arranging objects, hand washing, counting, and others. Two studies in adults also suggested a possible reduction of 50% or greater in these behaviors.[94,95]

The preliminary evidence is suggestive that clomipramine might be effective in reducing self-injurious and stereotypic behaviors in autism and other developmental disabilities. One seizure occurred in the 35 patients in the two child studies.[92,93] Since seizures are frequently seen in autism, the need for informed consent, extreme caution, and careful monitoring is self-evident if clomipramine is used.

9. Contraindications, Drug Interactions, and Toxicity

Contraindications for the use of TCAs in children and adolescents should include a previous history of hypersensitivity to TCAs. These drugs are toxic and even fatal in overdosage, and parents need to be instructed to be careful with the medication since inadvertent poisoning could occur if medication falls into the hands of younger siblings. If such care cannot be guaranteed, TCAs may be contraindicated.

There is only one study in children or adolescents of interaction of antidepressants with other drugs[26]; but adult studies suggest that interactions include the following: (1) combining neuroleptics with TCAs requires lower doses of TCAs[26]; (2) in adults, if TCAs are added to MAOIs, a toxic reaction may occur, although the combination is reported to be safe when both drugs are started simultaneously or the TCA is started first[96]; (3) desipramine antagonizes the antihypertensive effect of clonidine[97] and guanethidine[98]; (4) phenothiazines can elevate TCA plasma levels; (5) imipramine can increase phenytoin concentrations[99]; (6) barbiturates decrease TCA levels[100]; and (7) methylphenidate increases imipramine plasma levels.[101]

10. Treatment of Overdosage of TCAs

Overdosage with TCAs is one of the commonest causes of poisoning in children under the age of 18 in the United States, and TCA toxicity carries with it a significant probability of death. Treatment of TCA overdose depends on an understanding of which effects of TCAs have the greatest potential for causing morbidity and mortality. The main toxic

TABLE 8. Four Cardiovascular Effects of TCAs in Overdose

TCA effect	Cardiovascular effect	Treated with
1. Quinidine effect	Cardiac conduction blocks	Alkalinization (bicarb),
	Increased refractory period	phenytoin, lidocaine
	Increased stimulation threshold	
	Decreased cardiac conduction velocity (particularly in the intraventricular bundles of HIS)	
	Severely decreased ventricular automaticity	
2. Peripheral effect	Hypotension	Vasopressors
3. Blocking the reuptake of norepinephrine effect	Tachycardia	β-Blockers
	Sinus tachycardia	
	Mild hypertension	
	Slight increase in cardiac output	
	Ventricular ectopic beats	
4. Anticholinergic effect	Increased heart rate	**Physostigmine—not**
	Slightly increased blood pressure	**recommended in**
	Agitation, delirium	**TCA overdose.**

effects of TCAs which cause problems are the cardiovascular effects. Table 8 lists the four main cardiovascular effects of TCAs.

Overdose with TCAs causes tachycardia, hypotension, premature ventricular contractions (PVCs), and prolonged PR, QRS, and QT_c intervals. Conduction defects and hypotension are the most common reasons for morbidity and mortality. The most severe disturbances are due to bundle branch blocks, ventricular arrhythmias, atrioventricular (AV) conduction defects, profound bradycardia with variable conduction defects, and cardiac arrest.[102,103]

The anticholinergic effects of TCAs cause increased heart rate and blood pressure, and mental status changes; however, the anticholinergic effect does not contribute significantly to the severe cardiotoxic effects of a TCA overdose. Treatment with physostigmine does not change the outcome of the overdose, and it can produce serious side effects and even death. It is not recommended in treatment of TCA overdose.[104–106]

The blockage of reuptake of norepinephrine is responsible for tachycardia, sinus tachycardia, mild hypertension, slightly increased cardiac output, and ventricular ectopy. These all can be reversed by β-blockers.

The quinidine effect is responsible for the conduction defects and the arrhythmias and, along with the hypotensive effect, is a major contributor to the morbidity and mortality of TCA overdoses. The following recommendations are general recommendations for managing overdose of TCAs[105,106] and not specific to children and adolescents.

Recommendations for Managing Overdose of TCAs*

1. If ventricular arrhythmias, conduction disturbances, seizures, or mental status alterations occur during the first 6 hours of observation, the patient should be admitted to an ICU. Serum blood levels of TCAs have no predictive value, and

*This information is for emergency use only. In general, overdosage is best managed by emergency medicine experts, not by psychiatrists.

ECG monitoring should continue for at least 24 hours if there is any prolongation of the QRS.[105]

2. Absorption should be prevented by gastric lavage with a large-bore orogastric tube (32 French—children, 40 French—older adolescents or adults). *Ipecac or apomorphine should be avoided because of the possibility of seizures and aspiration.*

3. Initially, give 60–100 g (older adolescents or adults) or 1 g/kg (children) of activated charcoal in an aqueous slurry, followed by 20 g (older adolescents or adults) or half the dose (children) administered every 2 hours for several doses. Single doses do not significantly affect the clearance of TCAs, so repeated doses are necessary.

4. Give a cathartic such as magnesium sulfate, 30 g (older adolescents or adults), or magnesium citrate, 4 mL/kg (children).

5. Manage hypotension with crystalloid infusion and alkalinization. If a vasopressor is needed, norepinephrine, 4 μg/mL, may be given at 0.1–0.2 μg/kg per minute.

6. Monitor for ventricular arrhythmias (multifocal PVC, ventricular tachycardia, flutter, and fibrillation), and if they occur, admit the child to an ICU to be treated by the appropriate specialists.

7. Use diazepam, 10 mg IV, and then phenobarbital to treat seizures.

8. Monitor input, output, and electrolytes and correct any problem.

9. Insert an artificial airway if needed and keep tidal volume at 10–15 mL/kg.

Neither dialysis nor forced diuresis is effective in TCA overdoses because TCAs are highly protein-bound (>70%) and have a large tissue distribution. Sinus tachycardia does not need to be treated.

Maprotiline overdoses can be managed in the same way as TCA overdoses. Amoxapine overdoses can also be managed in the same way as TCA overdoses except renal failure can occur days after the overdose.[107] Because of the possibility of renal failure with amoxapine, hydrate the patient with isotonic saline at 500 mg/L per hour for the first 3–4 hours of hospitalization and force diuresis using mannitol or loop diuretics such as furosemide. The mechanism of renal failure is not known. Bupropion overdosage can cause seizures, so treat to prevent seizures as under TCA overdosage recommendations.

C. Monoamine Oxidase Inhibitors (MAOIs)

There are no controlled studies of MAOIs with pediatric populations. There are anecdotal reports that MAOIs like tranylcypromine, phenelzine, and isocarboxazid may be useful in the treatment of bipolar or unipolar depressed children and adolescents who do not respond to antidepressants.[108] However, because the dietary constraints associated with the use of MAOIs may not be followed, given the impulsivity of many children and adolescents, great caution should be exercised in prescribing these medications. Newer MAOIs (e.g., moclobemide), which are both reversible and unaffected by dietary amines, may offer advantages over current MAOIs.[109]

1. Definitions and Classes

MAOIs are divided into two classes, the hydrazine and nonhydrazine types. Phenelzine (Nardil®) and isocarboxazid (Marplan®) are both hydrazine MAOIs; tranylcypromine (Parnate®) is a nonhydrazine MAOI resembling amphetamine.

Monoamine oxidase exists in two forms, monoamine oxidase A (MAO-A) and monoamine oxidase B (MAO-B). MAO-A deaminates norepinephrine, serotonin, and normetanephrine. MAO-B deaminates dopamine and phenylethylamine. MAOIs prevent the metabolism and deactivation of these monoamine neurotransmitters. Some MAOIs are selective and inhibit only MAO-A or MAO-B, but most in current use are nonselective. Clorgyline and moclobemide are examples of MAO-A inhibitors, and selegiline (Deprenyl®) is an example of a MAO-B inhibitor. Only the MAO-A inhibitors have been shown to have antidepressant effect.[110]

2. Pharmacology

MAOIs increase the availability of the monoamines by inhibiting their degradation. MAOI-A increases the availability of norepinephrine, normetanephrine, and serotonin, and MAOI-B increases the availability of dopamine and phenylethylamine. The effect of these actions is basically sympathomimetic. The MAOIs also affect organ systems other than the brain, since MAO occurs in the liver, gastric mucosa, and other areas. Because of their presence in liver, they may interfere with the hepatic metabolism of other drugs.[111] A hypertensive crisis ("blue cheese effect") can be produced when substances high in tyramine are ingested, due to the pressor effect of tyramine. Tyramine is normally inactivated by MAO-B. Selective inhibitors like moclobemide or clorgyline, which inhibit only MAO-A, do not produce this hypertensive effect.

At a given dosage of MAOI, full MAO inhibition occurs in about 5 days. Most MAOIs (with the exception of newer agents like moclobemide) cause an irreversible monoamine oxidase inhibition that reverses only as new monoamines are produced, so their effects generally last up to 2 weeks after medication is discontinued. Moclobemide has a very short half-life (2 hr), is a reversible inhibitor of MAO-A, and is the only MAOI in which no washout period is necessary before starting another medication.[113] Hydrazine MAOIs are inactivated to their hydrazine metabolites primarily by acetylation.[110] About 50% of the population are *slow acetylators* and thus may have prolonged responses to hydrazine MAOIs. MAO inhibition can be evaluated by a blood test to assess the MAO inhibition in platelets. A platelet MAO inhibition of 85% is felt to be a therapeutic level.[110]

3. Clinical Effects

MAOIs typically produce a stimulant effect before developing a full antidepressant effect. As mentioned, the antidepressant effect seems to be related to the drug's capacity to inhibit MAO-A, but while the effects of MAO inhibition are seen immediately, the antidepressant effect does not appear for several weeks. The stimulant actions may be perceived as therapeutic (as in ADHD) or as side effects, depending on clinical symptomatology. For example, MAOIs also inhibit REM sleep and may cause problems with insomnia and produce the sensation of not having slept well.

4. Clinical Indications

Clorgyline, moclobemide, selegiline, phenelzine, and tranylcypromine have all been used in children, but studies are few.[111] Because of the potential problems with compliance and side effects, these medications should be used sparingly, and only after others have been tried. Moclobemide has fewer side effects and does not require dietary restrictions so it has a greater margin of safety. The MAOIs are not the treatments of choice for the disorders listed below. Though they are reportedly useful for some children, their use should require justification by special clinical imperatives. If MAOIs are used, the parents and child should be amply prepared. The clinician should have the parents sign consent forms spelling out the potential dangers of the medication and supply them with a list of medications and foods to be avoided. As always, the parents, not the child, should be responsible for administering and monitoring the medication.

a. Affective Disorders

It has been claimed that MAOIs are more effective than other antidepressants in adults with atypical depressions, usually associated with anxiety, fatigue, overeating, and oversleeping.[112] Mocolobemide (available outside the United States) has been studied in adults and has been demonstrated to be effective in depression and well tolerated with minimal side effects.[113] One study of MAOIs in children who had been unresponsive to TCAs found a fair to good response, although compliance was a problem.[114] The use of MAOIs in child and adolescent depression at the current time should be reserved for more serious and unresponsive cases and requires proper study.

b. Attention-Deficit Disorders

The effects of MAO-A and MAO-B inhibitors and the selectivity of their action have been studied in ADHD.[115,116] Clorgyline (MAO-A inhibitor) and tranylcypromine (MAO-A/MAO-B inhibitor) were both as effective as dextroamphetamine. Moclobemide has been studied in children with ADHD at a dosage of 100 mg b.i.d. (2.3–5 mg/kg body weight).[117] The children showed a 40% improvement in target symptom severity, and side effects were minor. Selegiline (MAO-B inhibitor) was not found to be effective in ADHD. This supports the hypothesis that the symptoms in ADHD are mainly affected by changes in the levels of norepinephrine and serotonin. Because of the difficulties with MAOIs and the small number of studies with newer agents, they should only be used in ADHD as agents of last resort.

5. Side Effects

The most common side effects of MAOIs are hypotension and orthostatic hypotension. These effects are predictable and controllable. In fact, the MAOI pargyline (Eutonyl®) was marketed in the past primarily as an antihypertensive. Other common effects include insomnia, afternoon sleepiness, dry mouth, fatigue, hyperreflexia, drowsiness, constipation, and nighttime myoclonic jerking. Adolescent males may experience a decrease in sex drive and impairment in erection and ejaculation. Usually, they will not reveal these troubles unless asked about them. Occasionally, weight gain and edema may occur. Hepatotoxicity may occur with hydrazine types and is usually associated with a period of anorexia, malaise, fatigue, and a slowly developing jaundice. Mania has been precipitated in adults, and confusion has been reported.

6. Contraindications, Drug Interactions, and Toxicity

MAOIs are contraindicated if the patient has a known allergy to them or if there is a pheochromocytoma. They must not be used with serotonergic antidepressants (fluoxetine, fluvoxamine, sertraline, clomipramine, paroxetine, or venlafaxine) or adrenergic drugs.

When administering MAOIs with a TCA, the **antidepressant** (TCA) should be adminis-tered **before** the **MAOI** ("a" before "m"), and not the reverse. They should not be started if the patient or family is unlikely to follow dietary and medication restrictions. If started, they should be stopped if the patient or family is noncompliant with dietary and medication restrictions.

The interaction of MAOIs (except moclobemide) with tyramine-containing foods resulting in inactivation of gut MAO can cause a *hypertensive crisis*. Patients may experi-ence a pounding headache, palpitations, chest pain, tachycardia, and flushing. This was called the *blue cheese and Chianti wine effect*, since aged cheeses and some wines and liquors are high in tyramine. Other foods containing aged proteins such as summer sausage and pickled herring are also high in tyramine. Generally, foods that are aged or overripe should be avoided. MAOIs should not be administered with stimulants (e.g., amphetamine, methylphenidate, and cocaine) or other sympathomimetic medications. Over-the-counter cold preparations, antihistamines, and compounds containing pseudoephedrine, epi-nephrine, phenylephrine, or phenylpropanolamine should be avoided. Many of the foods that children and adolescents like to eat are foods to be avoided, so dietary noncompliance rates may range from 30 to 50%.[114] As noted earlier, patients should be given a list of foods and all medications to be avoided.[30]

In the event of a hypertensive crisis, chlorpromazine (an adrenolytic antipsychotic; see Chapter 10) from 25 to 100 mg PO can be used to treat and abort such a crisis. Nifedipine (Procardia®) capsules have also been used. A 10-mg capsule of nifedipine is bitten open in the mouth, and this achieves more rapid vasodilation than if swallowed.

If the crisis is severe, then emergency room treatment is necessary. Treat hypertensive crises with phentolamine, 2.5–5 mg IV q5min, until blood pressure is under control, or with nitroprusside, 1 mcg/kg IV per minute titrated to 10 mcg/kg per minute as needed. Methyl-dopa and guanethidine are contraindicated as they may potentiate hypertension.

A *serotonin hypermetabolic crisis* (the **"serotonin syndrome"**) can occur if com-pounds high in serotonin or serotonin-elevating compounds are taken with MAOIs, and hence such combinations must be avoided.[118] The symptoms of the serotonin syndrome are extreme hyperthermia, CNS irritability, hyperreflexia, coma, seizures, and death. Seroton-ergic antidepressants such as fluoxetine and clomipramine, the analgesic meperidine (Demerol®/Pethedine®), and tryptophan have been associated with hypermetabolic crisis as have other medications. The antispasmodic dantrolene (Dantrium®) has been used to treat this crisis starting at 0.5 mg/kg and increasing to 2.0 mg/kg b.i.d. or t.i.d. until the crisis resolves. It should be continued for 1 or 2 days after the crisis has ceased. The serotonin syndrome and its treatment will be discussed more thoroughly in Section III.D.7.

7. Treatment of MAOI Overdosage

MAOI overdosage produces cardiovascular and central nervous system toxicity. Cardiovascular toxicity includes profound hypotension, dizziness, hypertension, headache, tachycardia, precordial pain, bradycardia, and cardiac arrest. Severe hypertension may occur if the MAOI has been taken with sympathomimetic drugs or high tyramine-containing foods. Central nervous system toxicity includes hypothermia, diaphoresis, tachypnea, neuromuscular weakness, mental confusion, miosis, coma, and signs of CNS excitation such as tremors, agitation, increased deep tendon reflexes, involuntary move-ments, and seizures. Treatment is focused on correcting the cardiovascular and CNS disturbances and eliminating the MAOI from the body as soon as possible (based on adult data).[106]

Recommendations for Managing Overdose of MAOIs*

1. In treating hypotension, *vasopressors should be avoided because they may cause severe hypertension*. However, if a pressor must be used, use norepinephrine since the dosage can be more easily controlled. Treat hypotension positionally by placing the patient in the Trendelenburg position and give IV fluids.
2. Treat hypertensive crises with phentolamine, 2.5–5 mg IV q5min, until blood pressure is under control, or with nitroprusside, 1 mcg/kg IV per minute, titrated to 10 mcg/kg per minute as needed. The β-blocker labetalol has also been successfully used. Methyldopa and guanethidine are contraindicated since they can exacerbate hypertension.
3. Treat CNS excitation, if severe, with diazepam, 2–10 mg IV. Avoid using low-potency antipsychotics like chlorpromazine because they may exacerbate hypotension.
4. Hyperthermia should be managed with a cooling blanket or other external cooling. Phenothiazines should not be used because they can cause irreversible shock.
5. Decrease the urinary pH from 8 to 5 to increase the excretion of tranylcypromine about sevenfold.[119] Consider hemodialysis since it can provide rapid recovery from overdoses of both tranylcypromine and phenelzine.[120,121]

D. Selective or Specific Serotonin Reuptake Inhibitors (SSRIs)

1. Definition

SSRIs are a class of antidepressants which inhibit the reuptake of serotonin (5-HT) into the presynaptic neuron terminal. They are selective because they are not equally potent at inhibiting serotonin reuptake at all serotonin receptor-subtype sites in the central nervous system. Selective stimulation of the 5-HT receptors has differential effects on affect, appetite, energy, sleep, aggressiveness, libido, anxiety, body temperature, heart rate, blood pressure, concentration, and learning. Many serotonin receptor subtypes have been identified. Table 9 shows the behaviors and physiological functions believed to be regulated by some of the commonly mentioned serotonin receptor subtypes.[122,123]

2. Pharmacology and Pharmacokinetics

The primary mechanism of action of SSRIs is to increase the presence of the monoamine serotonin by inhibiting its reuptake into the presynaptic nerve terminal. SSRIs are believed to be effective in depression because of the increased levels of brain serotonin which they produce.[124] Reuptake inhibitors are referred to as "selective" because the degree of reuptake inhibition various among SSRIs and different serotonin receptor subtypes.[125] It has been theorized that a relative deficiency of the monoamine serotonin (5-HT) is related to the symptoms of depression, including insomnia, anorexia, irritability, anxiety, fatigue, psychomotor retardation, and suicidal thoughts and behavior.

The pharmacokinetics of SSRIs vary depending on the specific SSRI. As shown in Table 3, the half-lives of SSRIs vary from 4 hr (venlafaxine) to 10 days (fluoxetine). Fluoxetine's long half-life includes the 10-day half-life of its active major metabolite,

*This information is for emergency use only. In general, overdosage is best managed by emergency medicine experts, not by psychiatrists.

TABLE 9. Serotonin (5-HT) Receptor Subtypes and Their Clinical Significance[a]

5-HT receptor subtype	Behaviors and functions regulated by subtype
1A	Anxiety, depression, sexual behavior, food intake, aggression, impulsivity, hypothermia, lowering of blood pressure and heart rate, pain
1C	Anxiety, mood, learning, aversion, CSF absorption, food intake, temperature, locomotion.
1D	Anxiety, appetite, cerebral vasoconstriction
2	Anxiety, depression, confusion, suicide, sleep, hyperthermia, sweating, motor function, coordination, hallucinations, vasoconstriction, raising of blood pressure and heart rate
3	Emesis, diarrhea, mesolimbic dopamine release (antianxiety)
4	Muscle contraction, learning

[a]Refs. 122 and 123.

norfluoxetine. Most SSRIs have long enough half-lives that they can be administered once daily. Venlafaxine requires administration twice a day because of its 4-hr half-life. The half-lives of SSRIs, with the exception of sertraline, increase with repeated dosing due to autoinhibition (i.e., they inhibit their own metabolism).[126] Both fluoxetine and paroxetine inhibit their own metabolism, which is why their kinetics are nonlinear (small increases in dose can produce large increases in blood level). For example, fluoxetine's half-life increases from about 1.9 days with a single dose to 5.7 days after multiple doses. Sertraline does not inhibit its own metabolism, and its half-life is essentially unchanged with multiple doses. The kinetics of sertraline are linear within the therapeutic dosage range.

SSRIs can inhibit the cytochrome P450 isoenzymes and increase the blood levels of medications that are metabolized by the P450 isoenzymes. Table 10 lists the specific cytochrome P450 isoenzymes inhibited by the SSRIs and some common classes of medication metabolized by the isoenzymes.[127,128] The effect of isoenzyme inhibition is to increase the concentration and effect of the classes of medications mentioned.

3. Clinical Effects

The SSRIs in therapeutic doses reduce anxiety, improve mood and relaxation, decrease aggressiveness, and produce a sense of well-being. Often, patients report feeling better within the first few days of treatment; however, a full antidepressant effect is not usually seen for 4–8 weeks. The SSRIs may have initial stimulating effects, antianxiety effects, sedative effects, or relaxant effects depending on the SSRI, initial dosage, and patient individuality. The initial effects depend on the side-effect profile of the specific SSRI (see Table 11). Excessive dosing can produce side effects of anxiety and "behavioral activation," and overdosages or drug interactions can produce toxic symptoms.

4. Clinical Indications

a. Affective Disorders

There have been seven uncontrolled studies[129–135] and two controlled studies completed[136,137] evaluating the effectiveness of the SSRIs in child and adolescent depression. One controlled study[136] failed to find a difference between placebo and fluoxetine; however, a recent placebo-controlled study[137] with 96 patients demonstrated the effectiveness of

TABLE 10. Degree of Inhibition of Cytochrome P450 Isoenzymes by SSRIs[a]

Isoenzyme inhibition	Fluoxetine (Prozac®)	Sertraline (Zoloft®)	Fluvoxamine (Luvox®)	Paroxetine (Paxil®)	Venlafaxine (Effexor®)
2D6 inhibition (2D6 metabolizes Type 1C antiarrhythmics, secondary-amine TCAs, and antipsychotics)	+++++	+++	+	+++++	+
3A4 inhibition	+++	+	+++++	+/−	Unknown
2C inhibition (2C metabolizes benzodiazepines)	+++++	+/−	+++	Unknown	Unknown
1A2 inhibition (1A2 metabolizes tertiary-amine TCAs)	+	+	+++++	+	Unknown

[a]Refs. 127 and 128.

fluoxetine. The effectiveness in child and adolescent depressions approached the 60% effectiveness seen with adults. The majority of children responded to 20 mg daily of fluoxetine, and the side effects were minimal. Three children dropped out because of manic excitement. Between 5 and 20 mg daily seems the best dosage for most children and adolescents, and it decreases the likelihood of side effects. However, some children may require 5-, 10-, or 40-mg dosages.[130]

The open studies with sertraline showed that children and adolescents respond to dosages of sertraline in the 25–200 mg daily range.[132,134,135] The average dosage in the studies was about 100 mg daily. None of the studies were controlled; characteristically, the rates of response and doses were higher than in the controlled studies with fluoxetine.

Children and adolescents may respond better to SSRIs than to TCAs because of developmental differences. Animal studies of the development of the monoamine neurotransmitter systems have found a developmental difference in the rate at which neurotransmitter systems mature.[138] Children's dopamine (DA) or norepinephrine (NE) systems

TABLE 11. Selected Side Effects of SSRIs[a,b]

Side effect	Fluoxetine	Sertraline	Paroxetine	Fluvoxamine	Venlafaxine
Nausea	+++	++++	++++	++++++	++++++
Nervousness	+++	+	+	++	+++
Anorexia	++	−	+	+	++
Insomnia	++	++	++	+++	++
Drowsiness	+	++	++++	+++	+++
Tremor	+	++	++	+	+
Fatigue	+	+	+++	++	+
Dry mouth	+	++	+	+	+++
Dizziness	+	+	++	++	+++
Sweating	+	++	++	+	++
Diarrhea	+	++	+	+	−
Constipation	−	−	+	+/−	++
Sexual dysfunction	+	+++	+++	++	++++

[a]Refs 15 and 157.
[b]Each + represents about a 4% incidence of the side effect after adjusting for placebo effect; a − represents a decreased incidence of the side effect relative to that reported for placebo.

may not be fully developed until late adolescence or adulthood while their serotonin (5-HT) systems may be more mature. If this is the case, then children might not respond to TCAs because of their immature DA and NE systems. They might respond like adults to SSRIs because their 5-HT system is more adultlike.

b. Attention-Deficit Disorders

A preliminary trial with fluoxetine in children and adolescents with attention-deficit disorders[139] showed about a 60% improvement rate. However, the use of fluoxetine as a primary treatment for ADHD should be viewed as experimental only, particularly in light of case reports of memory impairment from fluoxetine.[140,141]

Because venlafaxine inhibits the reuptake of NE similarly to TCAs (Table 2), it has been tried in ADHD in adults[142] and in children.[143] In all, 73% of the adults and 44% of the children responded. The dropout rate due to intolerable side effects ranged from 25 to 40%. The dosage range for the children was 37.5–75 mg daily, and the dosage for adults was about twice as much. Based on these preliminary open studies, it would appear that venlafaxine would be a poor choice for children and adolescents because of its side effects.

c. Anxiety Disorders and Obsessive–Compulsive Disorder (OCD)

There have been eight studies of SSRIs in anxiety disorders[144–151] and three controlled studies.[152–154] One controlled study did not show any significant difference between placebo and fluoxetine for the obsessive–compulsive symptoms in Tourette syndrome.[152] Another rigorous double-blind crossover study of children with OCD[153] found a 45% decrease in the severity of symptoms over 8 weeks.

A controlled study[154] of selective mutism failed to show significant group differences, probably due to a small number of patients. However, other uncontrolled studies of selective mutism[146,151] showed fluoxetine to be effective.

Fluoxetine appears to be helpful in separation anxiety, social phobia, and generalized anxiety disorders.[144,145,150] However, these results are preliminary, and the evidence comes from uncontrolled studies. No controlled studies have yet been done.

The dosage range of fluoxetine is from 10 to 60 mg daily, and that of fluvoxamine is from 100 to 300 mg daily. There is a tendency for OCD to be treated with higher dosages of medication; however, the most well-controlled study was conducted with a fixed 20-mg dosage and achieved significant results. The other anxiety disorders generally were treated with doses averaging between 20 and 30 mg daily of fluoxetine.

d. Autism and Developmental Disabilities

Children (and some adults) with autism or mental retardation were treated in an open trial with fluoxetine, 10–80 mg daily.[155] About 65% of the patients had a significant reduction of target symptoms (perseverative behavior, irritability, and so forth). Another study treated transition anxiety and agitation in autistic disorder with low dosages of sertraline, 25–50 mg daily.[156] Reduction in the anxiety and agitation due to transitional change was seen in about 2–8 weeks. Controlled studies are needed; however, since the symptoms of autism are so difficult to treat, a trial of an SSRI might be clinically warranted.

5. Side Effects and Drug Interactions

The SSRIs differ primarily in terms of their side effects. They probably are all equally effective in children and adolescents, so the most suitable SSRI can be picked based on its side-effect profile. Table 11 contains the relative frequencies of common side effects observed with the various SSRIs in adults.[157] The percentages are arrived at by adjusting for side effects due to placebo.

The side-effect profiles are similar, so specific SSRIs can be picked to minimize the chances of an undesirable side effect. Compliance is important in children, and noncompliance after side effects are experienced (particularly nausea) may be due to "bait poisoning."[158] The term *bait poisoning* comes from a technique used to prevent animals from attacking and eating their natural prey, based on having the animals eat bait composed of meat from their prey and a substance producing nausea and vomiting (like apomorphine or lithium). Since SSRIs can produce nausea, they may cause "bait poisoning" in children and adolescents and cause them to be noncompliant and avoid taking their medication. This is another reason to use a low initial dosage when starting treatment.

One of the most common reasons for children and adolescents to drop out of SSRI treatment is due to "behavioral activation" and disinhibition.[129,159] One study employed high doses (up to 80 mg daily) and had a high (23%) incidence of "mania,"[129] and in case reports of five adolescents with mania from SSRIs,[159] three of the five were on dosages greater than 20 mg. This effect seems to be just another SSRI side effect and not mania. There is no evidence yet to support this hypothesis. A study of the side effects of fluoxetine (20 or 40 mg daily) showed behavioral activation and other side effects to be dose-dependent. Lowering the dosage reduced or eliminated the side effects.[160] "Mania" actually seems to be behavioral activation due to excess medication. **"Start low and go slow"** and reduce the dosage to avoid dose-dependent side effects.

Venlafaxine can produce an increase in blood pressure. Because the blood pressure side effects can be significant, blood pressure monitoring is necessary if treating with venlafaxine.

Abrupt withdrawal from SSRIs due to discontinuation, missing doses, or too rapid tapering of the SSRI can cause an **SSRI discontinuation syndrome**.[161] The symptoms of the SSRI discontinuation syndrome are dizziness and problems with balance, nausea and vomiting, fatigue, myalgias, chills, paresthesias, sleep and dreaming disturbances, increased levels of anxiety, irritability, and crying spells. The syndrome occurs when the dosage is rapidly decreased. It is mild and short-lived; however, it is upsetting to children and their parents. It occurs more often with SSRIs with short half-lives. In adults, at least one symptom occurred in 31% with clomipramine, 20% with paroxetine, 14% with fluvoxamine, 2% with sertraline, and none with fluoxetine.[162] The SSRI discontinuation syndrome can be avoided by slowly tapering the SSRIs by reducing the dosage every 5 to 7 days. It can be reversed within 24 hours by reintroducing the SSRIs at lower doses and tapering.[163]

Because SSRIs inhibit the cytochrome P450 isoenzymes, a number of specific medications have their metabolism affected or have the potential to have their metabolism affected by the SSRIs. Table 12 lists the relative potency of the SSRIs in inhibiting the metabolism of selected medications. Most of the data are based on pharmacological and in vitro data. Case reports of actual blood-level elevations have been reported for desipramine, diazepam, tolbutamide, phenytoin, alprazolam, carbamazepine, trazodone, theophylline, clozapine, haloperidol, imipramine, and amitriptyline.[128] Until in vivo data are available on all medications mentioned in Table 12, the table can be used by physicians to estimate the probable degree to which the medication's metabolism might be affected by a given SSRI.

6. Contraindications

Contraindications include a prior history of hypersensitivity to the SSRI. It is contraindicated to add MAOIs to an SSRI or vice versa because the **serotonin syndrome** can

TABLE 12. Effect of SSRIs on the Metabolism of Medications through Cytochrome P450 (CYP450) Isoenzymes[a]

Medication	Metabolized by CYP450	Fluoxetine (Prozac®)	Sertraline (Zoloft®)	Fluvoxamine (Luvox®)	Paroxetine (Paxil®)	Venlafaxine (Effexor®)
Alprazolam (Xanax®)	3A4	+++	+	+++++	+/−	Unknown
Amitriptyline (Elavil®)	2C, 3A4, 1A2	+++++	+++	+++++	+++++	+
Astemizole (Hismanal®)	3A4	+++	+	+++++	+/−	Unknown
Brofaromine	2D6	+++++	+++	+	+++++	+
Caffeine	1A2	+	+	+++++	+	Unknown
Carbamazepine (Tegretol®)	3A4	+++	+	+++++	+/−	Unknown
Citalopram	2C	+++++	+/−	+++	Unknown	Unknown
Clomipramine (Anafranil®)	2C, 3A4, 1A2	+++++	+++	+++++	+++++	+
Clozapine (Clozaril®)	1A2, 2D6	+++++	+++	+++++	+++++	+
Codeine	2D6	+++++	+++	+	+++++	+
Desipramine (Norpramin®)	2D6	+++++	+++	+	+++++	+
Dexamethasone (Decadron®)	3A4	+++	+	+++++	+/−	Unknown
Dextromethorphan	2D6, 3A4	+++++	+++	+	+++++	+
Diazepam (Valium®)	2C	+++++	+/−	+++	Unknown	Unknown
Encainide	2D6	+++++	+++	+	+++++	+
Erythromycin	3A4	+++	+	+++++	+/−	Unknown
Flecainide (Tambocor®)	2D6	+++++	+++	+	+++++	+
Fluoxetine (Prozac®)	2D6	+++++	+++	+	+++++	+
Fluvoxamine (Luvox®)	1A2	+	+	+++++	+	Unknown
Haloperidol (Haldol®)	2D6, 1A2	+++++	+++	+++++	+++++	+
Hexobarbital	2C	+++++	+/−	+++	Unknown	Unknown
Imipramine (Tofranil®)	2C, 3A4, 1A2	+++++	+++	+++++	+++++	+
Lidocaine	3A4	+++	+	+++++	+/−	Unknown
Maprotiline (Ludiomil®)	2D6	+++++	+++	+	+++++	+
Mephobarbital (Mebaral®)	2C	+++++	+/−	+++	Unknown	Unknown
Metoprolol (Lopressor®)	2D6	+++++	+++	+	+++++	+
Mianserin	2D6	+++++	+++	+	+++++	+
Midazolam (Versed®)	3A4	+++	+	+++++	+/−	Unknown
Moclobemide (Aurorix®)	2C	+++++	+/−	+++	Unknown	Unknown
Nefazodone (Serzone®)	3A4	+++	+	+++++	+/−	Unknown
Norfluoxetine	2D6	+++++	+++	+	+++++	+

TABLE 12. (*Continued*)

Medication	Metabolized by CYP450	Fluoxetine (Prozac®)	Sertraline (Zoloft®)	Fluvoxamine (Luvox®)	Paroxetine (Paxil®)	Venlafaxine (Effexor®)
Nortriptyline (Pamelor®)	2D6	+++++	+++	+	+++++	+
Omeprazole (Prilosec®)	2C	+++++	+/-	+++	Unknown	Unknown
Paroxetine (Paxil®)	2D6	+++++	+++	+	+++++	+
Perphenazine (Trilafon®)	2D6	+++++	+++	+	+++++	+
Phenacetin	1A2	+	+	+++++	+	Unknown
Phenytoin (Dilantin®)	2C, 1A2	+++++	+	+++++	+	Unknown
Propafenone (Rythmol®)	2D6	+++++	+++	+	+++++	+
Propanolol (Inderal®)	2D6	+++++	+++	+	+++++	+
Protriptyline (Vivactil®)	2D6	+++++	+++	+	+++++	+
Quinidine	3A4	+++	+	+++++	+/-	Unknown
Remoxipride	2D6	+++++	+++	+	+++++	+
Risperidone (Risperdal®)	2D6	+++++	+++	+	+++++	+
Sertraline (Zoloft®)	3A4	+++	+	+++++	+/-	Unknown
Tacrine (Cognex®)	1A2	+	+	+++++	+	Unknown
Terfenadine (Seldane®)	3A4	+++	+	+++++	+/-	Unknown
Theophylline (Theodur®)	1A2	+	+	+++++	+	Unknown
Thioridazine (Mellaril®)	2D6	+++++	+++	+	+++++	+
Timolol (Timoptic®)	2D6	+++++	+++	+	+++++	+
Tolbutamide	2C	+++++	+/-	+++	Unknown	Unknown
Trazodone (Desyrel®)	2D6	+++++	+++	+	+++++	+
Triazolam (Halcion®)	3A4	+++	+	+++++	+/-	Unknown
Venlafaxine (Effexor®)	2D6	+++++	+++	+	+++++	+
Verapamil (Calan®, Isoptin®)	1A2, 3A4	+++	+	+++++	+	Unknown
Warfarin	2C	+++++	+/-	+++	Unknown	Unknown

[a]Refs. 127 and 128.

occur and death can result. Other medications added to an SSRI, such as L-tryptophan, dihydroergotamine, and sumatriptan, can also cause the serotonin syndrome.

7. Treatment of SSRI Overdosage and the Serotonin Syndrome

The SSRIs are basically safe in overdosage. Treat with gastric lavage, emesis, and supportive care.

The **serotonin syndrome** is potentially fatal if not diagnosed and rapidly treated. With

TABLE 13. Criteria for the Serotonin Syndrome[a]

A. Coincident with the addition of or increase in a known serotonergic agent to an established medication regimen, at least 3 of the following clinical features are present:
   1. Mental status changes (confusion, hypomania)
   2. Agitation
   3. Myoclonus
   4. Hyperreflexia
   5. Diaphoresis
   6. Shivering
   7. Tremor
   8. Diarrhea
   9. Incoordination
   10. Fever
B. Other etiologies (e.g., infectious, metabolic, substance abuse, or withdrawal) have been ruled out.
C. A neuroleptic had not been started or increased in dosage prior to the onset of the signs and symptoms listed above.

[a]Ref. 118.

treatment, it can resolve rapidly. Treatment is based on experience in adults; adjust dosages as needed for children. The differential diagnosis of the serotonin syndrome includes neuroleptic malignant syndrome (NMS), malignant hyperthermia, lethal catatonia, psychostimulant or MAOI overdose, anticholinergic syndrome, drug withdrawal, and CNS disease (infection, infarction, bleed).[118] In NMS there is almost always severe muscle rigidity, elevated creatine phosphokinase (CPK), a slower evolution (24–72 hr), and a slower onset—typically within 2 weeks after adding a neuroleptic or increasing the dosage of the neuroleptic. In the serotonin syndrome the onset is usually acute within a few hours after the medication change, rigidity is seldom present, and the CPK is not elevated. Criteria for diagnosing the serotonin syndrome in adults are shown in Table 13.

Treat the serotonin syndrome as follows*:

1. Immediately discontinue the offending agents.
2. In mild cases, send the patient home with close follow-up and a PRN of lorazepam, propranolol, or cyproheptadine.
3. In moderate to severe cases, hospitalize with close monitoring and appropriate supportive care.
4. Give lorazepam 1–2 mg slow IV push q30min until improvement or sedation occurs (however, up to 16 mg has been given IV within 1 hr with rapid resolution and without significant side effects[123]).
5. If no help, give propranolol 1–3 mg q5min up to a dosage of 0.1 mg/kg.
6. If no help, give cyproheptadine 4 mg PO q4h, not to exceed 20 mg per 24 hr.
7. If no help, consider experimental approach such as nitroglycerin.

E. Combinations

In the past few years, clinicians have used combinations of medications more often in child and adolescent psychiatric disorders. Some clinicians view this as fine-tuning neurochemistry to compensate for hypothetical biochemical deficits. That level of biological

*This information is for emergency use only. In general, overdosage is best managed by emergency medicine experts, not by psychiatrists.

treatment sophistication is not yet available. Polypharmacy should be avoided if possible (for details, see Chapter 1). However, an empirical target symptom approach attentive to effects on children's and adolescents' functioning can be clinically justifiable.

1. TCAs Combined with Stimulants and SSRIs

TCAs have been combined with stimulants and with SSRIs.[164-166] Two studies were case reports,[164,166] and one was a controlled study.[165] Because of the likelihood of the serotonin syndrome, combining fluoxetine and clomipramine as in one study[166] would not currently be recommended.

The combination of therapeutic doses of methylphenidate (MPH) and desipramine in a well-designed placebo-controlled study of 16 hospitalized children with ADHD and mood disorders suggested that the combination was more effective than Ritalin for attention, hyperactivity, oppositional–defiant, and aggressive behavior,[165] but not more helpful for mood. Also, a case report of three children with Tourette syndrome treated with MPH and imipramine (IMI) suggested that they seemed to respond to the combination.[164] These findings are tentative and need to be replicated in other controlled studies.

2. SSRIs Combined with Stimulants

The combination of methylphenidate or amphetamines used openly with fluoxetine, trazodone, or sertraline was reported to be helpful in seven adolescents with ADHD and comorbid major depression in an uncontrolled series of cases.[167] Another uncontrolled open study reported that 30 of 32 children with ADHD and comorbid anxiety and depression improved when treated with a combination of methylphenidate and fluoxetine.[168] Of note, the dosage of fluoxetine in this study was *gradually* increased, and none of the children developed "behavioral activation." One child developed agitation and restlessness after 3 months of treatment. As ever, uncontrolled studies are therapeutically optimistic about the benefits of combined treatment. These findings are merely suggestive.

F. Other

The use of St. John's wort is discussed in Chapter 15 under "Hypericin."

G. Summary of Antidepressant Treatment of Children and Adolescents

Antidepressants have been used to treat children and adolescents with depression, ADHD, enuresis, selective mutism, anxiety disorders, aggressiveness, and autism.

SSRIs show some promise in treating affective disorders, anxiety disorders (including OCD and selective mutism), and possibly features of autism in children; however, studies are still few, and their results should be viewed with caution. One well-designed study exists indicating effectiveness in depression.[137] The effectiveness in this study approached that seen with adult depression. The SSRIs also seem to be helpful in treating anxiety disorders. Other than their interactions with the cytochrome P450 system and the potential for adverse drug–drug interactions, SSRIs are generally well tolerated. Because of their safety and possible effectiveness, they are a first choice in child and adolescent depression.

In ADHD, combining SSRIs with stimulants may help offset the side effects seen when severe ADHD is treated with stimulants alone. When mood swings, appetite loss, depression, and insomnia become disabling, they may be helped by the combination. Venlafaxine may be useful for ADHD; however, its side effects are poorly tolerated.

If a child or adolescent develops side effects to one SSRI, it does not mean that he or she will *not* respond to a different SSRI. In adults who switched from fluoxetine to sertraline because of side effects, 76% responded to sertraline and tolerated it well.[169]

While open trials with TCAs in depression indicated that antidepressants might be effective, subsequent double-blind studies have failed to demonstrate a clear superiority over placebo. Thus, given this and their toxicity, there is little to justify use of TCAs as a first choice in child depression. In selected severely depressed children, antidepressants may be justifiably tried as part of a comprehensive treatment plan, but the reasons for their use and potential effectiveness must be carefully considered and documented.

In ADHD, TCAs are helpful but are second-choice medications after stimulants. Also, they tend to produce more side effects. They are effective in reducing restlessness and anxiety and may improve attention but cannot be expected to help conduct symptoms. They may be helpful in combination with stimulants to augment the effect of stimulants and enhance compliance.

In enuresis, TCAs are symptomatically effective, but relapse is high on cessation of the medication. The "bell and pad" is the treatment of choice since it can be curative. The role of TCAs in anxiety disorders is unestablished. The more serotonergic TCAs may be helpful in OCD and trichotillomania.

The serotonergic TCA clomipramine and SSRIs may be helpful in treating stereotypic and self-injurious behaviors in autism and developmental disabilities. The potential for toxicity and seizures needs to be kept in mind when deciding to treat developmental disabilities in children and adolescents with TCAs.

Because of the large variability in plasma levels of TCAs, plasma levels should be measured whenever possible to prevent toxic levels from occurring. With any type of antidepressant, pretreatment workup should include the usual laboratory tests, including tests of cardiac, liver, thyroid, and kidney function as indicated (see Chapter 4). Antidepressants are major psychoactive agents, and much more research is needed to continue to define indications and contraindications in pediatric psychopharmacology.

MAOIs may be helpful, as they are in adults, in depressions that show atypical features such as hypersomnia and overeating, but controlled studies in children are needed. They may be helpful in ADHD as a last resort. However, they should be prescribed only sparingly after other treatments have failed. The new reversible MAOI, moclobemide, shows promise because of its greater safety.

Combination treatment with antidepressants and stimulants shows some promise. Further controlled studies of combinations need to be done to assess their potential risks and benefits.

IV. ANTIMANICS

A. Introduction

In the DSM-IV, the diagnosis of "manic syndrome" requires a distinct period of abnormally elevated, expansive, or irritable mood and at least three (four in the case of irritable mood) of the following: inflated self-esteem, decreased need to sleep, talkativeness, flight of ideas, distractibility, psychomotor agitation, and excessive involvement in pleasurable activities with a high potential for painful consequences.[8] While mania clearly occurs in typical form in adolescents,[170] it has also been reported, though much less frequently, in children.[171,172] A monograph on manic–depressive disorder[173] summarizes knowledge of this disorder in adults (and in children) and is recommended for further reading (see also Chapter 7).

1. Epidemiology of Mania

The incidence of manic episodes (ever) in 14- to 16-year-olds is 0.6% and 0.6–1% in adults.[174] Twenty percent of adults have their first symptoms before age 20 (0.5% between the ages of 5 and 9, 7.5% between 10 and 14, and 12% between 15 and 19), and the peak onset is in late adolescence and early adulthood.[174]

2. Antimanic Drugs

The antimanic medications used in adults[173] include lithium, carbamazepine (Tegretol®), valproic acid (Depakene®, Depakote®/Epilim®), clonazapem (Klonopin®, Rivotril®), verapamil (Calan®, Isoptin®), nifedipine, and diltiazem. There have been a few studies of these medications in manic children and adolescents. The available studies need replication with larger samples.

B. Lithium

1. Definition

Lithium is a naturally occurring alkali metal, situated above sodium in the periodic table, and is found in mineral deposits and in seawater. In the past, lithium chloride was used as a salt substitute in cardiac patients; however, toxicity occurred and its use was discontinued. The preparations that are used in psychiatry are the lithium salts, primarily lithium carbonate or citrate. Cade first described the use of lithium salts to quiet acute agitated and psychotic manic patients, but toxicity discouraged its use for many years.[175] Currently, lithium is considered as the primary prophylactic maintenance treatment to prevent or reduce the likelihood of subsequent manic episodes,[176] and as the preferred treatment for acute manic episodes after the first 5 days,[172] which is the time it takes to become effective.

2. Cellular Actions

Lithium has effects on electrolytes, central nervous system (CNS) neurotransmitters, and cellular transport mechanisms. Sodium and potassium excretion initially increase and then return to normal within about 1 week in adults. Calcium excretion decreases and serum levels may increase slightly.[177] The CNS effects of lithium are thought to be caused by altered membrane transport mechanisms related to effects on the distribution of sodium, calcium, and magnesium and on glucose metabolism. Lithium has been noted to inhibit release of norepinephrine and dopamine in calcium-dependent neurons, but it may enhance serotonin release. These effects have been suggested as possible causes of lithium's mood-stabilizing and antiaggressive effects[110] though its action is not fully understood.

3. Pharmacokinetics

Lithium elimination is almost entirely dependent on renal mechanisms.[19] By the first year of life, kidney function in children approaches that of adults (Chapter 2). As children have a higher glomerular filtration rate than adults, they typically require higher doses of lithium than adults to achieve therapeutic blood levels.[178,179] Lithium appears to affect cells by ionic substitution. It can replace calcium, magnesium, sodium, and potassium ions intracellularly and hence change the properties of cells and interfere with membrane transport.[180]

Apart from the higher excretion rate, the pharmacokinetics of lithium in children are assumed to be qualitatively similar to those in adults,[181] i.e., first-order linear kinetics are present (see Chapter 2).[182] Thus, as the dose increases or decreases, the steady-state serum lithium concentration increases or decreases proportionately.[183] Lithium is rapidly absorbed when taken orally, and maximum blood levels are achieved 1–3 hr following ingestion. Lithium does not bind to protein, is distributed throughout the total body water, and is not metabolized but excreted unchanged.[184,185]

4. Behavioral and Emotional Effects

There have been no studies on the behavioral and emotional effects of lithium in children who do not have a psychiatric diagnosis. The effects on children with conduct disorders, affective disorders, and psychosis seem to be a decrease in aggressiveness, explosive outbursts, anger, and mood fluctuations. Cycles of behavioral excesses may be attenuated or blunted. Untoward effects of slurred speech, drowsiness, ataxia, and confusion may occur and are more common in young children.[186–191]

5. Cognitive and Learning Effects

Studies in adults suggest that lithium may cause some degree of cognitive impairment.[173] There has been some study in children, and available information suggests little effect (good or bad) at therapeutic blood levels;[186,192] however, drowsiness and confusion can occur in younger children as mentioned above.

6. Adverse Effects

There have been three studies of the side effects of lithium in children.[191,193,194] The most common side effects of lithium in children include tremor, drowsiness, ataxia, confusion, nausea, vomiting, diarrhea, headache, polyuria, and weight gain.[171,191,195] These are infrequent in older children and adolescents[171] but more frequent in children under the age of 6.[191] Comparison of the frequency of these side effects in children treated with lithium and those given placebo showed that these side effects occurred more frequently in the lithium-treated group and that they occur often at therapeutic levels.[194] Weight gain occurred often in both groups, but there was no significant difference. Lithium side effects may be less than side effects encountered with stimulants.[192] Leukocytosis and a decrease in thyroxine-iodine have also been reported.[189] In addition to durable side effects, peak lithium level is sometimes associated with transient vomiting and nausea, muscle weakness, and a dazed feeling. Table 14 shows the side effects (corrected for placebo) for children on lithium. However, since studies in children are still few, the data on side effects in adults will be reviewed; presumably, children are at similar risk.[196]

**TABLE 14. Frequency of Selected Side Effects
of Lithium in Children after Correcting
for Side Effects Due to Placebo[a]**

Side effect	Frequency (%)[b]	Side effect	Frequency (%)[b]
Vomiting	32	Drowsiness	2
Headache	17	Anorexia	9
Stomachache	−3[c]	Diarrhea	5
Nausea	24	Polyuria	5
Tremor	19		

[a]Ref. 194.
[b]Based on 5- to 12-year-old children receiving lithium ($n = 46$) or placebo ($n = 45$).
[c]Three percent more children on placebo have stomachaches than children on lithium.

a. Dermatologic

Lithium has been associated with both exacerbation and precipitation of acne.[197] Possible treatments include reduction or discontinuation of lithium or addition of tetracycline.[198] The appearance of acne is especially distressing to adolescents.

b. Osseous

Lithium deposition in bones, which has been noted in adults, theoretically might cause problems in bone metabolism in a growing child.[199] However, many years of lithium treatment in adults suggest that lithium does not pose any increased risk for osteoporosis.[200]

c. Endocrine

Lithium can induce hypothyroidism as indicated by elevated thyroid-stimulating hormone (TSH).[201] Therefore, pretreatment assessments of thyroid function are necessary to provide estimates of function and a baseline by which to assess any subsequent changes. Lithium-induced hypothyroidism and goiter are reversible with thyroid hormone replacement,[183] which may need to be prescribed for only a limited time. Weight gain is a common complication with lithium therapy in adults and is directly related to duration of treatment.[202] The etiology is unclear. If an adolescent female is on lithium, she should be monitored carefully to avoid pregnancy, as lithium may be teratogenic.

d. Neuromuscular

Muscular weakness and hand tremor are common neuromuscular side effects.[203] Hand tremor can occur at therapeutic lithium levels as well as at elevated serum levels. Lowering of lithium dose usually helps this problem. Propranolol is also helpful.[204]

e. Hematologic

Hematologic side effects include low-grade leukocytosis ($9000–13,000/mm^3$) and thrombocytosis.[205,206]

f. Urinary

Nephrotic syndrome has been reported in one adolescent,[207] but four 13- to 15-year-olds had unimpaired tubular and glomerular renal function after being treated with lithium carbonate for 3–5 years.[208]

7. Clinical Indications and Usage

a. General Diagnostic Considerations

The U.S. Food and Drug Administration (FDA) advises against the use of lithium in children under 12.[178] Recent evidence suggests that lithium maintenance treatment may increase the chance of mania occurring upon lithium withdrawal.[209,210] This suggests that it may not be advisable to start maintenance lithium treatment in children and adolescents until the second episode to avoid precipitating manic episodes sooner than they would naturally occur.[210] When treating children and adolescents with maintenance lithium, it is important to explain this to parents and guardians and keep lithium blood levels at the lowest clinically effective level and continue maintenance treatment for at least 2 years.[210] Written consent from the parents and assent from the youngster should be obtained. As with other pharmacologic interventions in children, use of lithium should be part of an overall comprehensive treatment plan including a range of treatment modalities (see Chapter 1).

Lithium carbonate has been prescribed for children and adolescents with a variety of diagnoses and/or behavioral problems. It has been recommended that lithium be considered in aggressiveness, manic–depressive illness, childhood depression, refractory depression, high-risk offspring of lithium responders, and emotionally unstable personality disorder.[187,211] As will be seen, the few studies available generally confirm these indications.[170,212–215] Other disorders, such as ADHD or unipolar depressive disorder, do not seem to respond so well.

b. Medical Workup

A careful medical history including a detailed history of any kidney problems, cardiovascular disease, or use of medications that interfere with sodium regulation in the body should be done (see Chapter 4). Questions about low-salt (or idiosyncratic) diet or diuretic treatment should be asked. Laboratory tests should include baseline complete blood count (CBC) with differential, thyroid function tests, electrolytes, kidney function tests including 24-hr urine collection for creatinine clearance, blood urea nitrogen, creatinine levels, and ECG (see Chapter 4).

c. Treatment in Bipolar Disorders

Bipolar disorder is rare or infrequent in children. As in adults,[173] 50% of adolescent (and child) patients ultimately diagnosed as manic according to DSM-III-R criteria originally will have received another diagnosis, primarily schizophrenia.[172,216,217] As a result, there are few studies of lithium in childhood bipolar disorder; most are controlled and include doubtful cases and other diagnostic groups as well.[171,192,212,215] There are no well-designed double-blind, placebo-controlled studies of lithium's effectiveness in mania in childhood bipolar disorder. Although results of available studies to date are not entirely in agreement, there is evidence that lithium may be helpful and that relapses can be reduced, particularly where the diagnosis is clear-cut or there is a strong family history. Thus, lithium treatment should be considered for treatment of child and adolescent bipolar disorder at some point after the onset of the illness. This is particularly important given that 50% of children and adolescents with bipolar disorder have an unfavorable long-term outlook.[217] This figure is similar to that seen in adults.[173] However, given the chance for inducing early manic cycling upon discontinuation of lithium, lithium maintenance should probably not be undertaken until after the second episode and then continued for at least 2 years.[210]

The following are suggested indications for lithium treatment in juvenile bipolar disorder: (1) episodes of mania and depression; (2) history of hypomania with severe depression; (3) severe depression with psychomotor retardation, hypersomnia, psychosis, and family history of bipolar disorder[218,219]; (4) an acute psychotic disorder with affective features; and (5) disruptive behavior disorders with family history of good response to lithium or of mood disorders.[181]

d. Effects on Aggressive Behavior and Conduct Disorder

A common reason for a referral to a child psychiatric clinic and for hospital admission is explosive/aggressive behavior and conduct disorder.[220] Antipsychotics (neuroleptics) are useful in the treatment of aggressive behavior, but they may be sedating, have potential to interfere with learning, and can cause dyskinesia (see Chapter 10).[188,221] There are three controlled studies of lithium in aggressive behavior and conduct disorder.[195,222,223] One found that lithium was as effective as haloperidol and caused fewer side effects than haloperidol.[195] In another study, lithium, 600–1800 mg daily (average 1200 mg daily) for 6 weeks, in children aged 5 to 12 years produced marked improvement in aggression (bullying, fighting, and temper outbursts) in 40% and moderate improvement in 28%.[222] Serum lithium levels were 0.5–1.8 mEq/L (mean 1.1 mEq/L). Another study failed to find any difference in aggressiveness between placebo- and lithium-treated adolescents aged 12 to 17 years treated for 2 weeks.[223] Lack of a difference may be due to the short duration of treatment or a difference in response between children and adolescents. Uncontrolled studies showed a beneficial effect of lithium on aggression (Chapter 7).[187,212–214] However, aggressive children and adolescents and their families are often among the least compliant, so that lithium monitoring and supervision requirements may limit this use.

e. Attention-Deficit Hyperactivity Disorder

It has been suspected that ADHD may be a precursor or an analogue of bipolar disorder. Consequently, lithium has been tried in several, mostly uncontrolled or diagnostically dubious studies.[192,212,224] The evidence is mostly against any useful effect unless there are affective symptoms. Augmentation of the effect of stimulants in some cases is a possibility, but this needs further study and should be regarded as experimental.

f. Unipolar Major Depression

In the few studies in children and adolescents,[212,225,226] there is no good evidence that lithium is effective either as a single treatment or as an augmentation of antidepressant treatment.

g. Dosage

One study[227] systematically tested a lithium dosage schedule for prepubertal children based on weight to determine the dose of lithium that would give a serum lithium level within the presumed therapeutic range for adults (0.6–1.2 mEg/L). Lithium was given in approximately equal doses three times daily. Dividing the daily dosage into three mealtime doses may reduce gastrointestinal side effects like nausea and vomiting,[228,229] as these are related to the rate of the rise of the serum lithium level.[230] The total daily doses were determined by body weight as follows: Less than 25 kg, 600 mg/day; 25–40 kg, 900 mg/day; 40–50 kg, 1200 mg/day; 50–60 kg, 1500 mg/day. Almost 90% of the subjects on this regimen were within therapeutic range (0.6–1.2 mEq/L) after 5 days of lithium treatment. Side effects were minimal.

h. Contraindications and Drug Interactions

Patients with preexisting cardiovascular disease taking diuretics or on a low-salt diet are at increased risk for lithium intoxication and require careful monitoring.[231] Although lithium is contraindicated in acute renal failure, chronic renal failure is not an absolute contraindication.[232] Also, severely ill and dehydrated patients should not be treated with lithium[233] until medically stable.

There are no studies of the interaction of lithium and other drugs in children. However, studies in adults indicate some likely interactions. For example, thiazide diuretics decease lithium clearance within several days of initiation of the diuretic,[234] and can raise lithium levels. Carbamazepine and neuroleptics may also increase the potential for lithium toxicity,[235,236] and theophylline increases lithium clearance (about 20%).[237] Other adverse drug interactions are possible since lithium may have an effect on all organs in the body.

i. Treatment of Lithium Toxicity and Overdosage

The symptoms of lithium toxicity are nausea, vomiting, diarrhea, restlessness, tremor, fasciculations, ataxia, confusion, dysarthria, renal dysfunction, electrolyte imbalance, apathy, convulsions, and coma. ECG changes like those in hypokalemia can occur.

Recommendations for Treatment of Lithium Toxicity and Overdosage*

1. Treat with gastric emesis or lavage after acute overdose, as mentioned previously. Lithium is not adsorbed to charcoal.
2. Monitor I & O, hydration, electrolytes (especially potassium levels), and lithium blood levels.
3. Plasma lithium levels greater than 2.5–3.0 mEq/L require hemodialysis. Forced diuresis does not work and can result in serious electrolyte imbalance. Hemodialysis is the treatment of choice for severe lithium intoxication, since lithium is rapidly removed by dialysis. Plasma levels may increase if redistribution and/or continued gastrointestinal absorption occurs. Repeat dialysis if needed.

C. Carbamazepine

1. Pharmacology

Carbamazepine (CBZ) is an anticonvulsant drug chemically related to the TCAs[184] (see Chapter 12). It is useful in generalized, simple, and complex partial seizures, as discussed in detail in Chapter 12. It exerts an anticonvulsant effect by blocking the posttetanic potentiation and reducing postsynaptic responses but, unlike other anticonvulsants, has a stimulating adrenergic action as well (Chapter 12). It has been found to be helpful in treating mania in adults,[238,239] and it is now being studied for similar use in mania and agitated states in children and adolescents.[240] Pharmacology is detailed in Chapter 12.

2. Clinical Effects

a. Behavioral Effects

Carbamazepine has some weak stimulantlike actions that help reduce some of the typical depressant effects of anticonvulsants. CBZ is used for treating epilepsy, trigeminal

*This information is for emergency use only. In general, overdosage is best managed by emergency medicine experts, not by psychiatrists.

neuralgia, pain syndromes, diabetes insipidus, and temporal lobe epilepsy (Chapter 12), in addition to its use in mania.[238] In 23 open and double-blind controlled studies in adults, 53% of subjects with acute mania showed a marked or moderate response to CBZ.[239] There is only one report of CBZ in child or adolescent mania.[240] As in adults, lithium-resistant patients may respond to CBZ, and it may augment lithium response at blood levels of 8–9 mg/L.

b. Pharmacokinetics, Dosage, and Blood Levels

CBZ has linear kinetics; i.e., an increase in the dose of CBZ linearly increases CBZ blood levels.[241] However, CBZ causes autoinduction of enzymes that metabolize it. This process continues for over a 4- to 6-week period and may lead to the decline of CBZ serum levels[242] (see Chapter 12). The half-life in adults is 25–65 hr; however, since CBZ induces its own metabolism, this may decease to 12–17 hr on repeated dosages. The usual dosage in children is 200–600 mg/day in divided doses. The therapeutic level of CBZ for seizure disorders is 5–10 mg/L, and studies in psychiatric disorders in adults and adolescents[241,242] have generally kept to this range. Blood levels need to be followed in children to avoid toxicity and because of potential increases in metabolism.

3. Clinical Indications

Currently, there are no proven indications for carbamazepine in child and adolescent psychiatry other than epilepsy (Chapter 12) and trigeminal neuralgia. However, clear-cut mania not responsive to lithium could receive a trial of carbamazepine alone or in combination with lithium, on the not unreasonable assumption that it is the same disorder at any age.

It has been claimed that CBZ is useful for treating emotional lability, aggressive dyscontrol states, and ADHD in children, particularly when associated with an abnormal EEG. An open study[243] and a metaanalysis of 10 studies[244] suggested a response to CBZ in doses ranging from 100 to 800 mg daily. Epilepsy and abnormal EEGs were present in a significant percentage of children. The improvement was sometimes comparable to that seen with methylphenidate; however, CBZ's usefulness in ADHD is still speculative until more controlled studies are available.

It is not clear if CBZ improves or adversely affects cognitive functioning. Some studies suggest that CBZ improves cognition, and others do not (see Chapter 12). Moderate doses of CBZ were shown in one study to have an adverse effect on memory and learning.[245] Although CBZ may be an alternative in ADHD treatment, the potential for adverse effects on learning requires careful monitoring.

4. Side Effects

Adverse effects of CBZ include leukopenia and maculopapular rash with edema. Agranulocytosis and aplastic anemia have occurred in adults. The leukopenia in children is time-limited and fortunately usually does not progress to aplastic anemia.[172] Vertigo, drowsiness, unsteadiness, nausea, vomiting, and dizziness may occur transiently at the start of therapy. Systemic lupus erythematosus, neutropenia, and proteinuria have also occurred.[246,247] Tics or myoclonic body movements may be triggered. Cases of hepatitis have been reported, and a fatal case of eosinophilic myocarditis has been reported.[248] Both CBZ and valproate may predispose women to polycystic ovaries and hyperandrogenism.[249] As with all anticonvulsants, carbamazepine may cause or exacerbate the symptoms of aggressivity, inattention, emotionality, and irritability in some children[246,250] (see Chapter 12).

Adverse effects should be treated by tapering CBZ slowly to prevent rebound seizures.

Benzodiazepines can be used prophylactically if CBZ needs to be abruptly discontinued because of toxicity.

5. Treatment of Overdosage of Carbamazepine

The recommendations for treatment of overdosage of carbamazepine are the same as those for TCAs (Section III.B.10), except seizures should be treated with benzodiazepines and phenobarbital. Phenytoin use is discouraged.

D. Valproate

1. Pharmacology

Valproate (see Chapter 12) is an anticonsulvant believed to work by increasing the brain levels of γ-aminobutyric acid (GABA). Like CBZ, it has been used in mania and agitated states in adults. It has been employed much more frequently in children and adolescents in the past few years for controlling agitation and aggressiveness; however, the evidence for its effectiveness is limited.

2. Clinical Effects

The main clinical effects are antiepileptic. Valproate also has a quieting, antiagitation, and sedating effect.[250-252] The daily dosage of valproate for adults is 15–60 mg/kg. The half-life in adults is 6–16 hr, and the therapeutic blood levels for seizure disorders are in the range of 50–100 mg/L. Since there are no established ranges for dosage, half-life, or blood levels for the psychiatric use of valproate in children and adolescents, it is recommended that the guidelines for its use in epilepsy be followed (Chapter 12).

3. Clinical Indications

There are three open studies of the use of valproate in adolescent mania.[253-255] Valproate, 750–1250 mg daily (mean 1000 mg), was used for 7 weeks in an open trial with 6 adolescents with bipolar disorder aged 17 to 22 years.[253] Blood levels were 350–750 μmol/ L. Five of six showed a marked improvement. Valproate, 500 to 2000 mg daily (mean 1000 mg), was also used in 11 adolescents aged 12 to 17 years who were refractory to lithium and/ or neuroleptics.[254] Blood levels were 34–94 μg/mL. Nine of the eleven showed "a moderate or better" response. The range of treatment was 6–26 days (mean 17). Because giving oral loading doses to rapidly achieve therapeutic blood levels of valproate has been successful with adults,[256] five adolescents with bipolar disorder were similarly treated with an oral loading dose of 20 mg/kg (initial dosage, 750–1500 mg).[255] Blood levels were 46–84 mg/L (mean 64). It was well tolerated, and three of five patients responded. All studies suffered from the limitations of an open design, and two of three allowed significant doses of concomitant neuroleptics.[253,254]

There are no controlled studies of valproic acid in the treatment of childhood and adolescent disorders. Owing to limited experience with these medications in adults, their psychiatric use in children and adolescents should be considered experimental at present. Potential indicators include mania not responsive to lithium or carbamazepine, and possibly disorders where there is a clearly abnormal EEG.

4. Side Effects

Valproate can be sedating and can cause gastrointestinal side effects such as nausea, vomiting, and indigestion. Fatal hepatotoxicity has occurred,[257,258] usually during the first 6 months of treatment and particularly in young children. It is usually preceded by malaise, weakness, lethargy, facial edema, anorexia, vomiting, and escape from seizure control. It seems to occur less with monotherapy.[250] Neutropenia can occur in 20% of adults, and a fulminating pancytopenia and aplastic anemia have occurred.[250] Blood cell counts and platelet, coagulation, and liver function tests should be done at baseline and throughout drug treatment.[250] Valproate causes elevation of the plasma levels of other anticonvulsant drugs, raising the concentration of phenobarbital by as much as 40%. Contraindications would be known significant hepatic disease or dysfunction or hypersensivity to the drug. Valproate treatment requires monitoring CBC and liver enzymes at least q 3 months; however, hepatotoxicity usually has a rapid onset, and monitoring may not identify it.

A recent study found an 80% incidence of polycystic ovaries in females under the age of 20 who were treated with valproate for epilepsy.[249] Interestingly, another study observed one such adverse event which was thought to be unrelated to valproate treatment.[253] Data are presented in Table 15. Until this is explained, valproate should be limited to investigative use only.

5. Treatment of Overdosage of Valproate

Valproate overdosage signs and symptoms include nystagmus, headache, ataxia, tremor, and hallucinations or changes in vision. Cardiac effects may progress to heart block and can result in a deep coma.

Recommendations for Treatment of Overdosage of Valproate

1. Valproate is rapidly absorbed—use gastric lavage or emesis depending on mental status and time since ingestion.
2. General supportive measures as previously mentioned.
3. Maintain adequate urinary output.
4. Naloxone may reverse coma; however, it may also reverse anticonsulvant effect, so use cautiously if patient has a seizure disorder.

E. Clonazepam

1. Pharmacology

Clonazepam (see Chapters 12 and 15) is a benzodiazepine and has anticonvulsant activity based on its ability to enhance and augment the effect of GABA. Clonazepam has also been used in manic and agitated adults.[172,259]

2. Clinical Effects

All benzodiazepines have three clinical effects that are present to a lesser or greater degree: antianxiety effects, anticonvulsant effects, and muscle-relaxing effects (see also Chapters 11, 12, and 15). The usual dosages of clonazepam have been in the range of 2–5 mg/day, though dosages as high as 10–15 mg/day have been used in adults.[252] The half-life

TABLE 15. Incidence of Polycystic Ovaries and Menstrual
Disturbances in Women Treated with Valproate and Carbamazepine[a]

	Valproate ($N = 29$)	Carbamazepine ($N = 120$)	Controls ($N = 51$)
Polycystic ovaries	68%	45%	18%
Polycystic ovaries in women less than 20 years old	80%	27%	—
Menstrual disturbances	45%	19%	16%

[a]Ref. 249.

in adults is 20–80 hr. The half-life has not been determined in children and adolescents, and therapeutic blood levels have not been established.

3. Clinical Indications

There are no studies of the use of clonazepam in children and adolescents for mania or agitated states, although it has been used in panic attacks and anxiety disorders (see Chapter 15).[260,261] It may also prove to be helpful in acute mania that does not respond to more usual treatments (antipsychotics and lithium). In adults, it has been shown to reduce the amount of antipsychotic needed.[172] Sedative side effects are notable, however, and may preclude its use by most clinicians.

4. Side Effects

Like all benzodiazepines and CNS depressants, the side effects of clonazepam are mainly those of CNS depression. Sedation, drowsiness, and lethargy may interfere with learning. Clonazepam potentiates other CNS depressants such as alcohol, hypnotics, narcotics, and barbiturates. It may produce dependence and possible withdrawal symptoms if abruptly discontinued (Chapter 11). Because the half-life is so long, the withdrawal syndrome may not become apparent for days or weeks after discontinuing the medication.[250]

Clonazepam is basically safe in overdosage. Treat with gastric lavage, emesis, and supportive care.

F. Summary of Antimanics in Child and Adolescent Disorders

Lithium may be helpful in bipolar illness and managing severe aggressiveness in children. Children most likely to respond are those with a history of mania, a family history of bipolar disorder, or a history of a first-degree relative having a disorder that responded to lithium. If children with clear-cut bipolar disorder require lithium maintenance after their second manic episode, it should be continued for at least 2 years to prevent early recurrence of mania when lithium is withdrawn. Lithium may also be helpful in an occasional child with mood lability and antidepressant-resistant unipolar depression, although data are scant. The use of carbamazepine shows some promise in adolescent bipolar disorder and possibly in ADHD in the presence of abnormal EEGs. The use of valproate and clonazepam in children at the current time is experimental and is discouraged except in intractable cases.

Making the diagnosis of a mood disorder in children and adolescents is a complicated process that may require several evaluations before the final diagnosis is made. The physician should obtain information from several sources, including parents, teachers, siblings, and friends, as well as the child, who should be the primary source of information. If the mood disorder appears durable or severe, the child should preferably be referred to a child and adolescent psychiatrist who is trained and experienced in the diagnosis and treatment of mood disorders. There is reason to suggest that the depressions seen in children and adolescents may not be exactly the same as depressions see in adults even though they can be diagnosed using the same criteria. Comorbidity with adjustment, anxiety, or conduct disorder and drug abuse is high, and the depression may be secondary to one of these diagnoses. Depression may be transitory and, except in cases of clear-cut bipolar depression, should be managed conservatively. There is somewhat more justification for pharmacologic treatment of mood states in children and adolescents from current studies. The severity of bipolar disorder justifies extrapolation from adults to adolescents and children and invocation of appropriate treatment.

Multicenter, double-blind, placebo-controlled treatment studies with large numbers of children and adolescents are still needed to determine the efficacy of antidepressants and antimanics in children and adolescents with mood disorders. As ever in the history of medicine, therapeutic zeal continues to get considerably ahead of currently available treatment studies.

ACKNOWLEDGMENTS. The author wishes to thank Elizabeth Weller, M.D., Ronald Weller, M.D., and Shanour Yaylayan, M.D., for their contributions to the first edition of this chapter, many of which are still a basis for this edition.

REFERENCES

1. Quinn PO, Rapoport JL: One-year follow-up of hyperactive boys treated with imipramine or methylphenidate. *Am J Psychiatry* 132:241–245, 1975.
2. Rapoport JL, Quinn PO, Bradbard G, et al: Imipramine and methylphenidate treatments of hyperactive boys: A double-blind comparison. *Arch Gen Psychiatry* 30:789–793, 1974.
3. Werry JS, Aman MG, Diamond E: Imipramine and methylphenidate in hyperactive children. *J Child Psychol Psychiatry* 21:27–35, 1980.
4. Pliszka SR: Antidepressants in the treatment of child and adolescent psychopathology. *J Clin Child Psychol* 20:313–320, 1991.
5. Pliszka SR: Review article—Tricyclic antidepressants in the treatment of children with attention deficit disorder. *J Am Acad Child Adolesc Psychiatry* 26:127–132, 1987.
6. Werry JS, Dowrick PW, Lampen EL, et al: Imipramine in enuresis—Psychological and physiological effects. *J Child Psychol Psychiatry* 16:289–299, 1975.
7. Blackwell B, Currah J: The psychopharmacology of nocturnal enuresis, in Kolvin I, McKeith RC, Meadows SR (eds): *Bladder Control and Enuresis.* London, Heinemann, 1973, pp 231–257.
8. American Psychiatric Association: *Diagnostic and Statistical Manual of Mental Disorders*, Fourth Edition. Washington, DC, American Psychiatric Association, 1994.
9. Kashani JH, Sherman DD: Childhood depression: Epidemiology, etiological models, and treatment implications. *Integrative Psychiatry* 6:1–21, 1988.
10. Ryan ND: Heterocyclic antidepressants in children and adolescents. *J Child Adolesc Psychopharmacol* 1:21–31, 1990.
11. Spencer T, Wilens T, Biederman J: Psychotropic medication for children and adolescents. *Child Adolesc Clin North Am* 4(1):97–121, 1995.
12. De Boer T: The pharmacologic profile of mirtazapine. *J Clin Psychiatry* 57(suppl 4):19–25, 1996.

13. American Hospital Formulary Service Drug Information. Bethesda, American Society of Hospital Pharmacists, 1991.
14. Baldessarini RJ: Current status of antidepressants: Clinical pharmacology and therapy. *J Clin Psychiatry* 50(4):117–126, 1989.
15. *Physicians' Desk Reference.* Oradell, NJ, Medical Economics Data, 1997.
16. Baldessarini RJ, Cole JO: Chemotherapy, in Nicholi AM (ed): *The New Harvard Guide to Psychiatry.* Cambridge, Mass, Harvard University Press, 1988, pp 481–533.
17. Richelson E: Pharmacology of antidepressants—characteristics of the ideal drugs. *Mayo Clin Proc* 69:1069–1081, 1994.
18. Morselli PL: *Drug Disposition during Development.* Jamaica, NY, Spectrum Publications, 1977.
19. Jatlow PI: Psychotropic drug disposition during development, in Popper C (ed): *Psychiatric Pharmacoscience of Children and Adolescents.* Washington, DC, American Psychiatric Press, 1989, pp 29–44.
20. Briant RH: An introduction to clinical pharmacology, in Werry JC (ed): *Pediatric Psychopharmacology: The Use of Behavior Modifying Drugs in Children.* New York, Brunner/Mazel, 1978, pp 3–82.
21. DeVane CL, Jarecke CR: Cyclic antidepressants, in Evans WE, Schoentag JJ, Jusko WJ (eds): *Applied Pharmacokinetics. Principles of Therapeutic Drug Monitoring.* San Francisco, Applied Therapeutics, 1992, vol 33, pp 1–34.
22. Geller B, Cooper TB, Schluchter MD, et al: Child and adolescent nortriptyline single dose pharmacokinetic parameters: Final report. *J Clin Psychopharmacol* 7:321–323, 1987.
23. Moriselli PL, Bianchetti G, Dugas M: Therapeutic drug monitoring of psychotropic drugs in children. *Pediatr Pharmacol* 3:149–156, 1983.
24. deGatta MF, Garcia MJ, Acosta A, et al: Monitoring of serum levels of imipramine and desipramine and individuation of dose in enuretic children. *Ther Drug Monit* 6:438–443, 1984.
25. Preskorn SH, Bupp SJ, Weller EB, et al: Plasma levels of imipramine and metabolites in 68 hospitalized children. *J Am Acad Child Adolesc Psychiatry* 28:373–375, 1989.
26. Geller G, Cooper TB, Chestnut EC, et al: Preliminary data on the relationship between nortriptyline plasma level and response in depressed children. *Am J Psychiatry* 143:123–126, 1986.
27. Biederman J, Baldessarini RJ, Wright V, et al: A double-blind placebo controlled study of desipramine in the treatment of ADD: I. Efficacy. *J Am Acad Child Adolesc Psychiatry* 28:777–784, 1989.
28. Wilens TE, Biederman J, Geist DE, Steingard R, Spencer T: Nortriptyline in the treatment of ADHD: A chart review of 58 cases. *J Am Acad Child Adolesc Psychiatry* 32:343–349, 1993.
29. Biederman J, Baldessarini RJ, Wright V, Keenan K, Faraone S: A double-blind placebo controlled study of desipramine in the treatment of ADD: III. Lack of impact of comorbidity and family history factors on clinical response. *J Am Acad Child Adolesc Psychiatry* 32:199–204, 1993.
30. Gelenberg AJ, Schoonover SC: Depression, in Gelenberg AJ, Bassuk EL, Schoonover SC (eds): *The Practitioner's Guide to Psychoactive Drugs,* ed 3. New York, Plenum Press, 1991, pp 23–89.
31. Biederman J, Faraone SV, Baldessarini RJ, Flood J, Meyer M, Wilens T, Spencer T, Chen L, Weber W: Predicting desipramine levels in children and adolescents: A naturalistic clinical study. *J Am Acad Child Adolesc Psychiatry* 36:384–389, 1997.
32. Oesterheld JR: Erythromycin and clomipramine: Noncompetitive inhibition of demethylation. *J Child Adolesc Psychopharmacol* 6:211–213, 1996.
33. Bernstein JG: *Handbook of Drug Therapy in Psychiatry,* ed 2. Boston, PSG Publishing Co, 1988.
34. Hollister LE: Antidepressant drugs, in Dukes MNG (ed): *Meyler's Side Effects of Drugs, VIII.* New York, American Elsevier Publishing, 1975, pp 31–46.
35. Klein DF, Gittleman R, Quitkin F, et al: *Diagnosis and Drug Treatment of Psychiatric Disorders: Adults and Children.* Baltimore, Williams & Wilkins, 1980.
36. Klein RG, Koplewicz HS, Kanner A: Imipramine treatment of children with separation anxiety disorder. *J Am Acad Child Adolesc Psychiatry* 31:21–28, 1992.
37. Gualtieri CT: Imipramine and children: A review and some speculations about the mechanism of drug action. *Dis Nerv Syst* 38:368–375, 1977.
38. Casat CD, Pleasants DZ, Schroeder DH, et al: Bupropion in children with attention deficit disorder. *Psychopharmacol Bull* 25:198–201, 1989.
39. Barrickman LL, Perry PJ, Allen AJ, Kuperman S, Arndt SV, Herrmann KJ, Schumacher E: Bupropion vs methylphenidate in the treatment of attention-deficit hyperactivity disorder. *J Am Acad Child Adolesc Psychiatry* 34:649–657, 1995.
40. Conners CK, Casat CD, Gualtieri CT, Weller E, Reader M, Reiss A, Weller RA, Khayrallah M, Ascher J: Bupropion hydrochloride in attention deficit disorder with hyperactivity. *J Am Acad Child Adolesc Psychiatry* 35:1314–1321, 1996.
41. Aman MG: Psychotropic drugs and learning problems—a selective review. *J Learn Disabil* 13:87–97, 1980.

42. Preskorn SH, Weller EB, Weller RA, et al: Plasma levels of imipramine and adverse effects in children. *Am J Psychiatry* 140:1332–1335, 1983.

43. Kuekes ED, Wigg C, Bryant S, Meyer WJ: Hypertension is a risk in adolescents treated with imipramine. *J Child Adolesc Psychopharmacol* 2:241–248, 1992.

44. Task Force on Blood Pressure Control in Children: Report of the second task force on blood pressure control in children. *Pediatrics* 79:1–25, 1987.

45. Riddle MA, Nelson JG, Kleinman CS, et al: Sudden death in children receiving Norpramin: A review of three reported cases and commentary. *J Am Acad Child Adolesc Psychiatry* 30:104–108, 1991.

46. Biederman J: Sudden death in children treated with a tricyclic antidepressant. *J Am Acad Child Adolesc Psychiatry* 30:495–498, 1991.

47. Riddle MA, Geller B, Ryan N: Another sudden death in a child treated with desipramine. *J Am Acad Child Adolesc Psychiatry* 32:792–797, 1993.

48. Popper CW, Zimnitzky B: Sudden death putatively related to desipramine treatment in youth: A fifth case and a review of speculative mechanisms. *J Child Adolesc Psychopharmacol* 5:283–300, 1995.

49. Varley CK, McClellan J: Case study: Two additional sudden deaths with tricyclic antidepressants. *J Am Acad Child Adolesc Psychiatry* 36:390–394, 1997.

50. Saraf KR, Klein DF, Gittelman-Klein R, Groft S: Imipramine side effects in children. *Psychopharmacologia* 37(3):265–274, 1974.

51. Wagner KD, Fershtman M: Potential mechanism of desipramine-related sudden death in children. *Psychosomatics* 34:80–83, 1991.

52. Leonard HL, Meyer MC, Swedo SE, Richter D, Hamburger SD, Allen AJ, Rapoport JL, Tucker E: Electrocardiographic changes during desipramine and clomipramine treatment in children and adolescents. *J Am Acad Child Adolesc Psychiatry* 34:1460–1468, 1995.

53. Fletcher SE, Case CL, Sallee FR, Hand LD, Gillette PC: Prospective study of the electrocardiographic effects of imipramine in children. *J Pediatr* 122:654–654, 1993.

54. Jackson WK, Roose SP, Glassman AH: Cardiovascular toxicity of antidepressant medications. *Psychopathology* 20:64–71, 1987.

55. Elliott GR, Popper GW: Tricyclic antidepressants: The QT interval and other cardiovascular parameters. *J Child Adolesc Psychopharmacol* 1:187–189, 1990/1991.

56. Alderton HR: Tricyclic medication in children and the QT interval: Case report and discussion. *Can J Psychiatry* 40:325–329, 1995.

57. Blackwell B: Adverse effects of antidepressant drugs. Part I: Monoamine oxidase inhibitors and tricyclics. *Drugs* 21:201–219, 1981.

58. Sovner R, DiMascio A: Extrapyramidal syndromes and other neurological side effects of psychotropic drugs, in Lipton MA, DiMascio A, Killam DF (eds): *Psychopharmacology: A Generative of Progress.* New York, Raven Press, 1978, pp 1021–1032.

59. Petti TA, Law W: Abrupt cessation of high-dose imipramine treatment in children. *JAMA* 246:768–769, 1981.

60. Viesselman JO, Weller EB, Weller RA, Yaylayan S: Current psychopharmacologic treatment research of depressed children and adolescents, in Sholevar GP (ed): *The Transmission of Depression in Families and Children: Assessment and Intervention.* Northvale, NJ, Jason Aronson Inc., 1994.

61. Preskorn SH, Weller EB, Hughes CW, et al: Depression in prepubertal children: Dexamethasone non-suppression predicts differential response to imipramine vs placebo. *Psychopharmacol Bull* 23:128–133, 1987.

62. Puig-Antich J, Perel JM, Lupatkin W, et al: Imipramine in prepubertal major depressive disorder. *Arch Gen Psychiatry* 44:81–89, 1987.

63. Geller B, Cooper TB, Graham DL, et al: Pharmacokinetically-designed double-blind, placebo-controlled study of nortriptyline in 6–12 year olds with major depressive disorder. *J Am Acad Child Adolesc Psychiatry* 31:34–44, 1992.

64. Puig-Antich J, Perel JM, Lupatkin W, et al: Plasma levels of imipramine (IMI) and desmethylimipramine (DMI), and clinical response in prepubertal major depressive disorder. A preliminary report. *J Am Acad Child Psychiatry* 18:616–627, 1979.

65. Petti TH, Conners CK: Changes in behavioral ratings of depressed children treated with imipramine. *J Am Acad Child Adolesc Psychiatry* 22:355–360, 1983.

66. Kashani JH, Shekim WO, Reid JC: Amitriptyline in children with major depressive disorder: A double-blind crossover pilot study. *J Am Acad Child Psychiatry* 23:348–351, 1984.

67. Hazell P, O'Connell D, Heathcote D, Robertson J, Henry D: Efficacy of tricyclic drugs in treating child and adolescent depressions: A meta-analysis. *Br Med J* 310:897–901, 1995.

68. Kramer A, Feiguine R: Clinical effects of amitriptyline in adolescent depression. *J Am Acad Child Psychiatry* 33:686–644, 1981.

69. Geller B, Cooper TB, Graham DL, et al: Double-blind placebo-controlled study of nortriptyline in depressed adolescents using a "fixed plasma level" design. *Psychopharmacol Bull* 26:85–90, 1990.

70. Ryan ND, Puig-Antich J, Cooper T, et al: Imipramine in adolescent major depression: Plasma level and clinical response. *Acta Psychiatr Scand* 73:275–288, 1986.

71. Kye CH, Waterman CS, Ryan ND, Birmaher B, Williamson DE, Iyencar S, Dachille S: A randomized controlled trial of amitriptyline in the acute treatment of adolescent major depression. *J Am Acad Child Adolesc Psychiatry* 35:1139–1144, 1996.

72. Boulos C, Kutcher S, Marton P, Simeon J, Ferguson B, Roberts N: Response to desipramine treatment in adolescent major depression. *Psychopharmacol Bull* 27:59–65, 1991.

73. Robbins DR, Alessi NE, Colfer MV: Treatment of adolescents with major depression: Implications of the DST and the melancholic clinical subtype. *J Affect Disord* 17:99–104, 1989.

74. Strober M, Freeman R, Rigali J: The pharmacotherapy of depressive illness in adolescence, I: An open label trial of imipramine. *Psychopharmacol Bull* 26:80–84, 1990.

75. Ambrosini PJ, Bianchi MD, Metz C, Rabinovich H: Evaluating clinical response of open nortriptyline pharmacotherapy in adolescent major depression. *J Child Adolesc Psychopharmacol* 4:233–244, 1994.

76. Green WH: The treatment of Attention Deficit Hyperactivity Disorder with nonstimulant medications. *Child Adolesc Clin North Am* 4(1):169–195, 1995.

77. Psychotropics & seizure. *Just the Fax* 2(3):5, 1995.

78. Kaplan SL, Breit M, Gauthier B, et al. A comparison of three nocturnal enuresis treatment methods. *J Am Acad Child Adolesc Psychiatry* 28:282–286, 1989.

79. Berney T, Kolvin I, Bhate SR, et al: School phobia: A therapeutic trial with clomipramine and short-term outcome. *Br J Psychiatry* 138:110–118, 1981.

80. Bernstein GA, Garfinkel BD, Borchardt DM: Comparative studies of pharmacotherapy for school refusal. *J Am Acad Child Adolesc Psychiatry* 29:773–781, 1990.

81. Klein RG, Koplewicz HS, Kanner A: Imipramine treatment of children with separation anxiety disorder. *J Am Acad Child Adolesc Psychiatry* 31:21–28, 1992.

82. Flament MF, Rapoport JL, Berg CJ, et al: Clomipramine treatment of childhood obsessive–compulsive disorder. *Arch Gen Psychiatry* 42:977–983, 1985.

83. Leonard HL, Swedo SE, Rapoport JL, et al: Treatment of obsessive–compulsive disorder in children and adolescents: A double-blind crossover comparison. *Arch Gen Psychiatry* 46:1088–1092, 1989.

84. DeVeaugh-Geiss J, Moroz G, Biederman J, Cantwell, D, Fontaine R, Greist JH, Reichler R, Katz R, Landau P: Clomipramine in child and adolescent obsessive–compulsive disorder—A multicenter trial. *J Am Acad Child Adolesc Psychiatry* 31:45–49, 1992.

85. Hanna GL, Yuwiler A, Cantwell DP: Whole-blood serotonin during clomipramine treatment of juvenile obsessive–compulsive disorder. *J Child Adolesc Psychopharmacol* 3:223–229, 1993.

86. Swedo SE, Leonard HL, Rapoport JL, et al: A double-blind comparison of clomipramine and desipramine in the treatment of trichotillomania (hair pulling). *N Engl J Med* 321:497–501, 1989.

87. Riley WT, Sood A, Al-Mateen CS: Mixed effects of clomipramine in treating childhood trichotillomania. *J Child Adolesc Psychopharmacol* 3:169–171, 1993.

88. Weller EB, Weller RA, Carr S: Case study—imipramine treatment of trichotillomania and coexisting depression in a seven-year-old. *J Am Acad Child Adolesc Psychiatry* 28:952–953, 1989.

89. Sheikha SH, Wagner KD, Wagner RF: Fluoxetine treatment of trichotillomania and depression in a prepubertal child. *Cutis* 51(1):50–52, 1993.

90. Zubieta JK, Alessi NE: Acute and chronic administration of trazodone in the treatment of disruptive behavior disorders in children. *J Clin Psychopharmacol* 12:346–351, 1992.

91. Ghaziuddin N, Alessi NE: An open clinical trial of trazodone in aggressive children. *J Child Adolesc Psychopharmacol* 2:291–297, 1992.

92. Garber HJ, McGonigle JJ, Slomka GT, Monteverde E: Clomipramine treatment of stereotypic behaviors and self-injury in patients with developmental disabilities. *J Am Acad Child Adolesc Psychiatry* 31:1157–1160, 1992.

93. Gordon CT, State RC, Nelson JE, Hamburger SD, Rapoport JL: A double-blind comparison of clomipramine, desipramine, and placebo in the treatment of autistic disorder. *Arch Gen Psychiatry* 50:441–447, 1993.

94. Lewis MH, Bodfish JW, Powell SB, Parker DE, Golden RN: Clomipramine treatment for self-injurious behavior of individuals with mental retardation: A double-blind comparison with placebo. *Am J Ment Retard* 100:654–665, 1996.

95. McDougle CJ, Price LH, Volkmar FR, et al: Clomipramine in autism: Preliminary evidence of efficacy. *J Am Acad Child Adolesc Psychiatry* 31:746–750, 1992.

96. Ponto LB, Perry PJ, Liskow BI, et al: Tricyclic antidepressant and monoamine oxidase inhibitor combination therapy. *Am J Hosp Pharm* 34:954–961, 1977.

97. Briant RH, Reid JL, Dollery CT: Interaction between clonidine and desipramine in man. *Br Med J* 1:522–523, 1973.

98. Mitchel L Jr, Arias L, Oates JA: Antagonism of hypertensive action of guanethidine sulfate by desipramine hydrochloride. *JAMA* 202:973–976, 1967.

99. Perucca E, Richens A: Interactions between phenytoin and imipramine. *Br J Clin Pharmacol* 4:485–486, 1977.

100. Ballinger BR, Presly A, Reid AH: The effects of hypnotics on imipramine treatment. *Psychopharmacologia* 39:267–274, 1974.

101. Wharton RN, Perel JM, Dayton PG, et al: A potential clinical use of methylphenidate with tricyclic antidepressants. *Am J Psychiatry* 127:1619–1625, 1971.

102. Langou RA, Van Dyke C, Tahan SR, et al: Cardiovascular manifestations of tricyclic antidepressant overdose. *Am Heart J* 100:458–464, 1980.

103. Dumovic P, Burrows G, Vohra J, et al: The effect of tricyclic antidepressant drugs on the heart. *Arch Toxicol* 35:255–262, 1976.

104. Frommer DA, Kulig KW, Marx JA, Rumack B: Tricyclic antidepressant overdose: A review. *JAMA* 257:521–526, 1987.

105. Barone MA (ed): *The Harriet Lane Handbook. A Manual for Pediatric House Officers*, ed 14. St Louis, Mosby, 1996.

106. Rumack BH: Poisondex, Rocky Mountain Poison Center, Denver, 1982.

107. Pumariega AJ, Muller B, Rivers-Bulkeley N: Acute renal failure secondary to amoxapine overdose. *JAMA* 248:3141–3142, 1982.

108. Puig-Antich J, Ryan ND, Rabinovich H: Affective disorders in childhood and adolescence, in Weiner J (ed): *Diagnosis and Psychopharmacology of Childhood and Adolescent Disorders*. New York, John Wiley & Sons, 1985.

109. Rudorfer MV: Monoamine oxidase inhibitors: Reversible and irreversible. *Psychopharmacol Bull* 28:45–57, 1992.

110. Baldessarini RJ: Drugs and the treatment of psychiatric disorders, in Gilman AG, Rall TW, Nies AS, et al (eds): *Goodman and Gilman's The Pharmacological Basis of Therapeutics*, ed 8. New York, Pergamon Press, 1990, pp 418–422.

111. Green WH. *Child and Adolescent Clinical Psychopharmacology*. Baltimore, Williams & Wilkins, 1991, pp 134–137.

112. Akiskal HS: Mood disturbances, in Winokur G, Clayton P (eds): *The Medical Basis of Psychiatry*. Philadelphia, WB Saunders Co, 1986.

113. Fitton A, Faulds D, Goa KL: Moclobemide. A review of its pharmacological properties and therapeutic use in depressive illness. *Drugs* 43:561–596, 1992.

114. Ryan N, Puig-Antich J, Rabinovich H, et al: MAOIs in adolescent major depression unresponsive to tricyclic antidepressants. *J Am Acad Child Adolesc Psychiatry* 27:755–758, 1988.

115. Zametkin AJ, Rapoport JL: Noradrenergic hypothesis of attention deficit disorder with hyperactivity: A critical review, in Meltzer HY (ed): *Psychopharmacology: The Third Generation of Progress*. New York, Raven Press, 1987.

116. Zametkin A, Rapoport JL, Murphy DL, et al: Treatment of hyperactive children with monoamine oxidase inhibitors: I. Clinical efficacy. *Arch Gen Psychiatry* 42:962–966, 1985.

117. Trott GE, Friese HJ, Menzel M, Nissen G: Use of moclobemide in children with attention deficit hyperactivity disorder. *Psychopharmacology* (Supplement) 106:134–136, 1992.

118. Sternbach H: The serotonin syndrome. *Am J Psychiatry* 148:705–713, 1991.

119. Turner P, Young JH, Paterson J: Influence of urinary pH on the excretion of tranylcypromine sulfate. *Nature* 215:881–882, 1967.

120. Matter BJ, Donat PE, Bril ML, et al: Tranylcypromine sulfate poisoning: Successful treatment with hemodialysis. *Arch Intern Med* 116:18–20, 1965.

121. Versaci AA, Nakamoto S, Koloff WJ: Phenelzine intoxication: Report of a case treated by hemodialysis. *Ohio State Med J* 60:770–771, 1964.

122. Sussman N: The potential benefits of serotonin receptor-specific agents. *J Clin Psychiatry* 55 [2(suppl)]:45–51, 1994.

123. Brown TM, Skop BP, Mareth TR: Pathophysiology and management of the serotonin syndrome. *Ann Pharmacother* 30:527–533, 1996.

124. Grimsley SR, Jann MW: Paroxetine, sertraline, and fluvoxamine: New selective serotonin reuptake inhibitors. *Clin Pharm* 11:930–957, 1992.

125. Loenard HL, March J, Rickler KC, Allen AJ: Pharmacology of the selective serotonin reuptake inhibitors in children and adolescents. *J Am Acad Child Adolesc Psychiatry* 36:725–736, 1997.

126. Clein PD, Riddle MA: Pharmacokinetics in children and adolescents. *Child Adolesc Clin North Am* 4(1): 59–75, 1995.

127. Riesenman C: Antidepressant drug interactions and the cytochrome P450 system: A critical appraisal. *Pharmacotherapy* 15(6 Pt 2):845–995, 1995.

128. Nemeroff CB, DeVane L, Pollock BG: Newer antidepressants and the cytochrome P450 system. *Am J Psychiatry* 153:311– 320, 1996.

129. Jain U, Birmaher B, Garcia M, Al-Shabbout M, Ryan N: Fluoxetine in children and adolescents with mood disorders: A chart review of efficacy and adverse effects. *J Child Adolesc Psychopharmacol* 2:259–265, 1992.

130. Boulos C, Kutcher S, Gardner D, Young E: An open naturalistic trial of fluoxetine in adolescents and young adults with treatment-resistant major depression. *J Child Adolesc Psychopharmacol* 2:103–111, 1992.

131. Ghaziuddin N, Naylor MW, King CA: Fluoxetine in tricyclic refractory depression in adolescents. *Depression* 2:287–291, 1995.

132. Tierney E, Paramjit JT, Leinas JF, Rosenberg LA, Riddle MA: Sertraline for major depression in children and adolescents: Preliminary Clinical experience. *J Child Adolesc Psychopharmacol* 5:13–27, 1995.

133. Colle LM, Belair J, DiFeo M, Weiss J, LaRoche C: Extended open-label fluoxetine treatment of adolescents with major depression. *J Child Adolesc Psychopharmacol* 4:225–232, 1994.

134. Sallee FR, Nesbitt L, Dougherty D, Hilal R, Nandagopal VS, Sethuraman G: Lymphocyte glucocorticoid receptor: Predictor of sertraline response in adolescent major depressive disorder (MDD). *Psychopharmacol Bull* 31:339–345, 1995.

135. McConville BJ, Minnery KL, Sorter MT, West SA, Friedman LM, Christian K: An open study of the effects of sertraline on adolescent major depression. *J Child Adolesc Psychopharmacol* 6:41–51, 1996.

136. Simeon J, Dinicola V, Ferguson HB, Copping W: Adolescent depression: A placebo-controlled fluoxetine treatment study and follow-up. *Prog Neuro-psychopharmacol Biol Psychiatry* 14:791–795, 1990.

137. Emslie GJ, Rush AJ, Weinberg WA, Kowatch RA, Hughes CW, Carmody T, Rintelmann J: A double-blind, randomized, placebo-controlled trial of fluoxetine in children and adolescents with depression. *Arch Gen Psychiatry*, 54:1031–1037, 1997.

138. Kye C, Ryan N: Pharmacologic treatment of child and adolescent depression. *Child Adolesc Clin North Am* 4(1):261–281, 1995.

139. Barrickman L, Noyes R, Kuperman S, Schumacher E, Verda M: Treatment of ADHD with fluoxetine: A preliminary trial. *J Am Acad Child Adolesc Psychiatry* 30:762–767, 1991.

140. Bradley SJ, Kulik L: Fluoxetine and memory impairment. *J Am Acad Child Adolesc Psychiatry* 32:1078–1079, 1993.

141. Bangs ME, Petti TA, Janus MD: Fluoxetine-induced memory impairment in an adolescent. *J Am Acad Child Adolesc Psychiatry* 33:1303–1308, 1994.

142. Hedges D, Reimherr FW, Rogers A, Strong R, Wender PH: An open trial of venlafaxine in adult patients with attention deficit hyperactivity disorder. *Psychopharmacol Bull* 31:779–783, 1995.

143. Olvera RL, Pliszka SR, Luh J, Tatum R: An open trial of venlafaxine in the treatment of attention-deficit/ hyperactivity disorder in children and adolescents. *J Child Adolesc Psychopharmacol* 6:241–250, 1996.

144. Manassis K, Bradley S: Fluoxetine in anxiety disorders [letter]. *J Am Acad Child Adolesc Psychiatry* 33:761–762, 1994.

145. Birmaher B, Waterman GS, Ryan N, Cully M, Balach L, Ingram J, Brodsky M: Fluoxetine for childhood anxiety disorders. *J Am Acad Child Adolesc Psychiatry* 33:993–999, 1994.

146. Dummitt ES, Tancer NK, Klein RG: An open trial of fluoxetine for children with elective mutism. *Psychopharmacol Bull* 30:667, 1994.

147. Geller DA, Biederman J, Reed ED, Spencer T, Wilens TE: Similarities in response to fluoxetine in the treatment of children and adolescents with obsessive–compulsive disorder. *J Am Acad Child Adolesc Psychiatry* 34:36–44, 1995.

148. Riddle MA, Hardin MT, King R, Scahill L, Woolston JL: Fluoxetine treatment of children and adolescents with Tourette's and obsessive compulsive disorders: Preliminary clinical experience. *J Am Acad Child Adolesc Psychiatry* 29:45–48, 1990.

149. Apter A, Ratzioni G, King R: Fluvoxamine open-label treatment of adolescent inpatients with obsessive–compulsive disorder or depression. *J Am Acad Child Adolesc Psychiatry* 33:342–348, 1994.

150. Fairbanks JM, Pine DS, Tancer NK, Dummitt ES, Kentgen LM, Martin J, Asche BK, Klein RG: Open fluoxetine treatment of mixed anxiety disorders in children and adolescents. *J Child Adolesc Psychopharmacol* 7:17–29, 1997.

151. Dummit ES, Klein RG, Tancer NK, Asche B, Martin J: Fluoxetine treatment of children with selective mutism: An open trial. *J Am Acad Child Adolesc Psychiatry* 35:615–621, 1996.

152. Kurlan R, Como PG, Deeley C, McDermott M, McDermott MP: A pilot controlled study of fluoxetine for obsessive–compulsive symptoms in children with Tourette's syndrome. *Clin Neuropharmacol* 16:167–172, 1993.

153. Riddle MA, Scahill L, King RA, Hardin MT, Anderson GM, Ort SI, Smith JC, Leckman JF, Cohen DJ: Double-blind, crossover trial of fluoxetine and placebo in children and adolescents with obsessive–compulsive disorder. *J Am Acad Child Adolesc Psychiatry* 31:1062–1069, 1992.

154. Black B, Uhde TW: Treatment of elective mutism with fluoxetine: A double-blind, placebo-controlled study. *J Am Acad Child Adolesc Psychiatry* 33:1000–1006, 1994.

155. Cook EH, Rowlett R, Jaselskis C, Leventhal BL. Fluoxetine treatment of children and adults with autistic disorder and mental retardation. *J Am Acad Child Adolesc Psychiatry* 31:739–745, 1992.

156. Steingard RJ, Zimnitzky B, DeMaso DR, Bauman ML, Bucci JP: Sertraline treatment of transition-associated anxiety and agitation in children with autistic disorder. *J Child Adolesc Psychopharmacol* 7:9–15, 1997.

157. Preskorn SH, Janicak PG, Davis JM, Ayd FJ: Advances in the pharmacotherapy of depressive disorders. *Principles and Practices of Psychopharmacotherapy*, Williams & Wilkins, Baltimore, 1(2):1–24, 1995.

158. Brody JF: Bait poisoning and why kids complain about their medication. *J Child Adolesc Psychopharmacol* 7:71–72, 1997.

159. Venkataraman S, Naylor MW, King CA: Mania associated with fluoxetine treatment in adolescents. *J Am Acad Child Adolesc Psychiatry* 31:276–281, 1992.

160. Riddle MA, King RA, Hardin MT, Scahill L, et al: Behavioral side effects of fluoxetine in children and adolescents. *J Child Adolesc Psychopharmacol* 1:193–198, 1990.

161. Schatzberg AF, Haddad P, Kaplan EM, Lejoyeux M, Rosenbaum JF, Young AH, Zajecka J: Serotonin reuptake inhibitor discontinuation syndrome: A hypothetical definition. *J Clin Psychiatry* 58(suppl 7):5–10, 1997.

162. Lejoyeux M, Ades J: Antidepressant discontinuation: A review of the literature. *J Clin Psychiatry* 58(suppl 7):11–16, 1997.

163. Rosenbaum JF, Zajecka J: Clinical management of antidepressant discontinuation. *J Clin Psychiatry* 58(suppl 7):37–40, 1997.

164. Parraga HC, Kelly DP, Parraga MI, Cochran M, Maxim LT: Combined psychostimulant and tricyclic antidepressant treatment of Tourette's syndrome and comorbid disorders in children. *J Child Adolesc Psychopharmacol* 4:113–122, 1994.

165. Carlson GA, Rapport MD, Kelly KL, Pataki CS: Methylphenidate and desipramine in hospitalized children with comorbid behavior and mood disorders: Separate and combined effects on behavior and mood. *J Child Adolesc Psychopharmacol* 5:191–204, 1995.

166. Simeon JG, Thatte S, Wiggins D: Treatment of adolescent obsessive–compulsive disorder with a clomipramine–fluoxetine combination. *Psychopharmacol Bull* 26:285–290, 1990.

167. Findling RL: Open-label treatment of comorbid depression and attentional disorders with co-administration of serotonin reuptake inhibitors and psychostimulants in children, adolescents, and adults: A case series. *J Child Adolesc Psychopharmacol* 6:165–175, 1996.

168. Gammon GD, Brown TE: Fluoxetine and methylphenidate in combination for treatment of attention deficit disorder and comorbid depressive disorder. *J Child Adolesc Psychopharmacol* 3:1–10, 1993.

169. Brown WA, Harrison W: Are patients who are intolerant to one SSRI intolerant to another? *Psychopharmacol Bull* 28:253–256, 1992.

170. Weller EB, Weller RA, Svadjian H: Mood Disorders, in Lewis M (ed): *Child and Adolescent Psychiatry: A Comprehensive Textbook*. Baltimore, Williams & Wilkins, 1996, pp 650–665.

171. Varanka TM, Weller RA, Weller EB, et al: Lithium treatment of manic episodes with psychotic features in prepubertal children. *Am J Psychiatry* 145:1557–1559, 1988.

172. Weller RA, Weller EB, Tucker SG, et al: Mania in prepubertal children: Has it been underdiagnosed? *J Affect Disord* 11:151–154, 1986.

173. Goodwin FK, Jamison KR: *Manic–Depressive Illness*. New York, Oxford University Press, 1990.

174. Robins LN, Helzer JR, Weissman MM, et al.: Lifetime prevalence of specific psychiatric disorders in three sites. *Arch Gen Psychiatry* 41:949–958, 1984.

175. Cade JF: Lithium salts in the treatment of psychotic excitement. *Med J Aust* 11:349–352, 1949.

176. Prien RF, Caffey EM, Klett CJ: Prophylactic efficacy of lithium carbonate in manic–depressive illness. Report of the Veterans Administration and National Institute of Mental Health Collaborative Study Group. *Arch Gen Psychiatry* 28:337–341, 1973.

177. Rapoport JL, Mikkelsen EJ, Werry JS: Antimanic, antianxiety, hallucinogenic and miscellaneous drugs, in Werry JS (ed): *Pediatric Psychopharmacology: The Use of Behavior Modifying Drugs in Children*. New York, Brunner/Mazel, 1978, pp 316–355.

178. Jefferson JW: The use of lithium in childhood and adolescence: An overview. *J Clin Psychiatry* 43:174–177, 1982.
179. Schou M: Lithium in psychiatric therapy and prophylaxis. *J Psychiatr Res* 6:67–95, 1971.
180. Jefferson JW, Greist JH, Ackerman DL, et al: Mechanism of action, in Jefferson JW, Greist JH, Ackerman DL, et al (eds): *Lithium Encyclopedia for Clinical Practice*, ed 2. Washington, DC, American Psychiatric Press, 1987, pp 436–441.
181. Carlson GA: Bipolar disorders in children and adolescents, in Garfinkel B, Carlson G, Weller E (eds): *Psychiatric Disorders in Children and Adolescents*. Philadelphia, WB Saunders Co, 1990, pp 21–36.
182. Amdisen A, Carson S: Lithium, in Evans WE, Schentag JJ, Jusko WJ (eds): *Applied Pharmacokinetics: Principles of Therapeutic Drug Monitoring*. Spokane, Wash, Applied Therapeutics, 1986, pp 97–100.
183. Perry PJ, Alexander B, Liskow BI: Antimanic agents, in Perry PJ, Alexander B, Liskow BI (eds): *Psychotropic Drug Handbook*, ed 5. Concinnati, Harvey Whitney Books, 1988, pp 85–112.
184. Appleton WS: Pharmacological treatment for affective disorders, in Appleton WS (ed): *Practical Clinical Psychopharmacology*, ed 3. Baltimore, Williams & Wilkins, 1988, pp 81–150.
185. Fetner HH, Geller B: Lithium and tricyclic antidepressants. *Psychiatr Clin North Am* 15:223–241, 1992.
186. Platt JE, Campbell M, Green WH, et al: Cognitive effects of lithium carbonate and haloperidol in treatment-resistant aggressive children. *Arch Gen Psychiatry* 41:657–662, 1984.
187. Campbell M, Schulman D, Rapoport J: The current status of lithium therapy in child and adolescent psychiatry. *J Am Acad Child Psychiatry* 14:717–729, 1978.
188. Campbell M, Cohen IL, Small AM: Drugs in aggressive behavior. *J Am Acad Child Psychiatry* 21:107–117, 1982.
189. Campbell M, Fish B, Korein J, et al: Lithium and chlorpromazine: A controlled crossover study of hyperactive severely disturbed young children. *J Autism Child Schizophrenia* 2:234–263, 1972.
190. Gram LF, Rafaelson OJ: Lithium treatment of psychotic children and adolescents. *Acta Psychiatr Scand* 48:253–260, 1972.
191. Hagino OR, Weller EB, Weller RA, Washing D, Fristad MA, Kontras SB: Untoward effects of lithium treatment in children aged four through six years. *J Am Acad Child Adolesc Psychiatry* 34:1584–1590, 1995.
192. Carlson GA, Rapport MD, Kelly KL, et al: The effect of methylphenidate and lithium on attention and activity level. *J Am Acad Child Adolesc Psychiatry* 31:262–270, 1992.
193. Campbell M, Silva RR, Kafantaris V, Locascio JJ, Gonzalez NM, Lee D, Lynch NS: Predictors of side effects associated with lithium administration in children. *Psychopharmacol Bull* 27:373–380, 1991.
194. Silva RR, Campbell M, Golden RR, Small AM, Pataki CS, Rosenberg CR: Side effects associated with lithium and placebo administration in aggressive children. *Psychopharmacol Bull* 28:319–326, 1992.
195. Campbell M, Small AM, Green WH, et al: Behavioral efficacy of haloperidol and lithium carbonate. A comparison in hospitalized aggressive children with conduct disorder. *Arch Gen Psychiatry* 41:650–656, 1984.
196. Campbell M, Green WH, Deutsch SI: *Child and Adolescent Psychopharmacology*. Beverly Hills, Sage Publications, 1985.
197. Deandrea D, Walker N, Nehlmauer M, et al: Dermatological reactions to lithium: A critical review of the literature. *J. Clin Psychopharmacol* 2:199–204, 1982.
198. Jefferson JW: Lithium and tetracycline. *Br J Dermatol* 107:370, 1982.
199. Herskowitz J: Developmental toxicology, in Popper C (ed): *Psychiatric Pharmacosciences of Children and Adolescents*. Washington, DC, American Psychiatric Press, 1987.
200. Birch NJ, Horsman A, Hullin RP: Lithium, bone and body weight studies in long-term treated patients and in the rat. *Neuropsychobiology* 8(2):82–92, 1982.
201. Wilson WH, Jefferson JW: Thyroid disease, behavior and psychopharmacology. *Psychosomatics* 26:481–492, 1985.
202. Vendborg PB, Bech P, Rafaelsen OJ: Lithium treatment and weight gain. *Acta Psychiatr Scand* 53:139–147, 1976.
203. Vestergaard P, Amdisen A, Schou M. Clinically significant side effects of lithium treatment: A survey of 237 patients in long-term treatment. *Acta Psychiatr Scand* 62:193–200, 1980.
204. Kirk L, Baastrup PC, Schou M: Propranolol treatment of lithium-induced tremor. *Lancet* 2:106–107, 1973.
205. Reisberg B, Gershon S: Side effects associated with lithium therapy. *Arch Gen Psychiatry* 36:879–887, 1979.
206. Joffe RT, Kellner CG, Post RM, et al: Lithium increases in platelet count [letter]. *N Engl J Med* 311:674–675, 1984.
207. Wood IK, Parmelee DX, Foreman JW: Lithium-induced nephrotic syndrome. *Am J Psychiatry* 146:84–87, 1989.

208. Khandelwal SK, Varma CK, Marthy RS: Renal function in children receiving long-term lithium prophylaxis. *Am J Psychiatry* 141:278–279, 1984.
209. Suppes T, Baldessarini RJ, Faedda GL, Tohen M: Risk of recurrence following discontinuation of lithium treatment in bipolar disorder. *Arch Gen Psychiatry* 48:1082–1088, 1991.
210. Goodwin GM: Recurrence of mania after lithium withdrawal. *Br J Psychiatry* 164:149–152, 1994.
211. Alessi N, Naylor MW, Ghaziuddin M, Zubieta JK: Update on lithium carbonate therapy in children and adolescents, *J Am Acad Child Adolesc Psychiatry* 33:291–304, 1994.
212. Delong R, Aldershof AL: Long-term experience with lithium treatment in childhood: Correlation with clinical diagnosis. *J Am Acad Child Adolesc Psychiatry* 26:389–394, 1987.
213. Youngerman J, Canino IA: Lithium carbonate use in children and adolescents: A survey of the literature. *Arch Gen Psychiatry* 35:216–224, 1978.
214. Lena B: Lithium treatment of children and adolescents, in Johnson FN (eds): *Handbook of Lithium Therapy*. Lancaster, Penn, MTP Press, 1980, pp 405–413.
215. Strober M, Morrel W, Lampert C, et al: Relapse following discontinuation of lithium maintenance therapy in adolescents with bipolar I illness. A naturalistic study. *Am J Psychiatry* 147:457–461, 1990.
216. Carlson GA, Kashani JH: Manic symptoms in a non-referred adolescent population. *J Affect Disord* 15:219–226, 1988.
217. Werry JS, McClellan JM, Chard L: Childhood and adolescent schizophrenic, bipolar and schizoaffective disorders. A clinical and outcome study. *J Am Acad Child Adolesc Psychiatry* 30:457–465, 1991.
218. Strober M, Carlson GA: Bipolar illness in adolescents with major depression: Clinical, genetic, and psychopharmacologic predictors in a 3 to 4-year prospective follow up investigation. *Arch Gen Psychiatry* 39:549–555, 1982.
219. Akiskal HS, Down SJ, Jordan P, et al: Affective disorders in referred children and younger siblings and manic depressives. *Arch Gen Psychiatry* 42:996–1004, 1985.
220. Stewart MA, Beblois CS, Meardon J, et al: Aggressive conduct disorder of children: The clinical picture. *J Nerv Ment Dis* 16:604–610, 1980.
221. Campbell M: Psychopharmacology, in Noshpitz JD (ed): *Basic Handbook of Child Psychiatry*. New York, Basic Books, 1979, vol 3, pp 376–409.
222. Campbell M, Adams PB, Small AM, Kafantaris V, Silva RR, Shell J, Perry R, Overall JE: Lithium in hospitalized aggressive children with conduct disorder: A double-blind and placebo-controlled study. *J Am Acad Child Adolesc Psychiatry* 34:445–453, 1995.
223. Rifkin A, Karajgi B, Dicker R, Perl E, Boppana V, Hasan N, Pollack S: Lithium treatment of conduct disorders in adolescents. *Am J Psychiatry* 154:554–555, 1997.
224. Licamele WL, Goldberg RL: The concurrent use of lithium and methylphenidate in a child. *J Am Acad Child Adolesc Psychiatry* 28:785–787, 1989.
225. Ryan N, Meyer VA, Dachille S, et al: Lithium antidepressant augmentation in TCA-refractory depression in adolescents. *J Am Acad Child Adolesc Psychiatry* 27:371–376, 1988.
226. Strober M, Freeman R, Rigali J, et al: The pharmacotherapy of depressive illness in adolescence: II. Effects of lithium augmentation in nonresponders to imipramine. *J Am Acad Child Adolesc Psychiatry* 31:16–20, 1992.
227. Weller EB, Weller RA, Fristad MA: Lithium dosage guide for prepubertal children: A preliminary report. *J Am Acad Child Adolesc Psychiatry* 25:92–95, 1986.
228. Campbell M, Small AM, Green WM, et al: Lithium and haloperidol in hospitalized aggressive children. *Psychopharmacol Bull* 1:125–130, 1982.
229. Siassi I: Lithium treatment of impulsive behavior in children. *J Clin Psychiatry* 43:42–44, 1982.
230. Persson G: Lithium side effects in relation to dose and to levels of lithium in plasma. *Acta Psychiatr Scand* 51:285–288, 1975.
231. Jefferson JW: Treating affective disorders in the presence of cardiovascular disease. *Psychiatr Clin North Am* 6:141–155, 1983.
232. Lippmann S, Wagemaker H, Tucker D: A practical approach to management of lithium concurrent with hyponatremia, diuretic therapy and/or chronic renal failure. *J Clin Psychiatry* 42:304–306, 1981.
233. Tyrer SP: Lithium in the treatment of mania. *J Affect Disord* 8:251–257, 1985.
234. Jefferson JW: Serum lithium levels and long-term diuretic use. *JAMA* 241:1134–1136, 1979.
235. Shulka S, Godwin CD, Long LE, et al: Lithium–carbamazepine neurotoxicity and risk factors. *Am J Psychiatry* 141:1604–1606, 1984.
236. Prakash R, Kelwala S, Ban TA: Neurotoxicity with combined administration of lithium with a neuroleptic. *Compr Psychiatry* 23:567–571, 1982.
237. Perry PJ, Calloway RA, Cook B, et al: Theophylline precipitated alterations in lithium clearance. *Acta Psychiatr Scand* 69:528–537, 1984.

238. Ballenger JC, Post RM: Carbamazepine in manic–depressive illness: A new treatment. *Am J Psychiatry* 137:782–790, 1980.
239. Stromgrew LS, Boller S: Carbamazepine in treatment and prophylaxis of manic–depressive disorder. *Psychiatry Dev* 4:349–367, 1985.
240. Hsu LK: Lithium-resistant adolescent mania. *J Am Acad Child Psychiatry* 25:280–283, 1986.
241. Trimble MR: Anticonvulsants in children and adolescents. *J Child Adolesc Psychopharmacol* 1:107–124, 1990.
242. Levy R, Pitlick WH: Carbamazepine: Interaction with other drugs, in Woodbury DM, Penry JD, Pippenger CD (eds): *Antiepileptic Drugs*. New York, Raven Press, 1982, pp 497–505.
243. Kafantaris V, Campbell M, Padron-Gayol MV, Small AM, Locascio JJ, Rosenberg CR: Carbamazepine in hospitalized aggressive conduct disorder children: An open pilot study. *Psychopharmacol Bull* 28:193–199, 1992.
244. Silva RR, Munoz DM, Alpert M: Carbamazepine use in children and adolescents with features of attention-deficit hyperactivity disorder: A meta-analysis. *J Am Acad Child Adolesc Psychiatry* 35:352–358, 1996.
245. Forsythe I, Butler R, Berg I, McGuire R: Cognitive impairment in new cases of epilepsy randomly assigned to carbamazepine, phenytoin and sodium valproate. *Dev Med Child Neurol* 33:524–534, 1991.
246. Livingston S, Pauli L, Berman W: Carbamazepine in epilepsy. Nine year follow-up with special emphasis on untoward reaction. *Dis Nerv Syst* 35:103–107, 1974.
247. Killam FM, Fromm CH: Carbamazepine in the treatment of neuralgia: Use and side effects. *Arch Neurol* 19:129–136, 1968.
248. Salzman MB, Valderrama E, Sood SK: Carbamazepine and fatal eosinophilic myocarditis. *N Engl J Med* 336:878–879, 1997.
249. Isojarvi JI, Laatikainen TJ, Pakarinen AJ, Juntunen KT, Myllyla VV: Polycystic ovaries and hyperandrogenism in women taking valproate for epilepsy. *N Engl J Med* 329:1383–1388, 1993.
250. Rall TW, Schleifer LS: Drugs effective in the therapy of the epilepsies, in Gilman AG, Rall TW, Nies AS, et al (eds): *The Pharmacological Basis of Therapeutics*, ed 8. New York, Pergamon Press, 1990, pp 436–462.
251. Calabrese J, Delucchi G: Spectrum of efficacy of valproate in 55 patients with rapidcycling bipolar disorder. *Am J Psychiatry* 47:431–434, 1990.
252. McElroy SL, Keck P, Pope HG: Sodium valproate: Its use in primary psychiatric disorders. *J Clin Psychopharmacol* 7:16–24, 1987.
253. Paptheodorou G, Kutcher SP: Divalproex sodium treatment in late adolescent and young adult acute mania. *Psychopharmacol Bull* 29:213–219, 1993.
254. West SA, Keck PE, McElroy SL, Strakowski SM, Minnery KL, McConville BJ, Sorter MT: Open trial of valproate in the treatment of adolescent mania. *J Child Adolesc Psychopharmacol* 4:263–267, 1994.
255. West SA, Keck PE, McElroy SL: Oral loading doses in the valproate treatment of adolescents with mixed bipolar disorder. *J Am Acad Child Adolesc Psychiatry* 5:225–231, 1995.
256. Keck PE, McElroy SL, Tugrul KC, Bennett JA: Valproate oral loading in the treatment of acute mania. *J Clin Psychiatry* 54:305–308, 1993.
257. Dreifuss FE, Santilli N, Langer DH, et al: Valproic acid hepatic fatalities: A retrospective review. *Neurology* 37:379–385, 1987.
258. Pope H, McElroy S, Keck P, et al: Valproate in the treatment of acute mania. *Arch Gen Psychiatry* 48:62–68, 1991.
259. Janicak PG, Bishes RA: Advances in the treatment of mania and other acute psychotic disorders. *Psychiatr Ann* 17:145–149, 1987.
260. Biederman J: The diagnosis and treatment of adolescent anxiety disorders. *J Clin Psychiatry* 51(suppl): 20–26, 1990.
261. Biederman J: Clonazepam in the treatment of prepubertal children with panic-like symptoms. *J Clin Psychiatry* 48:38–41, 1987.

10

Antipsychotics (Neuroleptics)

MONIQUE ERNST, M.D., Ph.D.,
RICHARD P. MALONE, M.D.,
AMY B. ROWAN, M.D.,
REGINA GEORGE, M.D.,
NILDA M. GONZALEZ, M.D.,
and RAUL R. SILVA, M.D.

I. DEFINITION, CLASSES, INDIVIDUAL DRUGS, AND GENERIC AND TRADE NAMES

Antipsychotic drugs form a large group of psychoactive agents mainly known for their antipsychotic clinical properties, though they are also effective in a variety of nonpsychotic disorders. Originally, these drugs were named neuroleptics, because of their ability to mimic neurological syndromes,[1] and this appellation is still in wide use, especially in the United States.

Presently, antipsychotics are divided into two groups, the typical (or classical) and the new atypical types. Several reasons led to the search for new antipsychotics: (1) 30% of patients are resistant to treatment with classical antipsychotics; (2) although typical (or classical) antipsychotics are effective on positive symptoms of schizophrenia, they are less so on negative symptoms; and (3) side effects can be severe and sometimes irreversible (e.g., tardive dyskinesia).

As shown in Table 1, there are six classes of classical antipsychotics: phenothiazines, butyrophenones, thioxanthenes, dihydroindolones, dibenzoxazepines, and diphenylbutyl-piperidines. Only one or two representative agents have been listed for each class, although

MONIQUE ERNST, M.D., Ph.D., and REGINA GEORGE, M.D. • Brain Imaging Center, National Institute on Drug Abuse, Baltimore, Maryland 21224. RICHARD P. MALONE, M.D. • Department of Mental Health Sciences, Philadelphia, Pennsylvania 19129. AMY B. ROWAN, M.D. • Child and Adolescent Psychiatry, The Children's Hospital of Philadelphia, Philadelphia, Pennsylvania 19104. NILDA M. GONZALEZ, M.D. • Department of Psychiatry, Henry Ittleson Center, Bronx, New York 10471. RAUL R. SILVA, M.D. • Child and Adolescent Psychiatry Department, St. Lukes/Roosevelt Hospital, New York, New York 10025.

Practitioner's Guide to Psychoactive Drugs for Children and Adolescents (Second Edition), Werry and Aman, eds. Plenum Publishing Corporation, New York, 1999.

**TABLE 1. Representative Classical Antipsychotic Drugs
and Dosages in Children and Adolescents**

Class	Generic name of drug (trade name) and chlorpromazine equivalents[a]	Daily dose in mg (mg/kg)	
		Children	Adolescents[b]
Phenothiazines			
Aliphatic	Chlorpromazine (Largactil®, Thorazine®), 100	10–200 (0.5–3.0)	50–600
Piperidine	Thioridazine (Mellaril®), 97	10–200 (0.5–3.0)	50–600
Piperazine	Trifluoperazine (Stelazine®), 2.8	2–20[c]	Not known
Butyrophenones	Haloperidol (Haldol®), 1.6	0.25–6.0 (0.016–0.15)[d]	1.0–16, mean 9.8
Thioxanthenes	Thiothixene (Navane®), 8.8	1.0–6.0, median 2.0 (0.1–0.3)	4.8–42.6 (0.3)
Dihydroindolones	Molindone (Moban®), 6.0	1.0–155 (0.1–2.0)	75–225, (mean 1.7 ± 1.03)
Dibenzoxazepines	Loxapine (Loxitane®), 17.4	Not known	25–200, mean 87.5
Diphenylbutylpiperidines	Pimozide (Orap®)	1–6 (0.12–0.3; not to exceed 0.3)[e]	1–9 (not to exceed 0.3)

[a]In milligrams; adapted from Davis et al.[2]
[b]For an acutely psychotic adolescent (e.g., weight of 70 kg), 300–600 mg per day (4–8 mg/kg per day) in chlorpromazine equivalents is indicated[4] (e.g., 1.0 mg haloperidol = 50 mg chlorpromazine). For maintenance and nonpsychotic disorders, dosage ordinarily should be at least 50% lower.
[c]Ref. 3.
[d]Up to 0.021 mg/kg per day in children with autistic disorder[5] and with conduct disorder.[6] Higher doses are for acutely psychotic and manic children only.
[e]Because of possible cardiotoxic effects, this dose should never be exceeded.

there may be more than one drug per class, especially in the case of phenothiazines.[2] The reason is that the behavioral effects of all antipsychotics are similar, and sound knowledge about the efficacy and safety of one or two drugs is more important than limited knowledge about an array of drugs. Table 1 contains both generic and trade names of representative antipsychotics, daily dose range in milligrams, and in milligrams per kilogram where available, and the chlorpromazine (CPZ) dose equivalent (the dose in milligrams that is equivalent to 100 mg of chlorpromazine). The latter is important because it allows ready comparisons among different antipsychotics. Antipsychotics are often grouped as high- and low-potency drugs, which tends to distinguish drugs with extrapyramidal side effects from those with atropinic side effects, respectively. These terms, however, are misleading because potency refers to milligram doses and not to efficacy, and all antipsychotics in common use seem equally effective. As pointed out in Chapter 2, efficiency might be a more accurate term than potency.

Table 2 lists atypical antipsychotics. The number of studies in children of atypical antipsychotics is even more limited than that of typical antipsychotics. Because they are not adequately investigated in children, dosage is given for adults; dosage for children and adolescents is given when available.

II. CLINICAL INDICATIONS

A. Introduction

The diagnostic categories of the fourth edition of the *Diagnostic and Statistical Manual of Mental Disorders* (DSM-IV)[11] will be used throughout this chapter. Like the

TABLE 2. Representative Atypical Antipsychotic Drugs
and Dosages in Children, Adolescents, and Adults

Class	Generic name of drug (trade name) and chlorpromazine equivalents	Daily dose in mg		
		Children	Adolescents	Adults
Dibenzodiazepines	Clozapine (Clozaril®, Leponex®)	Not known	Over 16 years of age: 100–700, mean 352[a]	300–600 in divided doses
Benzisoxazoles	Risperidone (Risperdal®)	Not known	Not known	4–10[b,c]
Thienobenzodiazepines	Olanzapine (Zypexa®)	Not known	Not known	5–15[d]
	Sertindole (Serlect®)	Not known	Not known	12–24[e]
Dibenzothiazepines	Quetiapine (Seroquel®)	Not known	Not known	75–750
Benzisothiazolyl piperazines	Ziprasidone (Zeldox®)	Not known	Not known	120–160[f]

[a]In Ref. 7.
[b]Refs. 8–10.
[c]Also available in an oral suspension form, enabling titration at very low dose. Most sources argue that not much is gained by increasing dosaage above 6–7 mg/day.
[d]Beasley CM Jr, Tollefson G, Tran P, et al: Olanzapine versus placebo and haloperidol: Acute phase results of the North American double-blind olanzapine trial [see comments]. *Neuropsychopharmacology* 14(2):111–123, 1996.
[e]Sertindole Consensus Meeting, 1995.
[f]Seeger TF, Seymour PA, Schmidt AW, et al: Ziprasidone (CP-88,059): A new antipsychotic with combined dopamine and serotonin receptor antagonist activity. *J Pharmacol Exp Ther* 275(1):101–113, 1995.

disorders defined in the DSM-III,[12] and its revision,[13] they do not always correspond to ICD-9 and ICD-10 categories.[14,15] In children and adolescents, antipsychotics are probably used in a wider range of disorders and symptoms than in adult psychiatric patients. In the latter, schizophrenia, other psychoses, mood disorders, and Tourette's disorder are the main indications. With the exception of Tourette's disorder, the frequency of these disorders is lower in children, though incidence increases sharply in adolescence. Antipsychotics are used in a variety of nonpsychotic conditions in children and adolescents to reduce disruptive behaviors. However, they should be given only in cases of severe psychopathology because of their potential neurotoxic effects in younger patients (see Section IV.).

Antipsychotics may reduce positive psychotic symptoms (delusions, hallucinations, and thought disorder), movement disorders (stereotypies and tics), disruptive behaviors [aggressiveness and self-injurious behavior (SIB)], temper tantrums, irritability, inattention, and hyperactivity. Decrease of negative symptoms like social withdrawal has also been reported.

1. Dosage

While handbooks and the *Physicians' Desk Reference* (PDR) (1998)[16] should serve as a guideline for dosage, the range of dosage and the mean or median dose may not be appropriate for some individuals. For example, children or adolescents with brain dysfunction or brain damage may be more sensitive to drugs and develop behavioral toxicity and/or extrapyramidal side effects on lower doses of antipsychotics than patients without central nervous system (CNS) damage. As a rule, every attempt should be made to maintain the child on a "minimum therapeutically effective dose", with minimal side effects, particularly on cognition and performance. In recent years, several studies of adult psychiatric patients have shown that high doses of typical antipsychotics are no more effective than much lower doses but are associated with more adverse effects.[17] Prescribing larger than necessary doses has resulted from a failure to distinguish between the need for rapid control of very disturbed behavior in adult psychotic patients and the relatively long time frame of the true antipsychotic effect (measured in days or even weeks). There has also been a failure to distinguish between acute (300–600 mg CPZ equivalents) and maintenance dosage, which can be quite low (100–300 CPZ equivalents).

While the usual effective dose will serve as a guide, the determination of the minimum therapeutically effective dose must be tailored to each child, except in acutely psychotic or manic patients. The dose should be started at a low, subtherapeutic level and be increased by small increments, less than twice a week, until therapeutic effect is achieved or side effects emerge, yet not to a level exceeding the maximum recommended dose. Some children and adolescents (up to one-third in schizophrenia) will not respond to any psychoactive agent, and very high doses are unjustifiable. In acutely psychotic adolescents who are more difficult to manage, the regimen can be greatly accelerated, starting with 4 mg/kg per day of CPZ equivalents.

When feasible, especially in maintenance, a single daily dose is recommended. At first, however, the antipsychotic should be administered in divided doses (two or three times a day), to allow early detection of side effects, particularly sedation, and finer tuning for maximum effectiveness. When sleep disturbance is an essential part of a psychiatric disorder such as agitated depression or mania, an evening (h.s.) dose may be given. However, antipsychotics should not be regarded as a medication for insomnia *per se* (see Chapter 15). A suggested dose regulation and increments in nonacutely ill children (which is generally the case), using haloperidol as an example, should begin with 0.25 mg/day and be gradually increased by 0.25 mg to a maximum of 3 mg/day. Dosages for adolescents in milligrams per day may be higher than those required for children.

Except in active psychotic states, medication should be discontinued every 6 months for 4 weeks, and assessment of abnormal movements should be carried out. A decision as to the need for continuation of pharmacotherapy should be made at this time .

2. Pretreatment Screening

Pretreatment routine screening (see Chapter 4 for full details) includes measurement of weight and height; neurological examination for tics, stereotypies, extrapyramidal disorders, and tardive dyskinesia; and laboratory tests including complete blood count, differential, and liver and kidney function tests. The Abnormal Involuntary Movements Scale (AIMS)[18], or similar standardized instrument, should be used to assess abnormal movements, following a schedule recommended for children.[19,20] These evaluations should be repeated as indicated, at least once every 6 months.

B. Schizophrenia

While schizophrenia is rare in children under 12, the rate of schizophrenia increases dramatically in adolescence.[21] Extensive research in adults showed that, while side effects differ, all antipsychotics (except clozapine) seem similarly effective in acute episodes at doses between 300 and 600 mg/day CPZ equivalents (approximately 4–8 mg/kg per day). Research also indicates that maintenance antipsychotic medication at lower doses (100–300 mg/day CPZ equivalents) can reduce frequency of relapses. Limited research has been conducted in younger age groups, but, as in adults, the high-potency (referring to the milligram equivalence of drug) antipsychotics seem to be preferred. Haloperidol has been the most studied, yet with only two double-blind studies, one in children[22,23] and one in adolescents.[24] In children, haloperidol in daily doses ranging from 0.02 to 0.12 mg/kg (mean 0.06 mg/kg) was therapeutically effective and superior to placebo.[22] By the end of the 4-week treatment period, hallucinations, ideas of reference, thought disorders, and particularly persecutory ideation were significantly reduced; frank delusions or blunted affect were not affected. In hospitalized adolescents with acute or chronic schizophrenia with acute exacerbation, loxapine (25–200 mg/day, mean 87.5) was compared with haloperidol (2.0–16.0 mg/day, mean 9.8).[24] Both drugs were highly effective in reducing psychotic symptoms, but haloperidol was less sedating.

However, most clinical trials were open and conducted in small samples. In these studies, thiothixene and thioridazine were equally effective in reducing psychotic symptoms within the first week of treatment; however, even though the reduction of symptoms was significant in half of the sample, overall improvement was only slight.[25] Daily doses ranged from 91 to 228 mg (mean 178 mg or 3.3 mg/kg) for thioridazine and from 4.8 to 42.6 mg (mean 16.2 mg or 0.30 mg/kg) for thiothixene.[25] Sedation was more prominent with thioridazine.

In general, despite the greater sensitivity of younger age groups to dystonic reactions, the high-potency antipsychotics are preferable to the low-potency drugs, mainly because they are less likely to cause sedation and adrenolytic effects like hypotension. Like adults, children may sometimes respond better to a low than to a high dose,[22] but more research is needed.

Clozapine is an atypical antipsychotic from the class of dibenzodiazepines. Its receptor blockade profile resembles that of chlorpromazine and thioridazine (anticholinergic, adrenolytic, serotoninolytic, and antihistaminic), but it differs from all other antipsychotics in its high affinity for D_1 receptors and low affinity for D_2 receptors. Extrapyramidal side effects are unusual, but sedation, salivation, and weight gain are more problematic. Only a few cases of tardive dyskinesia have been reported with clozapine.[3] Seizure threshold is reduced, and blood dyscrasias are quite high (up to 7%) but reducible to under 1% with weekly blood monitoring during the first 6 months of treatment. Clozapine may be useful in about one-third of adult schizophrenics who have failed to respond to other antipsychotics.[3] A preliminary report from a double-blind, placebo-controlled study indicates that clozapine is effective in the treatment of children with childhood-onset schizophrenia.[26] In this study of 21 previously neuroleptic-resistant subjects (mean age $\pm$ SD, 14 $\pm$ 2.3 years), clozapine was compared to haloperidol. Clozapine was rated superior to haloperidol on all measures and reduced both positive and negative symptoms. However, clozapine had to be discontinued in a number of subjects because of leukopenia, seizures, and weight gain.[27] Open trials of clozapine supported its therapeutic efficacy in the treatment of schizophrenia in children and adolescents[28-30]; dosages ranged from 75 to 800 mg/day (average doses range: 285–330 mg/day). Side effects included increased heart rate, sedation, salivation, orthostatic hypotension, hyperthermia, and leukopenia. Of note, 800 mg/day is an unusually high dose, and most adults respond on 300 mg/day or less.[31,32]

Another atypical neuroleptic, risperidone, has proven effective for the treatment of schizophrenia in adults.[33] Though controlled trials in children and adolescents are lacking, open-label studies suggest that risperidone is a promising treatment for schizophrenia in children and adolescents.[34-39] Armenteros et al.[34] reported that four schizophrenic subjects (mean age, 14.7 years) who completed a 6-week open trial of risperidone were significantly improved on the Brief Psychiatric Rating Scale (BPRS) and the Clinical Global Impressions (CGI) scale. Dosages ranged from 4 to 8 mg/day, and side effects included weight gain, sedation, acute dystonic reaction, and parkinsonian symptoms.

Other atypical antipsychotics, including olanzapine and sertindole, will soon be available on the market. Risperidone and the newer atypical antipsychotics may be preferable treatments to clozapine, particularly if they do not have potentially lethal side effects such as agranulocytosis.

In summary, there is evidence to suggest that neuroleptics are effective in the treatment of childhood schizophrenia. Dosage requirements may be different in prepubertal children and in adults, and side effects may be age-dependent.

C. Major Depression with Psychotic Features and Bipolar Disorder

1. Major Depression with Psychotic Features

Psychotic depression is rare in children[4] (see Chapter 7), and its treatment is primarily by antidepressants and/or electroconvulsive therapy (ECT), yet the psychotic symptoms require treatment in their own right.[40] The use of antipsychotic agents has been reported in only one study[41] of a small number of adolescents; remission of delusional ideation was achieved in all six adolescents with psychotic depression within 2 weeks of initiation of chlorpromazine treatment at 50–100 mg/day (mean plasma levels of 6–11 ng/mL). After 2–3 weeks, nortriptyline (20–35 mg/day; mean plasma levels, 52–137 ng/mL) was added; chlorpromazine plasma levels tended to decrease (to 3–8 ng/mL), probably through the induction of liver enzymes by nortriptyline. All but one patient responded to this combined treatment. Nortriptyline doses were significantly lower in this group of patients with combined treatment than in eight nondelusional depressed adolescents.[41] From a practitioner's perspective, this one study suggests that adolescents react similarly to adults, but more data are needed.

2. Bipolar Disorder

Bipolar disorder (i.e., manic or manic and depressive episodes) is unusual in children, although its frequency increases in adolescence.[4,42,43] There are no systematic reports on the use of antipsychotics in bipolar disorder in this age group. Both haloperidol and lithium are reported superior to chlorpromazine in adult manic patients, who are very difficult to treat when acutely ill. The onset of action is faster with haloperidol than with lithium,[44] yet the latter is considered the drug of choice (see Chapter 9). Haloperidol doses may need to be higher in acute bipolar disorder than in schizophrenia, whereas side effects seem less severe.[40,44] In adults, adding benzodiazepines can reduce the doses of antipsychotics required to treat acute manic states,[40] but there are arguments against combined therapy (see Chapters 1, 9, and 15).

Clozapine has been proposed for the treatment of refractory mania in adults.[45] There are several uncontrolled reports on the use of clozapine in children and adolescents.[46,47] Kowatch et al.[47] employed open-label clozapine for 6 weeks to treat 10 children and adolescents (aged 6–15 years) who had a variety of psychotic diagnoses, including five patients with bipolar disorder. No improvement was noted on the CGI and Children's Global Assessment Scale (CGAS) at doses ranging from 75 to 225 mg/day (mean daily dosage, 3.2 mg/kg).

In summary, studies on the safety and efficacy of neuroleptics in children with bipolar disorder are lacking. The clinical treatment of children with bipolar disorder continues to be guided by findings in adults, for whom neuroleptics can be used as a short-term adjunct to other mood stabilizers such as lithium.

D. Conduct Disorder and Conduct Problems

When conduct disorder includes severe aggressiveness and explosiveness, lower doses of antipsychotics like haloperidol may be useful in addition to psychosocial interventions.[48]

Several controlled studies assessed the efficacy of antipsychotics in conduct-disordered children. Most of these children were hospitalized[6,49–52] and were evaluated by various rating scales, including the Children's Psychiatric Rating Scale (CPRS).[53] These studies showed a reduction in aggression, hyperactivity, hostility, and social unresponsiveness. The most common side effects were sedation and dystonic reactions. Haloperidol was the most frequently used drug, but other antipsychotics were also effective. Gains were modest and achieved often at low dose (0.025–0.20 mg/kg), with little evidence that high doses would be more effective. In one study, haloperidol was as effective as lithium.[6] All of these trials were short-term; however, one report indicated diminution of side effects after a few days and efficacy remaining after 6 months.[54]

The effect of antipsychotics on cognition is of concern, particularly because learning disorders are often comorbid with conduct disorder. Several studies[49,50,55,56] have shown that when dosage of haloperidol was low (<0.06 mg/kg per day), apart from occasional initial sedative effects marked by psychomotor slowing, there was only a small, inconstant decrement in performance,[49,56] no evidence of cognitive impairment,[54] and even some improvement in one study at 0.025 mg/kg.[55] As in schizophrenic adults, long-term use seems to be associated with less cognitive impairment.[54]

At the present state of knowledge and availability of data on safety, antipsychotics like haloperidol may be prescribed in low dosage to a severely explosive and aggressive child and before other drugs (such as lithium or carbamazepine) are tried.

There are limited data on the treatment of aggression by atypical antipsychotics. In an open study, risperidone (at dosage up to 3 mg/kg) was shown to be effective for the treatment of aggression in six children (age range, 8–14 years) with a variety of psychiatric disorders.[57]

In summary, antipsychotics may be helpful in reducing severe aggression, particularly the explosive type, in conduct disorder. However, children with conduct disorder may be more susceptible to side effects such as sedation and adverse effects on cognition.

E. Autistic Disorder and Other Pervasive Developmental Disorders (PDD)

High-potency antipsychotics such as haloperidol, pimozide, and trifluoperazine have been found to be effective in reducing hyperactivity, aggressiveness, distractibility, temper tantrums, and stereotypies in autistic children.[3,5,58–61] In those autistic children who are mainly normoactive or hypoactive and anergic, haloperidol usually yields only sedation; pimozide may be more helpful.[62,63] A variety of antipsychotics have been tried, mostly in open studies. Chlorpromazine, a low-potency antipsychotic agent, seems sedating even at conservative doses, without significant decrease in target symptoms.[64,65] More importantly, chlorpromazine has been reported to lower seizure threshold and to worsen epilepsy.[66] Autism is associated with a relatively high rate of seizure disorder. Thioridazine seems less epileptogenic[67,68] but has not been studied in autism. This drug is unlikely to be preferable to chlorpromazine, given its similarity in side-effect profile. Trifluoperazine has been shown to be therapeutic in daily doses of 0.11–1.60 mg/kg, particularly in low-functioning autistic children[3] and in nonverbal, hypoactive, and anergic subjects. Thiothixene at doses of 1–2 mg/day decreased withdrawal, excitability, and stereotypies.[69] Side effects occurred only at doses 1.3–6 times higher than these lowest effective therapeutic doses and included excessive sedation, irritability, and parkinsonian signs. Molindone at daily doses of 1.0–2.5 mg (mean 1.5) produced a modest decrease of symptoms, particularly irritability, when administered over 6–12 weeks.[70]

However, of all these drugs, haloperidol is the only one that has been studied in a systematic fashion under double-blind conditions in this population. It was shown to be both clinically and statistically superior to placebo.[5,58,61] Conservative doses, individually regulated and ranging from 0.019 to 0.23 mg/kg per day,[5,59] markedly reduced sterotypies, withdrawal, hyperactivity, and irritability. Age was positively correlated with symptom reduction.[71] During up to 2 months' treatment, side effects were observed only above therapeutic doses and included excessive sedation and acute dystonic reactions.[5,58,59,61]

The data on autism suggest that children with other forms of PDD (e.g., with marked cerebral dysfunction, including Rett's syndrome[72]) might benefit from treatment with haloperidol or any other potent antipsychotic agent at the lowest possible dose (0.25–0.5 mg/day) and with small increments not more frequent than twice a week.

Because autism is a chronic disorder, long-term efficacy is very important. The one available long-term study of haloperidol (0.016–0.21 mg/kg) indicated that haloperidol was effective when administered over 6 months[73] or longer (M. Campbell, unpublished data). The severely disturbed autistic children treated in this study were able to remain with their families and in special-education classes in the public school system. Eleven of 60 children developed dyskinesias, three during haloperidol treatment and nine after discontinuation of the drug during the 4-week posttreatment placebo period;[73] there were no other side effects. The best responders were children whose behavior was characterized by angry and labile affect, irritability, and negativism. Social withdrawal, stereotypies, and speech abnormalities were significantly reduced, as was the sum of the 14 selected symptoms on the CPRS.[53] Clinically, aggressiveness and hyperactivity were diminished.

Reports indicated that haloperidol either did not differ from placebo in its effects on cognition[5,58] or facilitated performance in the laboratory[58,59]; when administered on a long-term basis, it had a positive effect on IQ performance.[74,75] The combination of haloperidol and behavior therapy (focusing on language acquisition by contingent reinforcement) facilitated imitative speech and was superior to either haloperidol alone or contingent reinforcement alone.[58]

In summary, haloperidol in low dosage has been shown to be a useful adjunct to the treatment of autistic children and sometimes a very important component of a comprehensive treatment program.

There are several reports on the use of risperidone in autistic adults[76,77] and children.[78] Perry et al.[78] conducted an open-label trial of risperidone in six children diagnosed with pervasive developmental disorder (aged 7–15 years). Risperidone dosages ranged from 1 to 6 mg/day, and the patients were treated for up to 5.2 months. Improvement was noted on CPRS items (angry affect and lability) and on the CGI scale. Side effects included weight gain, sedation, increased salivation, and stereotypies.

Overall, neuroleptics are an effective adjunctive treatment for many children with autism. Haloperidol, in low dosages, is the best established drug treatment in this population. The atypical neuroleptics show promise in this disorder, but more research is needed.

F. Tourette's Disorder

Haloperidol and pimozide in low doses are effective in the treatment of motor and vocal tics. Their use may be limited by sedation, adverse effects on cognition,[79] and extrapyramidal effects, although not all reports are in agreement.[80] Dysphoria or depression and school phobia were reported to occur in 16% and 4% of patients, respectively.[81] In a controlled study,[80] haloperidol (mean 0.08 mg/kg per day) seemed more effective than pimozide (mean 0.18 mg/kg).[80] The dosage of pimozide may have been too low: the pimozide/haloperidol ratio was 2.3:1, whereas others have employed a ratio of 4:1.[80] Of interest, this ratio is inconsistent with dopamine receptor blockade data where haloperidol and pimozide are approximately equipotent. A recent 24-week, placebo-controlled double crossover study of equivalent doses of haloperidol and pimozide was conducted in 22 subjects (7–16 years old) with Tourette's disorder.[82] Findings were a significant therapeutic effect for pimozide but not haloperidol compared to placebo, and a threefold higher frequency of serious side effects with haloperidol than with pimozide. Hence, pimozide may be superior to haloperidol in the treatment of Tourette's disorder. However, it is prudent to keep in mind that pimozide is alleged more cardiotoxic than haloperidol.

Open reports in the literature showed a therapeutic effect of risperidone in the treatment of Tourette's disorder or other tic disorders.[83,84]

Overall, haloperidol and pimozide are effective in decreasing vocal and motor tics. Dosage requirements are usually lower than those used in schizophrenia, and patients may be particularly vulnerable to the side effects of the neuroleptics. The atypical neuroleptic risperidone may prove to be a useful agent in the treatment of tics.

G. Mental Retardation Associated with Disruptive Behavior or Psychiatric Disorder

Psychiatric disorders (dual diagnosis) and certain behavioral symptoms are more common in mentally retarded individuals than in persons of normal intelligence.[85] Disruptive behavior characterized by aggressiveness against persons or property, impulsivity, and hyperactivity and self-injurious behavior (SIB) are of particular concern. When behavioral interventions fail or are difficult to implement, an antipsychotic agent may be helpful. Other disorders, such as anxiety and mood disorders, should receive the appropriate specific treatment.

Despite the large number of psychopharmacological studies in mentally retarded individuals,[86,87] the findings are difficult to interpret because the sample sizes are frequently small and many studies suffer from diagnostic vagueness and other methodological flaws.[87] Furthermore, most published reports involve adults or mostly adults, and their findings are not necessarily applicable to children and adolescents.

The use of atypical antipsychotics has not been carefully studied in patients with mental retardation, apart from the use of risperidone as an add-on therapy.[88]

1. Short-Term Efficacy

Antipsychotics are the drugs most frequently used to treat "behavioral" (i.e., disruptive) problems in mentally retarded individuals, even in community settings, where up to

42% of subjects under 19 years of age have been found to be on such medication.[89] However, there are increasing concerns that antipsychotics are either therapeutically ineffective or may have an adverse effect on adaptive functions, including cognition.[87,90]

In general, antipsychotic medications, mostly studied in institutional settings, produce modest clinical improvement[91,92]—in order of efficacy: reductions in stereotypies, hyperactivity, conduct problems, irritability, and self-injury as measured by the Aberrant Behavior Checklist.[93] Most antipsychotics (chlorpromazine, thioridazine, haloperidol, and pimozide) seem to be effective; however, there are *a priori* reasons for preferring high-potency drugs. Low-potency agents like chlorpromazine and thioridazine are strongly anticholinergic and more likely to impair cognition, cause sedation, and/or, in the case of chlorpromazine, lower seizure threshold in this vulnerable population.[68]

Dosage has not been well studied, but relatively low doses (e.g., 0.025 mg/kg in the case of haloperidol[94] or 2.5 mg/kg in the case of thioridazine[95]) are often as effective as higher doses (1.28–17.54 mg/kg; mean, 5.23).[95] Although controversial, it often seems that efficacy is inversely proportional to IQ;[96] in profoundly retarded subjects, little beyond reduction in stereotypies may be seen.

2. Effects on Cognition

Studies of the effect of antipsychotics on cognition are limited. Pimozide had no effect on learning[97] and only a slight positive effect on performance[98] in the laboratory. Thioridazine (1.75 mg/kg per day) did not influence cognitive–motor or IQ performance,[99] in contrast to methylphenidate.[99]

In summary, there is some evidence that neuroleptics, particularly high-potency neuroleptics, may be moderately helpful in reducing severely disruptive and destructive behaviors when they occur in mentally retarded youth. However, there are few well-controlled studies with this population.

H. Attention-Deficit Hyperactivity Disorder (ADHD)

Though stimulants (Chapter 8) and antidepressants (Chapter 9) are effective in ADHD, if a child fails to respond or has side effects, an antipsychotic drug may be useful. Such drugs should be used judiciously, because ADHD is a chronic disorder, and often[100,101] long-term drug maintenance is indicated, presenting a risk for tardive dyskinesia (see Section IV.A.2.d).

1. Short-Term Efficacy

a. Phenothiazines

The low-potency drugs chlorpromazine and thioridazine were among the first antipsychotic agents used in the treatment of hyperactivity in children of normal intelligence.[100,102] In controlled trials,[100,102,103] both drugs were shown to reduce hyperactivity and impulsivity at average daily doses of 5 mg/kg. Side effects included drowsiness, which declined with time,[102,103] photosensitization of skin (chlorpromazine[102]), enuresis (thioridazine[100]), and dry mouth. Of interest, an earlier placebo-controlled study reported a synergistic action of thioridazine with stimulants in hyperactive children.[100]

b. Butyrophenones

Among high-potency antipsychotics, haloperidol (0.025 mg/kg) was superior to placebo in reducing behavioral symptoms, including hyperactivity,[50] and was as effective as methylphenidate (0.3 mg/kg). A higher dose (0.05 mg/kg) of haloperidol was no more (less on some measures) effective in reducing behavioral symptoms and significantly increased side effects (especially dystonic reactions).

The effectiveness of thioridazine diminished between weeks 4 and 12 of treatment.[100] Hence, some level of tolerance, not usually seen with stimulants (Chapter 8), may develop with continued use of antipsychotics.

2. Effects on Cognition

The effects of antipsychotics on cognition and performance have been well researched in hyperactive children. Chlorpromazine (5 mg/kg per day) had either no effect or only a slight (nonsignificant) adverse effect on intellectual function, and no effect on distractibility measured by the number of shifts of playroom activities, which was significantly reduced by dextroamphetamine.[102,103] In addition to behavioral ratings, effects of drug on memory, vigilance, reaction time, and seat movements in the laboratory were critically assessed.[55] Haloperidol at 0.025 mg/kg per day over a 3-week period improved some cognitive functions slightly, whereas at 0.05 mg/kg per day it had an adverse effect on a short-term memory test.[55]

The results of these studies suggest that low doses of antipsychotics have little effect on cognitive function, and this may be secondary to better control of overactivity in these children. However, other studies indicate that not only the dose, but also the diagnosis, is an important factor,[6,58,59] and the above statement may not be true of other disorders (e.g., conduct disorder).

In summary, while not a first-line treatment, neuroleptics can be effective in treating hyperactivity and impulsivity in children with ADHD. They should be considered only after stimulants have failed and in severe cases. Neuroleptics do not appear to improve cognitive function significantly.

For more detailed discussion, reviews on this specific issue are recommended[55,104] (see also Chapters 5 and 8).

III. PHARMACOLOGY

A. Pharmacodynamics

There is evidence that abnormalities of neurotransmitter systems may underlie some psychiatric disorders, behavioral symptoms, and cognitive abnormalities. It follows that neuroreceptor-binding data may help the prediction of selective efficacy of antipsychotic and other therapeutic agents.[62] This may not only be of theoretical interest but also of practical/clinical value and may lead to rational pharmacotherapy.[62,63] However, except in one or two disorders such as schizophrenia or Tourette's disorder, the role of antipsychotic drugs is unknown and probably nonspecific.[2] Further, some problems in children and adolescents may stem from abnormal learning rather than abnormal brain function.

Antipsychotic drugs interact selectively with the receptors of a variety of classes of neurotransmitters in the brains of both laboratory animals and humans (Table 3).[62] These

TABLE 3. Receptor Affinities
of Representative Antipsychotic Drugs[a]

Drug	Neuroreceptor antagonized[b]				
	D_2	5-HT$_2$	α_1	ACh	H_1
Typical					
Chlorpromazine	++	+	++±	+	++
Thioridazine	++	+	++	++	+
Trifluoperazine	++±	±	±	±	±
Haloperidol	+++	±	+	−	−
Thiothixene	+++	+	+	−	±
Molindone	+	−	−	−	−
Loxapine	++	++±	−	−	++±
Pimozide	+++±	±	−	−	−
Atypical					
Clozapine	±	++	++	+++	++±
Risperidone	++++	+++++	+++	−	++
Olanzapine	+++	++++	+++	+++++	++++
Quetiapine[c]	++	+	++++	+++	++++
Sertindole[c]	+++++	++++	+++	+	+
Ziprasidone[c]	+++	++++	++	−	+

[a]Data are only illustrative—sources vary according to tissue used. Sources: Jann MW: *Pharmacotherapy* 11:179–195, 1991; Leysen JE: in Burrows GD, Werry JS (eds): *Advances in Human Psychopharmacology*. Greenwich, Conn, JAI Press, 1984, vol 3, pp. 315–356; Meltzer HY, Nash JF: *Pharmacol Rev* 43:587–604, 1991; Whitaker A, Rao U: *Psychiatr Clin North Am* 15:243–276, 1992.
[b]D_2 (*dopamine$_2$*): antipsychotic, extrapyramidal symptoms (EPS) ↑, chemoreceptor-induced emesis ↓, galactorrhea and other endocrine effects. *5-HT* (*serotonin*): ? antipsychotic, EPS ↓, ? negative symptoms ↓, ? arousal ↑, headaches, sexual dysfunction. α_1 (*adrenergic*): QT$_c$ prolongation (risk for cardiac arrhythmia in overdose), priapism, orthostatic hypotension, tachycardia, sedation. *ACh* (*cholinergic muscarinic*): EPS ↓, atropinic syndrome (sedation, dry mouth, delirium, constipation, urinary retention, blurred vision, sinus tachycardia, etc.), cognition ↓, motion nausea ↓. H_1 (*histaminergic*): ? sedation, ? hypotension, ? appetite stimulation, weight gain.
[c]Experimental drugs (not FDA approved), but close to clinical use. Sertindole is expected to be released in the near future.

include receptors of the dopaminergic, serotonergic, α-adrenergic, histaminergic, and cholinergic systems as well as of calcium channels.[62,105–109] Within the dopaminergic system, at least five types of receptors have been identified and different antipsychotics have differing affinities for these,[105,106] as they do for other types of receptors. Variations in receptor action differ between typical and atypical antipsychotics and influence their side-effect profiles. Binding to adrenergic and cholinergic receptors is particularly important in determining adverse effects. Both the effectiveness and side effects of antipsychotics have been related to their selective affinities and interactions with neurotransmitter receptors.[107–109] An understanding of these cellular effects can be helpful to the clinician and remove some empiricism in the choice of pharmacotherapy.

Atypical antipsychotics are defined in several ways. In preclinical research, the term atypical refers to compounds effective in psychosis models (i.e., dextroamphetamine-induced excitation model) but without effects in extrapyramidal syndrome (EPS) models (i.e., dopamine antagonist-induced catalepsy). In the clinical literature, an atypical antipsychotic indicates either (1) a drug effective against negative symptoms of schizophrenia, effective in treatment-resistant patients, and with reduced risk of producing EPS or (2) a drug as effective as haloperidol but with lower risk of producing EPS. The low incidence of EPS associated with clozapine treatment is probably the result of a low affinity for D_2

receptors.[110] Furthermore, Pilowsky et al.[111] showed that D_2 receptor occupancy was not the only factor contributing to antipsychotic effects, which would explain the therapeutic efficacy of clozapine despite its low affinity for D_2 receptors. A role for D_1 and particularly D_4 dopamine receptors, as well as for 5-HT$_2$ and 5-HT$_1$ serotoninergic receptors, has been hypothesized on the basis of their high occupancy rates by clozapine.[112–115] It was even suggested that clozapine's clinical action is not mediated by dopaminergic systems in light of findings that the destruction of dopamine terminals with 6-hydroxydopamine did not influence the pattern of cerebral activation indexed by c-fos induction after clozapine administration.[116] Meltzer[117] proposed that the low EPS profile and the efficacy in reducing negative symptoms reflect the combined action on 5-HT$_{2A}$ and D_4 receptors. The lower incidence of EPS with atypical antipsychotics is challenged in children by the recent report of high incidence of EPS in a group of 10 children (7–17 years) treated with low-dose risperidone.[118] This finding may reflect developmental changes in pharmacodynamics due to the maturation of neurotransmitter systems, particularly the dopaminergic system.[119]

The strong affinity of clozapine for cholinergic receptors[120] accounts not only for atropinic side effects but also possibly for behavioral symptoms "rebound psychosis or supersensitivity psychosis" associated with abrupt discontinuation.[121–124]

B. Pharmacokinetics

Studies of the pharmacokinetics of antipsychotics in children and adolescents are scarce, even though antipsychotics are commonly prescribed in young persons, particularly in those individuals with chronic disorder. It is thus necessary to extrapolate from the substantial data for adult patients, while recognizing the limitations of such inferences.

1. Oral Administration

Antipsychotics are differentially absorbed from the gastrointestinal (GI) tract. GI absorption depends on a large but individually variable first-pass effect, which presumably contributes to the wide interindividual variation (20-fold) of blood levels for a given dose. Antipsychotics are highly lipid-soluble, which both restricts the usefulness of blood level measurements and causes rapid entry into brain and other lipid tissues. Thioridazine is an anomaly; it is highly water-soluble, resulting in very high blood levels, which have been linked to reputed greater cardiotoxicity of this drug.

The half-life of these drugs varies but ranges between 20 and 40 hr in adults. However, because of their high lipid solubility, they take at least four times longer to reach a pharmacodynamic equilibrium (see Chapter 2) and at least several days to lose pharmacological effects after cessation of dosage. In short, they are long-acting drugs, both in achieving pharmacodynamic equilibrium and in clearing the body. Elimination is accomplished largely by deactivation in the liver to water-soluble derivatives like glucuronides; excretion is by the kidney, though biliary excretion is also important. Chlorpromazine, the first and best studied of the antipsychotics, produces almost 200 metabolites, some of which are active, so that effective elimination of effect may be even longer.

2. Parenteral Administration

Intramuscular or intravenous administration is not recommended for children or adolescents. Intravenous administration carries a risk of cardiotoxicity (cardiotoxic bolus) if the injection is too rapid; extravasation of the drug can result in tissue damage and even arterial spasm. Low-potency drugs like chlorpromazine and thioridazine are extremely irritating and cannot be recommended for parenteral use.

3. Depot Preparations

Depot preparations are not recommended for use in children and adolescents because of lack of knowledge about their efficacy and safety. However, in adolescents with schizophrenia, if there is good evidence of efficacy of antipsychotic but poor compliance and repeated psychotic episodes or progressive deterioration, depot preparations could be considered with due attention to the medicolegal issues involved.

4. Therapeutic Effect

Pharmacokinetic data speak only to the movement of the drug into, within, and out of the body. Therapeutic effect may not mirror these movements closely. In psychoses, the antipsychotic and antimanic effects may take several days or more to appear (see above).

5. Blood Levels

Because of the huge interindividual variations (up to 20-fold) in blood levels, and the lack of relationship between levels and therapeutic effect, measurement of blood levels has little value clinically except (1) when there is no therapeutic effect even with high dosage and (2) when there is unexpected toxicity at low dosage.

6. Pharmacokinetics in Children

In general, drugs are eliminated more rapidly in children than in adults[125] (Chapter 2). Age of subjects and half-life of chlorpromazine were found to be highly correlated.[126] As in adults, there is a 15-fold intersubject difference in haloperidol blood levels[127] and there is no correlation between blood levels and dosage.[128] Doses of 0.25–3.0 mg of haloperidol yielded levels of 0.5–8.3 ng/mL.[128]

Data on the relationship between plasma antipsychotic levels and clinical response in children and adolescents are sparse and controversial. While one study[129] found that plasma chlorpromazine levels of 40–80 ng/mL (at daily doses higher than 6 mg/kg) were required for a clinical response, another[125] showed a response to chlorpromazine at 6–11 ng/mL (50–100 mg/day) in six adolescents with psychotic depression. In autistic children, the higher the plasma levels, the greater was the reduction of symptoms in the short term but not over the longer term.[130] Induction of enzymes has been shown to occur with chlorpromazine, and, as a result, drug plasma levels diminished over time.[129] This effect may explain the greater clinical efficacy of thioridazine at week 4 than at week 12 in hyperactive children.[100] Knowledge of the individual activies of the cytochrome P450 enzymes that are responsible for metabolizing most psychotropics could be very useful for the clinician to predict response and risks from drug interactions.[131]

7. Interactions

Data on drug interactions with antipsychotics are limited. Plasma levels of antipsychotics are influenced by concurrent drug treatment.[132] For example, plasma levels of clozapine may be increased by concomitant cimetidine and reduced by phenytoin administration.[133] Plasma levels of nortriptyline appear unchanged when chlorpromazine is simultaneously administered and vice versa,[41] though this may not be true of imipramine. There are no other data for children. Studies in adult patients, however, suggest interactions with all other sedating drugs, antihypertensives, and cardiac medications. Carbamazepine (Tegretol®), sometimes used as an adjunctive agent in the treatment of "excited" states of treatment-resistant populations, lowers plasma levels of most antipsychotics by an average of 30%. Lithium, used in combination with antipsychotics for manic symptoms, may complicate fluid balance, particularly as antipsychotics increase sedation and loss of fluid. Benzodiazepines have potentially synergistic effects with clozapine in inducing respiratory depression and have been reported unsafe to use in combination with this agent. Many of the antipsychotics, including the newer atypical antipsychotics clozapine and risperidone, are metabolized by the P450 isoenzymes, including P450 CYP2D6.[134] Many other drugs are also metabolized by this enzyme system, leading to important drug interactions. For example, these enzymes are important in the metabolism of specific serotonin reuptake inhibitors (SSRIs), such that the use of the SSRIs can lead to elevations in antipsychotic blood levels and subsequent increased side effects.[135,136] Extrapyramidal side effects have been reported to occur after the addition of an SSRI to an antipsychotic treatment or the use of SSRIs in individuals who had received antipsychotics previously.[136] An alternative explanation for this interaction is a potential inhibitory influence of serotonergic activity on nigrostriatal function that is already impaired. In any case, blood levels of neuroleptics and EPS should be carefully monitored when an SSRI is combined with neuroleptics.

IV. SIDE EFFECTS

As already noted, antipsychotic drugs block differing but usually multiple combinations of receptors, which, in turn, leads to predictable side effects. A good knowledge of the relative receptor action profile of individual drugs will allow choice of side effects and their prevention. Few of these untoward effects are life-threatening. In fact, antipsychotics have one of the highest therapeutic-to-toxic ratios of any drug in medicine.

In general, antipsychotics can be grouped into two classes:

1. *Low-potency neuroleptics.* These drugs are more anticholinergic (generally also adrenolytic, antihistaminic, and serotoninolytic) than high-potency drugs. This group includes chlorpromazine, thioridazine, and clozapine. Because of their wide receptor action profile, they can cause many vegetative side effects. However, their anticholinergic action often prevents extrapyramidal symptoms.

2. *High-potency neuroleptics.* These drugs tend to have a somewhat "cleaner" profile and cause fewer side effects; especially, they have a lower incidence of sedation, atropinic symptoms, and hypotension. However, this group has a higher incidence of extrapyramidal symptoms.

Side effects of the antipsychotics will be described by systems.

A. Effects on the Central Nervous System

Anticholinergic (and possibly antihistaminic) actions result in a sedation unlike that produced by antidepressants (see Chapter 9), in that arousal is perhaps more readily achieved. Dopamine blockade in the nigrostriatal tract causes parkinsonian, dystonic, and other extrapyramidal side effects (see Section IV.A.2 below). In the chemoreceptor trigger zone of the vomiting center, dopamine blockade is antiemetic and is useful in toxic and chemotherapy conditions. It also inhibits the tuberoinfundibular system, leading to increased prolactin release and presumably galactorrhea and menstrual disturbances in some patients. In the mesolimbic and mesocortical systems, dopamine blockade is thought to produce ataraxis, a distinctive type of sedation characterized by arousable anhedonic indifference to environmental stimuli. In turn, this effect may mediate (however remotely) the fundamental antipsychotic effect, by reducing information flow and hence the "cognitive overload" thought to characterize schizophrenia. Serotonin blockade in the prefrontal region may reduce negative symptoms. Anticholinergic blockade can be useful in motion sickness, though drugs with fewer receptor-blocking actions such as scopolamine are preferable. Several antipsychotics, clozapine and chlorpromazine particularly, lower the seizure threshold. Central hypothalamic and peripheral adrenergic inhibition may lead to fluctuations in body temperature regulation.

Central nervous system adverse effects include behavioral toxicity, extrapyramidal side effects, sedation, seizures, and withdrawal symptoms.

1. Behavioral Toxicity

Behavioral toxicity occurs in children receiving antipsychotics often before the emergence of any extrapyramidal side effect (except dystonic reactions) or sedation.[5,58,59] It takes the form of either worsening of existing behavioral symptoms or the development of new ones, most commonly, irritability, depressive affect, apathy, and decreased or, paradoxically, increased motor activity (hyperactivity). Dysphoria, aggression, and school phobia have been reported with haloperidol in children with Tourette's disorder.[81,137] Behavioral toxicity is important to recognize, because it may lead either to the erroneous belief that the medication is ineffective or to the increase of dosage and subsequent appearance of other adverse effects. A stable pretreatment baseline behavioral evaluation is desirable to recognize behavioral toxicity.

2. Extrapyramidal Side Effects

Extrapyramidal side effects include acute dystonic reactions (muscle spasms), parkinsonian symptoms (muscle rigidity), akathisia (restless legs), and abnormal involuntary movements, such as dyskinesias and tardive dyskinesia. Acute dystonic reactions, parkinsonian symptoms, akathisia, and akinesia usually appear early, within hours, days, or weeks of onset of treatment; however, they can also appear later, particularly if there is a change in medication regimen or addition of a medication.

a. Acute Dystonic Reaction

An acute dystonic reaction usually develops early in treatment, within 1–12 hr[138] after drug administration or increase in dose; however, dystonic reactions can occur anytime, particularly within the first few weeks of an initial antipsychotic trial. An acute dystonic reaction may manifest itself as torticollis (neck twisted to the side), oculogyric crisis (eyes rolled back under lids), or dystonia of the tongue, esophagus, or trunk. It may be relieved quickly by oral or intramuscular administration of anticholinergic drugs such as benztropine (1–2 mg) or diphenhydramine (25 mg). To avoid acute dystonic reaction, antipsychotic drugs, particularly the high-potency agents, should be started at a low subclinical dose.

The two atypical antipsychotics currently marketed in the U.S. market, clozapine and risperidone, have both received attention because of the potential decreased incidence rate of dystonic reactions, as well as other EPS. However, it is unclear whether children and adolescents also experience a lower incidence of EPS with these drugs. Several open studies of risperidone and clozapine in children have indicated a relatively high incidence of extrapyramidal symptoms.[32,118,139] This heightened sensitivity to EPS in children is consistent with reports of higher incidence of EPS in children and adolescents[140] and with findings in laboratory animals showing an age-related decline in the neurochemical potency of various neuroleptics (up to 75- fold between the neonatal period and adulthood).

b. Parkinsonian Side Effects

Parkinsonian side effects may begin as early as the first 2–3 weeks of treatment and are manifested as fixed facial expression, drooling, pill rolling, tremor (6 cps), lack of arm swinging when walking, and the cogwheel or clasp-knife phenomenon in limbs. They may be rare in preschool-age children[59] but are seen quite frequently in older children[6] and adolescents. In one study, 34% of 61 children and adolescents (aged 10–18) developed parkinsonian side effects.[141] Further, in a fifth of those who did, the symptoms persisted for some time after discontinuation of the antipsychotic agent.[141] Unless symptoms are severe, decrease of dosage should be considered rather than administration of an antiparkinsonian agent, which may produce atropinic side effects such as behavioral disorganization and impairment of cognition; these latter drugs also aggravate tardive dyskinesia, although they probably do not contribute to its actual development.[142] Akinesia (or bradykinesia) usually develops as part of parkinsonism after 5–30 days of antipsychotic treatment. It is characterized by diminished gestures, movements, spontaneity, emotions, and speech.[143,144] Parkinsonism may be difficult to differentiate from depression, which is not uncommon after an acute schizophrenic psychotic episode. The rate of akinesia in this young age group is not known. Two studies of large samples of children and adolescents did not report occurrence of akinesia.[81,141]

c. Akathisia

Akathisia usually appears within 5–60 days. It is characterized behaviorally by motor restlessness and pacing and internally by the feeling of being driven. It is reported in 1.2%–11%[145] of children and in up to 75% of adults[146] who are on antipsychotics. Akinesia is difficult to differentiate from agitation or worsening of preexisting hyperactivity (behavioral toxicity), especially in psychotic children who may have difficulty verbalizing the characteristic discomfort. In a recent study of hospitalized children and adolescents aged 10–18, only 2% developed akathisia[141]; 4% of patients with Tourette's disorder (under 18 years of age), who are treated most commonly with haloperidol, developed akathisia.[81] Rate of occurrence of akathisia may be lower in children and adolescents than in adults. The etiology of akathisia is unclear since, unlike parkinsonism, it responds only unpredictably to antiparkinsonian drugs.[138] Propranolol (0.3–1.2 mg/kg per day) or benzodiazepines[138] may be more effective in treating this symptom. Reduction in antipsychotic dosage should be tried first, if feasible.

d. Abnormal Involuntary Movements (Dyskinesias) and Tardive Dyskinesia

i. **Dyskinesias**   These are another type of extrapyramidal disorder related to antipsychotic administration. They are most commonly associated with long-term treatment and thought to represent upregulation of dopamine receptors by chronic blockade. Dyskinesias are abnormal involuntary movements that can involve the muscles of any part of the body, but most frequently the muscles of the mouth, face, tongue and jaws, and upper extremities. The movements may be slow and rhythmical, vermicular (tongue), or irregular (athetotic, choreiform, ticlike), or they may take the form of ataxia and apraxia. As in adults, the topography of dyskinesias in children and adolescents is mainly orofacial and buccolingual.[147,148] The disorder may involve muscles of the diaphragm or larynx and be expressed as respiratory dyskinesias (grunts or other types of unusual vocalizations). A Tourette-like syndrome associated with long-term administration of haloperidol has also been reported.[149,150] Although most commonly associated with administration of antipsychotics, dyskinesias were reported with a variety of other drugs, including antihistamines[151,152] and antiseizure medication.[153] For a fuller review and discussion of methodological issues, the reader is referred to an American Psychiatric Association Task Force report[142] (see also Refs. 148 and 154–156). Drug-related dyskinesias are classified into tardive dyskinesia (of later onset during chronic treatment), covert dyskinesias (developing only upon lowering of the dose), and withdrawal dyskinesias (upon drug withdrawal).[142,157,158] The reported prevalence of tardive dyskinesias in children and adolescents varies from 8%[159] to 28%[160] to 51%.[161]

The differential diagnosis of drug-related dyskinesias includes tic disorders,[149] stereotypies,[145,148] and rocking in autism, mental retardation, and schizophrenia.[162] In some cases, dyskinesias cannot be distinguished from stereotypies (voluntary habits) by blind raters.[163] Drug-related dyskinesias should also be differentiated from other disorders associated with abnormal involuntary movements. To establish the diagnosis of drug-related movements, a reliable history of prior medication is important. Helpful criteria for more precise diagnosis of abnormal involuntary movements have been described.[164]

Prior to any psychoactive drug administration, each patient should be examined and rated on the AIMS[18] (or similar instrument) using procedures developed for children[19] (see also Chapter 4); patients should be monitored at fixed intervals during administration of the antipsychotic agent and weekly after its discontinuation. Two recent studies suggested that dose is not related to the development of dyskinesias[141,147]; these findings are controversial, and prudence recommends the use of the lowest therapeutically effective dose. Other risk factors in adults are female sex, mood disorder, and older age. Clozapine has a lower risk of tardive dyskinesia than do the other classical antipsychotics.

In a retrospective study, 12% of adolescents (14–18 years of age) developed tardive dyskinesia.[141] In a prospective long-term study of haloperidol, 29% of autistic children developed reversible dyskinesias,[147] 6% while receiving haloperidol; the remaining 23% developed withdrawal dyskinesias 4–34 days after drug withdrawal (mean, 14 days). Most movements ceased spontaneously within 7 days, but some lasted up to 7.5 months.[147] Cumulative haloperidol exposure prior to development of dyskinesias ranged from 56 days to 1875 days (median, 367 days).[147] In a sample of 104 children, 29 developed dyskinesias[165]; 15 of the 29 developed dyskinesias only once, and the remainder two to five times.[166] Children who had repeated dyskinesias could not be differentiated on any clinical or demographic characteristics from those who developed dyskinesias only once.[166]

Compared to the typical neuroleptics, clozapine has a low rate of occurrence of dyskinesias in adults.[167] It is too early to know whether the same will be true for children and adolescents. Hopefully, the rate of dyskinesias will be low also with risperidone, but again it is too early to be determined. Further research in this area is needed. Studies of risperidone have reported dyskinesias in adults[168] and withdrawal dyskinesias in children (Rowan, A. B. and Malone, R. P., unpublished).

ii. Tardive dystonia. This is an extrapyramidal side effect characterized by slow movements around the long axis of the body, ending in spasm, and is usually seen together with tardive dyskinesia.[142,169] It can be quite disabling,[142] and the spasms may also involve the facial muscles. A 15-year-old boy was shown to have both tardive dyskinesia and tardive dystonia; the latter involved 20- to 30-sec hypertonic episodes of neck, limb, and trunk posturings[170] while tardive dyskinesia comprised choreoathetotic movements, orofacial–lingual movements, and grimacing as well as dysarthria. The movement disorder lasted 5 months. Although young age and male sex are reported to be predisposing factors, no case of tardive dystonia was identified in 104 hospitalized patients aged 10–18 years, of whom two-thirds were boys.[141]

In conclusion, neuroleptic-related dyskinesias are the major long-term risk factor associated with neuroleptic administration. Children treated with neuroleptics should be carefully evaluated for abnormal movements already present at baseline (particularly in autism and mental retardation) and regularly during treatment. Periodic drug holidays should be considered to assess the need for continued drug treatment. Potential occurrence of withdrawal dyskinesias is to be carefully monitored during these drug discontinuation periods as they may change the risk/benefit ratio of the neuroleptic treatment. Withdrawal dyskinesias may indicate higher risk for tardive dyskinesia, and severe withdrawal dyskinesias may justify not resuming treatment.

Note: Rabbit syndrome[171] is a late-onset extrapyramidal side effect, characterized by rapid movements of the perioral muscles. Unlike tardive dyskinesia, these abnormal movements may be reduced by antiparkinsonian agents.

3. Sedation

The most common short-term side effect associated with antipsychotic treatment is excessive sedation (sleepiness or falling asleep), stemming from anticholinergic, adrenolytic, and, probably, dopaminolytic actions, implying that low-potency drugs will be most sedative. However, even with the high-potency antipsychotic haloperidol, sedation is the most common side effect, though at above therapeutic doses.[5,6,58,59,172] Pimozide may be less sedative.[63]

4. Seizures

Neuroleptics lower seizure threshold. Caution should be exercised in selecting antipsychotics for children with a known seizure disorder or EEG abnormalities, brain damage, or autism. As noted above, chlorpromazine is known to lower the seizure threshold and to increase the frequency of seizures in mentally retarded persons.[66] Thioridazine seems to carry less risk[68] and was even reported to decrease the frequency of seizures.[67] Clozapine warrants special consideration and is reviewed in Section IV.K, below.

5. Withdrawal Symptoms

Antipsychotics block neurotransmitter receptors of several types. Receptor blockade leads to receptor hypersensitivity as a compensatory mechanism. Consequently, withdrawal of the drug may lead to rebound symptoms, especially of a cholinergic type. Following discontinuation of antipsychotics, withdrawal phenomena rather similar to those seen with most drugs of dependence (see Chapter 11) may include vomiting, nausea, loss of appetite, diaphoresis, insomnia, agitation, destructiveness, and irritability.[160] These withdrawal phenomena cease within 8 weeks.[160] During a 4-week haloperidol withdrawal period, most autistic children gained weight, and only a few lost weight (under 1 kg).[173]

B. Effects on the Autonomic Nervous System

Anticholinergic actions produce an atropinic syndrome that is responsible for a number of minor side effects. Adrenolytic actions are most manifest in the cardiovascular system but may also affect other functions.

Anticholinergic side effects may include blurred vision, pupillary dilation, exacerbation of narrow-angle glaucoma, decreased salivation (dry mouth), decreased bronchial or other pulmonary secretions (which could lead to an exacerbation of asthma), tachycardia, decreased sweating, flushing, postural hypotension, constipation, paralytic ileus, retrograde ejaculation, and bladder paralysis.

C. Neuroleptic Malignant Syndrome

Neuroleptic malignant syndrome is a rare but serious condition. It is characterized by hyperthermia, extrapyramidal–parkinsonian symptoms, autonomic lability, and raised creatinine phosphokinase.[143,174–176] Onset is usually early in the treatment course, after dosage increase, change to another drug, or discontinuation of an antiparkinsonian agent. Persons of any age can be affected, including children and adolescents.[177,178] An emergency medical workup should be carried out immediately, the antipsychotic drug discontinued, and vigorous treatment in a critical care unit initiated. Treatment includes administration of an anticholinergic or a dopaminergic agent (e.g., bromocriptine) and life support (see Refs. 100–105).

For further discussion of acute side effects, their measurement, and laboratory monitoring, see Chapter 4 and Refs. 27, 104, and 109.

D. Cardiovascular Effects

The most common side effect is a benign tachycardia, but the most important clinically by far is orthostatic hypotension (i.e., faintness when standing up).[2,3,7,138,174]

Antipsychotics produce complex effects on cardiac conduction and excitability, primarily a quinidine-like slowing seen by a lengthening of the QTR interval beyond 0.44 sec on the electrocardiogram (ECG).[2,80,174] The cardiotoxic significance of these changes is disputed, and they may be transitory.[80] ECG may be considered especially when higher doses of antipsychotics are contemplated (e.g., >5 mg/kg per day CPZ equivalents) even though the risk is extremely low and contentious.[174] In cases of sudden death, it is difficult to determine whether an antipsychotic agent has a causal or contributory role or is merely coincidental. Sudden death in psychiatric patients was well described before the advent of antipsychotic drugs. A task force set up by the American Psychiatric Association[174] concluded that sudden cardiac death caused by antipsychotic drugs has not been firmly established and that, if it does occur, it must be rare; otherwise, it would have emerged clearly by now. Unlike patients on antidepressants, the overwhelming majority of patients on antipsychotics are unlikely to benefit from routine ECGs in the absence of cardiac disease and/or very high dosages. Pimozide is under particular scrutiny, and daily doses no higher than 0.3 mg/kg are recommended. Studies of ECG changes in children are limited. One study of eight autistic children failed to find any ECG changes with pimozide treatment.[63]

E. Endocrine Effects

Dopamine blockade in the tuberoinfundibular system can lead to increased prolactin release. As a result, breast enlargement, galactorrhea, menstrual abnormalities, and, in males, impotence may occur. Weight gain is frequent, especially with clozapine and low-potency neuroleptics, but can be controlled with diet and exercise. Some patients may experience hyperglycemia.

The long-term effects of neuroleptics on growth have not been widely investigated. During haloperidol treatment, autistic children (aged 2–7 years) showed a significant weight gain of 8 percentiles and a slight nonsignificant decrement in height (4.7 percentiles),[179] both measured by the growth charts of the National Center of Health Statistics.[180]

F. Effects on the Eye

Retinitis pigmentosa associated with very large doses of thioridazine (> 10 mg/kg) results in impairment of visual acuity and night vision by retinal deposits of brown pigment observable on fundus examination.[143] Corneal and lenticular opacities have been reported with chlorpromazine,[2] especially in young patients with mental retardation. However, in view of the widespread use of thioridazine and chlorpromazine, these eye complications seem to be rare.

G. Skin Reactions and Photosensitivity

Photosensitive skin reactions are seen with neuroleptics, especially chlorpromazine,[143] due to breakdown of the skin by ultraviolet light causing a histamine reaction in children.[102] Patients should be forewarned to use sun blockers and hats and to avoid sun exposure, especially at peak hours; a substitution of chlorpromazine is probably the best course to follow. Skin rashes may also occur with the use of antipsychotics as part of an allergic reaction; a change to a different type of antipsychotic drug is then advisable.

H. Blood Dyscrasias

Agranulocytosis may occur with any antipsychotic medication; the peak onset is between 3 and 8 weeks. It may appear acutely, in between routine blood tests. Practitioners should be alert for fever, sore throat, or other signs of infection that may indicate agranulocytosis. Agranulocytosis during clozapine treatment warrents special consideration and is discussed below in Section IV.K.

I. Hepatic Dysfunction

Abnormalities in liver function (e.g., elevated liver enzymes and cholestatic jaundice) have been reported infrequently, particularly with chlorpromazine and clozapine.[7]

J. Tissue Necrosis and Vasculitis

Intramuscular or intravenous injection of neuroleptics may result in local tissue necrosis and vasculitis, especially with the low-potency antipsychotics, possibly because of the higher concentration injected.

K. Clozapine: Special Considerations

The most serious side effect of clozapine is agranulocytosis which is life-threatening. Clozapine produces agranulocytosis (granulocyte count of <500/mm³) in approximately 1% of cases, which restricts the use of this drug to the treatment of severe and refractory cases of schizophrenia. It is recommended that clozapine be discontinued if the total white cell count falls below 2000/mm³, or if the granulocyte count is below 1000/mm³.[181] The most vulnerable period for developing agranulocytosis is between weeks 6 and 18 of clozapine administration. The white cell count should be monitored weekly in the first 18 weeks of treatment and monthly thereafter. For the management of clozapine-induced agranulocytosis, see Van Kammen and Marder.[181] The exact incidence of clozapine-induced agranulocytosis in children and adolescents is unknown, although some cases have been reported.[182] Clozapine-induced agranulocytosis appears to be associated with increased age and female gender. There is some evidence of a specific genetic predisposition [e.g., Ashkenazi Jews with human leukocyte antigen (HLA) haplotype B38, DR4, DQW3[183]].

Clozapine increases the incidence of seizures in adults, particularly at dosages above 600 mg per day.[184] This effect may be generalizable to the use of clozapine in adolescents.[185] Baseline EEGs may be indicated in children and adolescents before initiation of clozapine treatment.[185]

Other side effects of clozapine include sialorrhea (drooling), weight gain, orthostatic hypotension, sedation, liver function abnormalities, enuresis, gastrointestinal symptoms, constipation, ECG abnormalities, tachycardia, and fever.[186]

Clozapine withdrawal has been associated with "supersensitivity psychosis" or rebound psychosis.[121] Abrupt withdrawal produced anxiety, insomnia, motor restlessness or mute withdrawal, psychosis, tardive dyskinesia, altered consciousness, confusion, nausea, and diaphoresis.[110,121,187–190] These symptoms may be due to a cholinergic overdrive in response to clozapine's strong anticholinergic action.[122] Dosage should be slowly tapered, but if side effects necessitate rapid discontinuation, anticholinergics may be used to reduce withdrawal symptoms.

Despite the risks of blood dyscrasias, clozapine is a valuable drug in some cases of schizophrenia. Also, with careful monitoring, the risks are probably less than those of many other drugs used in medicine.

V. OVERDOSE AND MANAGEMENT

In assessing a neuroleptic overdose, the physician should determine whether other medications were also ingested because the use of multiple drugs is common in overdose situations, and adverse effects of drug interactions are possible.[134]

The antipsychotics have a high therapeutic index and are generally safe. Symptoms of an overdose are often an exaggeration of known pharmacological effects and adverse reactions. The most significant adverse reactions are neurological and cardiovascular.[191] Neurological adverse effects include extrapyramidal reactions, sedation, agitation, confusion, delirium, and seizures. Cardiovascular effects include hypotension and ECG abnormalities. Haloperidol has been reported to cause hypertension in children.[192] Urinary retention as a result of anticholinergic effects can also occur.

There is no specific antidote for a particular antipsychotic overdose. Treatment is primarily symptomatic and supportive. It is important to maintain an open airway as respiratory depression may occur. Additionally, extrapyramidal effects may produce dysphagia and respiratory difficulty. Activated charcoal may slow absorption in the first hours after intake, and gastric lavage may also be helpful up to several hours after ingestion because the anticholinergic effects of many antipsychotics can slow stomach emptying.[193] Although some manufacturers recommend emesis, others recommend against it because of the possibility that a dystonic reaction of the head and neck could result in aspiration of vomitus[16] Precautions against aspiration must be taken, especially in infants and children. Extrapyramidal symptoms may be treated with antiparkinson drugs or diphenhydramine.

Intravenous fluids, plasma, concentrated albumin, and vasopressor agents may be used to treat hypotension and circulatory collapse. However, epinephrine, dopamine, or other sympathomimetics with β-agonistic activity should not be used.[16] The antipsychotics can cause α-blockade, and the β-agonistic agents can actually lead to further hypotension. Stimulants, such as picrotoxin or pentylenetetrazol, may cause seizures, and their use should be avoided. Monitoring ECG for QRS and QT changes, tachycardia, bundle branch block, ventricular fibrillation, and cardiac arrest is important. ECG abnormalities are particularly noted with thioridazine.[194] The patient should also be monitored for shock and congestive heart failure. ECG monitoring is recommended for up to 24–72 hours because the effects of antipsychotic overdose can be delayed. The manufacturers of clozapine recommend 100 hours of respiratory and cardiac monitoring in cases of overdoses. The choice of antiarrhythmic agents varies, though many manufacturers recommend digitalis.[16] To control seizures initially, diazepam or lorazapam can be used, or the patient can be loaded with phenytoin.[195]

VI. SUMMARY/CONCLUSIONS

Antipsychotic drugs are useful in several psychiatric disorders in children and adolescents, notably in Tourette's disorder, schizophrenia, major mood disorders, autism, and conduct disorder with aggression. These drugs are also useful in the management of some behavioral symptoms such as hyperactivity, impulsivity, and aggressiveness in young persons of both normal and subnormal intelligence. The drug most frequently recommended for children and adolescents of normal intelligence and for those diagnosed with autistic disorder is haloperidol, and for persons of subnormal intelligence thioridazine. Except in acute psychotic disorders in adolescents, best results are obtained with low doses. There is some evidence that the greater the degree of CNS dysfunction, the lower the minimum effective dose required.

Antipsychotics must be used with caution and surveillance and, except in psychotic disorders and Tourette's disorder, should not be the treatment of choice, because of their short- and long-term side effects, which, though only very rarely life-threatening, can be uncomfortable and/or durable.[142] The emergence of behavioral toxicity, cognitive dulling, and extrapyramidal side effects (including dyskinesias) should be anticipated, carefully monitored, and dealt with by lowering the dosage if at all possible. However, when judiciously prescribed and clinically monitored, with periodic discontinuation, antipsychotics can help maintain a large number of severely disturbed children and adolescents with their families in the community.

REFERENCES

1. Hyman SF, Arana GW, Rosenbaum JF: *Handbook of Psychiatric Drug Therapy*. Boston, Little, Brown and Company, pp. 5–42, 1995.
2. Davis J, Barter J, Kane J: Antipsychotic drugs, in Kaplan H, Sadock B (eds): *Comprehensive Textbook of Psychiatry*. Baltimore, Williams and Wilkins, pp 1591–1621, 1989.
3. Fish B, Shapiro T, Campbell M: Long-term prognosis and the response of schizophrenic children to drug therapy: A controlled study of trifluoperazine. *Am J Psychiatry* 123:32–39, 1966.
4. McClellan J, Werry J: The psychiatric clinics of North America, in Shaffer D (ed): *Schizophrenia*. Philadelphia, WB Saunders, 1996, pp 131–148.
5. Anderson L, Campbell M, Adams P, et al: The effects of haloperidol on discrimination learning and behavioral symptoms in autistic children. *J Autism Dev Disord* 19:227–239, 1989.
6. Campbell M, Small A, Green W, et al: Behavioral efficacy of haloperidol and lithium carbonate: A comparison in hospitalized aggressive children with conduct disorder. *Arch Gen Psychiatry* 41:650–656, 1984.
7. Siefen G, Remschmidt H: Behandlungsergebnisse mit clozapin bei schizophrenen Jugendlichen. *Z Kinder-Jugendpsychiatr* 14:245–257, 1986.
8. Muller-Spahn F: The International Risperidone Research Group. Risperidone in the treatment of chronic schizophrenic patients: An international double-blind parallel-group study versus haloperidol. *Clin Neuropharmacol* 15:90A–91A, 1996.
9. Chouinard G, Jones B, Remington G, et al: A Canadian multicenter, placebo-controlled study of fixed doses of risperidone and haloperidol in the treatment of chronic schizophrenic patients. *J Clin Psychopharmacol* 13:25–40, 1993.
10. Marder S: Risperidone: Clinical development: North American results. *Clin Neuropharmacol* 15:92A–93B, 1992.
11. American Psychiatric Association: *Diagnostic and Statistical Manual of Mental Disorders*, ed 4. Washington, DC. American Psychiatric Association, 1994.
12. American Psychiatric Association: *Diagnostic and Statistical Manual of Mental Disorders,* ed 3. Washington, DC. American Psychiatric Association Press, 1980.
13. American Psychiatric Association: *Diagnostic and Statistical Manual of Mental Disorders*, ed 3, revised. Washington, DC. American Psychiatric Association, 1987.
14. International classification of diseases ICD–9, in: *Manual of the International Classification of Diseases, Injuries and Causes of Death*. Geneva, World Health Organization, 1977.
15. Thompson J, Green D, Savit H: Preliminary report on a crosswalk from DSM-III to ICD-9-CM. *Am J Psychiatry* 140:176–180, 1983.
16. *Physicians' Desk Reference*. Oradell, NJ. Medical Economics, 1992.
17. Simpson G. Pharmacology and treatment of the major psychoses. Paper presented at the 30th Annual Meeting of the American College of Neuropsychopharmacology, 1991.
18. Abnormal Involuntary Movements Scale. *Psychopharmacol Bull* 21:1077–1080, 1985.
19. Campbell M: Protocol for rating drug-related AIMS, stereotypies and CPRS assessments. *Psychopharmacol Bull* 21:1081, 1985.
20. Campbell M, Palij M: Measurement of untoward effects including tardive dyskinesia. *Psychopharmacol Bull* 21:1063–1082, 1985.
21. Campbell M, Spencer E, Kowalik S, et al: Schizophrenic and psychotic disorders, in Wiener J (ed): *Textbook of Child and Adolescent Psychiatry*. Washington, DC. American Psychiatric Association Press, pp 223–239, 1991.

22. Spencer E, Kafantaris V, Padron-Gayol M, et al. Haloperidol in schizophrenic children: Early findings from a study in progress. *Psychopharmacol Bull* 28:183–186, 1992.

23. Spencer E, Alpert M, Pouget E: Scales for the assessment of neuroleptic response in schizophrenic children: Specific measures derived from the CPRS. *Psychopharmacol Bull* 2:199–202, 1994.

24. Pool D, Bloom W, Mielke D, Roniger J, Gallant D: A controlled evaluation of loxitane in seventy-five adolescent schizophrenic patients. *Curr Ther Res* 19:99–104, 1976.

25. Realmuto G, Erickson W, Yellin A, et al: Clinical comparison of thiothixene and thioridazine in schizophrenic adolescents. *Am J Psychiatry* 141:440–442, 1984.

26. Kumra S, Jacobson L, Rapoport J: Childhood-onset schizophrenia: A double-blind clozapine trial. Paper presented at the 149th Annual Meeting of the American Psychiatric Association, 1996.

27. Gordon C, Frazier J, McKenna K, et al: Childhood-onset schizophrenia: An NIMH study in progress. *Schizophr Bull* 20:697–712, 1994.

28. Birmaher B, Baker R, Kapur S, Quintana H, Ganguli R: Clozapine for the treatment of adolescents with schizophrenia. *J Am Acad Child Adolesc Psychiatry* 31:160–164, 1992.

29. Frazier J, Gordon C, McKenna K, Lenane M, Jih D, Rapoport J: An open trial of clozapine in 11 adolescents with childhood-onset schizophrenia. *J Am Acad Child Adolesc Psychiatry* 33:658–663, 1994.

30. Remschmidt H, Schulz E, Martin M, Warnke A, Trott G: Childhood-onset schizophrenia: History of the concept and recent studies. *Schizophr Bull* 20:727–745, 1994.

31. Blanz B, Schimdt M: Clozapine for schizophrenia. *J Am Acad Child Adolesc Psychiatry* 32:223–224, 1993.

32. Remschmidt H, Schulz E, Martin P: An open trial of thirty-six adolescents with schizophrenia. *J Child Adolesc Psychopharmacol* 4:31–41, 1994.

33. Marder S, Meibach R: Risperidone in the treatment of schizophrenia. *Am J Psychiatry* 151:825–835, 1994.

34. Armenteros J, Whitaker A, Joachim N, Jaffer M, Gorman J: An open trial of risperidone in adolescents with schizophrenia. Paper presented at the workshop on: Critical Issues in the Treatment of Schizophrenia. Campaign on Schizophrenia 1995, pp 176–177.

35. Cosgrove F: Recent advances in pediatric psychopharmacology [letter]. *Hum Psychopharmacol* 9:381–382, 1994.

36. Cozza S, Edison D: Risperidone in adolescents [letter]. *J Am Acad Child Adolesc Psychiatry* 33:1211, 1994.

37. Greevich S, Findling R, Schulz S, Rowane W: Risperidone in the treatment of children and adolescents with psychotic illness: A retrospective review. Paper presented at the 148th Annual Meeting of the American Psychiatric Association, 1995.

38. Simeon J, Carrey N, Wiggins D, Milin R, Hosenbocus S: Risperidone effects in treatment-resistant adolescents: Preliminary case reports. *J Child Adolesc Psychopharmacol* 5:69–79, 1995.

39. Sternlicht H, Wells S: Risperidone in childhood schizophrenia [letter]. *J Am Acad Child Adolesc Psychiatry* 34:540, 1995.

40. Werry J, McClellan J, Chard L: Childhood and adolescent schizophrenic, bipolar, and schizoaffective disorder: A clinical and outcome study. *J Am Acad Child Adolesc Psychiatry* 30:457–465, 1991.

41. Geller B, Cooper T, Farooki Z, et al: Dose and plasma levels of nortriptyline and chlorpromazine in delusionally depressed adolescents and of nortriptyline in nondelusionally depressed adolescents. *Am J Psychiatry* 142:336–338, 1985.

42. Loranger A, Levine P: Age at onset of bipolar affective illness. *Arch Gen Psychiatry* 30:457–465, 1991.

43. Carlson G: Child and adolescent mania: Diagnostic considerations. *J Child Psychol Psychiatry* 31:331–341, 1990.

44. Shopsin B, Gershon S, Thompson H, et al: Psychoactive drugs in mania. A controlled comparison of lithium carbonate, chlorpromazine, and haloperidol. *Arch Gen Psychiatry* 32:34–42, 1975.

45. Calabrese J, Kimmel S, Woyshville M, et al: Clozapine for treatment-refractory mania. *Am J Psychiatry* 153:759–764, 1996.

46. Fuchs D: Clozapine treatment of bipolar disorder in a young adolescent. *J Am Acad Child Adolesc Psychiatry* 33:1299–1302, 1994.

47. Kowatch R, Suppes T, Gilfillan S, Fuentes R, Grannemann B, Emslie G: Clozapine treatment of children and adolescents with bipolar disorder and schizophrenia: A clinical case series. *J Am Acad Child Adolesc Psychopharmacol* 5:241–253, 1995.

48. Campbell M, Gonzalez N, Silva R: Shaffer D (eds): *The Pharmacologic Treatment of Conduct Disorders and Rage Outbursts*. Philadelphia, WB Saunders, 1992, pp 69–85.

49. Cunningham M, Pillai V, Rogers W: Haloperidol in the treatment of children with severe behavioural disorders. *Br J Psychiatry* 114:845–854, 1968.

50. Werry J, Aman M, Lampen E: Haloperidol and methylphenidate in hyperactive children. *Acta Paedopsychiatr* 42:26–40, 1975.

51. Greenhill L, Barmack J, Spalten D, et al: Molindone hydrochloride in the treatment of aggressive hospitalized children. *Psychopharmacol Bull* 17:125–127, 1981.
52. Greenhill L, Solomon M, Pleak R, et al: Molindone treatment of hospitalized children with conduct disorder. *J Clin Psychiatry* 46:20–25, 1985.
53. Children's Psychiatric Rating Scale (CPRS). *Psychopharmacol Bull* 21:765–770, 1985.
54. Wong G, Cock R: Long-term effects of haloperidol on severely emotionally disturbed children. *Aust N Z J Psychiatry* 5:296–300, 1971.
55. Werry J, Aman M: Methylphenidate and haloperidol in children: Effects on attention, memory and activity. *Arch Gen Psychiatry* 32:790–795, 1975.
56. Platt J, Campbell M, Green W, et al: Cognitive effects of lithium carbonate and haloperidol in treatment-resistant aggressive children. *Arch Gen Psychiatry* 41:657–662, 1984.
57. Fras I, Major L: Clinical experience with risperidone [letter]. *J Am Acad Child Adolesc Psychiatry* 34:833, 1995.
58. Campbell M, Anderson L, Meier M, et al: A comparison of haloperidol, behavior therapy and their interaction in autistic children. *J Am Acad Child Psychiatry* 17:640–655, 1978.
59. Anderson L, Campbell M, Grega D, et al: Haloperidol in the treatment of infantile autism: Effects on learning and behavioral symptoms. *Am J Psychiatry* 141:1195–1202, 1984.
60. Naruse H, Nagahata M, Nakane Y, et al: A multicenter double-blind trial of pimozide (Orap), haloperidol and placebo in children with behavioral disorders, using crossover design. *Acta Paedopsychiatr* 48:173–184, 1982.
61. Cohen I, Campbell M, Posner D, et al. Behavioral effects of haloperidol in young autistic children: An objective analysis using a within-subjects reversal design. *J Am Acad Child Psychiatry* 19:665–677, 1980.
62. Deutsch S, Campbell M: Relative affinities for different classes of neurotransmitter receptors predict neuroleptic efficacy in infantile autism. *Neuropsychobiology* 15:160–164, 1986.
63. Ernst M, Magee H, Gonzalez N, et al: Pimozide in autistic children. *Psychopharmacol Bull* 27:401–409, 1992.
64. Campbell M: Pharmacotherapy in early infantile autism. *Biol Psychiatry* 10:399–423, 1975.
65. Campbell M, Schopler E: Pervasive developmental disorders, in Karasu TB (chairperson) (ed): *Treatments of Psychiatric Disorders: A Task Force Report*. Washington, DC, American Psychiatric Association Press, 1989, pp 179–294.
66. Tarjan C, Lowery V, Wright S: Use of chlorpromazine in two hundred seventy-eight mentally deficient patients. *AMA J Disturbed Child* 94:294–300, 1957.
67. Pregelj S, Barkauskas A: Thioridazine in the treatment of mentally retarded children. A four-year retroactive evaluation. *J Can Psychiatr Assoc* 12:213–215, 1967.
68. Freeman R: Psychopharmacology and the retarded child, in Menolascino F (ed): *Psychiatric Approaches to Mental Retardation*. New York, Basic Books, 1970, pp 294–368.
69. Campbell M, Fish B, Shapiro T, et al: Thiothixene in young disturbed children: A pilot study. *Arch Gen Psychiatry* 23:70–72, 1970.
70. Campbell M, Fish B, Shapiro T, et al. Study of molindone in disturbed preschool children. *Curr Ther Res* 13:28–33, 1971.
71. Locascio J, Malone R, Small A, et al: Factors related to haloperidol response and dyskinesias in autistic children. *Psychopharmacol Bull* 27:119–126, 1991.
72. Rett A: Uber ein eingenartiges hirntrophicshes Syndrome bei Hyperammonamie in Kindersalter. *Wien Med Wochenschr* 166:723–738, 1996.
73. Perry R, Campbell M, Adams P: Long-term efficacy of haloperidol in autistic children: Continuous versus discontinuous drug administration. *J Am Acad Child Adolesc Psychiatry* 28:87–92, 1989.
74. Die Trill M, Wolsky B, Shell J, et al: Effects of long term haloperidol treatment on intellectual functioning in autistic children: A pilot study. Paper presented at the 31st Annual Meeting of the American Academy of Child and Adolescent Psychiatry, 1984.
75. Shell J, Perry R, Adams P, et al: Effects of long-term haloperidol treatment on intellectual functioning in autistic children. Paper presented at the 34th Annual Meeting of the American Academy of Child and Adolescent Psychiatry, 1987.
76. McDougle C, Brodkin E, Yeung P, Naylor S, Cohen D, Price L: Risperidone in adults with autism or pervasive developmental disorder. *J Child Adolesc Psychopharmacol* 5:273–282, 1995.
77. Purdon S, Lit W, Labelle A, Jones B: Risperidone in the treatment of pervasive developmental disorder. *Can J Psychiatry* 39:400–405, 1994.
78. Perry R, Pataki C, Munoz-Silva DM, Armenteros J, Silva RR: Risperidone in children and adolescents with pervasive developmental disorder: pilot trial and follow-up. *J Child Adolesc Psychopharmacol* 7(3):167–179, 1997.

79. Borison R, Ang L, Chang S, et al: New pharmacological approaches in the treatment of Tourette's syndrome, in Friedhoff A, Chase T (eds): *Gilles de la Tourette Syndrome*. New York, Raven Press, 1982, pp 377–382.
80. Shapiro E, Shapiro A, Fulop G, et al: Controlled study of haloperidol, pimozide, and placebo for the treatment of Gilles de la Tourette's syndrome. *Arch Gen Psychiatry* 46:722–730, 1989.
81. Bruun R: Subtle and underrecognized side effects of neuroleptic treatment in children with Tourette's disorder. *Am J Psychiatry* 145:621–624, 1988.
82. Sallee FR, Nesbitt L, Jackson C, et al: Relative efficacy of haloperidol and pimozide in children and adolescents with Tourette's disorders. *Am J Psychiatry* 154:1057–1062, 1997.
83. van der Linden C, Bruggeman R, van Woerkom T: Serotonin–dopamine antagonist and Gilles de la Tourette's syndrome: An open pilot dose-titration study with risperidone. *Mov Disord* 9:687–688, 1994.
84. Lombroso P, Scahill L, King R, et al: Risperidone treatment of children and adolescents with chronic tic disorders: A preliminary report. *J Am Acad Child Adolesc Psychiatry* 34:1147–1152, 1995.
85. Campbell M, Malone R: Mental retardation and psychiatry disorders. *Hosp Community Psychiatry* 42:374–379, 1991.
86. Aman M, Singh N: *Psychopharmacology of the Developmental Disabilities*. Berlin, Springer-Verlag, 1988, pp 1–28.
87. Aman M, Singh N: Pharmacotherapy and mental retardation, in Matson J, Mulick J (eds): *Handbook of Mental Retardation*. New York, Pergamon Press, 1991, pp 347–372.
88. Vanden Borre R, Vermote R, Buttiens M, et al: Risperidone as add-on therapy in behavioral disturbances in mental retardation: A double-blind placebo-controlled cross-over study. *Acta Psychiatr Scand* 87:167–171, 1995.
89. Intagliata J, Rimck C: Psychoactive drug use in public and community residential facilities for mentally retarded persons. *Psychopharmacol Bull* 21:268–278, 1985.
90. Aman M: Drugs and learning in mentally retarded persons, in Burrows G, Werry J (eds): *Advances in Human Psychopharmacology*. Greenwich, Conn, JAI Press; 1984, pp 121–163.
91. Aman M, White A, Field C: Chlorpromazine effects on stereotypic and conditioned behaviour of severely retarded patients—a pilot study. *J Ment Defic Res* 28:253–260, 1984.
92. Claghorn J: A double-blind comparison of haloperidol (Haldol) and thioridazine (Mellaril) in outpatient children. *Curr Ther Res* 14:785–789, 1972.
93. Aman M, Singh N: *Manual for the Abberant Behavior Checklist*. East Aurora, NY, Slosson Educational Publications; 1986.
94. Aman M, Teehan C, White A, et al: Haloperidol treatment with chronically medicated residents: Dose effects on clinical behavior and reinforcement contingencies. *Am J Ment Retard* 95:452–460, 1989.
95. Singh N, Aman M: Effects of thioridazine dosage on the behavior of severely mentally retarded persons. *Am J Ment Defic* 85:580–587, 1981.
96. Aman M, Marks R, Turbott S, et al: Clinical effects of methylphenidate and thioridazine in intellectually subaverage children. *J Am Acad Child Adolesc Psychiatry* 30:246–256, 1991.
97. White A, Aman M: Pimozide treatment in disruptive severely retarded patients. *Aust N Z J Psychiatry* 19:92–94, 1985.
98. Goldberg J, Kurland A: Pimozide in the treatment of behavioral disorders of hospitalized adolescents. *J Clin Pharmacol* 14:134–139, 1974.
99. Aman M, Marks R, Turbott S, et al: Methylphenidate and thioridazine in the treatment of intellectually subaverage children: Effects on cognitive–motor performance. *J Am Acad Child Adolesc Psychiatry* 30:816–824, 1991.
100. Gittelman-Klein R, Klein D, Katz S, et al: Comparative effects of methylphenidate and thioridazine in hyperkinetic children: I. Clinical results. *Arch Gen Psychiatry* 33:1217–1231, 1976.
101. Sleator E, von Neumann A, Sprague R: Hyperactive children: A continuous long-term placebo-controlled follow-up. *JAMA* 229:316–317, 1974.
102. Werry J, Weiss G, Douglas V, et al: Studies on the hyperactive child: III. The effect of chlorpromazine upon behavior and learning ability. *J Am Acad Child Psychiatry* 5:292–312, 1966.
103. Rapoport J, Abramson A, Alexander D, et al: Playroom observations on hyperactive children on medication. *J Am Acad Child Psychiatry* 10:524–534, 1971.
104. Aman M: Drugs, learning and the psychotherapies, in Werry J (ed): *Pediatric Psychopharmacology: The Use of Behavior Modifying Drugs in Children*. New York, Brunner/Mazel, 1978.
105. Davis K, Kahn R, Ko G, et al: Dopamine in schizophrenia: A review and reconceptualization. *Am J Psychiatry* 148:1474–1486, 1991.
106. Sokoloff P, Giros B, Martres M, et al: Molecular cloning and characterization of a novel dopamine receptor (D_3) as a target for neuroleptics. *Nature* 347:146–159, 1990.

107. Gould R, Murphy K, Reynolds I, et al: Antischizophrenic drugs of the diphenylbutylpiperidine type act as calcium channel antagonists. *Proc Natl Acad Sci USA* 80:5122–5125, 1983.
108. Peroutka S, Snyder S: Relationship of neuroleptic drug effects at brain dopamine, serotonin, alpha-adrenergic, and histamine receptors to clinical potency. *Am J Psychiatry* 137:1518–1522, 1980.
109. Richelson E: Neuroleptic affinities for human brain receptors and their use in predicting adverse effects. *J Clin Psychiatry* 45:331–336, 1984.
110. Farde L, Wiesel F, Stone-Elander S, et al: D2 receptors in neuroleptic naive schizophrenic patients. *Arch Gen Psychiatry* 47:213–219, 1990.
111. Pilowsky L, Costa D, Ell P, et al: Clozapine, single photon emission tomography and D2 dopamine receptor blockade hypothesis of schizophrenia. *Lancet* 340:119–202, 1992.
112. Farde L, Nordstrom AL, Wiesel F-A, Pauli S, Halldin C, Sedvall G: Positron emission tomographic analysis of central D_1 and D_2 dopamine receptor occupancy in patients treated with classical neuroleptics and clozapine: Relation to extrapyramidal side effects. *Arch Gen Psychiatry* 49:538–544, 1992.
113. Van Tol H, Bunzow J, Guan H, et al: Cloning of the gene for human D4 receptor with high affinity for the antipsychotic clozapine. *Nature* 350:610–619, 1991.
114. Altar C, Wasley A, Neale R, et al: Typical and atypical antipsychotic occupancy of D2 and S2 receptors: An autoradiographic analysis in rat brain. *Brain Res Bull* 16:517–525, 1988.
115. Canton H, Verriele L, Colpaert F: Binding of typical and atypical antipsychotics to 5HT1C and 5HT2 sites. *Eur J Pharmacol* 191:93–96, 1990.
116. Robertson G, Fibiger H: Neuroleptics increase c-fos expression in the forebrain: Contrasting effects of haloperidol and clozapine. *Neuroscience* 46:315–328, 1992.
117. Meltzer H: Role of serotonin in the action of atypical antipsychotic drugs. *Clin Neurosci* 3:64–75, 1995.
118. Mandoki M: Risperidone treatment of children and adolescents: Increased risk of extrapyramidal side effects. *J Child Adolesc Psychopharmacol* 5:49–67, 1995.
119. Baldessarini R, Teicher M: Dosing of antipsychotic agents in pediatric populations [editorial]. *J Child Adolesc Psychopharmacol* 5:1–4, 1995.
120. Synder S, Greenberg D, Yamamura H: Antischizophrenic drugs and brain cholinergic receptors. *Arch Gen Psychiatry* 31:58–61, 1974.
121. Ekblom B, Ericksson K, Lindstrom L: Super sensitivity psychosis in schizophrenic patients after sudden clozapine withdrawal. *Psychopharmacol Bull* 83:293–294, 1984.
122. Dilsaver S, Greyden J: Antidepressant withdrawal phenomena. *Biol Psychiatry* 19:237–256, 1984.
123. Dilsaver S, Feinberg M, Greyden J: Antidepressant withdrawal symptoms treated with anticholinergic agents. *Am J Psychiatry* 140:249–251, 1983.
124. Chouinard G: Severe cases of neuroleptic-induced super sensitivity psychosis. Diagnostic criteria for the disorder and its treatment. *Schizophr Res* 5:21–33, 1990.
125. Geller B: Psychopharmacology of children and adolescents: Pharmacokinetics and relationships of plasma/serum levels to response. *Psychopharmacol Bull* 27:401–409, 1991.
126. Furlanut M, Benetello P, Baraldo M, et al: Chlorpromazine disposition in relation to age in children. *Clin Pharmacokinet* 18:329–331, 1990.
127. Morselli P, Bianchetti G, Durand G, et al: Haloperidol plasma level monitoring in pediatric patients. *Ther Drug Monit* 1:35–46, 1979.
128. Poland R, Campbell M, Rubin R, et al: Relationship of serum haloperidol levels and clinical response in autistic children. Paper presented at the 13th CINP Congress (Collegium Internationale Psychopharmacologicum), Jerusalem, 1982.
129. Rivera-Camlimlin L, Griesbach P, Perlmutter R: Plasma chlorpromazine concentrations in children with behavioral disorders and mental illness. *Clin Pharmacol Ther* 26:114–121, 1979.
130. Campbell M, Poland R, Perry R, et al: Serum haloperidol levels and prolactin levels and clinical response in autistic children. Paper presented at the 35th Annual Meeting of the American Academy of Child and Adolescent Psychiatry, Seattle, 1988.
131. Brosen K: Recent developments in hepatic drug oxidation: Implications for clinical pharmacokinetics. *Clin Pharmacokinet* 18:220–239, 1990.
132. Rivera-Camlimlin L, Nasrallah H, Strauss J, et al. Clinical response and plasma levels: Effect of dose, dosage, schedules, and drug interactions on plasma chlorpromazine levels. *Am J Psychiatry* 133:652, 1976.
133. Devinsky O, Honigfeld G, Patin J: Clozapine-related seizures. *Neurology* 41:369–371, 1991.
134. Goff DC, Baldessarini RJ: Antipsychotics, in Ciraulo DA, Shader RA, Greenblatt DJ, Creelman W (eds): *Drug Interactions in Psychiatry*. Baltimore, Williams & Wilkins, 1995, pp 129–174.
135. Centorrino F, Baldessarini RJ, Frankenburg FR, Kando J, Volpicelli, Flood JG: Serum levels of clozapine

and norclozapine in patients treated with selective serotonin reuptake inhibitors. *Am J Psychiatry* 153:820–822, 1996.

136. Ciraulo DA, Shader RI: Fluoxetine drug–drug interactions: I. Antidepressants and antipsychotics. *J Clin Psychopharmacol* 10:48–50, 1990.

137. Mikkelson E, Detlor J, Cohen D: School avoidance and social phobia trigerred by haloperidol in patients with Tourette's disorder. *Am J Psychiatry* 138:1572–1575, 1981.

138. Baldasserini R: Drugs and the treatment of psychiatric disorders. in Gilman A, Rall T, Nies A (eds): *Goodman and Gilman's The Pharmacological Basis of Therapeutics*. New York, Maxwell/McMillan; 1991, pp 383–437.

139. Schmidt MH, Trott GE, Blanz B, Nissen G: Clozapine medication in adolescents, in *Psychiatry: A World Perspective*, Stefania CN, Rabavilas AD, Soldatos CR (eds). Amsterdam: Excerpta Medica, Proceedings of the VIII World Congress of Psychiatry, 1990, vol 1, pp 1100–1104.

140. Keepers G, Clappison V, Casey D: Initial anticholinergic prophylaxis for neuroleptic-induced extrapyramidal syndromes. *Arch Gen Psychiatry* 40:1113–1117, 1983.

141. Richardson M, Haughland G, Craig T: Neuroleptic use, parkinsonian symptoms, tardive dyskinesia, and associated factors in child and adolescent psychiatric patients. *Am J Psychiatry* 148:1322–1328, 1991.

142. Kane J, Jeste D, Barnes T, et al: *Tardive Dyskinesia: A Task Force Report*. Washington, DC, American Psychiatric Association Press; 1991.

143. Delay J, Deniker P: Drug-induced extrapyramidal syndromes, in Vinken P, Bruyn G (eds): *Handbook of Clinical Neurology*. Amsterdam, North-Holland Publishing Co, 1968, pp 248–266.

144. Rifkin A, Quitkin F, Klein D: Akinesia: A poorly recognized drug-induced extrapyramidal behavioral disorder. *Arch Gen Psychiatry* 32:672–674, 1975.

145. Van Putten T, Mutalipassi L, Malkin M: Phenothiazine-induced decompensation. *Arch Gen Psychiatry* 30:102–105, 1974.

146. Van Putten T, May P, Marder S: Akathisia with haloperidol and thiothixene. *Arch Gen Psychiatry* 41:1036–1039, 1984.

147. Campbell M, Adams P, Perry R, et al: Tardive and withdrawal dyskinesia in autistic children: A prospective study. *Psychopharmacol Bull* 24:251–255, 1988.

148. Campbell M, Grega D, Green W, et al: Neuroleptic-induced dyskinesias in children. *Clin Neuropharmacol* 6:207–222, 1983.

149. Perry R, Nobler M, Campbell M: Case report: Tourette-like symptoms associated with chronic neuroleptic therapy in an autistic child. *J Am Acad Child Adolesc Psychiatry* 28:93–96, 1989.

150. Klawans H, Nausieda P, Goetz C, et al: Tourette-like symptoms following chronic neuroleptic therapy, in Friedhoff A, Chase T (eds): *Advances in Neurology*. New York, Raven Press, 1982.

151. Smith R, Domino E: Dystonic and dyskinetic reactions induced by H_1 antihistaminic medication, in Fann W, Smith R, Davis J, et al (eds): *Tardive Dyskinesia: Research and Treatment*. Jamaica, NY, Spectrum Publications; 1980, pp 325–332.

152. Thach B, Chase T, Bosman J: Oral facial dyskinesia associated with prolonged use of antihistaminic decongestants. *N Engl J Med* 293:486–487, 1975.

153. Chadwick D, Reynolds E, Marsden C: Anticonvulsant induced dyskinesias. *J Neurol Neurosurg Psychiatry* 39:1210–1218, 1979.

154. Gardos G, Cole J, La Brie R: The assessment of tardive dyskinesia. *Arch Gen Psychiatry* 34:1206–1212, 1977.

155. Gerlach J: Pathophysiological mechanisms underlying tardive dyskinesia, in Casey D, Chase T, Christensen D, et al (eds): *Dyskinesia—Research and Treatment (Psychopharmacology Suppl 2)*. Berlin, Springer-Verlag, 1985, pp 99–103.

156. Kane J, Smith J: Tardive dyskinesia. *Arch Gen Psychiatry* 39:473–481, 1982.

157. Crane G, Naranjo E: Motor disorders induced by neuroleptics. *Arch Gen Psychiatry* 24:178–184, 1971.

158. Gardos G, Cole J, Tarsy D: Withdrawal symptoms associated with antipsychotic drugs. *Am J Psychiatry* 135:1321–1324, 1978.

159. McAndrew J, Case Q, Treffert D: Effects of prolonged phenothiazine intake on psychotic and other hospitalized children. *J Autism Child Schizophr* 2:75–91, 1972.

160. Gualtieri C, Quade D, Hicks R, et al: Tardive dyskinesia and other clinical consequences of neuroleptic treatment in children and adolescents. *Am J Psychiatry* 141:20–23, 1984.

161. Engelhardt D, Polizios P: Adverse effects of pharmacotherapy in childhood psychosis, in Lipton M, DiMascio A, Killam K (eds): *Psychopharmacology: A Generation of Progress*. New York, Raven Press; 1978.

162. Owens D, Johnstone E, Frith C: Spontaneous involuntary disorders of movement: Their prevalence, severity and distribution in chronic schizophrenics with and without treatment with neuroleptics. *Arch Gen Psychiatry* 39:452–461, 1982.
163. Meiselas K, Spencer E, Oberfield R, et al: Differentiation of stereotypies from neuroleptic-related dyskinesias in autistic children. *J Clin Psychopharmacol* 9:207–209, 1989.
164. Schooler N, Kane J: Research diagnoses for tardive dyskinesia [letter to the editor]. *Arch Gen Psychiatry* 39:486–487, 1982.
165. Campbell M, Locascio J, Choroco M, et al: Stereotypies and tardive dyskinesia: Abnormal movements in autistic children. *Psychopharmacol Bull* 26:260–266, 1990.
166. Malone R, Ernst M, Godfrey K, Locascio J, Campbell M: Repeated episodes of neuroleptic-related dyskinesias in autistic children. *Psychopharmacol Bull* 27:113–117, 1991.
167. Kane J, Honigfeld G, Singer J, Meltzer H: Clozaril Collaborative Study Group: Clozapine for the treatment-treatment resistant schizophrenic: A double-blind comparison with chlorpromazine. *Arch Gen Psychiatry* 45:789–796, 1988.
168. Woener M, Sheitman B, Lieberman J, Kane J: Tardive dyskinesia induced by risperidone? [letter]. *Am J Psychiatry* 153:843, 1996.
169. Crane G: Neuroleptics and their long-term effects on the central nervous system, in DeVeaugh-Geiss J (ed): *Tardive Dyskinesia and Related Involuntary Movement Disorders*. Boston, John Wright Publishing Co, 1982, pp 71–84.
170. McLean P, Casey D: Tardive dyskinesia in an adolescent. *Am J Psychiatry* 135:969–971, 1978.
171. Villeneuve A: The rabbit syndrome: A peculiar extrapyramidal reaction. *Can J Psychiatry* 17:69–72, 1972.
172. Campbell M, Cohen I, Small A: Drugs in aggressive behavior. *J Am Acad Child Psychiatry* 21:107–117, 1982.
173. Spencer EK, Campbell M: Children with schizophrenia: Diagnosis, phenomenology and pharmacotherapy. *Schizophr Bull* 20(4):713–725, 1994.
174. Simpson G: *APA Task Force on Sudden Death*. Washington, DC, American Psychiatric Association Press, 1987.
175. Silver J, Yudofsky S: Psychopharmacology and electroconvulsive therapy, in Talbott J, Hales R, Yudofsky S (eds): *The American Psychiatric Press Textbook of Psychiatry*. Washington, DC, American Psychiatric Press; 1989, pp 767–843.
176. Levinson F, Simpson G: Neuroleptic-induced extrapyramidal symptoms with fever. *Arch Gen Psychiatry* 43:839–848, 1986.
177. Geller B, Greydanus D: Haloperidol-induced comatose state with hyperthermia and rigidity in adolescence: Two case reports with a literature review. *J Clin Psychiatry* 40:102–103, 1979.
178. Klein S, Levinsohn M, Blumer J: Accidental chlorpromazine ingestion as a cause of neuroleptic malignant syndrome in children. *J Pediatr* 107:970–973, 1985.
179. Green WH, Campbell M, Wolsky BB: Effects of short and long term haloperidol administration on growth in young autistic children. Paper presented at the 31st Annual Meeting of the American Academy of Child Psychiatry, 1984.
180. Hamill PVV, Drizd TA, Johnson CL, et al: NCHS Growth Charts, 1976. Monthly Vital Statistics Report, Health Examination Survey Data, National Center for Health Statistics Publication (HRA) 76–1120, 25(3):1–22, 1976.
181. Van Kammen D, Marder S: Biological therapies: Clozapine, in Kaplan H, Sadock B (eds): *Comprehensive Textbook of Psychiatry VI*. Baltimore, Williams & Wilkins, 1995.
182. Rapoport J: Clozapine and child psychiatry [editorial]. *J Child Adolesc Psychopharmacol* 4:1–3, 1994.
183. Lieberman J, Yunis J, Egea E, Conoso R, Kane J, et al: HLA B38, DR4, DQW3 and clozapine-induced agranulocytosis in Jewish patients with schizophrenia. *Arch Gen Psychiatry* 47:945–948, 1990.
184. Haller E, Binder R: Clozapine and seizures. *Am J Psychiatry* 147:1069–1071, 1990.
185. Freedman J, Wirshing W, Russell A, Palmer Bray M, Unutzer J: Absence status seizures during successful long-term treatment of an adolescent with schizophrenia. *J Child Adolesc Psychopharmacol* 4:53–62, 1994.
186. Birmaher B: Clozapine for child and adolescent schizophrenia. *Child Adolesc Psychopharmacol News* 1:1–4, 1996.
187. Simpson G, Lee J, Shrivastava R: Clozapine in tardive dyskinesia. *Psychopharmacology* 56:75–80, 1978.
188. Alphs L, Lee H: Comparison of withdrawal or dose reduction of clozapine. *J Clin Psychiatry* 52:346–348, 1991.
189. Eklund K: Super sensitivity and clozapine withdrawal. *Psychopharmacology* 91:135, 1987.
190. Borison R, Diamond B, Sinha D, Gupta R, Prince Ajiboye A: Clozapine withdrawal rebound psychosis. *Psychopharmacol Bull* 24:260–263, 1988.

191. Allen MD, Greenblatt DJ, Noel BJ: Overdose with antipsychotic agents. *Am J Psychiatry* 137:234–236, 1980.
192. Cunningham DG, Challapalli M: Hypertension in acute haloperidol poisoning. *J Pediatr* 95:489–490, 1979.
193. Giannini AJ: *Psychotropic Drug Overdose*. New York, Hemisphere Publishing Corp., 1992, p 39.
194. Buckley NA, Whyte IM, Dawson AH: Cardiotoxicity more common in thioridazine overdose than with other neuroleptics. *Clin Toxicol* 33:199–204, 1995.
195. Krishel S, Jackimczyck K: Antidepressants, lithium, and neuroleptic agents. *Psychiatr Asp Emerg Med* 9:53–85, 1991.

11

Drugs of Abuse

ANDREA EISNER, M.D., and JON McCLELLAN, M.D.

I. INTRODUCTION

Substance abuse refers to the maladaptive use of any chemical, legal or illicit, to produce alterations in brain functioning, mood, behavior, and/or level of perception. There are at least three different ways in which substance abuse may result in substantial child and adolescent psychiatric morbidity: (1) exposure during gestation to substances with known behavioral teratogenicity; (2) psychosocial deprivation and/or physical harm as a result of caretakers' substance abuse disorders; and (3) substance abuse disorders and their consequences in children and adolescents themselves. This chapter will focus specifically on the child and adolescent psychopathology associated with substance abuse as well as the psychopharmacology of the substances involved.

Owing to space limitations, many issues will only be discussed briefly. For a more extensive review, readers are referred to the text by Schuckit.[1]

II. DEFINITIONS

Since the various terms relating to substance abuse are often used in an inconsistent or idiosyncratic fashion, both professionally and by media and the public, the following accepted definitions will be used in this chapter.

Drug of abuse: Any substance, either prescribed (e.g., morphine), available within the culture (e.g., alcohol), or illicit (e.g., phencyclidine), that is used to produce an alteration in brain functioning, mood, behavior, and/or level of perception. The mere use of such substances does not imply abuse, which must be further defined by specific patterns of dysfunctional behavior (see below).

Intoxication: The development of a substance-specific syndrome in which the current effect of the substance on the central nervous system (CNS) produces maladaptive behavior.[2]

ANDREA EISNER, M.D., and JON MCCLELLAN, M.D. • Departments of Psychiatry and Behavioral Science, University of Washington, Seattle, Washington 98195.

Practitioner's Guide to Psychoactive Drugs for Children and Adolescents (Second Edition), Werry and Aman, eds. Plenum Publishing Corporation, New York, 1999.

Tolerance: The need for escalating doses of the substance to produce the same desired effect. Tolerance is produced both by enzymatic changes in hepatic degradation of the agent (metabolic tolerance) and by changes in responsivity of target cells (i.e., CNS tissue). Tolerance to a single agent generally produces cross-tolerance to other drugs within the same class.

Withdrawal: The development of physiologic changes upon sudden cessation of the abused substance. The symptoms of withdrawal vary with the agent in question but frequently involve alterations in the functioning of the autonomic nervous system.

Substance use disorders, as defined by the fourth edition of the *Diagnostic and Statistical Manual of Mental Disorders* (DSM-IV), are subdivided into substance abuse and substance dependence.

Substance abuse disorder: A maladaptive pattern of substance use, recurrently during a 12-month period, where the substance use leads to clinically significant impairment or distress. If drug dependence is present, that diagnosis takes precedence.

Substance dependence disorder: A maladaptive pattern of substance use leading to clinically significant impairment or distress, as manifested by at least three of the following symptoms within a 12-month period: tolerance; withdrawal; using more or longer than intended; wishing or attempting unsuccessfully to cut back on use; spending a lot of time obtaining, using, or recovering from use of the substance; cutting back on important social, occupational, or recreational activities owing to substance use; and continuing substance use despite knowledge of physical or psychological problems likely caused or exacerbated by the substance.[2]

This change in diagnostic criteria from DSM-III-R indicates the importance of assessing loss of control over substance use, in addition to the physiologic symptoms of tolerance and withdrawal, in determining whether substance dependence is present. This diagnostic criterion change will likely mean that many adolescents, who often do not experience physiologic withdrawal symptoms, will now meet criteria for drug dependence.

III. EPIDEMIOLOGY

A. Frequency and Type of Substance Abuse

The abuse of illicit substances by adolescents in the United States rose sharply in the 1960s and early 1970s and subsequently underwent a steady decline until 1993, when it again rose sharply. While rates vary, similar trends have been found in studies of Canadian youth[3] and in descriptions of general patterns of use in Europe.[4]

In 1995, the 21st year of an ongoing survey of high school seniors in the United States, Johnston and colleagues[5] reported that 39% of those surveyed reported using an illicit drug at some time in the the preceding 12-months, compared to a peak rate of 54% in 1979, but up from 27% in 1992. (The study characterizes students by grade. Eighth graders are generally 13 and 14 years old, 10th graders are 15 and 16 years old, and 12th graders are 17 and 18 years old.) Among 10th graders surveyed, 33% reported illicit drug use in the preceding 12 months (up from 20% in 1992), and 21% of 8th graders surveyed reported such use (almost double the 11% in 1991).[5]

When examined by specific substances, the 1995 survey indicates that marijuana use has shown a particularly strong resurgence since 1992. Thirty-five percent of 12th graders, and 29% of 10th graders reported using marijuana in the previous 12 months compared to 22% and 15%, respectively, in 1992. Among 8th graders, 16% reported use in the previous 12 months, compared to 6% in 1991. Especially disturbing is the fact that 4.6% of high school seniors reported current daily marijuana use.

Use of other illicit drugs, including LSD, other hallucinogens, amphetamines, stimulants, and inhalants, has also increased since the early 1990s. However, the prevalence remains well below the level of use in the late 1970s.[5]

The use of alcohol has been fairly stable over the past several years. In 1995, the proportion of students having five or more drinks in a row during the two weeks preceding the survey were 15% of 8th graders, 24% of 10th graders, and 30% of 12th graders. Fifty-one percent of 12th graders reported some ingestion of alcohol over the 30 days prior to being surveyed, down from 57% in 1990 and 72% in 1980.[5]

Tobacco use has increased over the past few years. Of students surveyed, 19% of 8th graders, 28% of 10th graders, and 34% of 12th graders reported smoking tobacco in the 30 days prior to the survey. Almost 22% of high school seniors report daily cigarette use, up from 17% in 1992, but down from the peak of 29% in 1977.[5]

The increase in illicit substance and tobacco use is associated with a recent decline in adolescents' perception of risk associated with drug use and smoking. Peer disapproval of drug use, an important deterrent to use, has also been declining.[5]

The rise in self-reported substance abuse noted in the 1970s was associated with a lowering of the age of first experimentation. A small percentage of children first experiment with intoxicants before the 6th grade, with the frequency of first use then rising steadily from ages 12 through 18.[6] The prevalence of substance abuse, including alcohol abuse, peaks between ages 18 and 22, after which it declines. Among those who abuse, multiple drug abuse is common.[7]

B. Risk Factors for Abuse

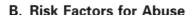

Characteristics that appear to place a youth at risk for substance abuse include: (1) family history of substance abuse; (2) history of sexual, physical, and/or psychological abuse or neglect; (3) dropping out of school; (4) teenage pregnancy; (5) low socioeconomic status; (6) mental health problems (especially suicidal behavior, depression, and anxiety); (7) physical handicaps; (8) learning and language disorders; (9) delinquency; and (10) male gender, as males have a higher rate of daily substance abuse (except for tobacco and stimulants, which female adolescents use at an equal to slightly higher rate).[8,9] Among ethnic groups, Native Americans have the highest rates of abuse, and blacks and Asian-Americans have the lowest. Among high school seniors, Hispanics have the highest lifetime and annual prevalence rates for cocaine, while whites in the 12th grade have the highest lifetime and annual prevalence rates for marijuana, inhalants, hallucinogens, opiates other than heroin, amphetamines, barbiturates, tranquilizers, and cigarettes.[9] Environmental factors, including substance abuse in peers and family members, also increase a child's vulnerability. Early age of onset of substance use predicts subsequent drug abuse.[8]

Of all the above risk factors, a family history of substance abuse (which invokes biological, psychological, and social etiologic mechanisms) is believed to be the greatest single predictor for the development of a substance abuse disorder.[10] The presence of one or more of these risk factors may also negatively influence the availability and effectiveness of treatment once a substance abuse disorder has developed.

IV. ETIOLOGY

The exact etiology of substance abuse and dependence is not known, and, in any case, the contributions of variables probably differ among individuals. Put another way, no one factor is likely to be the only or the inexorable cause. Furthermore, most persons with the traits, characteristics, or conditions mentioned below do not have substance abuse or dependence.

A. Predisposing Personality and Cognitive Traits

Personality traits have been identified which may increase one's vulnerability to substance abuse. Cloninger et al.[11] described in 11-year-olds two personality characteristics, high novelty seeking and low harm avoidance, that were associated with later (at age 27 years) alcohol abuse. Interestingly, children with exactly the opposite traits, i.e., low novelty seeking and high harm avoidance, also were found to have an increased risk for adult alcohol abuse.

In regard to comorbid or preceding psychiatric disorders, alcohol and substance abuse disorders frequently present during the course of disruptive externalizing behavior disorders, such as conduct, hyperactive, and oppositional disorders.[12] Weiss and colleagues found higher rates of substance abuse in adolescents diagnosed as hyperactive during childhood.[13]

Neuropsychological impairment, consisting of deficits in attention, memory, visual-perceptual motor performance, and language processing (associated with poorer reading achievement), has been described in the sons of alcoholic fathers.[11]

The above-described traits, characteristics, or conditions are probably not linked uniquely and necessarily to a specific substance abuse disorder. Rather, such associations are thought to represent some fundamental disturbance of behavioral self-regulation that manifests itself in a number of spheres of human activity. Substance abuse is involved only as a consequence of the general availability of the substances, especially in those environments where disordered behavior is common.

B. Biological "Markers"

Twin and adoption studies have supported the likely contribution of genetic or constitutional factors to the risk for substance use disorders.[14] Researchers have looked for biological markers or characteristics that may differentiate high-risk from low-risk individuals. When compared with controls, individuals at risk for alcoholism (drinking but not yet alcoholic 18 to 25 year-old children of alcoholics) report a decreaed intensity of subjective feelings of intoxication and show less static ataxia (body sway) in response to an ethanol challenge.[15]

Although it has been proposed that biochemical anomalies may lead to an inherited vulnerability for abusing specific substances ("pharmacogenetics"), only general associations between substance abuse disorders, personality or trait variables, and biochemical "markers" have been described.[1]

Cloninger has hypothesized that specific neuronal and neurotransmitter systems play a role in each of three heritable behavioral traits (two of which were mentioned above).[16] These are (1) midbrain dopaminergic neurons in novelty seeking; (2) dorsal raphe serotonergic neurons in harm avoidance; and (3) locus coeruleus noradrenergic neurons in reward dependence.

Attempts to refine clinical and biochemical subgroups of substance abuse disorders are currently under way in order to identify potential mechanisms of vulnerability. Findings from these investigations will allow the focus of substance abuse research to progress from studies that explore the mechanisms of psychotropic effects, which are uniformly demonstrable in all humans and many mammalian species, to those that explore the mechanisms by which psychotropic effects of substances produce maladaptive behaviors in certain individuals.

V. PATTERNS OF ABUSE AND OUTCOME

The outcome for adolescents who experiment with substances of abuse is quite variable, and most will not go on to develop serious substance abuse disorders. Even those who display patterns of abuse as teenagers will not necessarily abuse substances as adults.[7] However, substance abuse in adolescents still should not be ignored or considered merely a passing phase. Independent of any deleterious later outcome, substance abuse disorders clearly have significant psychological, physical, and social morbidity and are a significant contributor to teenage mortality. In the United States, approximately 8000 motor vehicle deaths of teenagers per year are alcohol-related, while approximately one-third of adolescent suicides and one-half of teenage homicides are associated with alcohol and drug use.[17,18] Evaluation and treatment must be undertaken when alcohol or other substance abuse is suspected.

The progression from casual experimentation to substance abuse disorder generally occurs in four stages[19]: (1) drinking beer and/or wine, (2) smoking cigarettes and drinking hard liquor, (3) smoking marijuana, and (4) abusing other illicit drugs. Because these stages are derived from clinical histories of adolescents presenting for treatment for substance abuse disorders, it is erroneous to assume that abuse of the early-stage substances always or even commonly leads to illicit substance abuse. Rather, the more readily available and socially acceptable agents, tobacco and alcohol, serve as gateway substances for certain vulnerable individuals who go on to develop overt patterns of abuse with alcohol, tobacco, and/or illicit drugs.[7] The majority of teenagers in any of these four stages will not have substance abuse problems as adults.

VI. PRINCIPLES OF DIAGNOSIS

A. Accurate History

The presence of a substance abuse disorder cannot be accurately diagnosed unless an appropriate history is taken. Such a history is all too often ignored, both in primary-care settings and in mental health evaluations. Insufficient or inaccurate information regarding patterns of abuse then leads to erroneous diagnostic and treatment decisions.

Inquiry about substance use and patterns of use should be included in routine pediatric and family medicine practice. All children and adolescents referred for emotional and behavioral problems must be evaluated for substance abuse disorders because they are particularly at risk. Questions should be direct and specific. Incorporating structured interviews and self-report instruments, which include specific inquiries regarding substance abuse history, into the routine assessment process may help prevent misdiagnosis.[7]

A thorough history should elicit information regarding (1) substances of abuse used, age of onset, frequency, patterns of use, quantities used, route of administration, and the presence of symptoms of either tolerance or dependence; (2) family history of substance abuse; (3) associated symptoms and/or comorbid conditions, such as mental status changes, conduct problems, affective symptoms, suicidality, or a deterioration in academic, social, or interpersonal functioning; (4) social risk factors, e.g., substance abuse in the home, history of abuse, or association with substance-abusing peers; and (5) psychological factors, i.e., attitudes toward substance abuse.[20]

The assessment of children and adolescents is, at best, complicated. Patients (or family members) often minimize or deny any symptoms of substance abuse. As in all other aspects of child and adolescent mental health, confirming history from other sources is almost always necessary. Alternatively, it is also common for practitioners to overinterpret a history of substance abuse when they find it. Many adolescents experiment with substances of abuse without meeting criteria for abuse disorder (i.e., significant impairment).[20] It is important that reasonably consistent techniques reflecting current diagnostic standards are used to review the individual's clinical presentation before applying a specific DSM-IV or similar diagnostic label.

B. Comorbid Psychiatric Conditions

The presence of related conditions must be considered if abuse and dependency disorders are diagnosed. Psychiatric conditions associated with substance abuse disorders in children and adolescents include affective disorders, conduct disorder, attention-deficit hyperactivity disorder (ADHD), anxiety disorders, post traumatic stress disorder (PTSD), bulimia nervosa, schizophrenia, personality disorders, and suicidal behaviors.[20] These conditions all have significant impact on treatment considerations.

C. Health Problems

If a history of "high-risk" behaviors such as intravenous drug administration or prostitution to support a dependency is elicited, an evaluation for and counseling regarding hepatitis and sexually transmitted diseases, especially those relating to human immunodeficiency virus (HIV), must be pursued.[20] The known negative effects of cigarettes, alcohol, and drugs (such as cocaine, marijuana, and some sedative–hypnotics) on a developing fetus require that all pregnant teenagers be properly evaluated for substance abuse disorders and receive extensive reproductive counseling and substance abuse treatment, as indicated.

Accidents and trauma in adolescents, including motor vehicle, bicycle, and skateboard accidents and drownings, commonly occur under the influence of substances. Clinicians should have a high level of suspicion for substance abuse when adolescents present following accidents or trauma. Other medical consequences of substance abuse are uncommon in adolescents, except in the case of inhalation of aromatic or halogenated hydrocarbons or other organic solvents (e.g., glue sniffing and gasoline "huffing"). These substances occasionally can produce neurotoxicity, cardiac arrhythmia, and renal toxicity. Smoking is associated with decreased exercise tolerance in adolescents.

D. Laboratory Evaluation

Laboratory screening tests, other than toxicology screens, have not been shown to be useful in the assessment of substance abuse disorders in adolescents. Toxicology screens are solely indicated for the assessment of acute intoxication or in monitoring patients' compliance with treatment for identified substance abuse disorders. Their usefulness beyond these indications is limited and, at best, controversial.

Typical urine drug abuse screens can detect several barbiturates and benzodiazepines, marijuana and its metabolites, phencyclidine, methaqualone, several opiates, amphetamine, methamphetamine, and cocaine and its metabolites (Table 1). It should be noted that solvents and other inhalants and LSD cannot be detected by routine screening.[21] Adulteration of the urine specimen, by addition of bleach, vinegar, lemon juice, salt, soap, or "Gold Seal" tea, can produce a false-negative result, as can diluting urine by drinking excessive fluids or use of a diuretic. Temperature, specific gravity, pH, measurements and urinary creatinine measurements are used to determine if samples are vaild. Other factors in false-negative results are related to the pharmacokinetics, such as the volume of distribution and the elimination half-life, as well as the quality control of the laboratory. False-positive results can occur due to antibody cross-reactivity with a substance bearing some structural similarity to a drug that is screened. Examples include poppy seeds, which can result in a positive result for opiates, and decongestants such as ephedrine, phenylephrine, and pseudoephedrine, which can result in a positive result for stimulants. Dextromethorphan, diphenhydramine, chlorpromazine, and thioridazine all show cross-reactivity in screening for phencyclidine.[21]

The period of time following drug use during which positive drug screens are obtained varies, depending on the specific drug, the sensitivity of the test, and the patterns of use. For example, some drugs taken chronically may redistribute in body stores and then be slowly released back into the bloodstream, thus enabling detection to occur later after last use.

E. Social Assessment

Social factors that frequently complicate substance abuse disorders, such as unemployment, lack of education, physical and sexual abuse, family discord, low socioeconomic status, and inadequate living situations, will greatly affect any treatment plans and require skilled social assessment and intervention.

VII. SUBSTANCES OF ABUSE

The different substances of abuse will be introduced by class (e.g., CNS depressants, stimulants, hallucinogens), followed by a brief discussion of their respective pharmacology, clinical effects, and specific pharmacologic treatment indications. Some of these agents also have therapeutic indications (i.e., CNS depressants and stimulants) and are

TABLE 1. Drug Screening in Children and Adolescents[a]

Class	When detectable in urine	Detectable duration of single dose	Detectable duration of prolonged use	Notes
Amphetamine/ methamphetamine	Within 20 min of administration	Less than 48 h	Up to 7–12 days	Longer duration in more acidic urine
Barbiturates	Within 30–40 min of administration	Short-acting: 1–3 days; intermediate-acting: up to 5 days; long-acting: up to 2–3 weeks	Phenobarbital for anticonvulsant use is constantly positive	
Benzodiazepines	*May only be detectable after prolonged use*	3 days; metabolites will be positive 3–4 days after start of medication	*Varies with labs and drug;* may remain positive 5–7 days after cessation of chronic use with some drugs, or even up to 4–6 weeks with some lab measures	May not be detectable with single dose use
Cocaine	Within 20 min	2–4 days	2 weeks after cessation	Metabolite benzoylecgonine present after cocaine no longer in urine
Opiates				
Codeine	Within 10 min	20–40 hr		Heroin immediately metabolizes into morphine; ratio of codeine to morphine changes: initially codeine > morphine; after 20–40 hr, morphine > codeine
Morphine	Within 10 min	4 days		
Heroin	Within 10 min	4 days as morphine		
Phencyclidine	Within 20–30 min	Unknown	May remain positive up to 30 days; average 14 days after cessation	Many false positives, cross reactivity with dextromethorphan and diphenhydramine
Cannabinols	Within 1 hr	5–10 days	10–20 days after cessation	

[a]Adapted from Harborview Chemical Dependency Project, International Clinical Laboratories, Seattle, Washington, from Clinical Toxicology for the Pediatrician, *Pediatrics Clinics of North America* 42(2):321, 1995.

discussed in greater detail in other chapters of this book. A more general guideline to treatment will follow this section.

A. CNS Depressants

CNS depressants include alcohol, sedative–hypnotics/anxiolytics (see Chapter 15), and inhalants. Although markedly different in their biochemistry, pharmacology, and toxicology, individual agents of this class produce similar physiologic, psychological, and behavioral effects, display cross-tolerance and cross-dependence, and have similar treatments for acute intoxication and withdrawal.

1. Alcohol

Alcohol is the most widely used CNS depressant and is a major contributor to morbidity and mortality within Western civilization.[1] It is readily available to many children and adolescents; in addition to alcoholic beverages, over-the-counter cold preparations, mouthwash, and even aftershave containing alcohol are also ingested by some youth in order to become intoxicated.

a. Pharmacology

Ethanol, the active agent in all alcoholic beverages (beer, wine, and liquor), has wide-ranging effects on most body systems. It acts by interfering with either cell membrane functioning, intracellular respiration, or cellular energy processing. While its main effect is to suppress CNS activity, at lower doses it may produce behavioral stimulation, possibly due to either direct stimulant effects or differential suppression of inhibitory neurons.[1]

The effects of alcohol on CNS functioning vary from impaired coordination and euphoria at lower blood alcohol levels (20–99 mg/dL) to coma and death at higher levels (400 mg/dL and greater). However, the impact of a particular blood level varies greatly between individuals and is dependent on a variety of factors, including age, sex, weight, prior exposure to alcohol, and the degree of tolerance.[1]

Alcohol is completely absorbed in the digestive tract. Approximately 85% is metabolized in the liver, mostly to acetaldehyde via the enzyme alcohol dehydrogenase, with the rest being excreted through the lungs, sweat, and urine. The genetic control of alcohol dehydrogenase and its isoenzymes may be an important contributor to the heritability of alcoholism.[1]

b. Patterns of Abuse

As with adults, alcohol use by adolescents begins in the context of social events or group activities. In many countries, alcohol consumption is actively promoted by advertising which depicts drinking as "cool" and "normal." Some individuals may then progress to the point where their use of alcohol becomes maladaptive.

c. Effects

Long-term alcohol use may have a deleterious impact on multiple body systems, including gastrointestinal (GI), cardiovascular, hematopoietic, peripheral, and CNS effects.[1] Only those changes specific to its psychoactive effect will be discussed here.

In small amounts, alcohol may induce euphoria and behavioral stimulation, whereas higher doses produce sedation, cognitive depression, dysphoria, irritability, anxiety, motoric dysfunction, and poor judgment. Chronic abuse ultimately results in more widespread psychosocial dysfunction.[1] Other noted effects include insomnia, "hangovers" (i.e., periods of malaise, nausca, hcadache, and tremulousness that occur frequently after bouts of drinking), and "blackouts" (periods of anterograde amnesia occurring during heavy intoxication). Adolescents rarely experience withdrawal symptoms of increased autonomic activity, seizures, or delirium tremens.

d. Tolerance and Dependence

Tolerance and dependence both develop after repeated ingestion of alcohol and stem from metabolic changes in the degradation of the ethanol and the direct adaptation of the CNS. Some individuals with tolerance may function with blood alcohol levels in the lethal range; thus, the clinician should be wary of trusting clinical impressions when trying to estimate degrees of intoxication. Cross-tolerance with other CNS depressants does occur; however, the concurrent use of these agents can also potentiate alcohol's effects.[1] As noted above, adolescents rarely demonstrate physiologic dependence.

e. Treatment

i. Acute Intoxication. The main risks in acute intoxication are due to CNS depression and inhalation of vomitus. Treatment should be directed to their prevention. Treatment of acute intoxication with alcohol includes maintenance of airway, electrolyte balance, fluid intake, and serum glucose concentration. Nutritional supplementation, including thiamine as prophylaxis against Wernicke's encephalopathy, is always indicated when abuse is suspected.[1]

ii. Withdrawal. Wheras mild symptoms of alcohol withdrawal may be managed supportively, the presence of severe withdrawal symptoms, i.e., delirium tremens, with autonomic instability, mental status changes, and possibly seizures, is a medical emergency and requires immediate medical attention, usually in a hospital setting. Fortunately, this condition is extremely rare in adolescent alcoholics.

Benzodiazepines are recommended for the treatment of moderate to severe alcohol withdrawal because of their relative safety compared with CNS depressants or anticonvulsants, including the limited risk of respiratory depression or hypotension, and the option to use them intramuscularly. The choice of benzodiazepine to be used should be made based on the agent's half-life (see Chapter 15), route of administration, hepatic functioning in the patient, history of previous treatment, and the physician's familiarity with the agent. The treatment should be short-term until the patient is stabilized from the withdrawal syndrome, after which the benzodiazepine should be tapered. Long-term use is not recommended because of cross-tolerance, and therefore cross-dependency.[1]

iii. Dependence. Only specific medical interventions are discussed here. General management issues are discussed later in this chapter. There has been some discussion regarding use of disulfiram (Antabuse®) for alcohol dependence in adolescents, although there are only a few case reports of such use, showing questionable efficacy.[22] Disulfiram markedly alters the metabolism of alcohol by irreversibly inactivating the enzyme acetaldehyde dehydrogenase, thus resulting in a marked increase of acetaldehyde in the blood. Symptoms and signs of this acetaldehyde syndrome include flushing, pulsating headache, nausea, vomiting, sweating, thirst, chest pain, significant drop in blood pressure, dizziness or fainting upon standing, weakness, vertigo, blurred vision, marked uneasiness, respiratory difficulties, and confusion. The ingestion of alcohol by an individual previously given disulfiram results in these aversive symptoms, which are then expected to be cognitively paired to alcohol consumption and thus negatively reinforce alcohol consumption. Because of ethical concerns, it is unlikely that aversive pharmacotherapy should be used much in treatment of adolescent alcohol dependence.[23] Some recent findings in the pharmacotherapy of alcoholism have suggested potential use of an opioid antagonist, such as naltrexone, or serotonin uptake inhibitors, such as fluoxetine,[23] but no such agent has a proven role yet in treatment of alcohol dependence.

2. Anxiolytics and Sedative–Hypnotics

For purposes of discussion, this class of compounds includes barbiturates, barbiturate-like anxiolytics (e.g., methaqualone), and benzodiazepines. The nonbenzodiazepine, non-barbiturate-like anxiolytics buspirone and hydroxyzine are not considered CNS depressants, have low abuse potential, and therefore will not be discussed. The pharmacology of sedative–hypnotics and anxiolytics, their adverse effects, and therapeutic indications in children and adolescents are reviewed in detail in Chapter 15.

a. Pharmacology

Sedative–hypnotics depress excitatory CNS activity. Barbiturates are proposed to bind to neuronal chloride channels; their binding then increases resting potential and prevents depolarization. Benzodiazepines potentiate the effects of γ-aminobutyric acid (GABA), an inhibitory amino acid neurotransmitter, by binding to a site on the chloride channel. When benzodiazepines bind to this site, the affinity of the GABA receptor for the neuronally secreted neurotransmitter is increased. The neuronal systems that utilize GABA are found diffusely throughout the brain, but the specific anxiolytic effects of these agents are thought to be mediated by cortical, hippocampal, septal, and amygdaloid GABAergic neurons.

The different sedative–hypnotics vary greatly in their length of action but are all generally metabolized hepatically, with subsequent renal excretion, and therefore blood levels depend on the degree of distribution among various body tissues as well as the rate of metabolic degradation.[1]

b. Patterns of Nontherapeutic Use

Group use is less typical with sedative-hypnotics. Since "recreational" use is masked by the lack of telltale signs (e.g., the distinct odor of alcohol or the injected conjunctiva and marijuana smoke on the breath or clothes), it is less "risky" for the individual to attend public functions such as dances or sporting events. If alcoholic beverages are then consumed at, or after, such social functions, intoxication occurs more readily and the risk of a "mixed" overdose is more imminent because of potentiation of alcohol's effects.[1]

c. Effects

Like alcohol, the sedative-hypnotics produce CNS depression, which may vary from mild lethargy to respiratory depression, coma, and death. A misnamed "paradoxical reaction" of extreme excitation and agitation also has been reported in children (see Chapter 15). The psychotropic effects of sedative-hypnotics that result in their abuse include sedation and disinhibition.[1]

Long-term abuse of the sedative-hypnotics, unlike that of alcohol, has not been shown to result in permanent organic impairment, although short-term memory impairment on neuropsychological testing has been reported.[1]

d. Tolerance and Dependence

Tolerance to the effects of the sedative-hypnotics appears to be mediated by the induction of catabolic enzymes. Rebound anxiety following their acute use has been proposed as a mechanism whereby dependence develops.[1]

e. Treatment

i. Acute Intoxication.   As with alcohol, acute intoxication produces CNS depression and the risk of aspiration, coma, and possibly death in the case of overdose. General supportive measures, including maintenance of airway, electrolyte balance, and fluid intake should be provided.

ii. Withdrawal.   Any CNS depressant may produce a withdrawal syndrome similar to that of alcohol. When significant symptoms (e.g., autonomic instability and mental status changes) are present, the treatment is also similar, i.e., short courses of benzodiazepines or longer-acting barbiturates. If the substance of abuse is a prescription drug, simply prolonging the taper of that agent will also reverse the withdrawal symptoms.[1]

3. Inhalants

Inhalants are lipid-soluble, volatile compounds and include petroleum distillates (such as gasoline, turpentine, toluene, xylene, and benzene), fluorinated hydrocarbons found in aerosols, and the preanesthetic agents ether and nitrous oxide (laughing gas). Common, readily available sources of these agents include model airplane glue, nail polish remover, and typewriter correction fluid.[1,24]

Some surveys have indicated rates of use of inhalants in young adolescents (6th to 8th graders) in the range of 11–13% for use in the past year or lifetime use;[24,25] the rates tend to decline in older adolescents. This has raised questions about such use being an early marker for later substance abuse.

a. Pharmacology

As their name suggests, these agents are inhaled rather than taken orally and thus enter the systemic circulation without first-pass hepatic metabolism. This results in a "high" of more rapid onset. No specific receptor interactions mediate the effects of these agents. Rather, these agents impact on the production and distribution of neurotransmitters within the lipid bilayer of the neuronal plasma membrane. They are generally metabolized both renally and hepatically.[1]

b. Patterns of Use

In most cases the agent is passed from one individual to another in a bag containing a rag soaked in the inhalant. Group use is the rule and often occurs in "fads" among teenagers with limited access to other drugs of abuse.[1] The abuse is generally intermittent, and long-term abuse is uncommon.

c. Effects

The effects are usually short-term (lasting for as little as 15–30 min without repeated use) and include an altered sense of consciousness, misperceptions, decreased inhibitions, and euphoria, followed by lassitude and sleep.[1,24] Following the acute effects, symptoms of GI distress, coughing, mucous membrane irritation, tinnitus, and photophobia may occur. Cardiac arrhythmias are more common (or, rather, less rare) with halogenated hydrocarbons, which can sensitize the myocardium to the effects of noradrenaline (see Chapter 15); arrhythmias are among the most common causes of death associated with inhalant abuse. It should be noted that glues usually do not contain halogenated hydrocarbons. Long-term, heavy use of inhalants may result in significant hepatic, renal, cardiac, and pulmonary toxicities, and both peripheral neuropathies and CNS toxicities.[24] Gasoline inhalation may result in lead poisoning, although such outcomes are rare.[1]

d. Tolerance and Dependence

While tolerance to the acute effects may develop with prolonged use, no characteristic withdrawal syndrome has been described.[24]

e. Treatment

Management of acute overdose is similar to that for other CNS depressants (see above), with supportive care and monitoring of cardiac, renal, and respiratory functioning.

B. Stimulants

Stimulants include (1) cocaine (both the hydrochloride salt and the esterified base), (2) the amphetamines (dextro-amphetamine and methamphetamine), and (3) methylphenidate. Common street names for cocaine include crack, freebase, or rock, while methamphetamine is called crank. The abuse of these agents, particularly cocaine, peaked in the early 1980s, and although such abuse in youth has subsequently declined, it remains a major public health concern.[1,6]

The stimulant medications dextroamphetamine and methylphenidate are used as a first-line treatment for attention-deficit hyperactivity disorder (ADHD) in children and adolescents. Use of these medications for treatment of ADHD must be distinguished from use of these drugs in nonprescribed ways. Numerous studies have shown that methylphenidate and dextroamphetamine are rarely abused by children and adolescents who are prescribed these drugs to treat ADHD symptoms. Additionally, while there are some side effects associated with amphetamines and methylphenidate when used as prescribed (especially decreased appetite), they do not produce the euphoric "high" that is associated with cocaine. (See Chapter 8 for further discussion of stimulant treatment of ADHD.)

1. Pharmacology

Stimulants act by increasing CNS catecholamine activity, either by causing the release of neurotransmitters from their storage sites in neuronal terminals, by blocking neurotransmitter uptake, or by mimicking the effect of the catecholamines (primarily norepinephrine and dopamine) on nerve terminals.[1] Repeated exposure decreases the availability of intrasynaptic catecholamines, and thus larger dosages are required to produce similar effects (i.e., tolerance).

The length and rapidity of action vary, depending on both the specific agent used and the route of administration. The onset of action when cocaine is administered intranasally, intravenously, or by smoking is within seconds. The effects of cocaine generally last several minutes to one hour, whereas those of amphetamine and methylphenidate last for several hours. Although some hepatic degradation occurs with the amphetamines, these agents are renally excreted.[1] Cocaine is mainly inactivated by serum and hepatic esterases.

2. Patterns of Nontherapeutic Use

Cocaine may be snorted, injected intravenously, or smoked (especially the crystallized form of cocaine known as crack or rock).[1] Cocaine is primarily abused for its euphoric effects, and while it once was considered a drug for the "elite," its use has become more prevalent in all socioeconomic groups. Intravenous cocaine is sometimes accompanied by the use of heroin in combination with the cocaine ("speedball") to buffer the stimulant effects of cocaine and reduce the effects of the post-use dysphoria, or "crash."

The amphetamines are usually ingested, but they may be taken intravenously. They produce euphoria but also are used to lose weight (i.e., diet pills) or to avoid sleep (e.g., when studying for exams). Care must be taken in prescribing and monitoring these agents since physician prescriptions are a primary source of illicitly used stimulants.

3. Effects

In some persons, stimulants produce a sense of euphoria while increasing cognitive arousal and energy. However, when they are used in clinically appropriate doses, primarily in treatment of ADHD, this euphoric effect is not usually seen. Some people experience dysphoria rather than euphoria. Physically, stimulants can produce tremors, tics, tachycardia, anorexia, and insomnia. At toxic levels, they may induce psychosis and cardiac arrhythmias.[1]

4. Tolerance and Dependence

Tolerance for the euphoric effect develops quickly with these agents, resulting in rapidly escalating dosage needs among abusers.[1] Physical dependence also occurs, with symptoms of malaise, depression, fatigue, anorexia, insomnia, and drug craving all noted on acute withdrawal. Cross-tolerance may develop between noncocaine stimulants, but it is unclear whether it generalizes to cocaine.[1]

5. Treatment

a. Acute Toxicity. Management of stimulant toxicity focuses on reduction of CNS irritability, sympathetic nervous system overactivity, and psychotic symptoms. High fevers can occur and should be treated vigorously. Seizures can be treated with diazepam, although care must be taken in case the diazepam causes respiratory depression or arrest (especially when multiple drugs may be present in overdose). Acidification of the urine may promote renal excretion of amphetamines.

Medications should be used judiciously in the treatment of panic reactions secondary to stimulants. When needed, benzodiazepines may be helpful. In treating stimulant-induced psychosis, antipsychotic therapy is a useful adjunct to supportive therapy. High-potency agents (e.g., haloperidol) are preferable to low-potency agents (e.g., chlorpromazine) to avoid hypotension and anticholinergic side effects. Also, chlorpromazine tends to increase the half-life of amphetamine. Benzodiazepines are recommended by some authors; however, others have expressed concern over their potential to increase violence secondary to disinhibition.[1]

b. Withdrawal. Pharmacologic treatment for cocaine abuse has focused primarily on minimizing the drug craving associated with cocaine withdrawal. Kaminer reviewed medication treatment for cocaine abuse[23]; there appeared to be some efficacy of desipramine in attenuating cocaine craving, although controlled trials of such treatment in adolescent cocaine abusers are lacking. A medication-free period is usually indicated prior to initiating antidepressant therapy since the withdrawal symptoms may abate quickly on their own.[1]

C. Nicotine and Tobacco

The abuse of tobacco (the sole source of nicotine) and its sequelae cost the United States billions of dollars annually in health care costs and loss of productivity and remains a worldwide public health care challenge.[1] Despite community and government efforts to decrease its availability and appeal, tobacco continues to be widely abused by teenagers, even as use in adults has declined.

1. Pharmacology

Nicotine affects multiple CNS sites. It stimulates the release of norepinephrine and dopamine. Depending on the dose, it may either increase or decrease the release of acetylcholine. The nicotine in cigarette smoke is rapidly absorbed into the pulmonary venous circulation, thus bypassing initial hepatic uptake and metabolism. Within seconds, nicotine can be detected in the brain and reaches peak serum concentrations (between 25 and 50 ng/mL) immediately following the smoking of a cigarette. An initial drop in nicotine's serum concentration after a cigarette is smoked occurs as the drug is distributed throughout the body, after which it is oxidized in the liver to cotinine, an inactive metabolite.

2. Patterns of Use

Smoking frequently begins in early adolescence (first experimentation usually occurs prior to 12 years of age). No particular social pattern of use is typical, although social adjustment difficulties are more common among teenage smokers. Tobacco is one of the so-called "gateway" drugs, its use often preceding that of other drugs of abuse.[1,19] There are limited data regarding the use of smokeless tobacco, with one survey indicating a 10% prevalence in the 30 days prior to being surveyed in 10th and 12th graders.[9] There is a significant increase in the incidence of head and neck cancer in users of smokeless tobacco, and thus its use is not benign.

3. Effects

Nicotine increases cognitive arousal via stimulation of acetylcholine receptors in the basal forebrain neuronal systems. Smokers report increased alertness and demonstrate enhanced attention and memory on visual surveillance tasks. Diminished irritability and aggression, enhanced relaxation, and increased euphoria appear to contribute to its reinforcing properties.

Nicotine's effects on multiple body systems are too extensive to outline in detail here. However, it does increase both heart rate and blood pressure, and the non-nicotine by-products of smoking impede respiratory function and contain carcinogenic substances.[1]

4. Tolerance and Dependence

Tolerance develops quickly to nicotine's psychological effects, whereas tolerance to its physiologic effects takes longer. Withdrawal from nicotine consistently results in craving for it (i.e. tobacco), irritability, anxiety, restlessness, decreased concentration, and weight gain.[1]

5. Treatment

a. Acute Toxicity. Nicotine overdoses are rare except in toddlers who ingest the leftover cigarette butts left out in an ashtray. The resultant toxic syndrome, which consists of vomiting, bradycardia, and respiratory arrest, can be life-threatening, and urgent medical attention in a hospital setting is essential. Gastric lavage and cardiopulmonary support are implemented as necessary.[1]

b. Withdrawal. Nicotine replacement therapy, using either nicotine gum or nicotine skin patches, is useful in relieving withdrawal symptoms. Nicotine nasal spray and nicotine inhalers are alternative forms of nicotine replacement therapy that are being developed. Nicotine patches and gum are the recommended initial therapies for smoking cessation.[26] Neither treatment should be used by an active smoker because of nicotine intoxication.[23]

Clonidine, a postsynaptic α_2-agonist that decreases sympathetic activity in the locus coeruleus, has been shown in some studies to improve the rate of smoking cessation and may be an alternative for smokers who prefer not to receive nicotine or who have failed nicotine replacement therapy. (See Chapter 15 for more information regarding treatment with clonidine.)

6. Therapeutic Uses

A number of reports have been published suggesting that cigarette smoking can alleviate the excessive sedation of the antipsychotic drugs and decrease tics in patients with Tourette syndrome. However, no controlled clinical trials of nicotine have been completed to date. The potential for abuse and health risks preclude any clinical use of this drug, especially in children and adolescents.

D. Dissociative Agents

Phencyclidine (PCP, commonly called angel dust) is the most commonly abused agent in this class. Other dissociative anesthetics, such as fentanyl, also have abuse potential.

1. Pharmacology

PCP is readily absorbed regardless of route of administration, is both hydrophilic and lipophilic, and therefore may have a very long half-life (several hours to days). Metabolism is primarily hepatic. It is a noncompetitive *N*-methyl-d-aspartate (NMDA) antagonist that binds to a site within the calcium-channel and blocks calcium influx. The psychotropic effects of PCP are thought to be mediated by hippocampal neurons, and one report suggests that they may be reversed using the calcium channel blocker verapamil.[27] However, PCP potentially interacts with multiple neurotransmitter systems, including the catecholamines, acetylcholine, GABA, serotonin, and/or opiates, all of which increase the complexity of its effects.[1]

2. Patterns of Use

PCP may be smoked, ingested, combined with other drugs (e.g., marijuana), or injected intravenously. Since it is relatively inexpensive to manufacture, it is often substituted for, or sold as, other more expensive street drugs [e.g., tetrahydrocannabinol (THC)].

3. Effects

The effects of PCP may vary greatly across different individuals, dosages, and settings in which it is used.[1] Furthermore, due to the lipophilic nature of the compound, it may be released episodically from fat stores, thereby increasing the duration of effects and decreasing the accuracy and utility of serum and urinary drug levels.[1]

At lower doses (1–5 mg), PCP produces euphoria, decreased coordination, increased emotionality, and mild tachycardia, diaphoresis, and lacrimation; higher doses (5–10 mg) lead to intoxication, perceptual illusions, and possible numbness in the extremities.[1]

Toxic reactions to PCP may include marked mental status changes, delirium, psychosis, catatonia, and autonomic changes, such as tachycardia, fever, hypertension, seizures, and respiratory depression. Some of these reactions are potentially life-threatening and require intensive medical evaluation and support.

4. Tolerance and Dependence

Tolerance to the psychotropic effects of PCP is noted. However, evidence regarding a distinct withdrawal syndrome is lacking.[1]

5. Treatment of Toxic Reactions and Overdose

Medical assessment of toxic reactions is essential because of potential life-threatening effects. For acute toxic reactions, intensive medical support in a hospital setting is required. The judicious use of low-dose benzodiazepines or high-potency antipsychotics may be useful adjuncts. However, because the side-effect profile of PCP and antipsychotics overlap considerably (anticholinergic effects, lowering of seizure threshold, increased muscle destruction and muscular rigidity), special care must be taken when administering antipsychotic agents to someone with a possible PCP intoxication.

E. Hallucinogens

Hallucinogens include the cannabinols, lysergic acid diethylamide (LSD or "acid"), mescaline (found in peyote), methylene dioxymethamphetamine (MDMA) ("ecstasy" or "XTC"), and psilocybin (found in some species of mushrooms). For the purposes of this discussion, the cannabinols will be considered separately from the other hallucinogens.

1. Cannabinols

Cannabinols include marijuana and its derivative, hashish, of which the chief intoxicant is tetrahydrocannabinol (THC). Common street names include reefer, grass, weed, pot, and hash (for hashish).[1] These agents are widely used by youth, and although they are classified as hallucinogens, they generally alter sensations of feelings and consciousness rather than causing outright hallucinations.

a. Pharmacology

The rapidity of onset and length of action depend on the route of administration. When smoked, subjective effects are noted within 30 min and may last 2–3 hr. These time frames are somewhat longer when the drug is ingested. THC is quite fat-soluble and has a prolonged half-life of approximately 7 days.[1] It is hepatically metabolized and excreted primarily in stool.

The mechanism of action of THC is not well understood, but its effects appear to be mediated through disruption of cellular metabolism and protein formation and may involve interactions with the dopamine system and benzodiazepine binding sites.

b. Patterns of Use

Marijuana and hashish are most often smoked but may be ingested. Many youth experiment with these agents, usually (like alcohol) in group situations. Solitary and heavier marijuana use is associated with other drug and alcohol use.[1]

c. Effects

THC has multiple psychological effects, including euphoria, relaxation, hunger, and an altered perception of time. Short-term memory is impaired. Anxiety symptoms, including panic attacks, and mild paranoia may occur. Physically, THC can produce tremors, decreased coordination, dry mouth, and bloodshot eyes.[1] Hallucinations can be seen in toxic reactions.

d. Tolerance and Dependence

Tolerance is not generally a problem with marijuana, although some cross-tolerance may occur with alcohol. It is questionable whether distinct withdrawal symptoms occur, but there are reports of mild sleep and appetite disturbances on cessation of the drug.

e. Treatment

Pharmacotherapy is generally not indicated for cannabinol abuse. A potential exception is use of antipsychotics for acute drug-induced psychosis (see Chapter 10). However, if the psychotic symptoms last for more than a few days, evaluation for other primary psychiatric disorders must be considered, since those with or developing psychotic disorders often use cannabis.

f. Therapeutic Indications

THC has been used to treat glaucoma and side effects of chemotherapy in cancer patients, and as an antinausea and appetite stimulant in AIDS patients but has no other uses in medicine now.

2. Other Hallucinogens

The hallucinogens (e.g., LSD, mescaline, and MDMA) are used to produce alterations in sensory perceptions, including visual illusions and hallucinations.

a. Pharmacology

The hallucinogens generally have similar chemical structures, are well absorbed orally, and tend to have adrenergic properties.[1] However, their relative potencies (regarding dosage requirements) and lengths of action may vary greatly.[1] While their exact mechanism of action is unknown, they are known to impact on many areas of CNS functioning, with predominate effects on serotonin brain receptors.[1]

b. Patterns of Use

The use of hallucinogens peaked in the 1960s and then subsequently declined with the increased popularity of other agents such as cocaine and PCP. LSD has had a resurgence over the last few years. Some Native American groups have used hallucinogens in religious rituals for centuries. However, most youth use them recreationally.

c. Effects

The primary psychotropic effects of hallucinogens include euphoria, altered perceptions, hallucinations, and an increased sense of introspection. Flashbacks—the reexperiencing of perceptual and emotional sensations similar to drug-induced symptoms—may occur for days or weeks after use of the drug. Physically, hallucinogens produce adrenergic effects, including dilated pupils, tremors, facial flushing, and an increase in blood pressure and body temperature.[1]

d. Tolerance and Dependence

Tolerance to increasing doses develops quickly and then abates when the abuse is stopped. Cross-tolerance exists between most of the hallucinogens except for marijuana. Physical dependence has not been described.[1]

e. Treatment

Medications are usually not necessary for the treatment of either acute panic reactions or drug-induced psychosis. If pharmacotherapy is needed, benzodiazepines are recommended, since the anticholinergic effects of antipsychotic agents may exacerbate the anticholinergic effects of hallucinogens.

f. Therapeutic Indications

Despite past claims that these agents may be useful adjuncts for psychotherapy, there is no evidence to support this use.[1]

F. Opiates

While opiates and opiatelike synthetic drugs are important medically for the management of pain, they also have a great potential for abuse. Included in this class of compounds are heroin (diacetylmorphine, often called smack or horse), morphine, meperidine, and codeine (3-methoxymorphine). These drugs constitute a serious problem in small, often inner-city, disadvantaged populations. Late adolescence and early adulthood are the times of greatest risk of abuse.

1. Pharmacology

The rapidity of onset, length of action, and relative potency vary greatly among the various opiate analgesics. They are metabolized hepatically and excreted through liver and bile.[1]

These agents act as agonists at a number of endogenous opiate receptor subtypes (μ, σ, δ, and κ) in the brain and spinal cord. The different receptor subtypes are associated with different clinical manifestations. Activity at the μ and σ sites seems to produce much of the psychoactive effects.[1]

2. Patterns of Use

Opiate abusers may either obtain drugs through medical sources (i.e., prescription drugs), use "street drugs," or be on legally obtained methadone maintenance. Youth most often use illicit (nonmedically obtained) opiates. All routes of administration are used, i.e., oral ingestion, intravenous, snorting, and/or smoking. Use generally begins as intermittent, but some individuals may then progress to daily use.[1]

3. Effects

These agents all produce analgesia, sedation, and euphoria. Associated symptoms include constricted pupils (except with meperidine), constipation, tremors, and confusion. Higher doses can produce fatal depression of CNS, respiratory, and cardiac functioning. The risk is increased with the use of street opiates because the strength varies greatly and is often unknown.

4. Tolerance and Dependence

Tolerance develops quickly, with some addicts being able to tolerate very high doses without signs of toxicity.[1] Cross-tolerance does occur among the various opiates. Dependence, both physical and psychological, develops very quickly with these agents. Withdrawal symptoms include malaise, runny nose, sweating, disrupted sleep and appetite, irritability, autonomic symptoms (e.g., dilated pupils, "goosebumps"), nausea, vomiting, and muscle aches, all of which may last up to a few weeks or more. Those agents with shorter half-lives tend to produce more marked and acute withdrawal syndromes.[1]

5. Treatment

a. Acute Intoxication and Overdose. Overdose of opiates is a medical emergency. Opiate antagonists are used clinically both for treatment of acute overdoses and as a maintenance drug to prevent relapse of abuse. Their clinical use in other psychiatric disorders is discussed in Chapter 15. Naloxone is the most commonly used antagonist for overdoses (used in conjunction with intensive medical support). Patients must be carefully monitored because naloxone has a short half-life and may lose its effectiveness while there are still toxic levels of opiate.

b. Withdrawal. Unlike withdrawal from alcohol and CNS depressants, opiate withdrawal states are seldom life-threatening despite being dramatic and uncomfortable. Acute opiate withdrawal should be treated with supportive care but may also require treatment with methadone or the α_2-adrenergic agonist clonidine. Polysubstance abuse is common, so other substances may aggravate the risk of withdrawal.

c. Dependence. Naltrexone, a long-acting opiate antagonist, has been successfully used for long-term drug-free maintenance, although the dropout rate in naltrexone treatment programs is greater than in methadone maintenance programs.[1] Methadone has been used successfully for long-term maintenance. Follow-up studies indicate that opiate addicts in methadone maintenance programs have lower rates of subsequent substance abuse and criminal behavior.[1] However, these programs have generally only included adults, and there is little information about the use of methadone in adolescents.

G. Miscellaneous Agents

Antitussive preparations as well as nonprescription anorexic agents and stimulants are primarily reviewed because of their availability, low abuse potential, and complex mechanisms of action. Many pharmacies in the United States keep "over-the-counter" antitussive preparations "behind the counter," where their purchase can be better monitored.

These complex pharmacologic cocktails frequently contain an antihistamine (see Chapter 15), which produces sedation and potentiates a narcotic analgesic; a non-narcotic cough suppressant, which nevertheless is an agonist for a subgroup of opiate receptors; a peripheral sympathomimetic; and sweetened syrup that is up to 10% ethanol. These preparations can be purchased legally without restriction. Although "mini"-epidemics of abuse with these cocktails have been reported, their general inability to cross the blood–brain barrier (see Chapter 2) results in weak psychotropic effects.

"Over-the-counter" or mail-order appetite suppressants and stimulants also have minimal psychotropic effects in comparison to their peripheral effects on sympathetic nervous system activity. Although they are infrequently abused, cardiovascular collapse and even stroke have been reported with these agents because of their cardiovascular effects.

A phenomenon that may contribute to the abuse of these above-mentioned, weakly psychotropic agents is conditioned abuse.[28] In animal paradigms, if substances of low abuse potential are repeatedly coadministered with a potent psychotropic substance of abuse, eventually the weakly psychotropic agent alone will produce similar behavioral effects. Such behavioral conditioning highlights the complexity of a psychotropic agent's effect on behavior and suggests that the effects of a substance of abuse may be partially reproduced by classical conditioning.

VIII. PRINCIPLES OF TREATMENT

This section will examine the more generic issues of substance abuse treatment common to all drugs. Drug-specific pharmacologic interventions were discussed in the previous section.

Most treatment interventions used for adolescents and children with substance abuse disorders are derived from therapies used with adults. There are many differing views as to what constitutes appropriate treatment, and unfortunately a data base supporting any one particular approach or philosophy is lacking. It is clear that a treatment plan must integrate a variety of factors, including specifics regarding the substance(s) of abuse, comorbid disorders, psychological and developmental attributes of the individual, family and peer dynamics, and the available resources and treatment programs within the community.[7,20]

The basic principles used in the treatment of substance abuse disorders are similar regardless of the specific substance(s) of abuse. Three major treatment goals must be addressed: (1) maximize the physical and mental health of the patient, (2) increase the likelihood of abstinence by enhancing the motivation of the patient through the use of patient and family education, psychotherapies, and behavior modification techniques, and (3) decrease social and environmental factors that act to facilitate further abuse by providing vocational and life-skills training, family counseling, and support for the development of non-substance-abusing peer groups and recreational activities. Treatment of adolescents must be peer-oriented and account for the developmental tasks and cognitive attributes of adolescents.[20]

A. Treatment Programs

Treatment programs generally are divided into four categories: outpatient, inpatient, residential, and aftercare. These share certain features, including (1) the goal of abstinence from substances of abuse, (2) the use of group therapies that include other substance abusers, (3) the use of self-help groups, i.e., Alcoholics Anonymous (AA) and Narcotics Anonymous (NA), and (4) the approach that substance abuse disorders are not cured but rather require ongoing treatment to maintain remission.

1. Outpatient Programs

Outpatient programs vary widely across different communities. This category of treatment programs includes counseling services, family therapies, educational programs, support (social, vocational, and legal) services, self-help groups, community mental health programs, day treatment programs, and halfway houses. Outpatient programs are the most common and cost-effective, although their effectiveness is controversial. Success in these programs generally depends on the motivation of the patient and family and is negatively influenced by comorbid psychiatric or medical disorders or other confounding social or environmental stresses.

2. Inpatient Programs

Inpatient programs usually provide more extensive diagnostic, psychosocial, academic, and family evaluations and therapies and are based in a hospital setting. Therapeutic modalities usually include a structured behavior program and milieu therapies; individual, group, and family therapies; self-help groups like AA; and academic and/or vocational programs. Inpatient treatment is generally reserved for those for whom outpatient treatment has failed or for whom confounding psychiatric, medical, family, or other social factors limit the ability to address the substance abuse issues on an outpatient basis. Inpatient treatment should be considered for those adolescents at risk for substance use withdrawal or with a past history of withdrawal problems, as well as adolescents with psychiatric disorders, symptoms, or behaviors such as psychosis or homicidal, suicidal, or other acutely dangerous behaviors. When inpatient treatment is utilized, lengths of stay should be kept short, since there is no evidence that longer hospital stays improve outcome as long as the hospitalization is followed by extended (6–12 months) aftercare services. One difficulty with inpatient programs is their expense. In the United States, they often require insurance and are frequently not available to public-sector patients.

3. Aftercare

Aftercare programs are an important component of inpatient treatment and contribute greatly to their success. These range from partial hospitalization programs to weekly counseling meetings and also include involvement in ongoing self-help groups. Strong case-management services are helpful in keeping patients involved in aftercare programs, thus decreasing attrition.

4. Residential Treatment

Residential treatment generally provides a level of treatment similar to inpatient treatment, although it is not necessarily hospital-based; it provides many of the same treatment modalities as inpatient programs but is generally less intensive, often does not provide the medical component of an inpatient program, and is considered more long-term. This kind of treatment may be indicated for a small number of patients whose comorbid psychiatric disorders and/or confounding social situations are so severe that success in less restrictive programs is not possible. These programs generally provide a multidimensional treatment approach, with an intensive structured milieu behavioral program, individual, group, and family counseling, self-help groups, and academic/vocational programs.

B. Pharmacotherapy

Specific pharmacologic interventions were discussed in the section on specific drugs of abuse. The primary role for pharmacotherapy in treating substance abuse disorders is for (1) managing withdrawal syndromes and acute toxicities and (2) treatment of comorbid psychiatric disorders. On a broader scale, the overall basic health requirements, including nutritional needs, of patients undergoing substance abuse treatment must be assessed. Unless there is a specific indication for their use, medications generally should be avoided once withdrawal is completed.

This recommendation extends to the use of psychotropics for apparent affective or anxiety syndromes, since the effects of the substance abuse and its withdrawal can mimic primary affective or anxiety disorders, and, as such, symptoms may clear with time. The exception to this is the use of antipsychotic agents necessitated by the emergence of psychotic symptoms. However, if the psychosis persists beyond the period of acute intoxication and withdrawal, the presence of a primary psychotic disorder must be considered.

Many adolescents presenting with substance use disorders do have comorbid psychiatric disorders; a period of abstinence from psychoactive substances and use of psychosocial interventions should be first used to address affective and anxiety symptoms. Factors that would suggest the need for additional pharmacotherapy for a comorbid psychiatric disorder include (1) history of psychiatric symptoms that clearly predate substance use or occur during definite periods of abstinence; (2) a significant family history of the psychiatric disorder; (3) past treatment failures and relapses; and (4) past success in using specific pharmacotherapeutics in treating the symptoms or disorder.[20] Even when pharmacotherapy is indicated, no medication on its own can be used to treat substance abuse/dependence; multimodal treatment is needed.

C. Treatment Outcome

The literature examining the effectiveness of treatment interventions for substance abuse disorders is confounded by a multitude of methodological problems, including insufficient follow-up periods and variations in defining the disorders, patient groups, treatment variables, and the outcomes themselves. Studies generally suggest beneficial effects of treatment but do not demonstrate superior efficacy with any specific approach. Several studies indicate that relapse rates are high.[29] More research is needed to examine the efficacy, specificity (with regard to defined groups of patients), and long-term impact of different treatment modalities. Comparison groups need to be incorporated into study designs since "spontaneous" improvement without treatment is not uncommon over time with adolescents, and factors that contribute to this outcome have not been systematically studied.

IX. CONCLUSIONS

Despite decreasing rates of substance abuse in youth, substance abuse disorders remain a major public health care concern and are associated with significant morbidity and mortality. Children and adolescents with substance use disorders require careful evaluation, including consideration of any comorbid psychiatric conditions and other confounding psychological, social, and interpersonal aspects of functioning. A clear understanding of the pharmacologic differences between substances of abuse is necessary, especially when treating acute intoxication and withdrawal. However, the clinician should also note that multiple-drug abuse is the rule rather than the exception and that the long-term management of substance abuse disorders is similar regardless of the specific characteristics of the particular agent. Alcohol and tobacco abuse remain the most serious of these disorders from an overall public health point of view.

REFERENCES

1. Schuckit MA: *Drug and Alcohol Abuse: A Clinical Guide to Diagnosis and Treatment*, ed 3. New York, Plenum Press, 1989.
2. American Psychiatric Association: *Diagnostic and Statistical Manual of Mental Disorders*, ed 4. Washington, DC, American Psychiatric Association Press, 1994.
3. Hindmarsh KW, Opheim EE: Drug abuse prevalence in Western Canada and the Northwest Territories: A survey of students in grades 6–12. *Int J Addict* 25:310–315, 1990.
4. Hartnoll R, Avico U, Ingold FR, et al: A multicity study of drug use in Europe. *Bull Narcotics* 41:3–27, 1989.
5. Johnston LD, Bachman J, O'Malley P: Press release from the "Monitoring the Future: A Continuing Study of the Lifestyles and Values of Youth" study. Ann Arbor, University of Michigan Institute for Social Research, December 11, 1995.
6. Oetting ER, Beauvais F: Adolescent drug use: Findings of national and local surveys. *J Consult Clin Psychol* 58:385–394, 1990.
7. Bailey GW: Current perspectives on substance abuse in youth. *J Am Acad Child Adolesc Psychiatry* 28:151–162, 1989.
8. Kumpfer KL: Prevention of alcohol and drug abuse: A critical review of risk factors and prevention strategies, in Shaffer D, Philips I, Enzer NB (eds): *Prevention of Mental Disorders, Alcohol and Other Drug Use in Children and Adolescents*. Rockville, Md, US Department of Health and Human Services, 1989.
9. Johnston LD, O'Malley PM, Bachman JG: *National Survey Results on Drug Use from The Monitoring the Future Study, 1975–1994, Volume 1*. The University of Michigan Institute for Social Research. Rockville, Md, US Department of Health and Human Services, 1995.

10. Bachman JG, Wallace JM Jr, O'Malley PM, et al: Press release from the "Monitoring the Future: A Continuing Study of the Lifestyles and Values of Youth" study. Ann Arbor, University of Michigan Institute for Social Research, February 25, 1991.
11. Cloninger CR, Sigvardsson S, Bohman M: Childhood personality predicts alcohol abuse in young adults. *Alcoholism Clin Exp Res* 12:494–505, 1988.
12. Halikas J: Substance abuse in children and adolescents, in Garfinkel BD, Carlson GA, Weller EB (eds): *Psychiatric Disorders in Children and Adolescents.* Philadelphia, WB Saunders Co, 1990.
13. Weiss G, Hechtman L, Perlman T, et al: Hyperactives as young adults: A controlled prospective ten-year follow-up of 75 children. *Arch Gen Psychiatry* 36:675–681, 1983.
14. Dinwiddle SH, Cloninger CR: Family and adoption studies in alcoholism and drug addiction. *Psychiatr Ann* 21:206–214, 1991.
15. Schuckit MA, Gold EO: A simultaneous evaluation of multiple markers of ethanol and placebo challenges in sons of alcoholics and controls. *Arch Gen Psychiatry* 45:211–216, 1988.
16. Cloninger CR: Neurogenetic adaptive mechanisms in alcoholism. *Science* 236:410–416, 1987.
17. Shaffer D, Garland A, Gould M, et al: Preventing teenage suicide: A critical review. *J Am Acad Child Adolesc Psychiatry* 26:675–687, 1988.
18. Macdonald DI: Patterns of alcohol and drug use among adolescents. *Pediatr Clin North Am* 34:275–288, 1987.
19. Kandel DB: Stages in adolescent involvement in drug use. *Science* 190:912–914, 1975.
20. Bukstein O: Practice parameters for child and adolescent substance abuse. *J Am Acad Child Adolesc Psychiatry*, in press.
21. Woolf AD, Shanon MW: Clinical toxicology for the pediatrician. *Pediatr Clin North Am* 42:317–333, 1995.
22. Myers WC, Donahue JE, Goldstein MR: Disulfiram for alcohol use disorders in adolescents. *J Am Acad Child Adolesc Psychiatry* 33:484–489, 1994.
23. Kaminer Y: Pharmacotherapy for adolescents with psychoactive substance use disorders. *NIDA Research Monograph* 156:291–324, 1995.
24. Meadows R, Verghese A: Medical complications of glue sniffing. *S Med J* 89(5):455–462, 1996.
25. Hansen WB, Rose LA: Recreational use of inhalant drugs by adolescents: A challenge for family physicians. *Fam Med* 27(6):383–387, 1995.
26. American Psychiatric Association: Practice guideline for the treatment of patients with nicotine dependence. *Am J Psychiatry* (suppl) 153(10):1–31, (1996).
27. Montgomery PT, Mueller ME: Treatment of PCP intoxication with verapamil. *Am J Psychiatry* 142:882, 1985.
28. Silverman PB: Direct dopamine agonist-like activity conditioned to cocaine. *Pharmacol Biochem Behav* 37:231–234, 1990.
29. Bukstein O: Treatment of adolescent alcohol abuse and dependence. *Alcohol Health Res World.* 18(4):296–301, 1994.

12

Antiepileptics (Anticonvulsants)

EILEEN P. G. VINING, M.D., RICHARD O. CARPENTER, M.D., and MICHAEL G. AMAN, Ph.D.

I. INTRODUCTION

Child mental health professionals should be interested in anticonvulsant drugs for three reasons. First, epilepsy is a relatively common disorder in children and adolescents with developmental disabilities and behavioral disorders. Second, anticonvulsant drugs, acting as they do to alter brain excitability, often have effects on behavior, emotions, and cognition. Third, the psychotropic effects of certain anticonvulsants, notably carbamazepine, valproate, and clonazepam, now are utilized in the treatment of certain psychiatric disorders such as bipolar and anxiety disorders, and this psychiatric use may well extend further in the future.

This chapter is organized in three parts. First, there is a discussion of epilepsy, its treatment, and the pharmacology of the commonly used anticonvulsant medications. This is followed by an overview of the cognitive and behavioral function of people with epilepsy, recognizing the contributions of factors such as the underlying seizure disorder, psychosocial setting, and the individual anticonvulsants. Finally, the psychiatric uses of these drugs are discussed; elsewhere in this book (Chapters 9 and 15), there is discussion of their efficacy in the treatment of specific psychiatric disorders.

II. THE USE OF DRUGS IN EPILEPSY

Unlike most of this book, this section is not meant to be a comprehensive guide to treatment (of epilepsy), which certainly initially should be left to specialists in the area.

EILEEN P. G. VINING, M.D. • Department of Neurology and Pediatrics, Johns Hopkins University School of Medicine, Baltimore, Maryland 21287. **RICHARD O. CARPENTER, M.D.** • Private practice, Atlanta, Georgia 30327. **MICHAEL G. AMAN, Ph.D.** • The Nisonger Center for Mental Retardation and Developmental Disabilities, Ohio State University, Columbus, Ohio 43210-1296.

Practitioner's Guide to Psychoactive Drugs for Children and Adolescents (Second Edition), Werry and Aman, eds. Plenum Publishing Corporation, New York, 1999.

Rather, its purpose is to inform those whose work brings them into association with children with epilepsy.

A. When to Prescribe

The prescription of antiepileptic drugs has undergone a change in the last 15 years as researchers have contributed to the knowledge of the natural history of seizures and as the spectrum of antiepileptic drug (AED) side effects has been better understood. With these data, physicians are better able to advise families concerning the risks and benefits involved in refraining from treatment or in prescribing medication for the child who has experienced a seizure.[1]

1. Risk of Recurrence of Seizures

The risk of recurrence of seizures is discussed in Ref. 2. In the past, if a child had a seizure, medication was immediately prescribed. This was done out of concern that "seizures beget seizures" and that great harm could result by permitting the child to have additional seizures. We now know that these fears are essentially unwarranted. It is clear from a variety of studies that individuals may have a single seizure and never have a recurrence. Depending on the study, the chance of recurrence after a single nonfebrile seizure ranges from 30 to 80%.[3,4] This wide range of possibility of recurrence is an epidemiologic reality, but what is the likelihood for a given patient? Few patients have a risk as high as 80%. It is important to know who is at greatest and who is at least risk, as this will influence the risk–benefit analysis. A recent study analyzed this issue prospectively in children.[5] After following 283 children for a mean of 30 months, a cumulative risk of seizure recurrence of 42% at 48 months was found. If the seizure was considered idiopathic, was generalized, and if the electroencephalogram (EEG) was normal, the cumulative risk of recurrence was only 26% at 36 months. On the other hand, if the seizure was symptomatic [presumably of a previous central nervous system (CNS) insult such as trauma or CNS infection], cumulative risk of recurrence was 60% at 36 months. Studies such as this are important in helping clinicians recognize that recurrence is not inevitable. Many children will experience only a single event, and the chronic use of potentially toxic medication to prevent something that will never happen is unwarranted at best and hazardous at worst. More information and better predictors of recurrence will make this element of decision making easier.

2. Consequences of Recurrence of Seizures

However, there will always be a chance of recurrence that is higher than in the population in general, and so the consequences of a recurrence must also be weighed (for additional discussion of this topic, see Refs. 2 and 6). These consequences vary with age.[6,7] In a young child who is generally well supervised, the consequence of recurrence may be small. That is, it is unlikely that the child will be seriously injured if another seizure occurs. On the other hand, an older, more independent child who ranges farther from home on a bicycle may be at a greater risk. The adolescent who is driving has still different risk parameters. This aspect of the decision making must be carefully individualized.

Another aspect of risk involves the potential danger to the nervous system from recurrent seizures. In children, the best information concerning this probably comes from the careful analysis of the impact of recurring febrile seizures (i.e., seizures occurring only in the setting of a febrile illness). In the National Collaborative Perinatal Project,[8] almost 1800 children were followed until age 7. Febrile seizures, even recurrent febrile seizures, were not linked to mental retardation, cerebral palsy, or learning problems. Even the risk of epilepsy (recurring afebrile seizures) was not substantially increased by recurring febrile seizures.

3. Cost/Benefit of AEDs

Unfortunately, benefit with the use of anticonvulsants cannot be guaranteed. Even when an appropriate AED is prescribed and levels are in the therapeutic range, 13–40% of children will experience a recurrence. Parents and professionals must realize that at least some risk of recurrence persists even when the child is treated. As with any medication, there are also risks of potential side effects. These are the focus of a major portion of this chapter. These side effects have become a major factor in the analysis of risk/benefit. If the risks of therapy outweigh the possible benefits, physicians and families should be more understanding of the decision to refrain from therapy when the likelihood of recurrence is small or when seizures are infrequent. This analysis also is reflected in the decision to tolerate partial control of seizures in order to minimize intolerable side effects.

B. Rationale for Prescription

1. Type of Seizure

The initial choice of an anticonvulsant medication is based on the type of seizure disorder a child has and the possible side effects or difficulties expected in using a particular medication.[6] Seizure classification is based on whether a seizure is believed to have a focal onset from a definable region of the brain (partial) or the onset is believed to be generalized, with bilateral and synchronous hemispheric involvement. Partial seizures can be either simple (motor, sensory, autonomic, psychic) or complex, which by definition means that consciousness has been impaired. Generalized seizures include absence seizures, myoclonic seizures, and tonic–clonic seizures (grand mal). A listing of seizure types is shown in Table 1 along with the old terms that were used prior to the adoption of the current International Classification in 1981.

2. Other Factors in Drug Choice

Once a seizure type has been determined, appropriate drugs are considered (see Table 2). After a review of possible side effects, cost of medication, and half-life (influencing the frequency at which drugs should be administered; see Chapter 2) as well as efficacy for a particular seizure type, a choice is made. For instance, partial complex seizures are probably equally well controlled by carbamazepine, phenobarbital, phenytoin, primidone, or valproic acid. Deciding which drug to prescribe depends on a variety of factors including the patient's age, social circumstances, and neurological function. The patient may have limited access to medical care or limited funds, and there may be a problem in administering medications multiple times a day. In that situation, phenobarbital might be an ideal drug. It is inexpensive and can be taken once a day. Although the physician should be concerned about possible side effects, particularly cognitive and behavioral (see below), it is the right medication if seizures are controlled and the child continues to feel well and perform at his or her baseline. If there are adverse changes in function, then it is probably the wrong medication, in spite of cost and ease of administration, and should be changed.

TABLE 1. Seizure Classification[a]

International classification	"Old terms"
I. Partial seizures	Focal or local seizures
A. Simple partial seizures (consciousness not impaired)	Focal motor seizures
1. With motor symptoms	Jacksonian seizures
2. With somatosensory or special sensory symptoms	Focal sensory seizures
3. With autonomic symptoms	
4. With psychic symptoms	
B. Complex partial seizures (with impairment of consciousness)	Psychomotor seizures
1. Simple partial onset	Temporal lobe seizures
2. With impairment of consciousness at onset	
C. Partial seizures that secondarily generalize	
II. Generalized seizures (convulsive or nonconvulsive)	
A. Absence seizures	Petit mal seizures
1. Absence	
2. Atypical	
B. Myoclonic seizures	Minor motor seizures
C. Clonic seizures	Grand mal seizures
D. Tonic seizures	Grand mal seizures
E. Tonic–clonic seizures	Grand mal seizures
F. Atonic seizures (astatic)	Akinetic, drop attacks

[a]Adapted from Rakel RE (ed): *Conn's Current Therapy*. Philadelphia, WB Saunders Co, 1990, p 803. Reprinted with permission of the publisher.

If the patient is very young, phenytoin might not be a good choice both in terms of the difficulty of maintaining therapeutic levels and because of potential cosmetic side effects. If a patient has hematologic problems, carbamazepine might be inappropriate. If there are underlying gastrointestinal problems, valproate may be inappropriate. Various factors are involved in deciding which drug should be recommended as initial therapy. There is as much art as there is science in making these judgments.

C. The Treatment Plan

Once the appropriate drug is chosen, the dosage should be increased until seizures are controlled or until clinical toxicity is seen. If a patient has infrequent seizures, it is reasonable to increase the dose until the patient has achieved a blood level within the therapeutic range, increasing subsequently only if there is seizure breakthrough. With AEDs, unlike most other drugs (except lithium) in this book, therapeutic monitoring of blood levels is very useful as a guideline to indicate subtherapeutic levels and possible problems with compliance. Blood levels also serve as a warning of impending toxicity, and, in more complex situations (polytherapy), blood levels may help determine which medication is more likely to be responsible for toxicity. Each patient must be monitored carefully and on an individual basis. This does not mean weekly blood drawing. It means looking at the impact of the therapy on the patient.

Finally, if seizures have been controlled for at least 2 years, consideration should be given to tapering the patient off medication. Epidemiologic studies indicate that 70–75% of patients who have had seizures successfully controlled can be weaned from medication without recurrence.

TABLE 2. Antiepileptic Drugs Therapy for Children[a]

Drug	Indications	Usual dose (mg/kg per day)	Usual dosage schedule	Half-life (hr)	Therapeutic range (μg/mL)	Side effects
Carbamazepine[c] (Tegretol®)	F, C, G	10–40	b.i.d.–q.i.d.	10–30	5–14	Headache, drowsiness, dizziness
Clonazepam (Klonopin®, Rivotril®)	M, A	0.05–0.10	b.i.d.–q.i.d	24–36		Drowsiness, ataxia, secretions, hypotonia, behavioral problems
Ethosuximide (Zarontin®)	A (? C, M)	20–40	b.i.d.	24–42	40–100	GI distress, rash, drowsiness, dizziness, blood dyscrasia, systemic lupus erythematosus
Gabapentin (Neurotin)	F, C	15–45	b.i.d.–q.i.d.	5–7		GI distress, dizziness, anxiety, change
Lamotrigine (Lamictal)	F, C (? others)	1–5 (on valproic acid), 5–15 (off valproic acid)	q.d.–b.i.d.	15–60		Rash, dizziness, diplopia, GI distress
Phenobarbital	F, C, G, S	2–8	q.d.–b.i.d.	48–100	10–25	Drowsiness, rash, ataxia, behavioral and cognitive problems
Phenytoin (Dilantin®)	F, C, G, S	4–8	q.d.–b.i.d.	6–30	10–20	Drowsiness, gum hyperplasia, rash
Primidone (Mysoline®)	F, C, G	12–25	b.i.d.–q.i.d.	6–12	6–12	Drowsiness, dizziness, rash, anemia
Topiramate (Topamax®)	F, C, (? others)	1–9	b.i.d.	19–23		Lethargy, dizziness, altered thinking
Valproic acid (Depakene®, Depakote®, Epilim®)	F, C, G, M, A	10	b.i.d.–q.i.d.	6–18	5–100	GI distress, hepatitis, alopecia, ataxia, tremors, pancreatitis, thrombocytopenia
Vigabatrin (Sabril®)	F, C, infantile spasms	40–100	b.i.d.	5–7		Lethargy, behavior changes, depression, abnormal vision, weight gain

[a]Adapted from Rakel RE (ed): Conn's Current Therapy. Philadelphia, WB Saunders Co, 1990, p 804. Reprinted with permission of the publisher.
[b]Safety and efficacy for use in children under age 6 have not been established.
[c]F, focal (partial–simple); G, generalized (tonic–clonic); C, partial-complex; A, absence; M, minor motor (akinetic, atonic, myoclonic); S, status.

III. PHARMACOLOGY OF DRUGS USED IN EPILEPSY

A. AEDs in General

It is reasonable to think about how AEDs work on a variety of levels: their effect on the whole brain, their effect on a variety of seizure models in experimental animals, their effect on neurons and neuronal interaction, and finally their effect at a molecular level. AEDs are tested traditionally by looking at their efficacy in animals in preventing naturally occurring photoconvulsive seizures in a baboon, *Papio papio*, with tonic–clonic seizures produced by maximal electroshock seizures, electrically induced or kindled seizures, and seizures produced by local cortical injury (freezing or locally applied convulsants).[9] Drugs vary in their ability to affect different types of seizures. For instance, benzodiazepines, valproic acid, and phenobarbital are effective against the natural seizures of *P. papio*. Phenytoin, phenobarbital, carbamazepine, and benzodiazepines are effective against maximal electroshock seizures.

At a neurophysiological level, the neuronal effects are studied (e.g., whether the drugs decrease epileptogenesis, propagation of discharge, transmission across synapses, or repetitive afterdischarges). For instance, valproic acid appears to decrease cortical spike activity (epileptogenesis), whereas phenytoin inhibits the spread of electrical activity.

Increasingly, action of AEDs is studied at the molecular level. At this level, the majority of AEDs act to decrease the spread of excitation across neurons, in particular, via alterations in ionic concentration gradients across cell membranes and alterations in synaptic transmitters [catecholamines, serotonin, acetylcholine, γ-aminobutyric acid (GABA), glycine, glutamate/aspartate, and adenosine]. Though many theoretical mechanisms have been proposed and various specific actions demonstrated, at therapeutic blood levels all AEDs seem to share a common action with all CNS depressants, which are thought to decrease ionic fluxes across the neuronal membrane, thereby decreasing excitability (see Chapters 11 and 15). Full discussion of these topics is beyond the scope of this chapter, but the reader is referred to specialized texts[10–12] and an excellent book that places these discussions in the intriguing framework of the actions of these drugs on neuronal networks.[13]

B. Bromides

Introduced in 1857, bromides are the oldest specific anticonvulsants. Simple salts, they are apparently useful in tonic–clonic as well as partial seizures. They have very long half-lives (approximately 12 days), the therapeutic range is narrow, and toxicity can become a real problem without careful monitoring of levels. Side effects include drowsiness and an acne-type rash. Psychotic reactions of a delirium type are rare, perhaps more frequently seen in the elderly. These drugs, usually administered as triple bromide elixir, are generally reserved for the most intractable seizures because of the frequency of side effects and difficulty in titrating the dose.

C. Barbiturates

1. Phenobarbital

Phenobarbital was introduced into clinical therapy of seizures in 1912 and has remained a mainstay of therapy ever since because of its ease of administration and low cost, though it has fallen into some disrepute recently.[14] It is readily absorbed and has a long half-life, 48–100 hr. The usual daily dose is 2–8 mg/kg, and generally, because of the long half-life, the medication can be given in a single daily dose. Neurotoxicity is probably the major side effect, with problems including drowsiness, irritability, changes in sleep patterns, attentional problems, and cognitive changes. Hematologic and hepatic problems are rare. Idiosyncratic drug rashes do occur and can be quite serious. Patients often show some evidence of toxicity when blood levels are over 25 mg/L.

2. Mephobarbital (Mebaral®)

Mephobarbital is demethylated to phenobarbital. Comparable levels of phenobarbital are achieved by using a 2:1 ratio (i.e., 2 mg of mephobarbital for each milligram of phenobarbital). It has received attention because of anecdotal evidence that it may have less neurotoxicity.

3. Primidone (Mysoline®)

Primidone is oxidized to phenobarbital and another metabolite, phenylethylmalonide (PEMA), which may also have anticonvulsant properties. Its initiation requires careful slow titration since early side effects may lead to discontinuation. If it is tolerated, many clinicians find that significantly higher levels of phenobarbital may be achieved without the sedation usually associated with the administration of phenobarbital itself. This drug is of interest because it may have additional anticonvulsant properties as well as less neurotoxicity.

D. Hydantoins (Phenytoin, Mephenytoin, Ethotoin)

The hydantoins are stereochemically related to the barbiturates.

1. Phenytoin (Dilantin®)

Since its introduction in the late 1930s, phenytoin has played an important role in seizure control because it was the first major anticonvulsant without significant sedating effects at doses able to control seizures. The pharmacology of the drug is somewhat complicated. Phenytoin inhibits its own biotransformation in a dose-dependent manner, and the enzyme system eliminating phenytoin can be completely saturated with usual therapeutic doses. In other words, it may take as long as 4–12 weeks for steady state to be actually achieved, although most drugs with its half-life would be predicted to reach steady state in about 5 days. In addition, when a patient is near or in the low end of the therapeutic range, a small increase in dosage may lead to very high serum concentrations, a function of the zero-order kinetics (see Chapter 2) seen with phenytoin.

There are significant age variables that also contribute to some difficulty in using phenytoin in children. In neonates, and even in young children, oral absorption of phenytoin is often incomplete and erratic. The elimination half-life also varies. It ranges from 20 to 60 hr in the newborn and diminishes to 5–18 hr in older children.

Dose-dependent side effects include drowsiness, ataxia, nausea, and vomiting. Idiosyncratic side effects include drug rashes, hepatitis, and lymphadenopathy. The chronic side effects of phenytoin are of particular concern in pediatrics. These include gingival hyperplasia, hirsutism (hair growth), and coarsening of facial features.

2. Other Hydantoins

There are several hydantoin derivatives that are occasionally used in the treatment of seizures. Mephenytoin (Mesantoin®) appears to be effective in controlling tonic–clonic and simple partial seizures. However, serious side effects (dermatitis, agranulocytosis, aplastic anemia, and hepatitis) occur more frequently than with phenytoin. Ethotoin (Peganone®) is probably less effective than phenytoin, though this may be related to the need to use high doses and to administer it three or four times a day. It does appear to have fewer side effects than phenytoin, particularly those of a cosmetic nature, which may be important in treating children.[15]

E. Succinimides

The succinimides are effective against pentylenetetrazol seizures, an animal model of absence seizures.

1. Ethosuximide (Zarontin®)

Ethosuximide is probably the most frequently prescribed drug for classical absence seizures (petit mal). It also appears to have some efficacy in myoclonic and atonic seizures. It has a long but variable half-life ranging from 20 to 60 hr, tending to be longer in older children and adults. Common side effects include gastrointestinal disturbances, headache, and drowsiness. More serious, but extremely rare, problems include leukopenia, rashes, and systemic lupus erythematosus.

2. Methsuximide (Celontin®)

Methsuximide is also useful in absence seizures but is probably not as effective as ethosuximide. Sometimes it is used as adjunctive therapy, and it is occasionally used in complex partial seizures. The side-effect profile is essentially similar to that of ethosuximide.

3. Phensuximide (Milontin®)

Phensuximide is rarely used because of reports of serious renal damage.

F. Carbamazepine (Tegretol®)

Carbamazepine (see Chapter 9) is widely used to control both partial and generalized tonic–clonic seizures. The average half-life with chronic administration is less than 20 hr and seems to decrease progressively, probably secondary to autoinduction of the metabolizing enzyme system. Because of the wide individual variability in half-life and problems with high peak levels similar to those seen with antidepressants (see Chapter 9), it is generally administered two or three times a day. A new sustained release formulation, Tegretol-XR, has recently become available and makes it possible to administer the medication on a twice-daily basis. Toxic symptoms, usually related to high levels, include dizziness, diplopia or blurred vision, drowsiness, and ataxia. Idiosyncratic reactions include exfoliative dermatitis, aplastic anemia, thrombocytopenia, pancytopenia, and jaundice. Fortunately, these symptoms are quite rare.

G. Valproic Acid (Depakene®, Depakote®, Epilim®)

Valproic acid (see Chapter 9) appears to be one of the more broad-spectrum anticonvulsants, effective in absence, myoclonic, tonic-clonic, and complex partial seizures. The average half-life is 8–9 hr when valproic acid is used with other enzyme-inducing comedications. It is longer when used as monotherapy. Generally, it is given two or three times a day. Common, often dose-related, side effects include gastrointestinal disturbance, sedation, tremor, and weight gain or loss. Idiosyncratic reactions include hepatic toxicity (markedly diminished when the drug is used as monotherapy), pancreatitis, thrombocytopenia, and alopecia.

H. Benzodiazepines (Diazepam, Clonazepam, Lorazepam, Clorazepate)

Both diazepam (Valium®) and lorazepam (Ativan®) are used intravenously in status epilepticus. Diazepam is not used as a chronic anticonvulsant, because it has a reputation for causing sedation, though most benzodiazepines are more alike pharmacologically than marketing strategies suggest (see Chapters 9, 11, and 15). Clonazepam (Klonopin®, Rivotril®) is used for absence, myoclonic, and atonic seizures and for infantile spasms where control with other drugs is difficult. It is also used as adjunctive therapy in a variety of other seizure disorders. The half-life is 20–40 hr. As with all benzodiazepines, tolerance may develop. Side effects include drowsiness, ataxia, and behavioral changes, such as irritability and hyperactivity. Difficulties in swallowing and handling of secretions in multiply handicapped children (epilepsy, mental retardation, and cerebral palsy) are noted. Clorazepate (Tranxene®) is used predominantly as adjunctive therapy in complex partial seizures. The half-life is approximately 40 hr. Side effects include drowsiness and dizziness as well as changes in personality. Lorazepam (Ativan®) is being used in some chronic seizure disorders, but adequate studies are not available.

I. Felbamate

Felbamate[16] (Felbatol®, a meprobamate analogue) was widely marketed as being efficacious as monotherapy or adjunctive therapy for partial seizures and was clinically effective in Lennox–Gastaut syndrome. It has a number of drug–drug interactions and requires careful titration of concomitant medications. Although originally believed to be virtually free of side effects, after about a year of clinical use (in 1994), an increased incidence of aplastic anemia and acute hepatic necrosis was noted, and careful instructions/warnings concerning its use have been issued. The risk of aplastic anemia may be as high as 1 in 4000 (possibly lower in children), and the risk of hepatic failure is approximately 1 in 7700. Other dose-dependent side effects included nausea, weight loss, insomnia, headache, and fatigue.

J. Gabapentin

Although gabapentin (Neurontin®) was formulated to function as a GABA agonist, its mechanism of action remains uncertain. This is a particularly important new medication since it is not hepatically metabolized and is cleared unchanged by the kidneys. Therefore, drug–drug interactions (with other antiepileptic medications or other concomitant medications) do not occur. It is licensed for use in adults as adjunctive therapy for partial seizures. Originally, it was believed that the maximal adult dose would be in the range of 1800 mg/day. Clinical use has expanded this dose range to as high as 4800 mg/day. It is thought that the body is unable to utilize doses exceeding this. It does have a short half-life and requires dosing three times a day.

Side effects include drowsiness, dizziness, ataxia, headache, nystagmus, tremor, and nausea/vomiting.

K. Lamotrigine

Lamotrigine[17] (Lamictal®) is a phenyltriazine and is chemically unrelated to other antiepileptic drugs. According to the package insert, one mechanism of action is an inhibitory effect on sodium channels; in vitro studies suggested that lamotrigine stabilizes neuronal membranes and thereby moderates the release of excitatory amino acids (e.g., glutamate and aspartate). Receptor binding assays showed a weak inhibitory effect on the serotonin 5-HT$_3$ receptor, but lamotrigine did not have high affinity for a variety of other receptors (dopamine D$_1$ and D$_2$, GABA, histamine H$_1$, κ-opioid, muscarinic acetylcholine, and serotonin 5-HT$_2$). Lamotrigine appears to have a wide spectrum of efficacy. It is currently licensed as adjunctive therapy in adults for partial seizures. However, clinical experience suggests that it is also useful in generalized tonic-clonic seizures, absence seizures, myoclonic seizures, and even infantile spasms.

Lamotrigine has a moderately long half-life, especially as monotherapy (24 h), and can generally be given two times a day. There are a number of drug interactions. When used with hepatic-enzyme-inducing medications such as phenytoin and carbamazepine, the half-life is reduced to 12 hr. There is some increased difficulty adding lamotrigine to valproic acid. Valproic acid markedly increases the half-life of lamotrigine (48–72 hr), and the concomitant use of these medications seems to increase the likelihood of developing severe drug rashes, including Stevens–Johnson syndrome. Therefore, lamotrigine is started at extremely low doses and increased slowly over 1–2 months. It can be increased at a somewhat faster rate if valproic acid is not present, but, in general, the initiation of this drug requires great patience to avoid drug rashes.

Side effects include dizziness, headache, diplopia, ataxia, nausea, somnolence, and vomiting. As noted above, severe rashes, Stevens–Johnson syndrome, hematologic abnormalities, and acute kidney failure have been reported.

L. Topiramate

Topiramate[18] (Topamax®) has recently been licensed, again as adjunctive therapy in adults for partial seizures. It appears to have multiple actions on sodium channel and non-

NMDA glutamate receptors making it efficacious against the spread of seizures and in the enhancement of GABA-mediated inhibition that may raise seizure threshold, making it effective in absence seizures. It has a long half-life (20–30 hr), is predominantly excreted by the kidneys, and has a relatively low potential for interacting with other antiepileptic drugs. It has only begun to be used in children but appears to have efficacy in tonic, atonic, atypical absence, and generalized tonic-clonic seizures.

The side-effect profile includes the usual problems of dizziness and somnolence but also more vague complaints like "abnormal thinking," confusion, and impaired concentration. Weight loss and kidney stones have also been reported.

M. New Drugs

Several new drugs are currently in various stages of testing in the United States, though licensed and approved for use elsewhere (see Ref. 18). Perhaps the most encouraging of these new drugs are γ-vinyl GABA (vigabatrin) and tiagabine. Several others are also being evaluated. Many of these reportedly are more specific and may have less toxicity with respect to the CNS.

IV. COGNITIVE AND BEHAVIORAL FUNCTION AND EPILEPSY

Interest in the cognitive and behavioral function of people with epilepsy has emerged gradually over the last 25 years as continued efforts are made to provide for comprehensive care and improved quality of life. Historically, an association between epilepsy and intellectual and emotional deterioration has been noted for millennia, beginning with observations of epileptic patients by physicians in ancient Greece. Nineteenth-century writers discussed defects in memory, loss of intellectual power, problems with attention, and "defective moral control" in individuals with severe epilepsy.[19] Numerous investigators in this century have attempted to characterize these earlier observations more rigorously. CNS lesions, seizure activity (frequency, type, duration, time of onset), environmental factors, parental attitudes, the child's temperamental and personality traits, and effects of AEDs contribute to a complex web affecting the cognitive and behavioral functioning of children with epilepsy. Untangling the individual threads has proved most challenging. The following section will focus on some of these individual factors.

A. The Role of Epilepsy

An extensive review of the literature on mental deterioration in epilepsy[20] revealed several important aspects of the role of epilepsy in cognitive and behavioral functioning. Factors including seizure type, age of seizure onset, seizure duration, and seizure severity are identified as impacting on the intellectual and emotional functioning of children. Lesser et al.[20] point out that more severe conditions such as infantile spasms and Lennox–Gastaut syndrome have high associations with mental retardation, while in less severe epilepsy syndromes, evidence for cognitive and behavioral dysfunction is more difficult to demonstrate scientifically. The Isle of Wight Study showed that 18% of children with epilepsy were reading two or more years below grade level, compared with 6.8% in the general population, and parental reports indicated emotional problems in 30% of children with epilepsy, compared with about 7% of children without epilepsy.[21]

Although many studies have attempted to sort out the relative contributions to cognitive function of age at seizure onset, duration of seizures, and seizure severity, conflicting findings seem to be the rule when focusing on the group of children with less severe forms of epilepsy. Methodological differences between studies, differing populations of children, and lack of appropriate control groups provide some explanation for the conflicting study results. In recent years, study methodologies have been refined, and the relative importance of these factors has become clearer. In a representative study,[22] 118 children with epilepsy were compared with a control group of 100 children without seizures, using detailed neuropsychological tests including the Wechsler Intelligence Scale for Children—Revised (WISC-R) and the age-appropriate Halstead–Reitan Battery. Overall, children with a history of seizures had a significantly lower Full Scale IQ (FSIQ) than children in the control group (FSIQ 93 versus 100, respectively). Children with minor motor seizures and those with atypical absence seizures fared most poorly (FSIQ 70 and 74 respectively), but all seizure types with the exception of classic absence type were associated with FSIQ scores below those of age-matched controls. Other findings included positive correlations between a higher degree of seizure control and higher FSIQ as well as a highly significant inverse correlation between years with seizures and FSIQ. This study[22] clarifies some points but remains flawed by not exploring the relative contributions of antiepileptic medication, psychosocial factors, and underlying etiology of the seizures.

B. The Role of Psychosocial Factors

Emotional and social factors have been noted by many investigators to play a significant role in the cognitive and behavioral functioning of children with epilepsy. Henriksen discussed the alteration in parental attitudes that occurs when a child develops a seizure disorder.[23] He noted that it is common for parents to watch their child closely, often chronically afraid of the next seizure and its consequences. Under these circumstances, parents can become overprotective, set lower standards for the child, and potentially upset normal family relationships by developing abnormal attachments to the child. The interplay between these biopsychosocial factors can adversely affect the child's behavioral and emotional functioning through a variety of mechanisms independent of the seizure disorder. The child might not be allowed to interact in a normal manner with peers. The child with epilepsy may become self-conscious, feel vulnerable, or believe that he or she is in some way flawed and unable to compete with peers. Lower standards for one child in a family could result in that child's academic underachievement, or it might engender feelings of jealousy or sibling rivalry. Abnormal attachments to a parent could interfere with the child's overall developmental progress.

C. The Role of AEDs

Prior to the early 1970s, research on the neurobehavioral effects of AEDs consisted of case reports and slightly more than 100 clinical trials focusing on the efficacy and toxicity of available AEDs. It has been pointed out[24] that these clinical trials suffered from a number of methodological flaws—only 3 involved a double-blind protocol or proper statistical analyses, 25 included EEG data, and only 5 included a proper psychological evaluation. Optimal treatment of patients prior to 1970 focused on control of the seizure disorder using drugs available at the time (bromides, barbiturates, and phenytoin). Attempts were made to minimize severe toxic side effects from the medications, yet there was less awareness of and regard for the more subtle changes in neurobehavioral functioning. In the mid-1970s, efforts of multidisciplinary teams evaluating patient responses to the newer AEDs (carbamazepine, valproate, and, more recently, vigabatrin, gabapentin, and lamotrigine) began to focus on achieving seizure control with fewer adverse effects on cognitive and behavioral functioning. New methodologies have contributed to the knowledge base: comparative studies of two or more AEDs, drug elimination studies, studies of AED effects in normal volunteers, and high-dose–low-dose AED comparative studies. (see Ref. 25).

Table 3 presents the results of a representative sample of these studies and illustrates the wide variation in methodologies as well as results. Few studies have been done in children. A discussion of some representative studies follows to illustrate details, study designs, and problems.

In one of the first double-blind, counterbalanced, crossover study designs,[26] adult patients with partial, complex partial, or generalized seizure disorders and normal IQ were initially stabilized on phenytoin (Dodrill and Troupin, 1977;[26] Table 3). They were then randomly assigned to a 4-month treatment regimen with either phenytoin or carbamazepine, with a crossover after 4 months to compare the cognitive and behavioral effects of phenytoin and carbamazepine. Results indicated no difference in seizure control between drug treatment regimens, but significant differences favoring carbamazepine were noted on a neuropsychological and personality test battery administered at the end of each 4-month period, specifically on subtests requiring attention and problem solving. Some improvement in emotional well-being as measured by the Minnesota Multiphasic Personality Inventory was noted, again favoring carbamazepine. Although this study was groundbreaking in terms of study design, controlling for variables other than individual AED effect, a subsequent brief communication[27] revealed that serum level differences (e.g., high phenytoin levels relative to therapeutic carbamazepine serum levels) accounted for all the reported differences in the study patients. In other words, the key issue was the difference between drug concentrations, perhaps not individual drug effect on cognition or behavior.

Another study[28] examined the cognitive and behavioral effects of phenobarbital and phenytoin versus carbamazepine using a study design that involved an attempt at eliminating the more sedating anticonvulsants and substituting carbamazepine (Schain et al., 1977; Table 3). Neuropsychological testing was performed initially and again after 4–6 months on carbamazepine and/or phenytoin. Substantial improvements were noted on tasks requiring problem solving, alertness, and attention. Seizure control was either improved or comparable to that achieved on the previous regimen in over 80% of the study patients.

The cognitive and behavioral effects of carbamazepine, sodium valproate, phenytoin, and clobazam were studied in normal volunteers using a 2-week double-blind, placebo-controlled, crossover design (Trimble and Thompson, 1983;[29] Table 3). All four drugs significantly impaired performance on some items of a battery of neuropsychological tests at serum drug levels in the commonly accepted therapeutic range, but the patterns of drug-induced impairments differed depending on which drug was studied. Largest impairments were seen with phenytoin, particularly with regard to memory functioning. Valproate and clobazam appeared to slow down mental functioning, and carbamazepine appeared to impair motor speed.

TABLE 3. Representative Comparative Studies of Antiepileptic Drugs in Adults and Children[a,b]

Study	Goal	Comments/study design	Epilepsy variables	Cognitive/behavioral variables
Dodrill and Troupin, 1977 (Ref. 26)	Compare "psychotropic effects" and neurophysiological functioning between PHT and CBZ.	40 adults in double-blind, prospective, crossover for 4 months each. WAIS and Halstead–Reitan Battery used to assess neuropsychological functioning. Mean serum levels high for PHT, normal levels for CBZ.	Partial, complex partial, or generalized Sz. Normal intelligence. No difference in Sz control between groups.	Most abilities similar between groups. Fewer errors noted with CBZ on tasks requiring attention and problem solving. Some minor emotional improvement with CBZ. Below-average IQ improved more with CBZ. Difference in serum levels accounted for differential drug effects.
Schain et al., 1977 (Ref. 28)	**Compare cognitive effects of CBZ, PB, and PHT.**	**45 children: 26 PHT/19 PB. Replace sedative anticonvulsant with CBZ over a 6-month period.**	**Partial, complex partial, or generalized Szs. Normal intelligence.**	**37/45 improved Sz control on CBZ. Substantial improvement on WISC—all measures dependent on problem solving. Improved attention and alertness.**
Nolte et al., 1980 (Ref. 42)	**Compare learning and school performance between PHT and PRM.**	20 children: high PHT (4) vs. low PHT (4) (pre and post 6 mo); pre and 6 mo post-discontinuation of long-term PHT (8) and PRM (4); 6 normal controls	**Normal intelligence. Sz-free.**	**Decrease in WISC, especially verbal, with high PHT. Other groups improved at 2nd testing.**
Trimble and Thompson, 1980 (Ref. 41)	Compare cognitive and behavioral effects of PHT, CBZ, PB, and PRM	Normal adults assigned separately to PHT, CBZ, VPA, or clobazam and placebo for 2 weeks each. Preassessment given before placebo or drug. Balanced crossover design.	Normal adult subjects, without epilepsy.	Test battery of memory and concentration performance, and perceptual, decision, and motor speed. Greatest number of changes occurred with PHT. CBZ, VPA, clobazam did not interfere with memory but variously reduced perceptual, decision or motor speed.

Reference	Purpose	Subjects/Methods	Patient characteristics	Results
Smith et al., 1987 (Ref. 24)	Compare efficacy of Sz control and toxicity of PB, CBZ, PHT, and PRM.	622 adults—either previously untreated or undertreated for Sz—in double blind prospective study. Extensive battery of neuropsychological tests given 1, 3, 6, and 12 mo after starting drug.	Normal intelligence. Simple, complex, primary, or secondary generalized Szs. Equal Sz control except for partial Sz, where CBZ better.	CBZ produced fewer adverse side effects on tests of attention/concentration and motor performance than other three drugs.
Vining et al., 1987 (Ref. 30)	Compare cognitive and behavioral effects of PB and VPA	21 children. Double-blind, counterbalanced, crossover for 6 mo; placebo-controlled.	Normal intelligence. Partial or tonic–clonic seizures. Medications in therapeutic range. Equal Sz control.	4/35 neuropsychological variables significantly worse on PB ($p < 0.01$).
Mitchell and Chavez, 1987 (Ref. 98)	Compare cognitive and behavioral effects of PB and CBZ.	33 children; 18 PB/15 CBZ × 12 mo (blind test). 19 studied at 12 mo (?N in each subgroup). No drug levels reported. No validation of testing methodology.	Normal intelligence, partial and/or secondary generalized Sz. Newly diagnosed. Trend to better seizure control with CBZ.	No difference on McCarthy Scales, WICS-R, and Raven's Matrices. Behavioral scale—no differences.
Gallassi et al., 1988 (Ref. 44)	Compare cognitive effects of CBZ and PHT.	25 adults; 13 CBZ/12PHT. 26 normal matched controls. Withdrawal of anticonvulsants by one quarter every 3 months.	Sz-free for 2 years. Patients who developed recurrent Szs were dropped from the study.	Both patient groups performed worse than controls on complex reaction times. PHT affects cognitive function more than CBZ. Cognitive deficits reversible with discontinuation of drug therapy.
Meador et al., 1990 (Ref. 46)	Compare neuropsychological effects of CBZ, PB, and PHT.	15 adults in double-blind, triple-crossover design × 3 mo each.	Complex partial epilepsy.	Significant differences only for digit symbol with decreased performance with PB.
Duncan et al., 1990 (Ref. 99)	Compare cognitive effects of PHT, CBZ, and VPA.	58 adults; 25 controls. Double-blind, placebo-controlled discontinuation study. Discontinued: PHT = 21, CBZ = 15, VPA = 22 over 1–7 weeks. Assessments at baseline, after drug gone, and 4 weeks later.	All patients receiving two or more AEDs.	All AEDs had deleterious effects on simple coordinated hand movements with immediate improvement with discontinuing meds. Improved attention and concentration with removal of PHT; no difference of CBZ or VPA.

(continued)

TABLE 3. (*Continued*)

Study	Goal	Comments/study design	Epilepsy variables	Cognitive/behavioral variables
Aman et al., 1990 (Ref. 53)	**Compare psychomotor effects of CBZ at high and low concentrations.**	**50 children; battery of cognitive and motor tests. Testing of each child at high and low CBZ concentrations.**	Normal intelligence. Partial and generalized Szs. Sz-free for 2 months.	Peak CBZ level associated with better attention span, seat activity, and motor steadiness. Improvement was greatest in children with partial Sz.
Farwell et al., 1990 (Ref. 35)	Compare cognitive effects of PB and placebo.	94 start placebo, 42 finish. 83 start PB, 53 finish. Psychological tests at baseline, at 2 yr, and at 6 mo off drug. Results based on intention to treat. Changes in IQ related to expected IQ.	Febrile Szs. Medication changed if intolerable side effects developed or Sz breakthrough.	PB-assigned group: IQ 8.4 points lower than placebo group at 2 years (95.54 vs. 103.95, $p = 0.0057$); IQ 5.2 points lower than placebo group at 6 mo after drug discontinued (100.94 vs. 106.17, $p = 0.052$). No effect on Sz recurrence.
Aman et al., 1994 (Ref. 43)	**Compare psychomotor effects of PHT at high and low concentrations.**	**50 children; battery of cognitive and motor tests. Assessment of each child at high and low PHT concentrations.**	Normal intelligence. Partial and generalized Szs. Sz-free for 2 months.	PHT concentrations and changes from trough to peak concentrations associated with very few differences in psychomotor performance; consistent with impression of no effect.

[a]Boldface type indicates child studies.
[b]Abbreviations: CBZ, carbamazepine; VPA, valproic acid; PB, phenobarbital; PRM, primidone; PHT, phenytoin; AED, antiepileptic drug; Sz, seizure; WAIS, Wechsler Adult Intelligence Scale; WISC, Wechsler Intelligence Scale for Children.

A large double-blind prospective study of 622 adults in the Veterans Administration system investigated the comparative effects of monotherapy with phenobarbital, phenytoin, carbamazepine, and primidone on seizure control and neurobehavioral functioning (Smith et al., 1987;[24] Table 3). The study design incorporated several improvements over earlier comparative studies: (1) double-blind, randomized prospective protocol, (2) monitoring of serum drug concentrations, (3) appropriate control population on which to standardize test procedures, (4) adequate sample sizes, (5) clarification of seizure type by EEG and imaging studies, and (6) quantified frequency and severity of seizures.

Results demonstrated equivalent seizure control for all four drugs, with the exception of clearly superior efficacy of carbamazepine in the treatment of partial seizures. Neuro-behavioral effects were demonstrated by comparing each participant's performance before starting medication and at 1 and 3 months on medication. The advantage of using study participants as their own controls became apparent when the authors were able to demon-strate that no AED improved performance on the test battery, but carbamazepine clearly caused the least deterioration in functioning on the combined total score for the test battery.

The psychological and behavioral effects of phenobarbital and valproic acid were compared in 21 children using a double-blind, placebo-controlled, counterbalanced, cross-over design.[30] Each medication was maintained in the commonly accepted therapeutic range for 6 months. No differences in seizure control between drugs were noted. Four tests of neuropsychological function (block design, performance IQ, FS IQ, and the Berkeley Paired Association Learning Task) were significantly adversely affected on phenobarbital compared with valproate. Parental assessments of their child's behavior indicated signifi-cantly more behavioral problems on three measures while the child was on phenobarbital ("fails to finish," "basically unhappy," and "unable to stop"). Additionally, children were more "hyperactive" while on phenobarbital. The authors noted that both parents and physicians felt that the children were faring well on medication but that the study results provided evidence that the drugs may have been adversely affecting cognitive functioning and behavior (see Vining et al., 1987;[30] Table 3).

Other studies from Table 3 are discussed in the relevant sections that follow.

V. UNINTENDED COGNITIVE/BEHAVIORAL EFFECTS OF AEDS

Accumulated evidence from multiple studies of AED treatment in adults and children, suggesting differential and potentially adverse behavioral and cognitive effects, prompted the Committee on Drugs of the American Academy of Pediatrics to formulate a statement in 1985 on anticonvulsant medication in seizure disorders in children.[31] This was revised in 1995 to reflect newly accumulated information, particularly in children.[32] The comprehen-sive, though poorly controlled, study of Herranz et al.[33] was cited to highlight the adverse impact of phenobarbital on behavior. The Committee on Drugs concluded that side effects may be subtle and discrete, affecting isolated functions rather than overall performance, and acknowledged that effective in-office screening procedures do not seem practical. Physicians were encouraged to extend monitoring of an antiepileptic medication's potential for side effects to include cognitive and behavioral functioning. Frequent parental, teacher, and office observations of a child's mood, cognitive functioning, and behavior while on AEDs were encouraged. Furthermore, physicians were advised that adverse changes in a child's cognitive and emotional functioning while on AEDs might suggest that the dose of medication should be reduced or the medication changed if no alternative explanations for the neurobehavioral effects were apparent. Their findings and more recent contributions from the literature are summarized below.

A. Phenobarbital

Behavioral disturbances in children taking phenobarbital are common; with the percentage of treated children showing difficulties ranging from 9% to 75%. Outside of obviously toxic ranges, behavioral disturbances do not appear to correlate with serum levels of barbiturate. Hyperactivity is most commonly reported by parents, but fussiness and sleep disturbances in younger children and lethargy, irritability, disobedience, stubbornness, and depressive symptoms in older children are noted as well. Investigators have reported that phenobarbital selectively impairs short-term memory functioning in a dose-dependent manner, and some studies have reported significant decreases in measures of cognitive functioning in children treated with phenobarbital. A representative sampling of these studies is presented below.

In a double-blind, placebo-controlled, randomized study[34] of phenobarbital in toddlers aged 6–36 months following a febrile convulsion, no significant differences in mean IQ scores were noted between groups after 8–12 months. However, memory function was found to decrease with increasing phenobarbital serum level, and children treated for 12 months with phenobarbital had significantly lower general comprehension subscale scores than those treated for 8 months. Additionally, children treated with phenobarbital were more prone to daytime fussiness and a nighttime sleep disturbance characterized by waking for some hours between 12 A.M. and 4 A.M.

In another double-blind, placebo-controlled, randomized study of children at risk following a febrile seizure,[35] half were assigned to placebo and half to phenobarbital for a 2-year treatment period. Analyzed on the basis of intention to treat, children assigned to the phenobarbital group had an average IQ score 8.4 points lower than that of children assigned to the placebo group. Serum levels of phenobarbital on the day of testing did not correlate with IQ scores. Seizure-free intervals did not differ significantly between the placebo and phenobarbital-assigned groups. Six months after discontinuation of the phenobarbital, the IQ difference between the phenobarbital and control groups showed a persistent difference of 5.2 points. The authors concluded that phenobarbital is associated with a depression of cognitive performance that may last months after the drug is discontinued. This study has provided a great deal of controversy regarding its methodology, specifically the "intention to treat" design. This methodology leads to an analysis of the functioning of patients assigned to a particular drug, not to an analysis of the patients taking a particular drug (see Farwell et al., 1990;[35] Table 3).

A significant association was found between treatment with phenobarbital and the development of a major depressive disorder and suicidal ideation in children with epilepsy aged 6–16 years who were being treated for a seizure disorder with either phenobarbital or carbamazepine.[36] As might be expected, family history of significant mental illness appeared to predispose to this effect. At follow-up 1–2½ years later,[37] the phenobarbital-treated group continued to show a higher rate of major depression than the carbamazepine-treated group (38% versus 0%, respectively). No differences in efficacy of seizure prophylaxis were noted. Patients who had discontinued therapy with phenobarbital recovered from their depression. Patients who were initially depressed on phenobarbital and continued taking it remained depressed at the time of follow-up.

In a recent study,[38] 73 children were assigned to carbamazepine, valproic acid, and phenobarbital in approximately equal-sized groups. Each child was tested prior to medication, assigned to monotherapy, and retested at 6 and 12 months. The carbamazepine and valproate groups had essentially static scores on the WISC-R and the Bender–Gestalt test, and their performance did not differ significantly from that of the phenobarbital group although the latter experienced a drop in FSIQ of 2.9 points. The subjects were also tested on an auditory evoked potential (AEP) test, and children receiving phenobarbital showed a significantly increased latency in the P300 composite as compared with subjects taking carbamazepine or valproate. The authors argued that prolonged P300 latency may reflect disturbed information processing in the children concerned and that this measure may be a particularly sensitive index of AED CNS effects.

Summary of Possible Cognitive and Behavioral Effects of Phenobarbital

1. Cognitive: Decreased performance on intelligence testing, impaired memory (dose-dependent?)
2. Behavioral: Hyperactivity, fussiness, sleep disturbance, lethargy, depressive symptoms, stubbornness, disobedience

In passing, it should be noted that these effects resemble those reported for CNS depressant drugs in general, not just AEDs (see Chapters 11 and 15).

B. Phenytoin

Not surprisingly, given the pharmacological similarity between phenytoin and ethanol, systemic effects of toxic serum levels of phenytoin can mimic the symptoms seen in ethanol intoxication, including nystagmus, ataxia, dysarthria, and mental changes.[39] Descriptions of mental changes at toxic serum levels include feelings of tiredness, difficulty concentrating, and emotional lability. Cognitive effects include deficits on neuropsychological tests, attentional difficulties, and difficulties with problem solving and visuomotor functioning. In more severe instances, children have been noted to have an illness resembling a degenerative neurological disease that abated when the phenytoin was discontinued.[40]

Over the years, investigators have had difficulty reaching a consensus about the degree of cognitive and behavioral impairment associated with therapeutic serum levels of phenytoin. One study[41] showed a decline in cognitive abilities associated with raised serum phenytoin levels in a subpopulation of children attending a special school for children with epilepsy. Another[42] found that verbal IQ scores in randomly assigned high- and low-serum-level phenytoin groups of children were lower in the high group after 6 months, with no significant differences between the low group and the control group (see Table 3). More recently, yet another group assessed the effect of high and low phenytoin concentrations in children with well-controlled epilepsy and relatively low phenytoin concentrations.[43] Transition from trough to peak drug concentrations within these children caused few discernible effects on an extensive cognitive–motor battery (26 variables in all), and the authors concluded that fluctuations in phenytoin concentrations had either no effect or immeasurably small effects in the subjects (see Aman et al., 1994;[43] Table 3).

Phenytoin was noted to have ongoing adverse cognitive effects in adults over a 12-month period relative to controls on tests of attention, visuomotor functioning, and intelligence.[44] When the medication was withdrawn toward the end of the study period, there were no differences between the medication withdrawal group and the control group (see Table 3). However, the results of several of these studies might be due to phenytoin's well-recognized adverse effects on motor performance, especially motor speed.[45] In a reanalysis of their data on 70 adult patients, Dodrill and Temkin covaried out motor speed[45] and found that all differences in cognitive function between the high- and low-serum-level phenytoin groups disappeared, suggesting that losses in cognitive abilities were not intrinsic to the ability to perform the task, but rather reflected slowed motor abilities. These findings were corroborated in a study of 15 adults with partial complex epilepsy (see Table 3).[46] They were also supported in a subsequent study with 21 healthy adult volunteers who received both phenytoin and carbamazepine.[47] The active drugs only appeared to differ at chance levels from one another. However, the subjects did appear to perform more poorly on an information recall task with both drugs as compared with a no-drug condition.

Summary of Possible Cognitive and Behavioral Effects of Phenytoin

1. Cognitive (related to motor speed?): Impaired attention, impairments of visuomotor functioning, impairments on problem-solving tasks
2. Motor coordination: Nystagmus, ataxia, dysarthria (toxic levels)
3. Behavioral: Emotional lability, tiredness

C. Carbamazepine

Much of the available literature on the use of carbamazepine in patients with epilepsy suggests facilitation of cognitive and behavioral functioning.[48] Improvements in intellectual capacities, in attention and concentration, and in perseverance have been noted. However, the basis for the carbamazepine-associated improvements often is unclear. Investigators have argued that the beneficial effects of carbamazepine might not be due solely to carbamazepine-specific enhancement of cognitive and emotional functioning; rather, the improvements may relate to the substitution or discontinuation of more sedating or otherwise impairing AEDs (and/or improved seizure control), as has been shown in the work of Schain et al.[28] and others (see Table 3). In this regard, some of the data from the Veterans Administration cooperative study,[49] involving 622 adults with epilepsy, are both interesting and provocative. No significant differences in sedation were reported by patients assigned to carbamazepine, phenytoin, phenobarbital, or primidone monotherapy.

However, treatment with carbamazepine is not without side effects. One study[50] reported adverse behavioral and cognitive side effects from treatment with carbamazepine at therapeutic serum levels in 7 of 200 children treated for epilepsy. Adverse behavioral effects included extreme irritability, combativeness, agitation, insomnia, and hyperactivity, while cognitive effects included delirium, difficulty thinking clearly, and "bewildered" and "spaced out" feelings. Effects of carbamazepine were more pronounced in children with mental retardation. All effects were reversed when carbamazepine was discontinued. In a recent multicenter study, 260 children were randomly allocated to carbamazepine and sodium valproate monotherapy.[51] Data for 126 of 130 children assigned to carbamazepine were available for analysis. The most commonly reported side effects for carbamazepine were somnolence (19.8% of subjects), fatigue (10.3%), headaches (7.1%), and dizziness (6.3%).

A study of the performance of children with newly diagnosed partial complex seizures using a battery of neuropsychological tests before and after beginning therapy with carbamazepine indicated that the children performed more poorly, in a concentration-dependent manner, than healthy age-matched controls on tests of efficiency of learning new information and on memory-scanning rate.[52] Inexplicably, children appeared to have a mild beneficial effect from carbamazepine on tests of eye–hand coordination in the nondominant hand. No changes were noted in attention, simple reaction time, behavioral adjustment, or motor performance in the dominant hand. A subsequent study[53] of children with well-controlled seizures receiving carbamazepine monotherapy indicated differential carbamazepine effects at peak and trough levels on a battery of cognitive–motor tests. Results showed no difference in overall functioning between low- and high-carbamazepine concentration groups of children. However, differences between low- and high-carbamazepine conditions within each child were significant. Small improvements in response tempo, seat activity, attention/impulsivity, and motor steadiness were noted with higher carbamazepine concentrations. Improvement was noted to be greatest in children with partial seizures (see Aman et al., 1990;[53] Table 3).

Summary of Possible Cognitive and Behavioral Effects of Carbamazepine

1. Cognitive: Impaired performance on learning and memory tasks (dose related?—possibly less so than for other AEDs)
2. Behavioral: Irritability, agitation, insomnia, sedation, emotional lability (possibly less than for other AEDs)

D. Valproate

When valproate was introduced as an anticonvulsant, as with carbamazepine, reports again appeared of a positive psychotropic effect. This impression was probably related to improved seizure control plus better observation and monitoring of drug effects and levels and the elimination of more sedative, cognitively impairing medications. Research into the effects of valproate on cognitive and behavioral functioning in children is sparse. Adult studies of valproate use in normal volunteers indicate that valproate has minimal adverse effects at low therapeutic levels but may have significant adverse effects on cognition at higher levels. In a comparison of phenobarbital and valproate in children,[30] valproate produced equal seizure control but fewer toxic cognitive and behavioral effects than phenobarbital (see Vining et al., 1987;[30] Table 3). In 46 children with well-controlled seizures receiving valproate monotherapy,[54] low-dose (<20 mg/kg per day) and high-dose (>20 mg/kg per day) groups were evaluated using a battery of cognitive–motor tests. Significantly more seat movements, poorer auditory–visual integration, and worse performance on a maze task were seen in children on higher doses of valproate compared with the lower-dose group. The study also assessed function with respect to high and low serum valproate concentrations over the day, but concentration differences had virtually no effect on performance. Thus, higher doses of valproate may impair performance on some cognitive and motor tasks in children, though results might be confounded by higher doses of valproate being given to children with more severe epilepsy.

Several reports of wide-ranging toxicity associated with valproate treatment have been noted in the literature. In one study,[55] 80% of children on valproate had some toxic effects, including anorexia, vomiting, hyperactivity, lassitude, sadness, or sleep alterations, with those on higher doses having more side effects. Acute delirium has been reported in patients with mental retardation and generalized seizures,[56] though not all cases could be attributed to valproate. In the multicenter study of carbamazepine and valproate referred to previously,[51] the data for 118 of 130 subjects assigned to valproate were usable. The most common CNS side effects associated with valproate were somnolence (9.3%), fatigue (5.1%), and headaches (5.1%).

Summary of Possible Cognitive and Behavioral Effects of Valproate

1. Cognitive: Impaired psychomotor performance (dose related?)
2. Behavioral: Restlessness, drowsiness, sadness (?), sleep alterations (?), delirium

E. Benzodiazepines

Benzodiazepines first became available in the United States in 1957 with the introduction of chlordiazepoxide (Librium®) to treat anxiety disorders (see Chapter 15). Other benzodiazepines including diazepam, clonazepam, and clorazepate were noted to have efficacy in the treatment of both anxiety disorders and epilepsy. Chronic use of benzodiazepines such as clonazepam can be associated with sedative-type behavioral side effects including drowsiness, irritability, and occasional aggressive behavior. One review showed the frequency of these problems to vary from 2 to 50%.[57] There may be a predisposition to these problems in children with underlying behavioral disorders.[58] Memory impairments have been demonstrated in short-term trials of diazepam in adult volunteers.[59] One uncontrolled investigation reported on the behavioral and neurological reactions of 115 children and adolescents (most of whom had mental retardation and/or cerebral palsy) who were treated with clobazam.[60] Among the 79 patients who were maintained on the drug for some time, 30 (38%) developed complete or partial tolerance for the drug's antiepileptic effect. In all, 83 subjects (72%) were said to improve and 30 (26%) to worsen on at least one of seven behavioral symptoms. Greatest improvement was reported for alertness, mood, attention span, appetite, and balance. However, many of these children were previously receiving 1, 4-benzodiazepines, so any changes may have been due, at least in part, to the discontinuation of more sedative drugs.

Summary of Possible Cognitive and Behavioral Effects of Benzodiazepines

1. Cognitive: Memory impairments (psychomotor slowing)
2. Motor coordination: Ataxia (dose-related)
3. Behavioral: Drowsiness, irritability, aggression

F. Felbamate

There is a paucity of data on felbamate because few large-scale studies have been conducted owing to concerns about toxicity that arose soon after its introduction. In a study of the efficacy of felbamate in childhood epileptic encephalopathy (Lennox–Gastaut syndrome), a global evaluation of quality of life (alertness, verbal responsiveness, general well-being, and seizure control) was made. Neuropsychological tests were also conducted. The global-evaluation scores were significantly higher in the felbamate group than in the placebo group from day 49 to the end of the study (day 70). The only statistically significant change noted in neuropsychological testing was an improvement in the digit-symbol test on day 70 in the felbamate group.[61] In one review of the newer AEDs, felbamate was described as structurally similar to meprobamate but without its sedative effects.[62] CNS side effects of felbamate include headache, somnolence, insomnia, dizziness, and fatigue.[62]

G. Gabapentin

There are very few reports available on the effects of gabapentin (GBP) on psychomotor and behavioral functioning in children. In adults, the primary CNS side effects are drowsiness and dizziness, although one controlled study failed to find any psychometric changes. (see Ref. 62). In a placebo-controlled study, GBP had no effect on composite psychomotor and memory scores. Higher doses did produce significantly increased drowsiness.[63] One report of the clinical experience with adults claimed that patients taking GBP add-on therapy actually experienced less nystagmus, tremor, and sedation than controls taking other forms of monotherapy.[64] A study of 55 children found that GBP had to be either reduced or discontinued in 7 youngsters (13%) who developed side effects characteristic of the disinhibition sometimes caused by the benzodiazepines.[65] All of the affected children had developmental delays. The most commonly reported problems were temper tantrums, hyperactivity, oppositional behavior, fighting, physical cruelty, proclivity to annoyance, and increased anger. These were usually an intensification of behaviors already present before therapy began, and all symptoms were reversible on reduction or elimination of medication. A report of a smaller series of children indicated similar behavior problems, as well as the emergence of some bizarre behaviors, with GBP therapy.[66] We are not aware of any studies in which GBP has been assessed for possible cognitive–motor effects in children.

Several studies have emerged in abstract and rather anecdotal form since GBP became readily available. In an abstract, 7 of 32 patients (22%) were reported to display irritability, fear, or anger.[67] Schantz et al. reported 20% with mood changes.[68] Significant behavioral changes (aggression, irritability, hyperactivity) occurred in four developmentally abnormal children, necessitating withdrawal of the medication.[69]

Summary of Possible Cognitive and Behavioral Effects of GBP

1. CNS/Cognitive: Drowsiness (?), dizziness (?)
2. Behavioral: Reversible symptoms characteristic of attention-deficit hyperactivity disorder, oppositional defiant disorder, or conduct disorder; reversible bizarre behaviors (?); irritability, fear, anger

H. Lamotrigine

Once again, there is a dearth of information regarding effects of this novel AED on the psychological and cognitive-motor response of pediatric populations. One report from a larger multisite study of lamotrigine (LTG) in adults reported "marginal" reductions on a cognitive–motor battery, but visual inspection of the findings by the present authors suggested that performance did in fact deteriorate.[70] CNS side effects of LTG in adults are said to include dizziness, headache, and somnolence.[62] One report commented on the response of 59 children in a residential school.[71] A dramatic reduction in spike and wave events, often independent of seizure control, was noted. The author noted anecdotally that there were improvements in the patients' feelings of well-being, and he speculated that this was due to the reduction in spike and wave events. Another report commented on a case series of 13 children and adolescents with severe intellectual impairments who received LTG for their epilepsy.[72] These workers observed no significant side effects, drug reactions, or behavior problems, and they speculated that the drug is especially useful in children having neurological impairments in addition to their epilepsy.

Summary of Cognitive and Behavioral Effects of LTG

It is too early to speculate what the cognitive and behavioral effects of LTG may be in children and adolescents, given the near absence of research. LTG is somewhat unusual, however, in that there are anecdotal reports of brightening of mood and possibly enhanced performance. Obviously, this needs scientific confirmation.

I. Topiramate

In a review of the double-blind trial of topiramate (TPM), Shorvon[73] reported that 27% of subjects receiving TPM reported somnolence, 25% abnormal thinking, 17% confusion, and 13% impaired concentration. These symptoms were more frequent at higher dosages.[73] In a very small series in which TPM was used in Lennox–Gastaut syndrome, parents reported that interaction with environment and alertness were very much or much improved in half of the patients. Sixty-three percent reported no change or minimal improvement in the children's response to verbal requests or activities of daily living. In the same paper, monotherapy substitution of TPM in children with partial onset seizures, who were controlled on a single medication but had intolerable side effects, showed that in one-third of the children the dosage could not be brought to a therapeutic level because of cognitive/behavioral side effects.[74]

Summary of Cognitive and Behavioral Effects of TPM

It is premature to assess completely the cognitive and behavioral effects of TPM. As usual, the beneficial effects may be related to seizure control. There is some concern about a higher frequency of loosely defined abnormal thinking and impaired concentration.

J. Vigabatrin

We were not able to locate studies of the effects of vigabatrin (VGB) on cognitive–motor performance or mood in children. However, there are several studies of this drug in predominantly adult populations (ages usually extending from the late teens into older age). Four of these studies[75–78] examined VGB as add-on therapy in patients who were already receiving one or more AEDs for epilepsy (most commonly, complex partial seizures). One of these enlisted nearly 150 subjects.[75] There was a progressive decline in performance on a cancellation task as dose rose from nil (placebo) to 6 g/day of VGB (2 of 13 cognitive–motor variables). A second study[76] reported decreases in hand tapping and memory for design (2 of 20 cognitive–motor variables) in subjects receiving 3 g/day of VGB. However, one open study reported improved reaction time on a computation test with 2 g/day of VGB (1 of 8 variables studied),[77] and another reported improvements on a cancellation task, a trail-making task, and on a verbal learning task.[78] One study employed a crossover design to compare placebo and 3 g/day of VGB and observed no changes on nine neuropsychological variables.[79] Another investigation compared VGB (50 mg/kg per day) and CBZ monotherapy and reported superior verbal fluency, verbal recall, mental flexibility, and finger tapping with VGB.[80] An important issue in these studies concerns variable seizure control; this applies especially to the add-on therapy studies. To the extent that VGB reduced seizures (as compared with no-drug conditions), this could create the impression of a direct drug-induced psychomotor benefit, whereas any cognitive improvement may be the *indirect* effect of improved seizure control.

In terms of VGB effects on mood and subjective state, one of these studies[76] reported severe depressive symptoms in 2 of 22 patients, mild depression in 4 (compared with 2 on placebo), and subjective reports of impaired memory in 2 (compared with 1 on placebo). Another investigation reported transitory sedation at 2 and 6 weeks, which was no longer present at 12 weeks.[79] Other studies reported actual improvements on a life satisfaction index and on depression scores[78] and reductions in negative life events with VGB.[77]

Ferrie et al.[81] reviewed severe behavioral reactions to VGB in children and adults. In a multisite European study of 135 children, 8.8% of participants had excitement or agitation and 2.2% experienced insomnia. In another study of VGB in 66 children, 26% of subjects had moderate to severe hyperkinesis and 3% had insomnia. Approximately 6% of children across the reviewed studies required a treatment change because of adverse behavioral changes. In studies of VGB in adults, 3.4% of subjects (summed across all studies) were regarded as having psychotic or other severe behavioral reactions. Ferrie et al. felt that preexisting behavioral disturbances were a predictor of behavioral reactions in children. Reynolds[82] has also synthesized impressions from clinical experience with adults treated with VGB. The most common side effect across studies was somnolence (27% of patients compared with 13% on placebo). Depression and confusion also featured prominently, although with prevalences below 5%. Depression was noted in about 4% of patients taking VGB, and psychosis was observed in a very small minority. Depression has always resolved after drug discontinuance. Reynolds urged caution in use of VGB in patients with a history of psychiatric disorder.

Summary of Possible Cognitive and Behavioral Effects of VGB

1. Performance on cancellation (vigilance), hand tapping (dexterity), and memory tasks may be impaired. Isolated reports also exist of psychomotor enhancement.
2. Reversible hyperactivity, excitement, agitation, and insomnia may occur in a minority of children.
3. Depression (reversible) and psychosis have been reported in adults.

VI. PSYCHOTROPIC EFFECTS OF AEDS

Investigators studying patients with epilepsy have long suggested that there might be an association between epilepsy and a variety of psychiatric disorders, and various attempts to define what this might be have ranged from "epileptic personality" to specific psychopathology linked to specific types of epilepsy or brain loci.[48] Subsequent research has failed to confirm these findings. Refinements in study methodology, better definition of observed phenomena in individuals with epilepsy, and more uniform control and study populations have shown that while persons with epilepsy have an increased risk of emotional and psychiatric problems compared with normal individuals and other patient groups with non-neurological disorders, this risk is about the same as in other neurological disorders.[83]

Postulated associations between brain dysfunction (including epilepsy) and psychiatric illness prompted clinicians to explore whether anticonvulsant drugs might have efficacy in the treatment of behavioral and emotional disorders in adults and children.

A. Carbamazepine

Studies of carbamazepine in animals have consistently demonstrated its ability to depress or abolish seizures in the limbic system and temporal lobes, areas of the brain long posited to have some link with psychiatric disorder(s). Findings in some highly dangerous individuals (without epilepsy) of EEG abnormalities in the temporal lobe were first described in the early 1940s. Investigators since that time have noted that some patients with psychomotor epilepsy (complex partial seizures) have episodic aggressive behavioral outbursts that are not truly ictal. In these patients, a personality constellation characterized by "affective overreaction," "episodic dyscontrol," slowness of thought and speech, perseverativeness, stubbornness, vagueness, and anxiety states emerged as defining characteristics of what has been termed an "epileptic personality."[84,85] It should be noted that the majority of people with complex partial seizures do not have an "epileptic personality."

The hypothesis that limbic system dysfunction might be characterized by certain personality changes and "episodic dyscontrol" prompted investigators to explore the possible role of carbamazepine in alleviating or improving these conditions. To date, numerous case reports suggest neuropsychological benefits from carbamazepine treatment in patients with such disorders as "episodic dyscontrol syndrome" (renamed intermittent explosive disorder in subsequent editions of the *Diagnostic and Statistical Manual of Mental Disorders*), "organic delusional disorder," "organic personality disorder," and borderline personality disorder, but unfortunately there are few scientifically rigorous data to support widespread use of carbamazepine for these conditions.

A more nebulous clinical indication for the use of carbamazepine has followed clinical reports such as one that reviewed studies of carbamazepine's psychotropic effects in over 2000 patients.[48] Effects noted were summarized as mostly changes in affect in areas such as irritability, aggressiveness, impulsivity, and dysphoric episodes giving way to an elevation of mood. This mood-stabilizing effect is important in treatment of bipolar mood disorder discussed in detail in Chapter 9 and elsewhere.[86,87]

The usefulness of carbamazepine in nonaffective, nonepileptic psychotic illness has been suggested, although studies of classically defined chronic schizophrenic patients have not shown carbamazepine to be better than placebo.[88] A review of available literature on the treatment-resistant nonresponsive psychosis in adults treated with carbamazepine[89] defined "nonresponsive psychosis" as that occurring in psychotic patients who have continuing symptoms like thought disorder, persistent hallucinations, or delusions despite adequate trials of neuroleptic medication. Some patients had a diagnosis of schizophrenia; others had atypical psychosis with aggressive tendencies and interpersonal difficulties. Of 11 patients with temporal lobe abnormalities on EEG but not true epilepsy, 8 were significantly improved with respect to their psychoses on carbamazepine compared with placebo. This suggests that carbamazepine may be worth studying in such carefully defined groups, although it is important to remember that psychotic manic patients are often misdiagnosed in their early episodes. Another review focused on carbamazepine's utility in managing aggression in adults and children.[90] Most of the studies were in adults with schizophrenia or schizoaffective disorder, and most of these investigations reported some benefit or extensive benefit. Two reports involved children who had attention-deficit hyperactivity disorder (ADHD) with aggression, and they were divided in outcome—one positive and one negative. The authors commented that the methodology of these studies was generally inadequate and that the number of investigations was small. They also stated that the usual cardiac precautions employed for tricyclic antidepressants should be employed with carbamazepine.[90]

Studies of the neuropsychiatric uses of carbamazepine in children are much less compelling than in adults. A review of 28 clinical trials (primarily in Europe) involving the treatment of over 800 children[91] found that few studies were double-blind or used diagnostically homogeneous groups. Conclusions were as follows. (1) Five of seven double-blind, placebo-controlled studies found improved behavioral functioning in children on carbamazepine compared with children on placebo. Three studies demonstrated significant improvements in "purposeful activity," mood, and social adaptation. (2) Seventeen non-comparative studies reported on carbamazepine's effect on specific behavioral target symptoms. Nine reported improvements in hyperactivity, and five in aggressiveness. Ten studies reported optimal benefits in patients with "nonspecific pathological EEG changes." (3) Side effects from carbamazepine treatment were noted in 26% of children and most commonly consisted of tiredness, skin reactions, dizziness, and nausea.

Another review[92] reported increasing use of carbamazepine to treat a number of neuropsychiatric disorders in children, including aggressive behavioral disorders, impulsivity, hyperactivity or episodic dyscontrol, and emotional disorders characterized by mood lability or dysphoria—despite the fact that there are currently no FDA-approved neuropsychiatric indications for the use of carbamazepine in children. Studies found consisted primarily of case reports and open trials with few double-blind, placebo-controlled investigations. Though early studies[93–95] suggested significant benefits from carbamazepine treatment in children suffering from emotional lability with aggressive features and other disruptive behavioral problems, rigorous further exploration of these interesting findings has not occurred. In particular, such studies need to take account of advances in psychiatric diagnosis and adhere to proper standards for clinical trials.

Summary of Possible Psychotropic Uses of Carbamazepine

1. Established efficacy: Bipolar mood disorders
2. Possible efficacy (worth studying further—not routine clinical use): (a) ADHD, (b) "intermittent explosive disorder" and aggressive disorders, (c) conduct disorder, (d) some mood disorders in children

B. Valproate

Valproate is discussed in Chapter 9, since it has so far only a foothold in psychopharmacology and that is in bipolar mood disorder,[96] although there are scattered reports of its use in panic, eating, and substance use disorders.

C. Other AEDs

Early workers suggested that a number of older AEDs, such as phenobarbital and phenytoin, might be helpful in managing certain disruptive disorders in children. Although there were several positive anecdotal reports to this effect, there is no good scientific evidence that phenobarbital, primidone, or phenytoin has any role to play in managing disruptive behavior in children or adolescents unless this is accompanied by epilepsy or, more doubtfully, intermittent explosive disorder.[97] In fact, phenobarbital, ethosuximide, and primidone are more identified with adverse behavioral changes.[97] Some recent studies of lamotrigine have suggested that this drug may have a mood-lifting effect in some dysthymic patients being treated for epilepsy.[17]

VII. SUMMARY

Children with seizure disorders requiring AEDs may experience adverse side effects from these drugs with respect to cognitive and behavioral functioning. Although there is a growing literature on the cognitive and behavioral effects of AEDs in adults and children, it is not clear that individual AEDs have specific toxic profiles in every patient. For instance, it is incorrect to assume that every child given phenobarbital will become hyperactive. Differences between individuals in their clinical response to AEDs as well as differences in research methodologies continue to confound research efforts to reach a broad consensus regarding psychoactive effects of individual AEDs. From a practical standpoint, physicians should be aware of the general therapeutic and toxic profiles of each AED and weigh the benefits and risks of specific AED use in each patient. Efforts to treat with monotherapy, to follow closely a child's school progress and behavioral functioning during treatment with AEDs, and to balance need for seizure control against side effects are a prudent course to follow.

Cumulative clinical experience and the proposed relationships between neuropathology and psychopathology have prompted the use of AEDs in a variety of neuropsychiatric disorders, but the range of AED efficacy in the treatment of childhood and adolescent psychopathological disorders remains to be established, except in those associated with true epilepsy and bipolar mood disorder (Chapter 9).

ACKNOWLEDGMENTS. Work on this chapter was supported in part by a research contract from the U.S. National Institute of Mental Health (Grant MH N01 MH80011) and MH48 to M.G.A.

REFERENCES

1. Freeman JM, Vining EPG, Pillas DJ: Seizures and Epilepsy in Childhood: A Guide for Parents. Baltimore, Johns Hopkins University Press, 1990.
2. Hauser WA, Hesdorffer DC: The natural history of seizures, in Wyllie E (ed): The Treatment of Epilepsy: Principles and Practice, ed 2. Baltimore, Williams & Wilkins, 1996, pp 173–178.
3. Hauser WA: Should people be treated after a first seizure? Arch Neurol 43:1287–1288, 1986.
4. Hart RG, Easton JD: Seizure recurrence after a first, unprovoked seizure. Arch Neurol 43:1289–1298, 1986.
5. Shinnar S, Berg AT, Moshe SL, et al: Risk of seizure recurrence following a first unprovoked seizure in childhood: A prospective study. Pediatrics 85:1076–1085, 1990.
6. Camfield CS, Camfield PR: General principles of antiepileptic drug therapy, in Wyllie E (ed): The Treatment of Epilepsy: Principles and Practice, ed 2. Baltimore, Williams & Wilkins, 1996, pp 763–770.
7. Shinnar S, Vining EPG, Mellits ED, et al: Discontinuing anticonvulsants in children with epilepsy after two years without seizures: A prospective study. N Engl J Med 313:976–980, 1985.
8. Nelson KB, Ellenberg JH: Prognosis in children with febrile seizures. Pediatrics 61:720–727, 1978.
9. French JA: Antiepileptic drug development and experimental models, in Wyllie E (ed): The Treatment of Epilepsy: Principles and Practice, ed 2. Baltimore, Williams & Wilkins, 1996, pp 693–699.

10. Rall TW, Schleifer LS: Drugs effective in the therapy of the epilepsies, in Goodman AG, Rall TW, Nies AS, et al (eds): *Goodman and Gilman's The Pharmacological Basis of Therapeutics*, ed 8. New York, Pergamon Press, 1990, pp 436–462.

11. Wyllie E (ed): *The Treatment of Epilepsy: Principles and Practice*, ed 2. Baltimore, Williams & Wilkins, 1996.

12. Engel J Jr, Pedley TA (eds): *Epilepsy: A Comprehensive Textbook*. Philadelphia, Lippincott-Raven, 1998.

13. Faingold CL, Fromm GH: *Drugs for Control of Epilepsy: Actions on Neuronal Networks Involved in Seizure Disorders*. Boca Raton, Fla, CRC Press, 1992.

14. Alvarez N, Kern RA, Cain NN, et al: Antiepileptics, in Reiss S, Aman MG (eds): *Psychotropic Medications and Developmental Disabilities: The International Consensus Handbook*. Columbus Ohio, The Nisonger Center UAP, 1998.

15. Browne TR, Pincus JH: Phenytoin (Dilantin) and other hydantoins, in Browne TR, Feldman RG (eds): *Epilepsy: Diagnosis and Management*. Boston, Little, Brown & Co, 1983, pp 175–189.

16. Fraught E: Felbamate, in Wyllie E (ed): *The Treatment of Epilepsy: Principles and Practice*, ed 2. Baltimore, Williams & Wilkins, 1996, pp 913–919.

17. Messenheimer J: Lamotrigine, in Wyllie E (ed): *The Treatment of Epilepsy: Principles and Practice*, ed 2. Baltimore, Williams & Wilkins, 1996, pp 899–905.

18. Fisher R: Newer antiepileptic drugs, in Wyllie E (ed): *The Treatment of Epilepsy: Principles and Practice*, ed 2. Baltimore, Williams & Wilkins, 1996, pp 920–930.

19. Gowers WR: *Epilepsy and Other Chronic Convulsive Diseases: Their Causes, Symptoms and Treatment*. London, William Wood, 1885.

20. Lesser RP, Luders H, Wyllie E, et al: Mental deterioration in epilepsy. Epilepsia 27:S105–S123, 1986.

21. Rutter M, Graham P, Yule W: *A Neuropsychiatric Study in Childhood*. London, Spastics International Medical Publications, 1970.

22. Farwell JR, Dodrill CB, Batzel LW: Neuropsychological abilities of children with epilepsy. *Epilepsia* 26:395–400, 1985.

23. Henriksen O: Specific problems of children with epilepsy. *Epilepsia* 29:S6–S9, 1988.

24. Smith DB, Mattson RH, Cramer JA, et al: Results of a nationwide Veterans Administration cooperative study comparing the efficacy and toxicity of carbamazepine, phenobarbital, phenytoin, and primidone. *Epilepsia* 28:S50–S58, 1987.

25. Devinsky O: Cognitive and behavioral effects of antiepileptic drugs. *Epilepsia* 36(Suppl. 2):S46–S65, 1995.

26. Dodrill CB, Troupin AS: Psychotropic effects of carbamazepine in epilepsy: A double blind comparison with phenytoin. *Neurology* 27:1023–1028, 1977.

27. Dodrill CB, Troupin AS: Neuropsychological effects of carbamazepine and phenytoin: A reanalysis. *Neurology* 41:141–143, 1991.

28. Schain RJ, Ward JW, Guthrie D: Carbamazepine as an anticonvulsant in children. *Neurology* 27:476–480, 1977.

29. Trimble MR, Thompson PJ: Anticonvulsant drugs, cognitive function, and behavior. *Epilepsia* 24:S55–S63, 1983.

30. Vining EPG, Mellits ED, Dorsen MM, et al: Psychologic and behavioral effects of antiepileptic drugs in children: A double blind comparison between phenobarbital and valproic acid. *Pediatrics* 80:165–174, 1987.

31. Committee on Drugs: Behavioral and cognitive effects of anticonvulsant therapy. *Pediatrics* 76:644–647, 1985.

32. Committee on Drugs: Behavioral and cognitive effects of anticonvulsant therapy. *Pediatrics* 96:538-540, 1995.

33. Herranz H, Armijo JA, Arteaga R: Clinical side effects of phenobarbital, primidone, phenytoin, carbamazepine, and valproate during monotherapy in children. *Epilepsia* 29:794–804, 1988.

34. Camfield CS, Chaplin S, Doyle A, et al: Side effects of phenobarbital in toddlers: Behavioral and cognitive aspects. *J Pediatr* 95:361–365, 1979.

35. Farwell JR, Lee YJ, Hirtz DG, et al: Phenobarbital for febrile seizures: Effects on intelligence and on seizure recurrence. *N Engl J Med* 322:364–369, 1990.

36. Brent DA, Crumrine PK, Varma RR, et al: Phenobarbital treatment and major depressive disorder in children with epilepsy. *Pediatrics* 80:909–917, 1987.

37. Brent DA, Crumrine PK, Varma R, et al: Phenobarbital treatment and major depressive disorder in children with epilepsy: A naturalistic follow-up. *Pediatrics* 85:1086–1091, 1990.

38. Chen YJ, Kang WM, So WCM. Comparison of antiepileptic drugs on cognitive function in newly diagnosed epileptic children: A psychometric and neurophysiological study. *Epilepsia* 37:81-86, 1996.

39. Vallarta JM, Bell DB, Reichert A: Progressive encephalopathy due to chronic hydantoin intoxication. *Am J Dis Child* 128:27–34, 1974.

40. Logan WJ, Freeman JM: Pseudodegenerative disease due to diphenylhydantoin intoxication. *Arch Neurol* 21:631–637, 1969.
41. Trimble M, Corbett J: Anticonvulsant drugs and cognitive function, in Wada JA, Penry JK (eds): *Advances in Epileptology: The Xth Epilepsy International Symposium.* New York, Raven Press, 1980, pp 113–120.
42. Nolte R, Wetzel B, Brugmann G, et al: Effects of phenytoin and primidone monotherapy on mental performance in children, in Johannessen SI, Morselli PL, Pippenger CE, et al (eds): *Antiepileptic Therapy: Advances in Drug Monitoring.* New York, Raven Press, 1980, pp 81–86.
43. Aman MG, Werry JS, Paxton JW, et al: Effects of phenytoin on cognitive–motor performance in children as a function of drug concentration, seizure type, and time of medication. *Epilepsia* 35:172–180, 1994.
44. Gallassi R, Morreale A, Lorusso S, et al: Carbamazepine and phenytoin: Comparison of cognitive effects in epileptic patients during monotherapy and withdrawal. *Arch Neurol* 45:892–894, 1988.
45. Dodrill CB, Temkin NR: Motor speed is a contaminating factor in evaluating the "cognitive" effects of phenytoin. *Epilepsia* 30:453–457, 1989.
46. Meador KJ, Loring DW, Huh K, et al: Comparative cognitive effects of anticonvulsants. *Neurology* 40: 391–394, 1990.
47. Meador KJ, Loring DW, Allen ME, et al: Comparative cognitive effects of carbamazepine and phenytoin in healthy adults. *Neurology* 41:1537–1540, 1991.
48. Dalby MA: Behavioral effects of carbamazepine, in Penry JK, Daly DD (eds): *Advances in Neurology.* New York, Raven Press, 1975, pp 331–343.
49. Mattson RH. Selection of antiepileptic drug therapy, in Levy R, Mattson R, Meldrum B, et al (eds): *Antiepileptic Drugs,* ed 3. New York, Raven Press, 1989, pp 103–115.
50. Silverstein FS, Parrish MA, Johnston MV: Adverse behavioral reactions in children treated with carbamazepine (Tegretol). *J Pediatr* 101:785–787, 1982.
51. Verity CM, Hosking G, Easter DJ: A multicentre comparative trial of sodium valproate and carbamazepine in paediatric epilepsy. *Dev Med Child Neurol* 37:97–108, 1995.
52. O'Dougherty M, Wright FS, Cox S, et al: Carbamazepine plasma concentration: Relationship to cognitive impairment. *Arch Neurol* 44:863–867, 1987.
53. Aman MG, Werry JS, Paxton JW, et al: Effects of carbamazepine on psychomotor performance in children as a function of drug concentration, seizure type, and time of medication. *Epilepsia* 31:51–60, 1990.
54. Aman MG, Werry JS, Paxton JW, et al: Effect of sodium valproate on psychomotor performance in children as a function of dose, fluctuations in concentration, and diagnosis. *Epilepsia* 28:115–124, 1987.
55. Herranz JL, Arteaga R, Armijo JA: Side effects of sodium valproate in monotherapy controlled by plasma levels: A study in 88 pediatric patients. *Epilepsia* 23:203–214, 1982.
56. Pakalnis A, Drake ME, Denio L: Valproate associated encephalopathy. *J Epilepsy* 2:41–44, 1989.
57. Browne TR: Clonazepam. *Arch Neurol* 33:326–332, 1976.
58. Bensch J, Blennow G, Ferngren H: A double blind study of clonazepam in the treatment of therapy resistant epilepsy. *Dev Med Child Neurol* 19:335–342, 1977.
59. Ghoneim MM, Mewaldt SP, Berie JL, et al: Memory and performance effects of single and 3 week administration of diazepam. *Psychopharmacology* 73:147–151, 1981.
60. Munn R, Farrell K: Open study of clobazam in refractory epilepsy. *Pediatr Neurol* 9:465–469, 1993.
61. The Felbamate Study Group in Lennox–Gastaut syndrome: Efficacy of felbamate in childhood epileptic encephalopathy. *N Engl J Med* 328:29–33, 1993.
62. Wilder BJ. How about the new antiepileptic drugs? *Can J Neurol Sci* 21(suppl.3):S17–S20, 1994.
63. Leach JP, Girvan J, Paul A, et al: Gabapentin and cognition: A double blind, dose ranging, placebo controlled study in refractory epilepsy. *J Neurol Neurosurg Psychiatry* 62:372–376, 1997.
64. Chadwick D: The role of gabapentin in epilepsy management, in Chadwick D, Browne TR (eds): *New Trends in Epilepsy Management. The Role of Gabapentin* (Proceedings of a satellite symposium held during Epilepsy Europe 1993). London, N Royal, 1993 pp 59–65.
65. Lee DO, Steingard RJ, Cesena M, et al: Behavioral side effects of gabapentin in children. *Epilepsia* 37:87–90, 1996.
66. Wolf SM, Shinnar S, Kang H, et al: Gabapentin toxicity in children manifesting as behavioral changes. *Epilepsia* 36:1203–1205, 1996.
67. Cugley AL, Swartz BE: Gabapentin associated mood changes? *Epilepsia* 36(suppl. 4):S72, 1995.
68. Schantz D, Towbin JA, Spitz MD: Changes in mood and affect in patients on gabapentin. *Epilepsia* 36(suppl 4):S73, 1995.
69. Zupanc ML, Schroeder VM: Behavioral changes in children on gabapentin. *Epilepsia* 36(suppl 4):S73, 1995.
70. Banks GK, Beran RG. Neuropsychological assessment in lamotrigine treated epileptic patients. *Clin Exp Neurol* 28:230–237, 1991.

71. Besag FM: Lamotrigine: Paediatric experience, in Richens A (ed): *Clinical update on Lamotrigine: A Novel Antiepileptic Agent.* Kent, England, Wells Medical Ltd, 1992, pp 53–60.

72. Leary PM, Allie S: A new drug suitable for children and young people with epilepsy and intellectual impairments. *Epilepsia* 34(suppl 6):371, 1995

73. Shorvon SD: Safety of topiramate: Adverse events and relationships to dosing. *Epilepsia* 37(suppl 2):S18–S22, 1996.

74. Glauser TA: Preliminary observations on topiramate in pediatric epilepsies, *Epilepsia* 38(suppl 1):S37–S41, 1997.

75. Dodrill CB, Arnett JL, Sommerville KW, et al: Effects of differing dosages of vigabatrin (Sabril) on cognitive abilities and quality of life in epilepsy. *Epilepsia* 36:64–173, 1995.

76. Grünewald RA, Thompson PJ, Corcoran R, et al: Effects of vigabatrin on partial seizures and cognitive function. *J Neurol Neurosurg Psychiatry* 54:1057–1063, 1994.

77. McGuire AM, Duncan JS, Trimble MR: Effects of vigabatrin on cognitive function and mood when used as add-on therapy in patients with intractable epilepsy. *Epilepsia* 33:128–134, 1992.

78. Provinciali L, Bartolini M, Mari F, et al: Influence of vigabatrin on cognitive performances and behaviour in patients with drug-resistant epilepsy. *Acta Neurologica Scand* 94:12–18, 1996.

79. Gillham RA, Blacklaw J, McKee PJW, et al: Effect of vigabatrin on sedation and cognitive function in patients with refractory epilepsy. *J Neurol Neurosurg Psychiatry* 56:1271–1275, 1993

80. Kalviainen R, Aikia M, Saukkonen AM, et al: Vigabatrin vs carbamazepine monotherapy in patients with newly diagnosed epilepsy. *Acta Neurol Scand* 52:989–996, 1995.

81. Ferrie CD, Robinson RO, Panayiotopoulos CP: Psychotic and severe behavioral reactions with vigabatrin: A review. *Acta Neurol Scand* 93:1–8, 1996.

82. Reynolds EH: γ-Vinyl GABA (vigabatrin): Clinical experience in adult and adolescent patients with intractable epilepsy. *Epilepsia* 33(suppl 5):S30–S35, 1992.

83. Dodrill CB, Batzel LW: Interictal behavioral features of patients with epilepsy. *Epilepsia* 27:S64–S76, 1986.

84. Tunks ER, Dermer SW: Carbamazepine in the dyscontrol syndrome associated with limbic system dysfunction. *J Nerv Ment Dis* 164:56–63, 1977.

85. Kessler AJ, Barklage NE, Jefferson JW: Mood disorders in the psychoneurologic borderland: Three cases of responsiveness to carbamazepine. *Am J Psychiatry* 146:81–83, 1989.

86. Small JG: Anticonvulsants in affective disorders. *Psychopharmacol Bull* 26:25–36, 1990.

87. Post RM, Altshuler LL, Ketter TA, et al: Antiepileptic drugs in affective illness. Clinical and theoretical implications. *Adv Neurol* 55:239–277, 1991.

88. Carpenter WT, Kurz R, Kirkpatrick B, et al: Carbamazepine maintenance treatment in outpatient schizophrenics. *Arch Gen Psychiatry* 48:69–72, 1991.

89. Neppe VM: Carbamazepine in nonresponsive psychosis. *J Clin Psychiatry* 49:22–28, 1988.

90. Young JL, Hillbrand M: Carbamazepine lowers aggression: A review. *Am Acad Psychiatry Law* 22:53–61, 1994.

91. Remschmidt H: The psychotropic effects of carbamazepine in non epileptic patients, with particular reference to problems posed by clinical studies in children with behavioural disorders, in Birkmayer W (ed): *Epileptic Seizures—Behaviour—Pain.* Bern, Hans Huber, 1976, pp 253–258.

92. Evans RW, Clay TH, Gualtieri CT: Carbamazepine in pediatric psychiatry. *J Am Acad Child Adolesc Psychiatry* 26:2–8, 1987.

93. Groh C: The psychotropic effect of Tegretol in non epileptic children, with particular reference to the drug's indications, in Birkmayer W (ed): *Epileptic Seizures—Behaviour—Pain.* Bern, Hans Huber, 1976, pp 259–263.

94. Puente RM: The use of carbamazepine in the treatment of behavioural disorders in children, in Birkmayer W (ed): *Epileptic Seizures—Behaviour—Pain.* Bern, Hans Huber, 1976, pp 243–252.

95. Kuhn-Gebhart V: Behavioural disorders in non epileptic children and their treatment with carbamazepine, in Birkmayer W (ed): *Epileptic Seizures—Behaviour—Pain.* Bern, Hans Huber, 1976, pp 264–267.

96. McElroy SL, Keck PE, Harrison GP, et al: Valproate in psychiatric disorders: Literature review and clinical guidelines. *J Clin Psychiatry* 50(suppl 3):23–29, 1989.

97. Trimble MR: Anticonvulsants in children and adolescents. *J Child Adolesc Psychopharmacol* 1:107–124, 1990.

98. Mitchell WG, Chavez JM: Carbamazepine versus phenobarbital for partial onset seizures in children. *Epilepsia* 28:56–60, 1987.

99. Duncan JS, Shorron SD, Trimble MR: Effects of removal of phenytoin, carbamazepine, and valproate on cognitive function. *Epilepsia* 31:584–591, 1990.

13

Psychoactive Effects of Medical Drugs

**L. EUGENE ARNOLD, M.Ed., M.D.,
IGOR JANKE, M.D.,
BRENT WATERS, M.D., F.R.C.P.,
F.R.A.N.Z.C.P.,
and ANTONY MILCH, M.B.B.S.,
F.R.A.N.Z.C.P.**

I. INTRODUCTION

This chapter addresses the psychoactive effects of general medical drugs used in the treatment of children and adolescents with physical illnesses rather than psychotropic drugs prescribed for psychiatric or behavioral indications. "Psychoactive effects" will refer to acute or subacute effects in the behavioral, emotional, or cognitive domain. Anticonvulsant (antiepileptic) drugs are covered in Chapter 12. To avoid wordy repetition, the term "children" will mean "children and adolescents" unless otherwise indicated.

A. Use of Medical Drugs by Children

Medical drugs are widely administered to children. They may be prescribed for the child, obtained over the counter, or opportunistically commandeered from leftovers prescribed for another family member.

In Germany, the annual per capita consumption of medical drugs for the year 1985 averaged 11.7 prescriptions for all persons. The 0–5-year age group had approximately the average rate; however, the 6–14-year age group received half this rate. The elderly received the majority of all prescribed medications.[1] In Australia in a 2-week period in 1983, 60% of

L. EUGENE ARNOLD, M.Ed., M.D. • Ohio State University, Columbus, Ohio 43210. **IGOR JANKE, M.D.** • Department of Psychiatry, Ohio State University, Columbus, Ohio 43210. **BRENT WATERS, M.D., F.R.C.P., F.R.A.N.Z.C.P.** • Edgecliff Centre, Edgecliff, New South Wales 2027, Australia. **ANTONY MILCH, M.B.B.S., F.R.A.N.Z.C.P.** • Queenscliff Health Centre, Manly Hospital and Community Health Services, North Manly, New South Wales 2100, Australia.

Practitioner's Guide to Psychoactive Drugs for Children and Adolescents (Second Edition), Werry and Aman, eds. Plenum Publishing Corporation, New York, 1999.

infants to 4-year-olds took one or more drugs, compared with 49% of 5- to 14-year-olds and 84% of those 65 years and older. Males were slightly more likely than females to have been given drugs. More than half of the drugs given to the Australian children were not prescribed. For both prescription and over-the-counter drugs, respiratory problems were the commonest indication.[2] Finally, in a study of a representative sample of 1590 children aged 0–16 years in the United Kingdom, surveyed over a 6-month period during 1984 and 1985, drugs were used on 9% of days.[3] About 45% of the drugs were not prescribed. Of the prescriptions, most were prescribed on weekends. Again, medications acting on the respiratory tract were the most common (42%), followed by analgesics (14%) and antibiotics (12%). The prevalence of drug use peaked at the beginning of primary school and dropped steadily into adolescence. Thus, studies in three developed countries showed a consistent pattern of frequent administration of drugs to children, especially for respiratory illness, almost half of which were not prescribed, with children below age 5 being administered drugs more often than older children and adolescents.

B. Prevalence of Psychoactive Effects of Medical Drugs in Children

There are no systematic data on the psychoactive effects of medical drugs on children. However, the World Health Organization (WHO) Collaborating Center for International Drug Monitoring (Uppsala, Sweden) tabulates clinical reports about suspected adverse drug reactions from national centers in countries participating in a Collaborative Program (Tables 1–4)* While useful, these data are incomplete for several reasons:

1. Compliance with notification to the WHO Center likely varies several hundredfold from country to country.
2. The two categories that include possible psychoactive effects ("CNS effects" and "psychiatric effects") may be construed differently from country to country (Table 2).
3. Compliance with nominating one of the four categories of likelihood of causality (certain, probable, possible, unlikely) is less than 40%.

Given the prevalence of medication of children and gross underreporting of side effects other than severe ones, the WHO figures undoubtedly represent only a fraction of the actual rates. Nevertheless, several important trends emerge from the data in the 5-year period sampled:

1. Reports of central nervous system (CNS) and psychiatric effects closely parallel the overall medication patterns noted earlier in that males slightly outnumber females and those below age 5 are more likely to be affected than older children.
2. Antibiotics (anti-infective agents) were implicated in 58% of reports on children followed by respiratory (6%), gastrointestinal and metabolism (5%), and dermatological (5%) preparations (Table 3). This differs from the relative rates of indications in the three studies cited at the beginning of this chapter, in which respiratory problems predominated.[1–3] Either respiratory drugs are more psychoactively benign than other drug categories or else many of the antibiotics in the WHO data were for respiratory indications and were classified as respiratory drugs in the earlier data.

---

*These data are not homogeneous, at least with respect to origin or likelihood that the pharmaceutical product caused the adverse reactions. Moreover, the information does not represent the opinion of WHO.

**TABLE 1. World Health Organization (WHO) Reports of All Forms
of Adverse Drug Reactions in Children Aged 0–15 Years (1985–1989[a])
by Country[b] and Age Group**

| Country | Number of reports | | | | |
| | Age (years) | | | | |
	<1	1–5	6–10	11–15	Total
Australia	335	455	273	388	1,451
Belgium	24	74	25	34	157
Bulgaria	6	106	70	45	227
Canada	5,956	3,747	488	486	10,677
Czechoslovakia	—	—	—	—	—
Denmark	90	262	112	152	616
Finland	1	89	48	45	183
France	229	471	237	245	1,182
Germany, Federal Rep.	53	199	148	145	545
Greece[b]	2	8	1	1	12
Hungary[b]	—	—	2	1	3
Iceland[b]	—	—	—	—	—
Indonesia	11	37	33	30	111
Ireland	29	128	106	97	360
Israel	22	38	13	13	86
Italy	38	98	79	61	276
Japan	24	74	62	56	216
Malaysia[b]	—	6	3	6	15
Netherlands	29	86	63	47	225
New Zealand	637	155	42	56	890
Norway	9	29	37	38	113
Poland	1	17	13	10	41
Romania	61	56	46	41	204
Spain	108	412	250	238	1,008
Sweden	237	824	302	340	1,703
Thailand	16	52	44	54	166
Turkey[b]	10	15	9	6	40
United Kingdom	1,061	3,162	765	1,237	6,225
USA	2,823	5,139	2,113	2,315	12,390
Yugoslavia	57	131	93	84	365
Total	11,869	15,870	5,477	6,271	39,487
(Relative incidence ratio)	4.81	1.29	0.44	0.51	1.00

[a]The figures are based on the year of onset of reaction or, if onset date is not stated, on the year the notification
was stored in the WHO database.
[b]The following countries joined the program after 1984: Greece (1990), Hungary (1989), Iceland (1989),
Malaysia (1990), and Turkey (1987).

Antibiotics not only may cause a high rate of CNS and psychiatric effects in
themselves but also may interact with psychiatric medication. For example, Csik
and Molnar[4] reported that a schizophrenic 17-year-old successfully maintained on
clozapine became sleepy, appeared distractible, showed psychomotor retardation,
and hypersalivated 1 day after receiving ampicillin for sinusitis.

3. Eighteen percent of the reports concerning children aged 0–15 years were of CNS
and psychiatric effects, compared to 16% for the full age span.

**TABLE 2. World Health Organization (WHO) Reports
on Adverse Drug Reactions
in Children Aged 0–15 Years (1985–1989) by Therapeutic
Group and System Affected**

	System affected[a]	
Drug therapeutic group	CNS	Psychiatric
Alimentary tract and metabolism	570	263
Blood and blood-forming organs	63	40
Cardiovascular system	156	90
Dermatologicals	221	173
Genitourinary system, including sex hormones	119	78
Systemic hormonal preparations, excluding sex hormones	91	56
General anti-infectives, systemic	4078	2690
Antineoplastic and immunomodulating agents	202	36
Musculoskeletal system	115	31
Central nervous system	926	583
Antiparasitic products	42	12
Respiratory system	599	573
Sensory organs	223	200
Various	73	26

[a]Selected as most likely to encompass psychoactive side effects.

There are few citations in the scientific literature concerning psychoactive effects of medical drugs. Further, little in the way of a systematic review can be found in standard texts on child psychiatry or pediatric psychopharmacology. There are several possible explanations why the issue has been so poorly documented:

1. It is possible—but unlikely—that medical drugs may rarely produce psychoactive effects in children. An extensive literature on the psychoactive effects of medical drugs, mainly in the elderly but spanning the entire adult age span,

**TABLE 3. Distribution of Reports of CNS and
Psychiatric Effects (1985–1989) Classified
According to Main Groups of Drugs**

Drug therapeutic group	All ages (% of total)	Age 0–15 years (% of total for age)
GI and metabolism drugs	7.8	5.1
Blood and blood products	3.2	0.9
Cardiovascular drugs	16.9	2.1
Dermatologicals	5.1	5.0
Genitourinary drugs and sex hormones	6.1	1.7
Hormones, systemic	1.3	1.1
Anti-infectives, including vaccines	18.2	58.4
Antineoplastic agents	2.6	1.5
Musculoskeletal drugs	10.1	1.9
CNS drugs	14.9	9.8
Antiparasitic products	0.5	0.5
Respiratory system drugs	3.7	6.0
Sensory organs	5.5	4.2
Various	4.1	1.7

TABLE 4. Distribution of Reports of CNS and Psychiatric
Effects (1985–1989) Classified According
to System–Organ Classes

System–organ class	All ages (% of total)	Age 0–15 years (% of total for age)
Skin and appendage disorders	16.3	17.9
Musculoskeletal disorders	2.0	1.8
Collagen disorders	0.3	0.1
Central nervous system disorders	9.8	10.6
Autonomic nervous system disorders	6.1	0.0
Vision/hearing/sensory disorders	3.0	1.5
Psychiatric disorders	6.2	7.5
Gastrointestinal disorders	10.4	7.3
Liver and biliary disorders	2.9	1.3
Metabolic disorders	3.8	1.9
Endocrine disorders	0.6	1.3
Cardiovascular and heart disorders	5.4	3.1
Vascular disorders	2.4	0.9
Respiratory disorders	4.5	3.6
Blood cell and clotting disorders	4.7	3.5
Urinary system disorders	2.9	2.1
Reproduction disorders	1.5	0.3
Fetal and neonatal disorders	0.5	1.0
Neoplasms	0.3	0.1
General disorders	12.8	22.9
Application site disorders	3.1	9.8
Resistance mechanism disorders	0.6	1.3

appears to be confirmed by the WHO data, which suggest that psychoactive effects constitute nearly a fifth of reported adverse drug reactions. Though children metabolize and excrete most drugs more efficiently than adults and are somewhat less susceptible to some common side effects, they are not likely to escape clinically significant and often dangerous side effects; these may affect all organ systems, including the brain.[5]

2. Altered behavior or emotions may be misidentified as normal variation in mood or behavior or as a normal psychological reaction to the stress of the illness for which the drug is being prescribed.

3. Younger children may not be sufficiently mature to perceive or report more subtle psychoactive effects, such as those on mood, perception, or motivation.

4. Parents may not identify psychoactive effects because they are not attuned to their child's mood or behavior.

5. When parents administer drugs to their child that have been prescribed for someone else, they may fear that reporting a reaction could cause trouble for them.

6. Doctors are generally unfamiliar with psychoactive effects of medical drugs and, therefore, may not anticipate or recognize such effects when they do occur.

7. Some of the drugs that cause psychoactive effects in adults (such as cardiovascular and musculoskeletal drugs) are prescribed for children much less, and pediatricians may be unfamiliar with the full range of psychoactive effects, which are outside their usual experience.

8. Psychiatrists, who would be expected to know most about psychoactive effects of drugs, may be asked to see and assess very few children who are suspected of suffering psychoactive effects of medical drugs.
9. Psychoactive effects may be correctly identified but presumed trivial and mundane, and not worth reporting.
10. Reports for a particular drug will be influenced by the extent of use of the drug, publicity, nature of psychoactive effect, and other factors that vary from time to time, from drug to drug, and from country to country.

For these reasons, it has been necessary to extrapolate from the literature on adults to provide a meaningful review.

C. General Principles of Managing Psychoactive Effects

The management of psychoactive effects of drugs includes acute treatment as well as prevention of future episodes. Acute treatment addresses specific antidotes and the likely course of resolution of the adverse psychoactive effect with or without withdrawal of the offending drug. Prevention addresses issues such as why the child took the medication and whether there is a risk of recurrence. Medical drugs may be taken in a variety of different contexts that have implications for management of unwanted effects:

1. The drug may have been prescribed for the child by a medical practitioner. Here the management strategy depends on consultation with the prescriber as to the need for the drug, possible substitutes or alternatives, balancing the psychoactive side effect against the benefit and need, and the availability of "coverage" drugs to treat the side effect. For example, a child who becomes hyperactive with an anticonvulsant needs treatment for the seizure disorder but may respond to a different anticonvulsant without hyperactivity or may respond only to the anticonvulsant that caused hyperactivity. In the latter case, addition of a stimulant or other psychiatric medication might treat the side effect and allow continuation of the successful anticonvulsant regimen.
2. The child may accidentally ingest a drug intended for another family member (usually an adult). This raises issues of adequate supervision of the child, of too easy access to dangerous substances, and of the family's drug-taking philosophy.
3. Children may deliberately ingest an overdose of their own or another's drugs in an attempt at suicide or other self-harm. This demands an inquiry into depression, suicidal behavior, stress, recent loss, etc.—a standard psychiatric assessment.
4. The drug may have been given to the child deliberately with good intention, but was not prescribed for the child. This raises issues such as public education, standards of child care, and poor judgment by the parent. On an individual case level, education and counseling of the parents is indicated.
5. The drug may have been obtained over-the-counter and considered safe and free of psychoactive effects. Here an important issue is education of parents as to the facts that (1) over-the-counter status does not guarantee safety and (2) many over-the-counter drugs, including those frequently used for children, such as antihistamines and decongestants, can cause various side effects such as sedation, excitement, and even hallucinations. Further, they can interact with prescribed medication, including psychiatric drugs. In many cases the conditions for which over-the-counter remedies are used can be treated alternately—or even not at all, being self-limited.

6. The drug may be deliberately or covertly given to the child by an adult with the intention of simulating or producing illness in the child—Munchausen syndrome by proxy.[6]

D. Attribution of Psychoactive Effects

Whitlock[7] pointed out that it is often difficult to decide when a given psychoactive effect should be attributed to a given drug, because of a number of problems. It may be difficult to decide whether a symptom or syndrome is caused by the drug or by the disease being treated. Distinguishing a psychiatric symptom from an extreme variant of the child's normal mood or behavior may be difficult. Other complicating factors include the dose of drug, other concurrent drugs, the age at exposure and the developmental stage of the child, the child's expectations of and attitudes toward illness, and the social and family background.[5] It is also relevant whether the effect has been produced by normal dosage, high dosage, or overdosage and whether the drug's metabolism or excretion has been altered by the underlying medical condition in such a manner as to lead to unexpectedly high blood levels. Finally, some drugs produce psychoactive effects when they are withdrawn abruptly rather than while they are being administered.

In addition to high dosage, there are three other factors that increase the probability that a psychiatric symptom is indeed a psychoactive side effect:

1. Drugs acting directly on the nervous system and drugs that easily cross the blood–brain barrier are more likely to cause psychoactive effects.
2. The state of the brain and its degree of reserve capacity are important. For example, elderly persons and patients with brain damage, degenerative brain disorders, or developmental disabilities may be more susceptible to the psychoactive effects of medical drugs.[8]
3. Even with presumed normal brain reserve, children with preexisting emotional or behavioral disorders associated with "difficult" temperament may be more susceptible, because of lack of psychological reserve.

While some psychoactive effects are readily explicable from knowledge of the likely action of the drug on brain function, others are inexplicable with our current knowledge. Moreover, some drugs affect the brain only indirectly through their actions on basic metabolic processes, ion balance, or fluid tissue compartments.

In some cases the psychoactive effect may be illusory. The child may have developed a psychiatric condition coincident with, or secondary to, a medical condition for which medical drugs are being prescribed. Making this distinction requires a careful history and familiarity with the usual secondary psychopathology of medical conditions, the typical pathogenesis of primary psychiatric disorders, and the usual and possible psychoactive effects of the prescribed drugs. For example, a child whose beloved grandparent was buried on Tuesday, whose beloved pet was run over on Wednesday, who took kaopectate for gastroenteritis on Wednesday night and Thursday morning, and who manifested tearfulness, irritability, loss of zest, and suicidal ideation on Thursday could safely have a diagnosis of adjustment disorder with depressed mood because neither gastroenteritis nor kaopectate is known to cause such effects and there is a plausible psychological explanation with credible pathogenesis of the psychiatric condition.

Though in some cases diagnosis or nondiagnosis of a psychoactive side effect of a medical drug may be clear, in many cases it will be a matter of reasonable suspicion. Sometimes the judgment can be made only after seeing the results of drug withdrawal.

E. Classification of Psychoactive Effects of Medical Drugs

A number of reviews of psychoactive effects of drugs administered to adults have been published.[9,10] Most have been simply unelaborated compendia classified either by drug, by drug group, or by the nature of the psychoactive effect. Several are updated regularly (notably the biweekly *Medical Letter on Drugs and Therapeutics* and *Meyler's Side Effects of Drugs*).[11,12]

One approach toward a rational classification could be to categorize drugs according to their likely mode of action. However, many drugs are pleiotropic, i.e., they have a variety of actions and potentially affect a number of neurotransmitter systems or other levels of organization within the brain. Thus, isolating one action is at best an oversimplification of the likely mechanisms and at worst may turn out to be incorrect. It is quite likely that any action-based classification would soon be obsolete, given that neuropsychopharmacology is still in its infancy. A second approach may be to separate effects into those that represent a neurotoxic process and are largely irreversible and those that are reversible. The third, a clinical approach, classifies psychoactive effects according to the mental state produced; this is the one adopted here.

Of the reviews organizing the data along diagnostic lines, most have distinguished between short-lived symptoms (often dose-dependent) and more prolonged changes in emotions and behavior that take the form of recognizable psychiatric syndromes and that may not remit immediately after the drug is stopped.[13–15] A frequent inclusion in these classifications that is particularly pertinent to children, but that has generally attracted little attention, has been a separate syndrome of behavioral toxicity, or intoxication, that falls within the acute group of symptoms. The classification that we have used here resembles that of McClelland[15] and utilizes DSM criteria.[16] It includes: (1) intoxication and withdrawal, (2) substance-induced delirium, (3) substance-induced psychosis, including delusional syndrome and hallucinosis, (4) substance-induced mood disorder (manic and depressive types), and (5) substance-induced anxiety.[15,16]

Distinguishing among the various psychoactive effects summarized in the following tables can be difficult, and likely they include substantial overlap. Although the fourth edition of the *Diagnostic and Statistical Manual of Mental Disorders* (DSM-IV) assumes that diagnostic categories are distinctive, the differentiation is often more difficult in practice. This is most clearly seen in the differentiation between delirium (an acute toxic brain disorder) when there are associated psychotic symptoms, and other psychotic states, such as secondary mania or hallucinosis. It is perhaps more realistic to view many effects as lying on some continuum of generally impaired brain function.

II. TYPES OF PSYCHOACTIVE EFFECTS

A. Intoxication

1. Diagnosis and General Features

DSM-IV defines intoxication as a reversible substance-specific syndrome due to recent ingestion of a psychoactive substance, characterized by maladaptive behavior or cognitive impairment resulting from the CNS effect of the substance and not better explained by another mental diagnosis.

Intoxication begins with slight impairment of normal functions and exaggeration of existing tendencies and includes deleterious alterations in perception, cognition, psychomotor performance, motivation, mood, activity, sleep, interpersonal relationships, and intrapsychic processes short of psychotic states like delirium (see below). Children with neurological dysfunction may already have some of these symptoms, so intoxication may be reflected in either worsening of existing symptoms or recruitment of additional symptoms or both. Minimal intoxication is unlikely to be noticed by other than the keenest observer. Subtle changes noticed by parents, often described in terms of personality or temperament changes, are frequently dismissed by professionals.

2. Drugs Causing Intoxication

Research on the effects of drugs on learning and cognitive function in children has largely focused on the effects of psychotropic drugs, particularly stimulants, antipsychotics, and lithium. With the exception of anticonvulsants, general medical drugs have been neglected. Yet many groups of medications can cause such effects. Most reports concerning children have been single case reports. However, notable exceptions are more systematic studies on asthma medication, corticosteroids, interferon, and antineoplastic chemotherapy (particularly for children with acute lymphoblastic leukemia).

The medical drugs (excluding anticonvulsants) that most commonly cause intoxication in children are antihistamines, anti-motion-sickness medications (often containing antihistamines), and narcotic analgesics.[15] Most such drugs are described in more detail in Chapters 11 and 15. Psychomotor impairment, as indicated by dysphoria, drowsiness, and listlessness, is a common side effect of these medications. (Note that these drugs may also cause delirium; see below.) However, sedation may occur with any medication that causes psychoactive effects. Other offenders are such antihypertensives as methyldopa, α_2-agonists, and β-blockers and the analgesic indomethacin, but these are not frequently used in children for medical indications. (However, α_2-agonists and β-blockers are increasingly used by child psychiatrists and pediatricians for their psychoactive effects.)

a. Theophylline

Theophylline has been implicated in behavioral problems and poor school performance in some studies, but more recent data have cast considerable doubt on this.[17,18] In a sibling-control study, Lindgren et al.[19] found no decrement of academic performance with either theophylline or corticosteroids for asthma. A placebo-controlled lab study actually found improved alertness and auditory vigilance task improvement despite subjective reports of dizziness.[20] One problem has been in separating the effects of the drug from possible neuropsychological effects of asthma itself. For instance, behavioral changes may be secondary to repeated episodes of hypoxia, resulting in minor brain damage,[21] or may be secondary to the psychological stress. A naturalistic study of 392 asthmatic children found that severity of asthma but not use of theophylline correlated with behavior problems.[22] Several other studies suggest that theophylline itself has no predictable effect on attention, activity level, mood, or cognitive processing.[23–26] However, the focus of study and chronicity of administration could affect study results. For example, a placebo-controlled healthy-adult lab study found significant improvement on 2 of 9 cognitive tests with theophylline and no difference on the other 7 tests; it also found that chronic, but not acute, dosage impaired mood.[27] Individual differences in sensitivity to theophylline have been reported, and children with preexisting attentional or achievement problems may be more vulnerable to adverse effects.[25]

b. Sympathomimetic Bronchodilators

Sympathomimetic bronchodilators, such as albuterol, isoproterenol, metaproterenol sulfate, and terbutaline sulfate, may cause mild symptoms of anxiety such as palpitations, tremor, and nervousness.[11] These effects are dose-related and reversible on cessation of medication.

c. Corticosteroids

Corticosteroids have become an integral part of chemotherapy regimes for a wide variety of systemic illnesses. Over the past four decades, numerous psychoactive effects have been documented, ranging from mild changes in mood to acute psychotic reactions and delirium. In adults, doses of prednisone over 40 mg/day may result in significant psychopathology, commonly triggered by a change in dose, but also occurring on stable dosage. It has been suggested that attention, and indirectly memory, are specifically impeded by the resultant suppression of ACTH.[28]

Recently, some studies have focused on the use of steroids in children, in particular in the treatment of asthma. High doses of corticosteroids (e.g., 40–80 mg/day of prednisone) have been associated with decreased verbal memory and increased depressive and anxious feelings.[29] In a controlled study, Suess et al.[30] demonstrated that hospitalized asthmatic patients treated with steroids experienced impaired verbal memory. Bender et al.,[29] in a study of severely asthmatic children aged 8–16 years, found that there were significant differences on measures of attention, impulsivity, hyperactivity, or motor control between high and low steroid doses. Increased depressive and anxious symptoms and impairment in long-term verbal memory were associated with high-dose steroids but not with theophylline or with pulmonary function.

Inhalation of corticosteroids in aerosol form has been introduced to obtain a local effect on the airways in asthmatic patients and minimize systemic side effects. However, psychoactive effects of hyperactive behavior and impaired coordination have been described in pediatric case reports even with this route of administration.[31,32] Asthmatic children requiring long-term inhalation treatment may be at particular risk of systemic side effects such as mood swings and impaired school performance.[33]

d. Interferon

Interferon commonly causes flulike symptoms of fatigue, malaise, anorexia, nausea, somnolence, confusion, and paresthesia.[34] It is estimated that one-third of interferon-treated patients develop mental and behavioral changes, with severe effects in 7%.[35] The incidence of toxicity appears to be related to the dose and age of the patients, with both the elderly and children being particularly sensitive.

e. Antineoplastics

Antineoplastic drugs that are lipophilic are likely to cross the blood–brain barrier, particularly if CNS radiotherapy has been previously or is concurrently administered. However, the more severe and persistent CNS side effects found in the latter cases are probably related to high-dose CNS radiotherapy and are often irreversible. They include decline in IQ, attention deficits, neuroendocrine axis dysfunction (resulting principally in growth retardation), and social withdrawal.[36,37]

f. Withdrawal Symptoms

Sudden withdrawal of certain drugs may precipitate significant behavioral symptoms or psychiatric disorder. This is seen most particularly with anticonvulsants and substances of abuse discussed in Chapters 8, 11, 12, and 15, but also with the muscle relaxant baclofen, autonomically active drugs, and corticosteroids. Note that the DSM-IV definition of "withdrawal" is restricted to addictive withdrawal, which we feel leaves a gap in clinical diagnosis, since nonaddictive drugs can also cause symptoms upon cessation.

3. Management of Intoxication and Withdrawal Symptoms

Even when drugs have relatively long half-lives, bunching most or all of the dosage into the evening may minimize some school-day symptoms. When these drugs have to be taken on a continuing basis, the behavioral effects may diminish as tolerance develops. Therefore, a wait-and-see attitude may be the best management for symptoms that are not incapacitating. However, if the intoxication is handicapping, dose reduction or discontinuation of the drug may be necessary. Specific treatment of symptoms is rarely necessary, as symptoms generally abate. If a withdrawal syndrome is suspected, reintroduction of the drug and a gradual stepwise reduction in dose may be necessary.

B. Delirium

1. Diagnosis and General Features

An acute toxic confusional state, or delirium, is the most prevalent drug-induced true psychiatric disorder. In contrast to intoxication, impairment is substantial, with disturbance of consciousness and cognition or perception. The principal symptoms are impaired ability to sustain attention, disorganized thinking, and rambling, incoherent speech. Other important features include impaired or fluctuating level of consciousness, perceptual disturbances such as hallucinations or illusions, changes in psychomotor activity, disorientation, cognitive and memory impairment, delusions, sedation, insomnia, and disinhibition.[16]

In children, these delirious states are often misdiagnosed as other psychiatric disorders such as schizophrenia, mood disorder, anxiety, or brief reactive psychosis or merely as oppositional or naughty behavior.[38] Clues to a possible delirium rather than one of the other psychotic disorders include negative family history, acuteness of onset, good premorbid function, intensity of sensorium disturbance or fluctuating consciousness, and especially recent initiation or dosage increase of a drug that could cause psychoactive effects.

High prevalence rates of delirium have been found in the adult hospitalized population, and it is reasonable to extrapolate from these data to indicate a particular risk for hospitalized children, especially those suffering from metabolic disorders, high fever requiring parenteral fluids, or neurological disorders[38] or receiving polypharmacy in intensive care.[39,40] It has been suggested that children are "more apt than adults to respond to fever and infection with delirious and hallucinatory states."[41] It is likely, although not empirically established, that this applies to the effects of medication as well. Prugh et al. reported that it was often difficult to detect delirium in children.[38] They also demonstrated that there may be a persistence of disturbed perceptual–motor performance in the recovery stages of a delirium. Of course, if a delirium already exists because of illness, medical drugs may exaggerate it.

TABLE 5. Drugs Causing Delirium

Anticholinergics	Miscellaneous drugs
Anticonvulsants	Aminocaproic acid
Antihistamines	Aprotinin
Antiparkinsonian drugs	Boric acid
Antibacterial, antifungal, and antiviral drugs	Coumarin
Antineoplastics	Deet
Cardiovascular and antihypertensive drugs	Disulfiram
General anesthetics	Flurothyl
Nonsteroidal anti-inflammatory drugs	Meclofenamic acid
Radiodiagnostic agents	Metoclopramide
Corticosteroids	Niridazole
Analgesics (especially meperidine)	Podophyllum resin
	Vitamin A

2. Drugs Causing Delirium

a. Central Anticholinergics

The drugs most commonly associated with delirium are the specific central anti-cholinergics like atropine and belladonna derivatives described in Chapters 11 and 15 (see Table 5). However, many other drugs also possess central anticholinergic properties. Children are particularly affected by the use of over-the-counter cough mixtures containing oxolamine citrate, atropine, or hyoscine.[42] Other agents such as antihistamines (most of which are anticholinergic as well) and mydriatic eyedrops may also produce delirium.[43]

b. Histamine-2 Receptor Blockers

Histamine-2 (H_2) receptor blockers such as cimetidine and ranitidine cause CNS changes, including acute confusional states, in up to 30% of cases; however, if renal or hepatic function is impaired, this rate nearly triples.[44,45] Of the H_2 blockers, cimetidine is the most likely to cross the blood–brain barrier, and the most likely to cause delirium.

c. Cardiovascular Drugs

The cardiovascular and antihypertensive drugs are well known to cause neuropsy-chiatric side effects. In approximately 25% of cases, digoxin causes confusion, dizziness, drowsiness, bad dreams, restlessness, nervousness, and agitation that may lead to delirium. Disopyramide, presumably through its anticholinergic effects, is also likely to produce delirium.[46] Delirium has been precipitated by diltiazem.[47] Other antiarrhythmic agents, such as procainamide and quinidine, have been reported more rarely to cause acute delirious states.[48] β-Blockers, notably atenolol and timolol eyedrops, also may induce delirium.[49]

d. Dopaminergic Agents

Dopaminergic agents such as levodopa and amantadine have been associated with the development of delirium, with associated visual hallucinations and psychotic symp-toms.[50,51]

e. Anti-Infective Agents

Anti-infective agents may cause a delirium that is unrelated to the preexisting systemic illness. An acute nonallergic confusional state termed Hoigne's syndrome[52] has been described in reaction to penicillin depot preparations. Associated symptoms described in children include fear of death, confusion, auditory and visual hallucinations, palpitations, cyanosis, and generalized seizures. The symptoms are typically of short duration and are now believed due to embolic–toxic reactions rather than procaine intoxication as first suspected.[52,53] Cephalosporins, gentamicin, nalidixic acid, antifungals, and antimalarials, notably chloroquine, may also result in delirium. Encephalopathic changes with lethargy, tremor, confusion, and seizures may occur in 1% of recipients of acyclovir. Preexisting hepatic, renal, or CNS disorders or concurrent use of intrathecal methotrexate or interferon may increase the risk of such effects.[54]

f. General Anesthetic Agents

General anesthetic agents are CNS depressants. Most of them are described in Chapters 11 and 15. However, ketamine is not, and it has been particularly associated with emergent delirium in children. Its chemical structure is related to that of phencyclidine, a common psychotogenic substance of abuse.[55] Other agents such as enflurane, halothane, and cyclopropane may also have psychoactive effects, including delirium, cerebral irritability, and dysphoria.[56]

g. Antineoplastic Agents

Antineoplastic agents have been associated with delirium and include methotrexate (particularly intrathecally), vincristine, vinblastine, bleomycin, 5-fluorouracil, carmustine, cytarbine, cisplatin, procarbazine, L-asparaginase, and prednisone.[57,58]

h. Nonsteroidal Anti-Inflammatory Drugs

The nonsteroidal anti-inflammatory drugs (NSAIDs) such as ibuprofen, naprosyn, and salicylates commonly cause CNS side effects, especially dizziness, vertigo, and headache. Delirium with associated sleep disruption has also been described, and salicylates have induced delirium with psychotic features.[59,60]

i. Organ Imaging Agents

Organ imaging agents may cause a range of psychiatric symptoms, particularly delirium. This may occur with the use of metrizamide as a neurological contrast agent for ventriculography and myelography, particularly in the cervical region.[61] Neurotoxic complications of contrast used in computed tomography (CT scans) have also been noted in children.[62]

j. Others

Many drugs that can cause intoxication symptoms, such as corticosteroids, can also cause delirium. Narcotics and mixed opiate agonist/antagonist agents can cause delirium; a frequent cause is meperidine.

Sudden withdrawal of some drugs will commonly result in a wide variety of symptoms, including delirium.

3. Management of Delirium

Children who have previously experienced delirium or who have a neurological dysfunction may be more susceptible, and special care is needed, with an eye on prevention and early detection. When delirium occurs, the dose of the relevant drug(s) should be reduced or stopped if possible. Delirium is a self-limiting disorder and ceases when the offending drug is withdrawn, so specific treatment beyond good nursing care is usually not required. Sedation with a *small* dose (to avoid dystonic reactions) of a high-potency antipsychotic with minimal anticholinergic action, such as haloperidol, may be useful in more severe cases.[9] Care should be exercised to prevent self-injury, either in reaction to an imagined threat or as a nonspecific action such as pulling out IV lines or rolling out of bed. The provision of orienting cues, including regular visits from family members, favorite toys, and transitional objects, is helpful. Using a night-light helps to minimize misperceptions. The reassuring presence of a consistent adult, either a family member or a nurse, may help the child with impaired reality testing and ensure that there is neither sensory deprivation nor overstimulation.[9]

C. Substance-Induced Psychotic Disorder with Delusions

1. Diagnosis and General Features

The distinction between psychotic delusional reactions of drug origin and delirium with associated psychotic features is made on the presence of a relatively clear sensorium in the former (i.e., the child is alert, coherent, and has no memory defect or disorientation). DSM-IV criteria include prominent delusions in excess of what would be expected from intoxication or withdrawal, evidence of specific medication related to the disturbance, occurrence not confined to the course of delirium, and inability to explain the disorder better by a psychotic disorder that is not substance-induced.

2. Drugs Causing Substance-Induced Psychotic Disorder with Delusions

Dopaminergic drugs such as levodopa, amantadine, and bromocriptine may induce paranoid delusional states; the elderly are more prone to the development of such reactions than either other adults or children.[63] However, a very large number of other medications may have such effects, though the reason is unclear (see Table 6).

3. Management of Substance-Induced Psychotic Disorder with Delusions

Antipsychotic medications are indicated if the reaction is severe when the offending drug is discontinued or eliminated. Usually, treatment needs only be brief because discontinuation of the offending drug leads to prompt remission.[9] If psychosis persists, preexisting or emergent schizophrenia or bipolar disorder with psychosis should be suspected (see Chapters 7, 9, and 10). Occasionally, a specific antidote, physostigmine given subcutaneously, intramuscularly, or intravenously, may be required for psychosis associated with anticholinergic poisoning.[64]

TABLE 6. Drugs Causing Organic Delusional Syndrome[a]

Corticosteroids	Miscellaneous drugs (*Cont.*)
Antibacterial drugs	Methantheline
Narcotic analgesics	Metrizamide
Histamine (H$_2$) receptor antagonists	Norephedrine
Cardiovascular drugs	Pergolide
Nonsteroidal anti-inflammatory drugs	Quinine
Miscellaneous drugs	Retinol
Aluminum	Sydnocarb
Aprindine	Thyroid hormones
Baclofen (on withdrawal)	CNS medications
Bupropion (Amphebutamone)	Amantadine
Cannabis	Amphetamine
Cathinone	Anticholinergics
Cyclopentolate	Anticonvulsants
Cyproheptadine	Bromocriptine
Desmopressin	Levodopa
Diethylpropion (Amfepramone)	Methylphenidate
Diphenhydramine	Scopolamine
Dronabinol	Stimulants
Isosafrole	PCP
Mepacrine	Cocaine

[a]After *Meyler's Side Effects of Drugs 1972, 1988* and *Annuals 1977–1979, 1989* and the *Medical Letter on Drugs and Therapeutics 1989.*

D. Substance-Induced Psychotic Disorder with Hallucinations (Hallucinosis)

1. Diagnosis and General Features

A diagnosis of substance-induced psychotic disorder with hallucinations requires persistent or recurrent hallucinations beyond what is ordinarily expected during intoxication or withdrawal, occurring outside delirium and not better explained by a psychotic disorder that is not substance-induced.

2. Drugs Causing Substance-Induced Psychotic Disorder with Hallucinations

a. Anticholinergics

Anticholinergics are particularly prone to cause hallucinations, which may occur even after topical (local) administration of cycloplegic eyedrops (pupil dilators) used in ophthalmological diagnosis.[43] Cyclopentolate, a rapid-onset, short-acting cycloplegic agent, has been particularly identified as resulting in hallucinations and psychotic episodes in children. In addition to its anticholinergic effect, it has a dimethylated side chain similar to certain hallucinogens.[12]

The antiasthma drug salbutamol has also been reported to induce hallucinations in susceptible children.[65] However, hallucinations have been described among adults administered numerous other medications (see Table 7), suggesting that individual susceptibility is more important than the drug involved.

TABLE 7. Drugs Causing Organic Hallucinosis[a]

Antiparkinsonian drugs	Miscellaneous
Antibacterial, antifungal, and antiviral drugs	Aminocaproic acid
Antiasthma drugs	Aprindine
Antineoplastic agents	Benzodiazepines
Cardiovascular and antihypertensive drugs	Baclofen (on withdrawal)
Sympathomimetic stimulants	Methysergide
Antihistamines	Pergolide
Analgesics and anti-inflammatory drugs	Vitamin D
Narcotic analgesics	

[a]After *Meyler's Side Effects of Drugs 1972, 1988* and *Annuals 1977–1979, 1989* and *The Medical Letter on Drugs and Therapeutics 1989.*

In some countries, over-the-counter cough preparations such as oxalamine citrate are commonly involved.

3. Management of Substance-Induced Psychotic Disorder with Hallucinations

Usually withdrawal of the offending drug is all that is required. However, if the child is very fearful, a low dose of a high-potency neuroleptic such as haloperidol may be useful.[9] The specific antidote physostigmine, given subcutaneously, intramuscularly, or intravenously, may be required for hallucinosis associated with anticholinergic poisoning.[64]

E. Substance-Induced Mood Disorder

The criteria for a Substance-Induced Mood Disorder require a prominent and persistent mood disturbance caused by drug use, causing clinical distress, not occurring only during delirium, and not better explained by a mood disorder that is not substance-induced. DSM-IV requests specification of manic, depressed, or mixed features. The manic and depressed types will be considered separately. The only difference from ordinary mood disorder is that substance use can be identified as the cause. In practice, the distinction may not be easy to make, although cessation of the offending drug must lead to alleviation of the syndrome.

1. Substance-Induced Mood Disorder with Manic Features (Manic Reaction)

a. Diagnosis and General Features

Manic reaction is characterized principally by euphoria, irritability, overactivity, grandiosity, and reduced need for sleep.

b. Drugs Causing Manic Reaction

Medications that result in manic reactions (Table 8) typically have central monoaminergic action. They may have a spectrum of psychiatric effects, including delirium and schizophrenia-like reactions. Drugs reported to cause mania include isoniazid and procarbazine, which share some qualities of monoamine oxidase inhibitors (MAOIs), over-the-

TABLE 8. Drugs Causing Manic Reaction[a]

Corticosteroids	Miscellaneous drugs (*Cont.*)
Antiparkinsonian drugs	Diltiazem
Antiasthma drugs	Isoniazid
Stimulants	Metrizamide
OTC sympathomimetics[b]	Metoclopramide
Miscellaneous drugs	Niridazole
Anticholinergics	Procainamide
Baclofen	Procarbazine
Bromide	Quinacrine
Cimetidine	Thyroid hormones
Cyclobenzaprine	Yohimbine
Cyclosporine	Zidovudine
Deet	

[a]After *Meyler's Side Effects of Drugs 1972, 1975, 1988* and *Annual 1989* and
The Medical Letter on Drugs and Therapeutics 1989.
[b]OTC, Over-the-counter.

counter sympathomimetic decongestants, levodopa, bromocriptine (dopamine agonist), and metoclopramide (dopamine antagonist).[66–68] Yohimbine, an α_2-adrenergic antagonist, and cyclobenzaprine, a structural analogue of amitriptyline, have resulted in manic reactions in patients with a previous history.[69]

Corticosteroids have already been described above as resulting in a wide variety of psychiatric symptoms. Most commonly, depressive and manic reactions have been described.[70] A 5-year-old girl was noted to develop a manic state consequent to budesonide inhalation.[23] There have also been nine case reports describing hypomanic reactions to the combination of ACTH and prednisone in the treatment of multiple sclerosis.[71]

Cimetidine, a histamine-2 antagonist, has had similar effects. Other medications, including thyroid preparations, bromides, baclofen (a chlorophenyl derivative of GABA, a naturally occurring inhibitory neurotransmitter), procainamide, metrizamide (contrast for myelography), and anticholinergic medications, have also precipitated manic episodes.[69] There have been a number of recent reports of adults with HIV infection or AIDS and no past psychiatric history developing a maniclike illness soon after commencing treatment with zidovudine (AZT).[72,73]

c. Management of Manic Reaction

Discontinuation of the possible offending drug should be tried before considering specific treatment with antipsychotics or lithium.[9] Nevertheless, the possibility should be considered that a manic reaction in a child reflects a predisposition to bipolar disorder.[74]

2. Substance-Induced Mood Disorder with Depressive Features (Depressive Reaction)

a. Diagnosis and General Features

In addition to meeting the DSM criteria for substance-induced mood disorder, the most prominent pervasive mood disturbance must be dysphoria or anhedonia. Such reactions are, however, dimensional or quantitative rather than categorical, and a wide spectrum of varying severity of depressed mood may result even from the same drug. Depression is

TABLE 9. Drugs Causing Depressive Reaction[a]

Analgesics and anti-inflammatory drugs	Miscellaneous drugs (*Cont.*)
Antibacterial and antifungal drugs	Diphenoxylate
Antineoplastics agents	Disulfiram
Antiparkinsonian drugs	Lysergide
Anticonvulsants	Mebeverine
Cardiovascular and antihypertensive drugs	Meclizine
Corticosteroids and hormones	Mesulergine
Stimulants and appetite suppressants	Methysergide
Miscellaneous drugs	Metoclopramide
Acetazolamide	Pizotiyline
Albuterol (salbutamol)	Primaquine
Anticholinesterases	PUVA therapy
Buflomedil	Theophylline
Choline	Total parenteral nutrition
Cimetidine	
Cyproheptadine	

[a]After *Meyler's Side Effects of Drugs 1972, 1975, 1988* and *Annuals 1977–1979* and *The Medical Letter on Drugs and Therapeutics 1989.*

often seen as an intermediate state before and after overt delirium, suggesting its position on a continuum.

b. Drugs Causing Depressive Reaction

i. Antihypertensive Drugs. Numerous medications are implicated (see Table 9). Antihypertensive drugs have been particularly associated with depression although they are not commonly used in children and adolescents for medical reasons. Reserpine was noted to cause depression in around 20% of adult hypertensive patients, possibly because of depletion of biogenic amines.[75] Although it has been recommended that patients with a history of depression should not be treated with α-methyldopa,[76] a 1983 literature review found only 30 cases of depression among 752 adult patients treated with the drug.[77] Symptoms of depression were equally common in patients treated with α-methyldopa and those treated with other antihypertensive agents. Other effects included sedation, drowsiness, forgetfulness, fatigue, and nightmares. Clonidine and guanfacine (see Chapter 15), like methyldopa, act to interfere with the release of noradrenaline and may result in sedation, at times mimicking depressive episodes. In children it is probable that these drugs are used more commonly in the treatment of attention-deficit hyperactivity disorder and Tourette syndrome than in any medical–surgical context (see Chapter 15).[78]

ii. β-Blockers. β-Blockers, particularly propranolol, have been suspected of causing depression (see Chapter 15). A 1990 metaanalysis found that propranolol caused depression as a side effect at a frequency greater than that of control medications.[79] Use was associated with fatigue, diminished libido, anorexia, and poor concentration. Depression could result from β-blocker-induced reduction of melatonin secretion.[80] This may be particularly so in the case of sleep disturbance and hallucinations. Lipophilic β-blockers, such as propranolol and oxprenolol, seemed to produce more neuropsychiatric adverse effects than hydrophilic β-blockers, such as atenolol and nadolol, which are less likely to cross the blood–brain barrier. All of this has been questioned by a large 1992 retrospective case-control study of Medicaid recipients with depression markers.[81] The expected significant association between depression and prior β-blocker use was found (odds ratio, 1.45) when no confounders were controlled for but disappeared (odds ratio, 0.98) when the investigators controlled for benzodiazepine use, frequent outpatient visits, and frequent use of drugs other than β-blockers. Thus, the previous reports of β-blockers causing depression may be spurious findings based on failure to control for confounding clinical factors.[81]

Other cardiovascular drugs may be involved in causing depression, however, such as in calcium-channel blockade for hypertension.[82] Diuretics may cause hypoglycemia or hypovolemia, lead to possible depression.

iii. Steroids. Steroids have been widely implicated as a cause of depression in adults. However, a family history of psychiatric disorder is found in 80–100% of patients experiencing such effects.[83] Children with inflammatory bowel disease treated with steroids have been reported at increased risk for development of depression. However, a study of 13 children with recent-onset inflammatory bowel disease found no association between steroid use or the severity of illness and depressive symptomatology.[84] Corticotropins such as ACTH have a side-effect profile similar to that of corticosteroids.[85] Mood disturbance may also be precipitated by steroid withdrawal.[86]

At times, it can be difficult to differentiate between the effect of steroids and the underlying disease. The effect varies with dosage, duration of treatment, and the personality of the patient. Higher doses have been noted to cause behavioral and personality changes. It has been suggested that the psychomotor stimulant effect is more significant with dexamethasone and less so with 6-methylprednisolone and methyleneprednisolone. Long-term treatment with corticosteroids may result in cerebral atrophy, which would be predicted to increase the risk of psychoactive side effects.[87] Psychoactive effects of topical corticosteroid preparations have also been described.[88] Alternate-day dosing of corticosteroids is associated with fewer mood (and cognitive) changes.

Pope and Katz[89] have suggested that the use of anabolic steroids has been underestimated in the medical literature despite their common use by athletes, typically starting in adolescence as part of competitive training. In their study of bodybuilders and football players, 22% had experienced a manic or depressed mood syndrome, and a further 12% had experienced psychotic symptoms during steroid use. Symptoms resolved a few weeks after cessation of steroids.

Oral contraceptive use is widespread among adolescents. but there have been no adolescent studies of mood change with oral contraceptives. A review of reports and studies in adults found a 15–56% frequency of depression. However, these studies have been criticized on the basis of selection bias, poor assessment of pretherapeutic mood state, and lack of clear definitions of depression.[90] Possibly, oral contraceptives induce tryptophan oxygenase, leading to pyridoxine deficiency, which results in depressed mood. However, a large prospective study concluded that the incidence of depression among users of oral contraceptives was no higher than that among matched controls.[91] Further, another review refers to a mood-stabilizing effect and ability to relieve premenstrual syndrome.[92] Thus, the question of any psychoactive effects from oral contraceptives remains open, despite individual convincing instances.

c. Management of Depressive Reaction

Removing possible offending drugs should alleviate the depression. If symptoms persist, other supportive treatment may be necessary. Occasionally, if the depressive syndrome is severe and persists well after the discontinuation of the offending drug, or if continued administration of the drug is required, antidepressants (Chapter 9) need to be considered.[9] With an eye to prevention, the possibility should also be considered that the child is predisposed to depression and should avoid known depressogenic drugs in the future or use them with caution.

In the case of oral contraceptives, if continued use is desirable, it is possible to use alternative preparations with varying estrogen or progesterone components. It has also been suggested that pyridoxine, 20 mg twice a day, is a useful supplement.

F. Substance-Induced Anxiety Disorder

1. Diagnosis and General Features

For diagnosis of substance-induced anxiety disorder, DSM-IV requires clinically stressful anxiety, panic attacks, or obsessions/compulsions, related to use of a drug, not occurring exclusively during delirium, and not better explained by an anxiety disorder that is not substance-induced. It should be diagnosed only when the anxiety symptoms are (1) the predominant clinical features (rather than mood or psychosis) and (2) in excess of those expected with intoxication or withdrawal. Since anxiety is commonly associated with illness, this diagnosis may be overlooked or difficult to distinguish.

2. Drugs Causing Substance-Induced Anxiety Disorder

A number of drugs may induce anxiety, as seen in Table 10. Prominent among these are sympathomimetic drugs, such as isoproterenol (isoprenaline), epinephrine, pseudo-ephedrine, caffeine, theophylline, and yohimbine. There has been much recent work using sympathomimetic agents such as yohimbine as experimental models for anxiety.[93] β-Adrenergic drugs, such as isoprenaline and albuterol (salbutamol), used to treat asthma, may also provoke anxiety when administered either orally or by aerosol. Corticosteroids have also been described as inducing anxiety.

Antihypertensive agents have been reported to have significant psychoactive effects. The angiotensin-converting enzyme (ACE) inhibitors, such as captopril and enalapril, may cause symptoms of anxiety, drowsiness, and irritability as well as depression.[94,95]

TABLE 10. Drugs Causing Organic Anxiety Syndrome[a]

Anticonvulsants	Miscellaneous drugs (*Cont.*)
Antibacterial and antiviral drugs	Cycloserine
Antihistamines	Dapsone
Antiasthma drugs	Dronabinol
Cardiovascular and antihypertensive drugs	Fluoxetine
Nonsteroidal anti-inflammatory drugs	Levodopa
Stimulants	Metrizamide
Miscellaneous drugs	Narcotics
Baclofen	Progabide
Bismuth salts	Quinacrine
Bromocriptine	Thyroid hormones

[a]After *Meyler's Side Effects of Drugs 1988* and *Annual 1989* and *The Medical Letter on Drugs and Therapeutics 1989*.

3. Management of Substance-Induced Anxiety

Discontinuation of the offending drug generally leads to resolution of symptoms. However, it may be necessary to continue the drug for medical reasons, in which case temporary use of an anxiolytic, such as a selective serotonin reuptake inhibitor (SSRI) or buspirone, may be considered. SSRI effects should be monitored closely for a paradoxical worsening of apparent anxiety from the occasional side effect of excitement. Where the medical treatment is continuous and chronic, behavioral treatment is preferable.

III. DEVELOPMENTAL CONSIDERATIONS

Much of the foregoing review was necessarily based on adult literature in the absence of relevant child and adolescent literature. In applying those findings to children and adolescents, we need to consider several developmental factors.

Age-Appropriate Vulnerability. Children, by virtue of their inexperience and dependent status, are more susceptible to situation-induced anxiety and depression than adults. It would not be surprising if their unsophisticated coping skills as well as less mature brain left them more vulnerable also to drug-induced disorders.

Effect of Underlying Illness. Children react more intensely to many illnesses than do adults (and also tend to recover quicker). This general biological increased reactivity to illness extends to the CNS, as illustrated in the fact that febrile seizures arc almost exclusively a childhood phenomenon. Therefore, the underlying illness is especially likely to induce psychiatric symptoms in children even without medication. In fact, a change in behavior and mood is often the first sign of illness in a very young child. This fact complicates the distinguishing of psychoactive drug side effects.

Impact on Developmental Trajectory. Children are in a state of dynamic change and growth biologically and psychologically. Chronic alteration of physiologic processes, and of the brain's chemical milieu, either by chronic illness (e.g., hypoxia from asthma) or by the drugs used to treat it (e.g., chronic corticosteroids) could conceivably impair development. For example, synaptic connections and other brain structures could be permanently affected by steroids.[96] This is in addition to the psychological effects (depression, anxiety) of having a chronic or severe illness.

Not only can the underlying illness or the drugs used to treat it have a direct effect on brain development, but also they can indirectly affect psychobiological development. If a chronic illness or its treatment interferes with education or peer relations (e.g., sedative side effect, activity restriction, or need for protective isolation), the child can "lose time" in the developmental trajectory and fall behind. Whether the child can ever make this up depends partly on the timing of optimal stages for learning certain skills. Since the brain depends on environmental input for its development, this chronic interference with such input could affect brain structure permanently and make the child more vulnerable to psychiatric disorders.[96]

Development versus Illness Effect versus Drug Effect. The foregoing poses a clinical puzzle whenever a child with a chronic illness develops an apparent psychiatric syndrome. Sometimes the normal (or illness-altered) course of development brings mood, anxiety, or behavioral symptoms (e.g, terrible twos, fearsome fours, adolescent turmoil). An intercurrent illness may delay a normal developmental stage to a time when it is not expected. For example, a child with a life-threatening congenital condition requiring numerous surgeries with frequent hospitalizations may have the autonomy surge with its attendant "terrible twos" delayed until age 3, when most children are expected to be their most charming. The illness itself may bring delayed emotional or behavioral symptoms, as the child wears down and despairs of a cure. An interaction of normal development and chronic illness can occur as the child matures enough cognitively to grasp the seriousness of the illness. Therefore, the appearance of new psychiatric symptoms in a child with a chronic illness treated with a drug known to cause psychoactive effects does not necessarily mean a drug-induced disorder.

In solving such a clinical puzzle, there is no substitute for careful history, examining the developmental trajectory, the timing of any drug initiation or dose changes relative to the symptom onset, any prior occurrences of the same symptoms, any over-the counter remedies used (as well as drugs prescribed for other family members), and the family history. The child should be carefully interviewed regarding feelings about the illness, subjective drug effects, plans for the future, age-appropriate fantasies, etc., in addition to standard mental status exam. If the medical condition permits, a trial discontinuation of suspected drugs may be needed to clarify the cause.

IV. IMPLICATIONS FOR CLINICAL PRACTICE AND FURTHER RESEARCH

Despite the high proportion of children receiving medication at least once a year and the apparent prevalence of psychoactive side effects, this area is relatively neglected scientifically. Although some overlap will remain between psychiatric and CNS effects, clear psychiatric diagnostic criteria (such as DSM or ICD) should be used when assessing the psychoactive effects of medication. For example, clearer differentiation between delirium and schizophreniform reactions, using the criteria cited, would be a significant improvement. A number of steps are indicated:

1. Medical students and hospital staff should be trained in the psychoactive effects of medication, including diagnostic and management skills. This would be particularly important for more subtle reactions, which are often missed. This would result in a more effective detection rate.
2. Continuing medical education for family physicians and pediatricians, from whom most children receive medical care, should also address such issues. This education would emphasize the interrelationship of polypharmacy, metabolism, and the preexisting medical state with the development of adverse reactions.
3. Greater psychiatric input, particularly in pediatric and general hospital settings via consultation-liaison, would promote improved diagnosis.
4. The reporting of adverse drug reactions should also be improved so that quantitative and qualitative data could be elicited in a more precise and comprehensive manner. The inadequacy of current reporting procedures is seen in the analysis of the WHO Collaborative Center data that are partly reported here.
5. There is need for good clinical research. The current state of knowledge is based on an accumulation of individual case reports. There are a number of avenues for more systematic evaluation. The Boston Collaborative Drug Surveillance Program has been the most significant study in this area to date.[1,70] However, an analysis of child and adolescent populations is long overdue. This could be done by surveying

psychoactive reactions in any or all of the different contexts where children are treated or receive medication, such as (a) family and primary pediatric practices, (b) general hospital pediatric wards, (c) specialist pediatric hospital settings, (d) special high-risk pediatric services, such as neonatal intensive-care units or asthma or oncology clinics, and (e) community studies (to detect nonprescribed drug effects).

6. Clinical diagnostic criteria and/or rating scales for substance-induced mental disorders (sensitive to drug-induced psychoactive effects yet simple for nonpsychiatrist physicians to use) must be developed for the pediatric population.

V. SUMMARY

A wide variety of medical drugs have been reported to have unwanted psychoactive effects. Drugs of particular concern are those with an anticholinergic action (potential to cause delirium) or that affect monoamines such as dopamine (with potential to cause psychotic states) or norepinephrine (with potential to cause mood disorder or anxiety). Other drugs of special note for children include corticosteroids, often used in asthma; antibiotics, used for the frequent respiratory infections of childhood; and antihistamines and over-the-counter decongestants, often used to prevent otitis media. Among adolescent athletes, anabolic steroid reactions may be more common than generally believed. High dosage, not allowing for the developmental stage and metabolic rate of the child, polypharmacy, rapid changes in dose, and not allowing for habituation all increase the risk.

REFERENCES

1. Elliger TJ, Trott GE, Nissen G: Prevalence of psychotropic medication in childhood and adolescence in the Federal Republic of Germany. *Pharmacopsychiatry* 232:38–44, 1990.
2. Australian Bureau of Statistics: Australian Health Survey Catalogue No. 4311.0, 1983.
3. Rylance GW, Woods CG, Cullen RE, et al: Use of drugs by children. *Br Med J* 297:445–448, 1988.
4. Csik V, Molnar J: Possible adverse interaction between clozapine and ampicillin in an adolescent with schizophrenia. *J Child Adolesc Psychopharmacol* 4:123–128, 1994.
5. Popper C: Developmental neurotoxicity, in Popper C (ed): *Psychiatric Pharmacosciences of Children and Adolescents*. Washington DC, American Psychiatric Press, 1989.
6. Rosenberg DA: Web of deceit: A literature review of Munchausen syndrome by proxy. *Child Abuse Neglect* 11:547–563, 1987.
7. Whitlock FA: Adverse psychiatric reactions to modern medication. *Aust N Z J Psychiatry* 15:87–103, 1981.
8. Harper CM, Newton PA, Walsh JR: Drug induced illness in the elderly. *Postgrad Med* 86:245–256, 1989.
9. Hollister LE: Drug-induced psychiatric disorders and their management. *Med Toxicol* 1:428–448, 1986.
10. Stoudemire A, Fogel BS: *Principles of Medical Psychiatry*. New York: Harcourt Brace & Jovanovich Publishers, 1989.
11. Dukes MNG: *Meyler's Side Effects of Drugs: An Encyclopaedia of Adverse Reactions and Interactions*, ed 11. Amsterdam, Elsevier, 1988.
12. Dukes MNG, Beeley L: *Side Effects of Drugs Annual 13: A Worldwide Yearly Survey of New Data and Trends*. Amsterdam, Elsevier, 1989.
13. Boston Collaborative Drug Surveillance Program: Side effects of non-psychiatric drugs. *Semin Psychiatry* 3:406–420, 1971.
14. Evans LES: Psychological effects caused by drugs in overdose. *Drugs* 19:220–242, 1980.
15. McClelland HA: Psychiatric disorders, in Davis DM (ed). *Textbook of Adverse Drug Reactions*. London: Oxford University Press, 1977, pp. 335–353.

16. American Psychiatric Association: *Diagnostic and Statistical Manual of Mental Disorders*, ed 4. Washington, DC, American Psychiatric Association Press, 1994.
17. Rachelefsky GS, Wo J, Adelson J, et al: Behavior abnormalities and poor school performance due to oral theophylline use. *Pediatrics* 78:1133–1138, 1986.
18. Weinberger M, Lindgren S, Linder B, et al: Effects of theophylline on learning and behavior: Reason for concern or concern without reason? *J Pediatr* 111:471–474, 1987.
19. Lindgren S, Lokshin B, Stromquist A, Weinberger M, et al: Does asthma or treatment with theophylline limit children's academic performance? *N Engl J Med* 327:926–930, 1992.
20. Tiplady B, Fagan D, Lamont M, Brockway M, Scott DB: A comparison of the CNS effects of enprofylline and theophylline in healthy subjects assessed by performance testing and subjective measures. *Br J Clin Pharmacol* 30:55–61, 1990.
21. Suess WM, Chai H: Neuropsychological correlates of asthma: Brain damage or drug effects? *J Consult Clin Psychol* 49:135–136, 1981.
22. Butz AM, Malveaux FJ, Eggleston P, Thompson L, et al: Social factors associated with behavioral problems in children with asthma. *Clin Pediatr* 34:581–590, 1995.
23. Creer TL, Gustafson KE: Psychological problems associated with drug therapy in childhood asthma. *J Pediatr* 115:850–855, 1989.
24. Furukawa CT, DuHamel TR, Weimer L, et al: Cognitive and behavioral findings in children taking theophylline. *J Allergy Clin Immunol.* 81:83–88, 1988.
25. Schlieper A, Alcock D, Beaudry P, et al: Effect of therapeutic plasma concentrations of theophylline on behavior, cognitive processing and affect in children with asthma. *J Pediatr* 118:449–455, 1991.
26. Creer TL, McLoughlin JA: The effects of theophylline on cognitive and behavioral performance. *J Allergy Clin Immunol* 83:1027–1029, 1989.
27. Bartel P, Delport R, Lotz B, Ubbink J, et al: Effects of single and repeated doses of theophylline on aspects of performance, electrophysiology, and subjective assessments in healthy human subjects. *Psychopharmacology* 106:90–96, 1992.
28. Schraa JC, Dirks JF: The influence of corticosteroids and theophylline on cerebral function. *Chest* 82:181–185, 1982.
29. Bender BG, Lerner JA, Kollasch E: Mood and memory changes in asthmatic children receiving corticosteroids. *J Am Acad Child Adolesc Psychiatry* 27:720–725, 1988.
30. Suess W, Stump N, Chi H, et al: Mnemonic effects of asthma medication in children. *J Asthma* 23:291–296, 1986.
31. Lewis LD, Cochrane GM: Psychosis in a child inhaling budesonide. *Lancet* 2:634, 1983.
32. Meyboom RHB, DeGraaf-Breederveld N: Budesonide and psychic side effects. *Ann Intern Med* 109:683, 1988.
33. Hollman GA, Allen DB: Overt glucocorticoid excess due to inhaled corticosteroid therapy. *Pediatrics* 81:452–455, 1988.
34. Rohatiner AZS, Proir PF, Burton AC, et al: Central nervous system toxicity of interferon. *Br J Cancer* 47:419–442, 1983.
35. Spiegel RF: The alpha-interferons: Clinical overview. *Semin Oncol* 14(suppl 2):1–12, 1987.
36. Cousens P, Waters BGH, Said J, et al: Cognitive effects of cranial-irradiation in leukemia: A survey and meta-analysis. *Child Psychol Psychiatry* 29:839–852, 1988.
37. Waters BGH, Said J, Cousens P, et al: Behavioral side effects of CNS prophylaxis. *J Am Acad Child Adolesc Psychiatry* 28:299–300, 1989.
38. Prugh DG, Wagonfeld S, Metcalf D, et al: A clinical study of delirium in children and adolescents. *Psychosom Med* 42(suppl):177–195, 1980.
39. Lipowski ZJ: Delirium (acute confusional states). *JAMA* 258:1789–1792, 1987.
40. Trzepacz PT, Teague GB, Lipowski ZJ: Delirium and other organic mental disorders in a general hospital. *Gen Hosp Psychiatry* 7:101–106, 1985.
41. Goodman JD, Sours JA: *The Child Mental Status Examination.* New York: Basic Books, 1967.
42. McEwen J, Meyboom RH, Thijs I: Hallucinations in children caused by oxolamine citrate. *Med J Aust* 150:449–450,452, 1989.
43. Kortabarria RP, Duran JA, Chacon JR, et al: Toxic psychosis following cycloplegic eyedrops. *Drug Intell Clin Pharm* 24:708–709, 1990.
44. Eisendrath SJ, Ostroff JW: Ranitidine-associated delirium. *Psychosomatics* 31:98–100, 1990.
45. Sax MJ: Clinically important adverse effects and drug interactions with H2-receptor antagonists: An update. *Pharmacotherapy* 7:110S–115S, 1987.
46. Ahamad S, Sheikh AI, Meerian MK: Disopyramide-induced acute psychosis. *Chest* 76:712–714, 1979.

47. Bushe VJ: Organic psychosis caused by diltiazem. *J R Soc Med* 81:296, 1988.
48. Johnson AJ, Day RO, Shaldon WA: A functional psychosis precipitated by quinidine. *Med J Aust* 153: 47–49, 1990.
49. Arbor N: Delirium induced by atenolol. *Br Med J* 297:1048, 1988.
50. Banergee AK, Falkai PG, Savidge M: Visual hallucinations in the elderly associated with the use of levodopa. *Postgrad Med J* 65:358–361, 1989.
51. Snoey ER, Bessen HA: Acute psychosis after amantadine overdose. *Ann Emerg Med* 19:668–670, 1990.
52. Silber TJ, D'Angelo L: Psychosis and seizures following the injection of penicillin G procaine: Hoigne's syndrome. *Am J Dis Child* 139:335–337, 1985.
53. Ilechukwu STC: Acute psychotic reactions and stress response syndromes following intramuscular aqueous procaine penicillin. *Br J Psychiatry* 156:554–559, 1990.
54. Arndt KA: Adverse reactions to acyclovir: Topical, oral, and intravenous. *J Am Acad Dermatol* 18:188–190, 1988.
55. Meyers EF, Charles P: Prolonged adverse reactions to ketamine in children. *Anesthesiology* 49:39–40, 1978.
56. Holm-Knudsen R, Nygard E, Laub M: Rectal induction of anesthesia in children: A comparison between ketamine–midazolam and halothane for induction and maintenance of anesthesia. *Acta Anaesthesiol Scand* 33:518–521, 1989.
57. Hurwitz RL, Mahoney DH Jr, Armstrong DL, et al: Reversible encephalopathy and seizures as a result of conventional vincristine administration. *Med Pediatr Oncol* 16:216–219, 1988.
58. Young D, Posner J: Nervous system toxicity of the chemotherapeutic agents, in Viken PJ, Bruyn GW (eds). *Handbook of Clinical Neurology*, vol 39, pt II. Amsterdam, Elsevier Biomedical Press, 1980.
59. Cuthbert MF: Adverse reactions to nonsteroidal antirheumatic drugs. *Curr Med Res Opin* 2:600–610, 1974.
60. Greer HD, Ward HP, Corbin KB: Chronic salicylate intoxication in adults. *JAMA* 193:555–558, 1965.
61. Elliott RL, Wilde JH, Snow WT: Prolonged delirium after metrizamide myelography. *JAMA* 252:2057–2058, 1984.
62. Haslam RHA, Cochrane DD, Amundson GM, et al: Neurotoxic complications of contrast computed tomography in children. *J Pediatr III* 6:837–840, 1987.
63. Montastruc JL, Rascol D, Rascol A: Comparison of bromocriptine and levodopa as first line treatment for Parkinson's disease: Results of a 3 year prospective randomized study. *Rev Neurol* 146:144–147, 1990.
64. Havener WH: *Ocular Pharmacology.* ed 4. St. Louis, CV Mosby Co, 1978.
65. Khanna PB, Davies R: Hallucinations associated with administration of salbutamol via a nebulizer. *Br Med J* 292:1430, 1986.
66. Krauthammer C, Klerman GL: Secondary mania: Manic syndromes associated with antecedent physical illness or drugs. *Arch Gen Psychiatry* 35:1333–1339, 1978.
67. Ritchie KS, Preskorn SH: Mania induced by metoclopramide: Case report. *J Clin Psychiatry* 45:180–181, 1984.
68. Vlissides DN, Gill D, Castelow MJ: Bromocriptine-induced mania? *Br Med J* 1:510, 1978.
69. Larson EW, Richelson E: Organic causes of mania. *Mayo Clin Proc* 63:906–912, 1988.
70. Boston Collaborative Drug Surveillance Program: Acute adverse reactions to prednisone in relation to dosage. *Clin Pharmacol* 13:694–698, 1972.
71. Minden SL, Orau J, Schildkraut JJ: Hypomanic reactions to ACTH and prednisone treatment for multiple sclerosis. *Neurology* 38:1631–1634, 1988.
72. Maxwell S, Scheftner WA, Kessler HA, et al: Manic syndrome associated with zidovudine treatment. *JAMA* 259:3406, 1989.
73. Wright JM, Sachdev PS, Perkins RJ, et al: Zidovudine-related mania. *Med J Aust* 150:339–341, 1989.
74. Waters BGH, Simeon J: Behavioral toxicity to medications in a six year old boy: A genetic marker? *J Am Acad Child Psychiatry* 22:492–494, 1983.
75. Shader RI: *Psychiatric Complications of Medical Drugs.* New York: Raven Press, 1972.
76. Editorial: *Br Med J* 180:119–120, 1966.
77. Demuth GW, Ackerman SH: Alpha-methyldopa and depression: A clinical study and a review of the literature. *Am J Psychiatry* 140:534–538, 1983.
78. Campbell M, Spencer EK: Psychopharmacology in child and adolescent psychiatry: A review of the past five years. *J Am Acad Child Adolesc Psychiatry* 27:269–279, 1988.
79. Patten SB: Propranolol and depression: Evidence from the antihypertensive trials. *Can J Psychiatry* 35:257–259, 1990.
80. Brismar K, Hylander B, Eliasson K, et al: Melatonin secretion related to side effects of beta blockers from the central nervous system. *Acta Med Scand* 223:525–530, 1988.
81. Bright RA, Everitt DE: Beta-blockers and depression: Evidence against an association. *JAMA* 267:1783–1787, 1992.

82. Hullett FJ, Potkin SG, Levy AB, et al: Depression associated with nifedipine-induced calcium channel blockade. *Am J Psychiatry* 145:1277–1279, 1988.

83. Caufman M, Kahner K, Paselow ED, et al: Steroid psychoses: Case report and brief overview. *J Clin Psychiatry* 43:75–76, 1982.

84. Burke P, Kocoshis SA, Chandra R, et al: Determinants of depression in recent onset paediatric inflammatory bowel disease. *J Am Acad Child Adolesc Psychiatry* 29:608–610, 1990.

85. Ruthgers AWF, Links TP, LeCoultre R, et al: Behavioral disturbances after effective ACTH treatment of the dancing eye syndrome. *Dev Med Child Neurol* 30:408, 1988.

86. Venkatarangam SH, Kutcher SP, Notkin RM: Secondary mania with steroid withdrawal. *Can J Psychiatry* 33:631–632, 1988.

87. Stiefel FC, Breitbart WS, Holland JC: Corticosteroids in cancer: Neuropsychiatric complications. *Cancer Invest* 7:479–491, 1989.

88. Gawkrodger D: Manic depression induced by dapsone in patients with dermatitis herpetiformis. *Br Med J* 30:860, 1989.

89. Pope HG Jr, Katz DL: Affective and psychotic symptoms associated with anabolic steroid use. *Am J Psychiatry* 145:487–490, 1988.

90. Slap GB: Oral contraceptives and depression. Impact, prevalence and cause. *J Adolesc Health Care* 2:53–64, 1981.

91. Fleming O, Seager CP: Incidence of depressive symptoms in users of the oral contraceptive. *Br J Psychiatry* 132:431–440, 1978.

92. Glick ID, Bennett SE: Psychiatric complications of progesterone and oral contraceptives. *J Clin Psychopharmacol* 6:350–367, 1981.

93. Shear MK: Pathophysiology of panic: A review of pharmacologic provocative tests and naturalistic monitoring data. *J Clin Psychiatry* 47(suppl):18, 1986.

94. Ministry of Health and Welfare, Tokyo: Angioneurotic oedema induced by enalapril maleate or captopril. Information on Adverse Reactions to Drugs, No. 84, 1987.

95. West Midlands Centre for Adverse Drug Reactions Reporting: ACE inhibitors and CNS adverse effects. Newsletter, June 1988.

96. Burns EM, Arnold LE: Biological aspects of stress: Effects on the developing brain, in: Arnold LE (ed): *Childhood Stress*. New York: John Wiley & Sons, 173–138, 1990.

14

Nootropics And Foods

C. KEITH CONNERS, Ph.D.,
and ELIZABETH P. SPARROW, M.A.

I. INTRODUCTION

Food, diet, vitamins, trace elements, minerals, and additives have been part of folk treatments for mental disorders dating back to itinerant peddlers of snake oil. Foods are often touted by those outside the traditional medical mainstream as substitutes for established treatments. Parents often besiege the practitioner with unproved remedies because they may sound more benign and "natural" than drugs or behavior modification. Unproved dietary remedies are frequently promoted by alternative practitioners seeking a competitive advantage in the marketplace of mental health services. These practitioners often target psychopharmacology as "unnatural" and dangerous compared to the beneficent natural use of foods and diet, thus playing upon parental anxieties and allegiances to holistic medicine.

The advent of a new class of pharmacological agents, the so-called "nootropics" or knowledge-enhancing drugs, offers the exciting prospect of pharmacological treatment of childhood disorders that have a significant cognitive component. It is fitting to consider nootropic drugs in the same category as foods. Much of the rationale for using foods as treatments comes from their roles as precursors of brain neurotransmitters. For example, choline, obtained from the diet, is a precursor for the neurotransmitter acetylcholine (ACh), suspected of having a pivotal role in memory processes and in the pharmacology of nootropics.

Possibilities for use of nootropics include developmental learning disorders, attentional disorders, organic brain syndromes, and mental retardation. Explorations with these agents are still in their infancy. To date, only one such compound (piracetam) has received extensive testing in adults and children. However, new and more potent versions are waiting in the wings, and clinicians will soon need a perspective on the issues surrounding this controversial new form of treatment.

Nootropics, like dietary remedies, have developed a subculture of enthusiasts who are prone to uncritical endorsements without substantive data to support them. The position is made even more complex by the deep populist suspicion among certain groups that the test

C. KEITH CONNERS, Ph.D. • Department of Psychiatry, Division of Medical Psychology, Duke University Medical Center, Durham, North Carolina 27710. **ELIZABETH P. SPARROW, M.A.** • Department of Psychiatry, Washington University, St. Louis, Missouri 63130.

Practitioner's Guide to Psychoactive Drugs for Children and Adolescents (Second Edition), Werry and Aman, eds. Plenum Publishing Corporation, New York, 1999.

of proof required in science is part of a medical conspiracy to keep remedies the profession cannot control out of the reach of the public. It is important for the clinician who uses pharmacological agents to understand fact and fiction surrounding nootropics and foods and to have a perspective on how to deal with these issues as they arise in clinical practice, with media, and in public education.

There *are* important facts and useful practices to be found in the literature on food, nootropics, and behavior. However, experimentation in the field is quite complex, and findings are easily misinterpreted, misused, or dismissed by cursory and uncritical reading of the literature. Several recent monographs attest to the vigorous activity in the field. This chapter will not attempt a comprehensive review of the entire field since several reports for lay[1,2] and professional audiences[3–5] are available. We will focus on those facts that seem relevant to current clinical practice or that have important implications for research.

II. NOOTROPICS

Nootropic agents are thought to enhance memory and learning. They have also been called "smart drugs" in the popular literature. The use of nootropics in research has increased considerably in the past 25 years, as shown in Fig. 1. In 1995 alone, almost 60 publications involved research with nootropics, whereas there were no publications dated pre-1972. Of the 544 medical articles to date mentioning nootropics, 213 pertain to humans. Clinical research with nootropics in humans has primarily involved piracetam. Piracetam has recently entered the public eye owing to national media focus on its use in a few children with Down's syndrome. It is important to note here that this use is thus far unsubstantiated by scientific research.

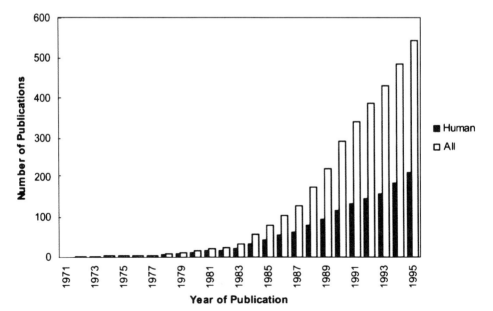

FIGURE 1. Cumulative frequencies of nootropics in medical journals, 1971–1995 (based on Medline search for "Nootropic").

A. Definition

Piracetam (Nootropil®, Nootropyl®, 2-oxo-1-pyrrolidone acetamide) was originally developed as a molecular analog of γ-aminobutyric acid (GABA) for the purpose of altering vestibular function in motion sickness, but it is probably neither a GABA agonist nor antagonist. A number of analogues of the piracetam molecule are currently under study, including oxiracetam (Neuromet®), pramiracetam, etiracetam, nefiracetam, aniracetam, and rolziracetam. This group of nootropics is commonly referred to as the "racetams."[6] Piracetam has virtually no detectable peripheral effects at any dose in animals or humans and does not affect cerebral blood flow, unlike other putative cerebral enhancers. It appears to alter cellular brain metabolism, however, since it increases levels of brain adenosine triphosphate (ATP). In normal volunteers, a single dose of piracetam was found to change brain global functional state as measured by multichannel electroencephalographic recordings.[7] It has been suggested that the defining characteristics of "nootropics" should include lack of peripheral effect, absence of action on blood flow, and an increase in brain metabolism.[8]

B. Mechanism of Action

Some evidence indicates that piracetam decreases ACh levels in the hippocampus without altering choline levels, suggesting that it causes an increased release of ACh stores.[9] Other data suggest that piracetam acts via ACh to alter norepinephrine (NE).[10] A close analogue, pramiracetam, increases firing rates from cholinergic neurons having their cell bodies in the medial septal area (MSA) and ventral globus pallidus (nucleus basalis).[11] Another acetam (nefiracetam) produces minor, restricted effects on monoamine systems in rats. A possible GABA-mediated mechanism has been suggested.[12] Yet another researcher has suggested that the effects of nootropics on memory are steroid-sensitive, with a resultant alteration in protein synthesis.[13,14]

Piracetam also blocks the effects of hypoxic amnesia, suggesting that its effects on memory may relate to cellular oxygen metabolism. However, these blocking effects seem more effective with earlier rather than late administration.[15] There is some suggestion that individual variance in children's metabolisms may alter the effectiveness of nootropics in treatment of mental retardation.[16]

C. Human Studies

Early studies by Dimond and Brouwers suggested that piracetam might facilitate transfer of information across the callosal pathways (which join the two cerebral hemispheres) and hence be a "super-connector" drug.[17] A number of studies with normal and dyslexic adults indicated that the drug might enhance verbal learning. These studies have been reviewed by Wilsher.[18] Conners and colleagues used event-related potentials to examine the effect of piracetam on verbal and spatial processing.[19,20] Piracetam only had effects on verbal targets, not nonverbal targets. This study was part of a multisite clinical study of piracetam over an entire academic year, in which there was a highly significant increase in reading age in a drug-treated sample of severe "dyslexia-pure" cases of about 1.5 years compared with about 0.4 years in placebo controls.[21] Another study involved use of aniracetam in humans with long-term chronic exposure to organic solvents.[22] Chronic administration of aniracetam did not significantly affect performance on most neuropsychological measures.

D. Conclusions

Despite some convincing data of efficacy and a lack of side effects, piracetam is not approved for use in the United States and is only approved for "emergency" use in Canada. It can be obtained as a nonprescription product from some countries, including England, Greece, Switzerland, and the Netherlands. Newer compounds are under study by American companies, and this class of drugs may be available eventually. Results regarding a clear benefit from use of piracetam with learning disabilities are inconsistent but show enough promise to warrant further study.[23] Other drugs involving cholinergic mechanisms, such as ergoloid mesylates (Hydergine®), or dietary treatments such as lecithin and choline have not been demonstrated to have efficacy for treatment of any cognitive function in children or adults (see below).

III. FOOD

Foods may be considered from the point of view of their *chemical constituents* and macronutrient content or in terms of their effects upon the *nutritional environment* through manipulation of meal structure and timing. There is a large and soundly based literature on the effects of nutrients on early brain growth and physical development and nutrient interaction with environmental variables. Such information has relevance to nutritional counseling in pregnancy and development and for health policy. We will not cover this topic since good summaries are available.[24,25] Rather, we will address the more commonly encountered controversial issues surrounding dietary constituents and diets as treatments.

A. Food Constituent Effects

1. Sweeteners

a. Sugar

One of the longest and most continuing controversies regarding food is whether sugar and other sweeteners promote adverse behavioral reactions in children. As early as 1922, observers described cases of hyperactive children who overindulged in candy and cookies and who apparently became calmer when sweet foods were removed from the diet.[26] Recent concerns over the role of sweeteners in general health[27] have increased the negative associations of sweeteners in the minds of both lay and medical groups. Almost half of pediatricians surveyed in 1983 believed that sugar plays a role in childhood hyperactivity.[28]

Evidence for the association of sugar and hyperactivity comes from correlational studies and from experimental studies in which sugar is used as a challenge. Methodologically sophisticated correlational studies support a relationship between carbohydrate intake (amount of sugar products consumed, ratio of sugar products to nutritional foods, and ratio of carbohydrate to protein intake) and destructive–aggressive and restless behaviors in hyperactive children, as well as restless behavior in normal 4- to 7-year-old children.[29] Unfortunately, in an otherwise careful study,[29] Prinz et al. based nutrient content on weight rather than calories. This would tend to inflate the amount of carbohydrate intake in such things as soft drinks. One well-controlled study purported to refute these associations because there were only 4 of 37 tests that were significantly correlated with sugar intake.[30] However, the four tests showed higher ankle actometer scores, more grid crossing in playroom activity, more attention shifts, and less time spent on-task to be correlated with increased sugar intake. One could well argue that these variables should have carried more weight in the hypothesis testing because of their direct relevance to attention-deficit symptomatology. Another well-designed study found that 5-year-old children who consumed excessive sugar were significantly poorer on tests of attention than those with low sugar intake.[31] A large correlational study[32] found that Wechsler IQ scores were significantly negatively correlated with the ratio of refined carbohydrate food calories to total diet calories and the ratio of carbohydrate to protein calories. The relationships were controlled for socioeconomic status (SES) and other demographic variables. Because of the inherent ambiguity of the causal direction in these correlational studies, experimental challenge studies have been undertaken to clarify whether high level of sugar consumption is a cause or a mere correlate of hyperactive and inattentive behavior. In a recent metaanalysis of the effects of sugar on behavior and cognition in children with attention-deficit hyperactivity disorder (ADHD), Wolraich et al.[26] determined that sugar does not significantly affect cognitive or behavioral performance in the majority of these children, although it may affect a small subset. Some studies show that a sugar diet is associated with an increase in errors on continuous performance tasks when compared with a placebo diet.[33] Several authors have suggested that parental expectancy effects may play a role in behavior ratings completed by parents regarding sugar-related behaviors.[26,34]

Natural experiments among diabetics whose glucose levels are radically altered by insulin show that both high and low levels of blood glucose lead to impaired cognitive function.[35–37] Some well-controlled studies show no effect of sugar challenges upon child behavior,[38,39] whereas others[5,40,41] show significant effects. The negative studies, reviewed elsewhere,[5] all involve short-term acute challenges and a failure to control for prior meal activity.

In a study by the senior author,[5] 83 normal and hyperactive children were randomly assigned to three different meal conditions, and within each meal condition they were given challenges of sucrose or aspartame on different days in a counterbalanced order. Deleterious effects of sucrose on attention occurred only when preceded by a carbohydrate meal, not after fasting or a protein meal. It is known that ingesting the large neutral amino acids (LNAAs) in protein counteracts the efflux of LNAAs from the blood caused by a carbohydrate-induced insulin reaction.[42,43] A higher concentration ratio of LNAAs to tryptophan prevents tryptophan from crossing the blood–brain barrier and increasing brain pools of serotonin. Therefore, the status of the protein/tryptophan concentration ratio should be critical in determining the behavioral effects of a sugar challenge. Following a high-protein meal, sugar should have little effect; when sugar is consumed following a carbohydrate meal, one would expect a large brain increase in serotonin levels, possibly with behavioral consequences involving sleep and relaxation.

We have hypothesized that the explanation for a more significant impact of sugar upon hyperactive children than normal children is due to a central dopamine defect which in turn leads to diminished control by counter-regulatory hormones such as growth hormone and cortisol. In our study,[5] the hyperactive children had significantly higher baseline blood glucose levels than normal controls, and when given the sugar challenge, they failed to respond by decreasing their output of cortisol and growth hormone as the normals did. Ordinarily, these hormones increase output when blood sugar is low and decrease output when blood sugar is high, serving to partially regulate blood sugar by increasing it when needed for active energy mobilization as in fight or flight.[44]

Although the challenge studies with sugar are inconclusive, the general health dangers of sugar, as well as studies that control for meal interactions, suggest that parents would be well advised to maintain limits on when and how much sugar is allowed in the diet. Our studies indicate the importance of sufficient protein in the diet to counteract the powerful carbohydrate-induced alterations of brain serotonin. Other studies, cited below in relation to vitamins, provide additional reasons for being cautious about the excess availability of sugar in the child's diet. **Clearly, the recommendation of maintenance of reasonable sugar intake in the presence of good nutrition and high protein intake is different from the exaggerated claims that sugar causes hyperactivity or that sugar-free diets are an effective treatment.**

b. Aspartame

This artificial sweetener has become a ubiquitous component of child and adult diets. Aspartame (trade names, Equal® and NutraSweet®) is a methyl ester of a dipeptide of aspartic acid and phenylalanine, both natural and essential components of ordinary food. Aspartame has eclipsed the use of saccharin and cyclamates, partly because the latter sweeteners have a history of concerns regarding carcinogenic effects and partly because of lack of an aftertaste and a superior sweetening power (180–200 times that of pure sucrose).

Aspartate can act as an excitatory neurotransmitter, and phenylalanine is an amino acid that serves as a precursor of brain tyrosine. Thus, aspartame has the potential for elevating blood levels of aspartate and phenylalanine to levels that could impair brain function. However, both acute experiments[45] and chronic feeding experiments appear to be reassuring that very high doses are safe as regards elevated blood levels of aspartame.[46] One recent study of children with seizures found that seizure activity was not associated with aspartame.[47] Also, no differences in behavior ratings completed by clinicians and parents or electroencephalographic measures were found.

Individuals with phenylketonuria (PKU) or those who are heterozygous for PKU are cautioned not to have high intakes of phenylalanine. Experiments suggesting that carbohydrates might significantly increase brain levels of orally ingested aspartame led to concern that individuals with PKU might be at risk in situations where they drink artificially sweetened colas in conjunction with cookies or cake, for example. While experiments on children with PKU indicate that a 12-oz beverage with 200 mg of aspartame does *not* elevate plasma phenylalanine significantly, with or without carbohydrate,[48] the long-term, cumulative effects of exposure have not been investigated in children.[49] A 12-week study of adult carriers of PKU genes found no change in cognitive function with chronic injection of aspartame.[50]

Individual case studies and single-case designs with children and adolescents have also raised concerns about psychotoxic effects of aspartame.[1] The senior author carried out a single-case design with double-blind challenges of a 4-year-old hyperactive boy and found increased aggression and poor compliance with parental commands in direct observation within a one-hour period of ingestion; significant later effects on sleep, mood, and activity level were also observed. This boy showed repeated severe behavioral episodes of hyperactivity and wild behavior when accidentally exposed to aspartame in school and restaurant situations over a period of many months of observation. Whether this represents a unique "allergic" response, a subtle conditioning effect from parental fears and expectations, or some other unexplained reactivity to aspartame cannot be determined. In a study of preschool-age children, no significant differences were found among children given sucrose, aspartame, or saccharin sweeteners over a 3-week period.[51] Wolraich et al.[51] also did not find significant differences in behavior associated with type of sweetener in a group of school-aged children labeled "sugar-sensitive." Researchers have failed to find significant differences on behavior ratings and cognitive measures in ADHD children who were given aspartame or placebo over a 2-week period.[52] **Although controlled studies do not implicate aspartame as a source of behavioral or cognitive deficits in children, moderation with children seems wise at this stage of our knowledge, particularly with young children.**

2. Caffeine

Caffeine, like theobromine and theophylline, is a methylxanthine. Its principal sources are coffee, cola drinks, chocolate, and tea. Depending upon the method of brewing, a 5-oz cup of coffee provides between 40 and 200 mg of caffeine. Children often consume large amounts of cola drinks. A 12-oz (355-mL) cola usually contains 30–60 mg of caffeine. Caffeine produces dose-dependent activation of the central nervous system (CNS) in children, as evidenced by increased amplitudes of evoked potentials.[53]

Animal research suggests that excessive maternal consumption of caffeine during gestation and lactation may lead to long-term effects on the child's sleep, learning ability, and anxiety, to name a few.[54] Caffeine intake, when combined with a low-protein diet, has been found to result in changes in brain composition in rodents.[55] However, caution should be taken in application of these results to humans until further research is conducted.

Caffeine-related disorders are recognized in the fourth edition of the *Diagnostic and Statistical Manual of Mental Disorders* (DSM-IV) by a group of diagnoses including caffeine intoxication, caffeine-induced anxiety disorder, and caffeine-induced sleep disorder.[56] Caffeine withdrawal has been included as a diagnosis under study. Restlessness, nervousness, and excitement are required symptoms of these diagnoses, along with other reactions characteristic of excess caffeine intake such as insomnia, psychomotor agitation, and flushed face. Several studies suggest that caffeine may be a cause of anxiety disturbances[57–59] though a large study conducted by the National Institute of Mental Health (NIMH) found no relationship.[60] Recent evidence links the action of caffeine to brain adenosine. Adenosine, a component of adenosine triphosphate, acts as a central depressant whose actions are opposite to those of caffeine, decreasing neuronal activity.[61]

Because caffeine is a CNS stimulant, the possibility that it might improve the behavior of hyperactive children, much as amphetamines and methylphenidate do, seems reasonable. However, early evidence from nonblind studies[62] has not been confirmed by controlled studies.[63] A recent review of the literature on behavioral effects of caffeine in children concluded that intake of *average* levels of caffeine does not affect hyperactive children.[64] Possible effects of caffeine on child behavior may depend upon prior levels of dietary intake, with high chronic users less affected by large doses than infrequent users.[65] Caffeine has no beneficial role as a pharmacotherapeutic agent, has known physical health risks, and, when consumed in large amounts, has potentially harmful effects on mood states. **Caffeine is suspected of contributing to unexplained anxiety disorders among children and adolescents who consume large amounts of cola drinks.**

3. Chocolate

Chocolate is a perennial favorite as a possible source of behavior problems in children. Perhaps this is because of its overwhelming attraction to both children and adults and its reputation as a source of sinful pleasure. Allergic reactions to chocolate are not uncommon in children; however, there are no hard data implicating it as a distinct etiologic agent in childhood mental disorders or symptomatic disturbances. Eaten in large amounts, it poses more of a threat to good nutrition than as a source of toxicity through excess intake of caffeine, theobromine, or theophylline.

B. Precursors of Essential Metabolic Substances

A number of dietary amino acids act as precursors for the synthesis of brain neuro-transmitters. For this reason, interest has been focused on their possible use as treatments and their potential role as inadvertent sources of problems.

1. Tryptophan

The most thoroughly studied precursor is tryptophan, which has long enjoyed a status among natural-food enthusiasts as a calming or antianxiety substance. Either as a pure amino acid or from food intake and stores in blood, tryptophan can exert marked effects upon brain function.

Normal carbohydrate intake may cause an increase in brain tryptophan, even though none is eaten directly. By causing an insulin response, carbohydrate causes an efflux of amino acids from the blood into interstitial fluid, thus reducing blood concentrations. However, because tryptophan is lightly bound to albumin, it is partially protected from this effect. As a result, carbohydrate loading causes tryptophan to gain precedence in crossing the blood–brain barrier into brain circulation. This occurs because the molecular carriers common to all protein transport respond to the concentrations of the various amino acids competing for transport into the brain. Since the relative concentrations of other LNAAs determine their access to a common carrier transport mechanism into the brain, either low intake of protein or high intake of carbohydrate may lead to a sudden increase in brain tryptophan. Because the amount of the rate-limiting enzyme in the brain for production of serotonin from tryptophan, tryptophan hydroxylase, is not regulated by feedback, an increase in brain tryptophan leads to an increase in brain serotonin content.[31,45] Serotonin is thought to exert effects on sleep and mood and modulatory effects on other brain amines, such as the catecholamines. As noted above, the tryptophan–serotonin link may play a role in the reaction of hyperactive children to sugar under certain conditions.

2. Choline and Tyrosine

Choline and tyrosine (precursors for acetylcholine and norepinephrine, respectively) have also been considered as possible dietary sources for changes in brain neurotransmit-ters. Animal studies suggest that pretreatment with tyrosine may serve as an important antistress measure through the regulation of brain norepinephrine,[66] though, unlike the biosynthesis of tryptophan, that of tyrosine is limited by a negative feedback upon the rate-limiting enzyme, and simply adding more tyrosine to the diet would not necessarily increase the output of brain tyrosine. In a single-blind study of the effect of oral tyrosine on seven children with attention-deficit disorder (ADD), tyrosine failed to produce any significant improvement.[67] Nevertheless, the role of tyrosine as a dietary precursor for norepinephrine raises possibilities of increased susceptibility to stress or mood disorders in children with low levels of protein intake.

There has been no documented use of other precursors such as choline for treatment of childhood disorders.

C. Vitamins

1. Deficiency States

From an international perspective, vitamin-deficiency states associated with malnutrition are a significant physical and mental health problem. Vitamin deficiencies affect neurotransmission, brain growth, myelinization, and neuronal excitability. Specific mental disturbances resulting from vitamin deficiencies are well known.[3] These include irritability, depression, and poor concentration associated with thiamine deficiency; hallucinations and catatonia associated with niacin deficiency; irritability and seizures in infants with pyridoxine (B_6) deficiency; memory loss and neurological symptoms associated with B_{12} deficiency; and irritability and psychosis associated with folic acid deficiencies. It has been suggested that children with ADHD may be deficient in vitamins, minerals, and essential fatty acids.[68] Furthermore, calcium, iron, and zinc deficiencies can enhance the negative effects of lead on development of cognition.[69] Other research has shown that vitamin B_6 (pyridoxine) is deficient in children with autism or Down's syndrome. When such deficiency states exist, vitamin and mineral supplementation is an accepted rational approach to treatment of both the physical and mental consequences of undernutrition. However, controversy arises when supplementation is proffered as a treatment for presumptively nutritionally normal children.

2. Supplementation in Normal Amounts

Early iron supplementation (ages 2–4) in children with iron-deficiency anemia appears to correct some associated cognitive deficits.[70] Vitamin and mineral supplements have also been touted as a means of improving intelligence. In 1988 Benton and Roberts[71] reported that the taking of a vitamin and mineral supplement over an 8-month period increased the nonverbal intelligence of 12-year-old British schoolchildren. The study was a well-designed, double-blind, placebo-controlled trial. This trial attracted considerable attention, and several replication studies appeared. The same multivitamin preparation was used with 61 12-year-olds, but there were no changes observed for a variety of intellectual measures.[72] A larger study with 227 7- to- 12-year-old children treated with a vitamin and mineral supplement over a 4-week period also found no changes.[73] In another study, 167 13-year-old Belgian schoolchildren were given a supplement or placebo for 5 months.[74] About one third of these boys with a typical diet low in vitamins and minerals showed increased nonverbal intelligence scores after receiving the supplement; boys receiving the placebo showed slightly declined scores. A recent large study involving 615 U.S. schoolchildren was carried out over a 12-month period of supplementation.[75] The tablets contained either placebo or vitamins and minerals at 50, 100, and 200% of the U.S. recommended daily allowance (RDA). Significant improvement in nonverbal intelligence was found for the 100% supplementation group compared with the placebo group.

Finally, Benton and Cook[76] reported a randomized double-blind study of 47 6-year-olds in which they found a 7.6-point IQ gain in the supplement group compared with a decline of 1.7 points in the placebo controls. Nutritional analyses revealed a strong positive relationship ($r = 0.55$, $P < 0.004$) between the amount of sugar in the diet and the change in IQ scores for three different IQ tests. The authors interpreted the findings to mean that high sugar intake is associated with vitamin deficiencies, which in turn result in lower IQ test results. The argument is supported by findings that micronutrient intake tends to be lower in children consuming higher amounts of sugar;[77] and fidgeting and frustratibility directly observed during the study showed a significant improvement in the supplemented group but not the placebo group.

The possibility that subtle vitamin-deficiency states result from excess sugar intake, and that nervous system functioning in children is thereby compromised, is an important finding worthy of serious consideration and further investigation. The fact of excess sugar intake among children presenting for clinical services is indisputable. The causal role of sugar in mental disturbances, however, has remained controversial. The present findings suggest that a subgroup of children with poor nutrition respond to a simple vitamin/mineral supplement. Both the findings regarding the role of adequate protein intake and the findings that supplements enhance nonverbal intelligence scores argue for a focus on adequate nutrition rather than an all-out struggle to get children to reduce their sugar intake. Sugar intake may only be relevant insofar as it prevents adequate nutrition, either in the form of adequate protein or adequate vitamins and minerals. **Although the mechanisms for impact upon attention/hyperactivity may be different, sugar excess and vitamin deficiencies have the same bottom line for parents; a well-rounded diet is the most sensible form of dietary "treatment."**

3. Megavitamins

The use of extremely large doses of vitamins ("megavitamin" or "orthomolecular" therapy) has been proposed for a number of childhood psychiatric disturbances, including autism, attention-deficit disorders, hyperactivity, and learning disabilities. Comprehensive reviews for both adult[78] and child[79] psychiatric disorders indicate little support for the hypothesis that special vitamin/mineral combinations or megadoses of vitamins have any beneficial value. Careful controlled studies[80-82] using the megavitamin formulary proposed by Cott for treating behavior and learning disorders[83] failed to confirm any positive benefits. Multiple studies have failed to replicate effects of megavitamin and mineral therapy for mentally retarded children as reported by Harrell and colleagues.[79] A study of vitamin C, vitamin B_6, niacinamide, and pantothenic acid in 200 autistic children by Rimland[84] reported benefits apparently attributable to B_6. A later study which removed and then added the B_6 back to the diet confirmed the B_6 effect.[85] Several other studies have also suggested improvement,[79] although such support is weak.[86] Unfortunately, a number of methodological flaws limit the interpretation of these and other studies of B_6 megadoses in autism. These include lack of control over the doses used and length of treatment (doses were administered by parents); confounding with a variety of other treatments including vitamin C and niacin; lack of comparison control groups; and lack of standardized measurement. In all such studies conducted by mail and telephone, there remains the issue of prior nutritional status. As with the Benton and Cook studies reported in the previous section, it is possible that there are subgroups of autistic children who are in fact deficient in certain vitamins or minerals. Pica, or the eating of a variety of non-nutritional substances, is very common among autistic children. Supplementation effects in that group might then be attributable to remedying a physical deficiency state.

Fragile X syndrome, a sex-linked genetic disorder, is usually associated with mental retardation. Although folic acid is not deficient in individuals with fragile X syndrome, there are some indications that supplementation of folic acid may produce a small therapeutic effect in prepubertal patients.[87] Observed benefits include improved attention span and concentration, suggesting that folic acid therapy may be helpful in other disorders. Side effects of folic acid (a water-soluble vitamin) include gastrointestinal symptoms, excitability, overactivity, and irritability.

It is very important to note that megavitamin therapy is not risk-free. Side effects of large doses of the fat-soluble vitamins (A, D, E, and K) include liver damage, changes in bone, and calcification of body tissues. Even water-soluble vitamins (e.g., folic acid, B_6) are associated with side effects. Megadoses of pyridoxine (B_6) can lead to peripheral neuropathy including numbness and lack of coordination, with some sensory–perceptual disturbances persisting after discontinuation.[79] Other potential side effects of B_6 megadoses are ulcers and seizures.[88]

D. Trace Minerals

Minerals are essential to a number of CNS functions. They are available in the diet by both intentional routes and unintentional routes. The amount present in the body varies from relatively high amounts to tiny traces. In order of amount, the macronutrient minerals (0.005% or more of body weight) are calcium, phosphorus, potassium, sulfur, sodium, chlorine, and magnesium. Trace amounts of iron, iodine, copper, zinc, manganese, and cobalt are also found in the human body.[3]

Iron is perhaps the most important dietary mineral in terms of worldwide problems associated with deficiency states. Fatigue, irritability, and short attention span have been clearly linked to subclinical deficiency states that are well short of frank anemia. Iron-deficient children are slower to learn laboratory tasks and perform more poorly on simple memory tests.[89] Though more controversial, a number of studies have suggested that iron supplementation improves cognitive behavior. Iron deficiency can result in poor storage and transport of zinc by means of its effects on cadmium.[69]

Zinc is thought to be marginally deficient in typical North American diets.[90] Behavioral deficits due to low zinc include irritability, mood disturbance, tremor, and some cerebellar postural–motor and fine-motor control problems. Some authors have suggested that zinc deficiency is responsible for ADHD.[91] Animal data indicate a possible effect of zinc status on brain catecholamines. Because of the presumed action of stimulant drugs on catecholamines, Arnold et al.[92] examined the hypothesis that zinc status would predict amphetamine improvement in ADHD. Eighteen subjects received a crossover treatment of dextroamphetamine or placebo for one month each. The difference between drug and placebo correlated significantly with baseline zinc levels ($r = 0.61$ for changes on the hyperactivity factor of the Conners Rating Scale). Patient baseline zinc was significantly below that of controls. **Though preliminary, these findings suggest the need for further investigation of the role of zinc in ADHD.**

E. Heavy Metals

Heavy metals such as lead, mercury, cadmium, and aluminum have no known nutritional value. They enter the body through the airways and through contamination of foodstuffs. The role of lead in producing hyperkinesis and cognitive deficits is now well established.[93–96] Lead has been shown to compete with calcium, thereby affecting release of neurotransmitters necessary for cognition.[69] Continuing lead exposure has been associated with cumulative losses in cognitive function during early childhood.[77] However, there have been exceptions reported.[97] Cadmium is frequently inhaled by children from sidestream smoke (i.e., smoke emitted as a by-product of smoking and inhaled by a bystander). A large dietary study found that children with high cadmium levels had lower IQ and poorer reading ability than those with low cadmium levels. Statistical controls ruled out demographic variables as causes. The cadmium effect was inversely related to the levels of zinc measured in the children. The authors concluded that dietary zinc protects against the toxic effects of cadmium. Dietary intake of carbohydrate was inversely related to the levels of zinc, showing once again that complex interactions between ordinary diet, protective, and harmful substances may account for a significant portion of variance in behavior and cognitive function. Even with SES and other background factors controlled statistically, a multiple regression indicated that 20% of variance in reading level was accounted for by the dietary factors.[98] In a study that examined the effects of prenatal exposure to heavy metals on the cognitive skills of children, higher amounts of cadmium, chromium, cobalt, lead, mercury, nickel, and silver in amniotic fluid were associated with lower scores on a measure of IQ.[99] In general, exposure to metal toxins has been found to negatively affect academic achievement, classroom behavior, and motor performance.[100]

F. Food Additives

Feingold was the first to propose that intentional food additives, particularly artificial colors and flavors, are a cause of hyperactivity in children.[101] This hypothesis spawned a large number of correlational and challenge studies to test the hypothesis.[102] Although most of the studies were unable to confirm the hypothesis, either by dietary exclusion or by challenge with artificial dyes,[103] some questions remain. First, one of the best studies found significant improvement in preschoolers treated with the Feingold diet (also known as the "Kaiser–Permanente" or "K-P" diet) compared with those receiving a carefully blinded control diet.[104] Second, critics of the various studies argued that they did not in fact test the hypothesis adequately.

A very rigorous trial was carried out in 1- to 3-year-old hyperactive children who had some signs of allergy, including rhinitis or rash, and who had sleep problems.[105] The investigators selected a group of 24 children who met criteria for ADD and used their regular diet over a 10-day period as a basis for selecting a control diet. The experimental diet ("back to basics") eliminated food dyes, flavors, preservatives, monosodium glutamate, chocolate, and caffeine. The children also received a multivitamin supplement containing no sugar or artificial colors or flavors. Most sources of sugar were eliminated, as were milk products for children who had some evidence of lactose intolerance. Food was provided in coded packages for the entire family and for the child on special occasions. This "family affair" approach ensured good compliance, which is otherwise a bugaboo of this type of research enterprise. Blood samples were taken at the end of each dietary phase.

Protein content of the control and experimental diets was kept equivalent. Blood studies showed a significant increase in the experimental group of 9 of the 11 vitamins assayed, and carbohydrates, sugar, and total calorie intake went down during the experimental diet. There was a highly significant improvement in daily ratings of hyperactivity and in sleep in the experimental group. There were also significant improvements in physical signs and symptoms, including chronic rhinitis, bad breath, headache, and sleep (earlier onset and fewer night awakenings). The broad nature of the exclusions makes it difficult to determine which variables might account for the improvement. However, the quality of the study makes it unlikely that the effects were spurious or placebo-related.

Boris and Mandel also conducted an elimination trial for foods, dyes, and preservatives in children with ADHD.[106] The majority of these children responded favorably. A double-blind, placebo-controlled food challenge showed significant differences between challenge and placebo days. Children with allergies generally showed more response than children without allergies.

Another study which also made a comprehensive elimination of offending foods by a systematic procedure of withdrawal and rechallenge also found quite striking levels of behavioral and physical improvement.[107] The subjects for this trial were not typical of attention-deficit hyperactivity disorders because a large number also had seizure or other neurological disorders, allergic conditions, or physical symptoms such as headache, abdominal discomfort, rhinitis, aches in limbs, skin rashes, and mouth ulcers. In the first phase of the study, lasting 4 weeks, the diet restricted foods to two meats, two carbohydrate sources, two fruits, a vegetable, water, calcium, and multivitamins. Patients showing improvement then went on to a second phase. In this phase, foods previously eliminated were reintroduced for one week at a time. If behavioral or physical symptoms recurred, the food was withdrawn again. The yellow food dye tartrazine and the preservative benzoic acid were given in a separate orange squash and in capsules, respectively, in a double-blind, placebo-controlled fashion. Of the 76 patients, only 14 did not show some adverse response to a suspected offending food reintroduced in phase two, confirming the improvement that occurred when it was first eliminated.

The third phase was a double-blind, placebo-controlled trial testing one of the specific foods that had caused a behavioral reaction in a child when reintroduced. Of the 31 children who entered this double-blind phase, 28 completed it. Multiple observers (parent, physician, testing psychologist) found that the children improved during the double-blind active phase compared to the placebo phase. The most common offending foods (79% of all children) were those containing benzoic acid and tartrazine, which were usually found to vary together. Over half of the children reacted adversely to cow's milk, chocolate, wheat, and grapes. Only cabbage, lettuce, cauliflower, celery, goat's cheese, and duck eggs showed no confirmed adverse reaction in any child.

This trial is important, both because of its comprehensiveness and rigor and because the effects were rather dramatic in most children. Forty-seven children ceased having headaches, and 13 who previously had seizures became seizure-free. Nevertheless, the authors point out the complexity of carrying out such dietary trials and argue that unsupervised trials could be dangerous. The diets were expensive and disruptive, and the authors noted the potential for using the diet as punishment or for attribution of all behavioral problems to the diet. Recently, the effects of various dose levels of tartrazine were investigated in a double-blind, placebo-controlled, repeated-measures study. Approximately half the children showed irritability, restlessness, and sleep disturbance with all dose levels of tartrazine.[108]

Both the "back to basics" diet and the oligoantigenic diets just discussed are extremely difficult to carry out in controlled trials because of the need for scrupulous monitoring and the possibilities of noncompliance. Nevertheless, both diets could be summarized as a combination of common sense and a well-balanced and nutritionally adequate approach. While there may well be specific offending agents (such as tartrazine and benzoic acid) that can readily be eliminated from children's diets, the rest of the diets usually approximated the recommendations of standard nutritional texts.

One alternative to changing diet in children with hyperactivity associated with food intolerance is "enzyme-potentiated desensitization" (EPD). EPD, an immunotherapy method, was developed in England in the 1960s. It involves injections of an enzyme, β-glucuronidase, with low levels of mixed allergens. Current theory states that EPD affects T-suppressor memory; therefore, after an initial round of injections, therapy can gradually be reduced or eliminated.[109] Hyperactive children who were previously found to be intolerant of certain foods were given several doses of EPD. The majority of the treated children became tolerant of foods that previously produced hyperactivity, while the majority of children in the control group continued exhibiting hyperactivity in response to the foods.[110] Although this approach is still viewed as experimental by many physicians in the United States, there are a few who apply EPD after diet modification fails.

The rather exciting findings of attentional and cognitive improvement obtained in the well-controlled trials of dietary control further underscore the likelihood that **much of the furor over dietary treatments may simply reflect the important role of good general nutrition for optimal cognitive and behavioral functioning in children.**

IV. SOME CLINICAL GUIDELINES FOR WORKING WITH PARENTS

A. Food Histories as Part of Regular History-Taking

In the authors' experience, it is rare for clinicians (except perhaps for pediatricians) to include food histories in the initial workup of new patients. Surprisingly, when this is done, extremes of dietary practice are quite frequently encountered in both inpatient and outpatient settings. For example, in one study on an inpatient service we found that one-third of the patients actually qualified for a diagnosis of pica based upon a 3-day diet diary and food history.[31] It is not unreasonable to ask parents to keep a 7-day diet diary during the first week of an evaluation. Software programs are available which make it quite easy to determine the nutrient intake of children. In many parts of the world, a specific history for lead exposure is important, with subsequent testing of lead levels as indicated by the findings. Guidelines for history taking and some appropriate forms may be found in Krieger[111] and Schwab and Conners.[107]

B. Ally with Parental Biases, Not Against Them

Many parents are more than willing to believe that dietary factors are important in their child's behavior. Rather than disputing this with the parents in an effort to get them to accept more conventional therapies, it seems wise to accept this belief system and use it to promote good general nutrition in the child. Telling the parent, "Yes, there is some evidence that too much sugar exacerbates hyperactivity, even though it doesn't cause it," and that

"Yes, there is some evidence that vitamins are important in attention and learning," does not mean committing to unproven and possibly harmful therapies. Rather, these statements can be used to promote a well-rounded diet, monitoring of food behavior, setting reasonable limits on when and how much the child eats, and awareness of harmful environmental conditions that interact with food. In the latter regard, elimination of second-hand smoke and prevention of toxicity from heavy metals by appropriate levels of calcium, iron, and zinc intake are well established as prophylactic approaches. Preschoolers are particularly vulnerable inasmuch as rapid CNS growth is occurring, and there is reasonable evidence that removing some of the food additives does have more than a placebo role in behavioral and somatic improvement.

C. Monitor Food Behavior during Treatment

Monitoring of child behavior is a powerful agent for change. During treatment, say, with pharmacological agents or other therapies, monitoring of food intake often makes parents more aware of food habits and results in adoption of better food habits. In Prinz and Riddle's survey of sugar intake in preschool children,[31] they found that children in the upper quartile of sugar intake were in the lower quartile for attentional function and that the only explanatory factor for the excess sugar intake was *ad lib* access to the refrigerator. Having parents monitor "refrigerator behavior" is a good way to begin positive changes that could have important nutritional consequences.

V. CONCLUSIONS

This review has shown that food and other nutritional substances can influence behavior and learning in children. However, once gross malnutrition, rare in most Western societies, is excepted, most effects are small, complex, infrequent, difficult to demonstrate, and more likely to affect disadvantaged children than those of the perpetually anxious middle class. Among the most probable are those relating to the balance between carbohydrate and other dietary components, although certain substances, such as metals like lead and cadmium, continue to cause concern. There is some evidence that children with true allergic disorders may show more dietary effects than others, although this requires replication.

There is little support for some of the more popular views that would assign the cause of major psychiatric disorders of children (such as ADHD, conduct disorder, or autism) often or exclusively to dietary factors. What interesting but grossly overblown theories like the Feingold or megavitamin hypotheses have achieved is to show that diet is an important, but difficult, area to research in child psychopathology. Also, although affluence may have (mostly) removed frank malnutrition from our children, it may have produced distortions of the natural balance of dietary components that helped to shape the metabolism of the hunter-gatherer *Homo sapiens*. The current obsession in the United States with cholesterol is but one example of such a distortion, far more valid and substantial than much of that which has occupied those concerned with the effect of diet on children's behavior. However, even if the latter theories have been largely wrong, like all good theories they have led to heuristic research and to more precise neurochemical ideas to advance our understanding of the relationships between brain and behavior.

As far as attempts to "feed" the brain and advance its development are concerned, apart from one such "nootropic" substance, piracetam, there has been little systematic research or encouragement to serious scientists. However, recent data indicate a marked upswing of research in this area, and breakthroughs are constantly being sought by pharmaceutical companies anxious to discover new markcts. The range of cognitive deficits between forgetfulness of normal aging and the dementia of Alzheimer's disease is so wide as to encourage remedies for all levels of the spectrum.

Regrettably, the lack of data has not prevented the growth of a huge popular mythology about nootropics and dietary and nutritional substances, fed (as it were) by an industry reaping huge profits from this quintessential human credulity and the perennial search for the elixir of life.

Practitioners, who (hopefully) are distinguished by a commitment to properly derived technical knowledge as their lodestar, should act as a buffer between parents and these mythology-derived treatments, which not only have very short half-lives, but often also cause parents both considerable inconvenience and expense as they try to change the family diet to match whatever tune the pied piper is currently playing.

REFERENCES

1. Conners CK: *Feeding the Brain: How Foods Affect Children.* New York, Plenum, 1990.
2. Millichap JG: *Nutrition, Diet, and Your Child's Behavior.* Springfield, Ill; CC Thomas, 1986.
3. Kanarek RB, Marks-Kaufman R: *Nutrition and Behavior.* New York, Van Nostrand Reinhold, 1991.
4. Conners CK: *Food Additives and Hyperactive Children.* New York, Plenum, 1980.
5. Conners CK: Sugars and hyperactivity, in Kretchmer N, Hollenbeck CB (eds): *Sugars and Sweeteners.* Boca Raton, Fla, CRC Press, 1991.
6. Gouliaev AH, Senning A: Piracetam and other structurally related nootropics. *Brain Res Brain Res Rev* 19: 180–222, 1994.
7. Wackermann J, Lehmann D, Dvorak I, Michel CM: Global dimensional complexity of multi-channel EEG indicates change of human brain functional state after a single dose of a nootropic drug. *Electroencephalogr Clin Neurophysiol* 86:193–198, 1993.
8. Giurgea C, Salama M: Nootropic drugs. *Prog Neuropsychopharmacol* 1:235–247, 1977.
9. Wurtman RJ, Magil SG, Reinstein DK: Piracetam diminishes hippocampal acetylcholine levels in rats. *Life Sci* 28:1091–1093, 1981.
10. Nyback H, Wiesel FA, Skett P: Effects of piracetam on brain monoamine metabolism and serum prolactin levels in the rat. *Psychopharmacology* 61:235–238, 1979.
11. Poschel BP, Marriott GG, Gluckman, MI: Pharmacology underlying the cognition-activating properties of Pramiracetam (CL-879). *Psychopharmacol Bull* 19:720–721, 1983.
12. Luthman J, Lindqvist E, Kojima H, Shiotani T, Tanaka M, Tachizawa H, Olson L: Effects of nefiracetam (DM-9384), a pyrrolidone derivative, on brain monoamine systems. *Arch Int Pharmacodyn Ther* 328:125–144, 1994.
13. Mondadori C: In search of the mechanism of action of the nootropics: New insights and potential clinical implications. *Life Sci* 55:2171–2178, 1994.
14. Mondadori C: The pharmacology of the nootropics; new insights and new questions. *Behav Brain Res* 59: 1–9, 1993.
15. Saletu B, Grunberger J, Anderer, R: On brain protection of co-dergocrine mesylate (Hydergine) against hypoxic hypoxidosis of different severity: Double-blind placebo-controlled quantitative EEG and psychometric studies. *Int J Clin Pharmacol Ther Toxicol* 28:510–524, 1990.
16. Turova NF, Ermolina LA, Baryshnikov VA, Kopaladze RA, Aziavchik AV: [Effect of nootropic agents on serum biochemical indices in intellectually deficient children.] *Zh Nevropatol Psikhiatrii Imeni S S Korsakova* 83:1558–1563, 1983.
17. Dimond S, Brouwers EYM: Increase in the power of human memory in normal man through the use of drugs. *Psychopharmacology (Berlin)* 49:307–309, 1976.
18. Wilsher C: A brief review of studies of piracetam in dyslexia. *J Psychopharmacol* 1:95–100, 1987.

19. Conners CK, Blouin AG, Winglee M, et al: Piracetam and event-related potentials in dyslexic males. *Int J Psychophysiology* 4:19–27, 1986.
20. Conners CK, Reader M, Reiss A, et al: The effects of piracetam upon visual event-related potentials in dyslexic children. *Psychophysiology* 24:513–521, 1987.
21. DiIanni M, Wilsher CR, Blank MS, Conners CK, et al: The effects of piracetam in children with dyslexia. *J Clin Psychopharmacol* 5:272–278, 1985.
22. Somnier FE, Ostergaard MS, Boysen G, Bruhn P, Mikkelsen BO: Aniracetam tested in chronic psychosyndrome after long-term exposure to organic solvents. A randomized, double-blind, placebo-controlled cross-over study with neuropsychological tests. *Psychopharmacology (Berlin) (QGI)* 101:43–46, 1990.
23. Aman MG, Rojahn J: Pharmacological intervention, in Singh NN, Beale IL (eds): *Learning Disabilities: Nature, Theory, and Treatment.* New York, Springer-Verlag, 1992, pp. 478–525.
24. Galler JR (ed): *Nutrition and Behavior.* New York, Plenum, 1984.
25. Wurtman RJ, Wurtman JJ (eds): *Nutrition and the Brain,* vols 1–4. New York, Raven Press, 1977–79.
26. Wolraich ML, Wilson DB, White, JW: The effect of sugar on behavior or cognition in children. A meta-analysis. *JAMA* 274:1617–1621, 1995.
27. National Academy of Sciences: *Sweeteners: Issues and Uncertainties.* Washington, DC: National Academy of Sciences, 1975.
28. Bennett FC, Sherman R: Management of childhood "hyperactivity" by primary care physicians. *J Dev Behav Pediatr* 4:88–93, 1983.
29. Prinz RJ, Roberts WA, Hantman E: Dietary correlates of hyperactive behavior in children. *J Consult Clin Psychol* 48:760–769, 1980.
30. Wolraich ML, Milich R, Stumbo P, Schultz F: Effects of sucrose ingestion on behavior of hyperactive boys. *J Pediatr* 106:675–682, 1985.
31. Prinz RJ, Riddle DB: Associations between nutrition and behavior in five-year-old children. *Nutr Rev* 44 (Suppl.):151–158, 1986.
32. Lester ML, Thatcher RW, Monroe-Lord L: Refined carbohydrate intake, hair cadmium levels, and cognitive functioning in children. *Nutr Behav* 1:3–13, 1982.
33. White JW, Wolraich M: Effect of sugar on behavior and mental performance. *Am J Clin Nutr* 62:242S–247S, 1995.
34. Hoover DW, Milich R: Effects of sugar ingestion expectancies on mother–child interactions. *J Abnorm Child Psychol* 22:501–515, 1994.
35. Flender J, Lifshitz F: The effects of fluctuations of blood glucose levels on the psychological performance of juvenile diabetics. *Diabetes* 25(Abstract):334, 1976.
36. Holmes CS, Hayford JT, Gonzalez JL, Weydert JA: A survey of cognitive functioning at different glucose levels in diabetic persons. *Diabetes Care* 6:180–185, 1983.
37. Lapp JE: Effects of glycemic alterations and noun imagery on the learning of paired associates. *J Learn Disabil* 14:35–38, 1981.
38. Behar D, Rapoport JL, Adams AJ, et al:Sugar challenge testing with children considered behaviorally "sugar reactive." *Nutr Behav* 1:277–288, 1984.
39. Milich R, Pelham WE: The effects of sugar ingestion on the classroom and playgroup behavior of attention deficit disordered boys. *J Consult Clin Psychol* 54:714–718, 1986.
40. Goldman JA, Lerman RH, Contois JH, et al: Behavioral effects of sucrose on preschool children. *J Abnorm Child Psychol* 14:565–577, 1986.
41. Conners CK, Glasgow A, Raiten D, et al: Hyperactives differ from normals in blood sugar and hormonal response to sucrose. Paper presented at the Annual Meeting of the American Psychological Association, New York, 1987.
42. Fernstrom JD, Wurtman RJ: Brain serotonin content: Physiological dependence on plasma tryptophan levels. *Science* 173:149–152, 1971.
43. Fernstrom JD, Wurtman RJ: Brain serotonin content: Increase following ingestion of carbohydrate diet. *Science* 174:1023–1025, 1971.
44. Luft R, Cerasi E, Madison LL, et al: Effect of a small decrease in blood-glucose on plasma-growth hormone and urinary excretion of catecholamines in man. *Lancet* 2:254–256, 1966.
45. Stegink LD: The aspartame story: A model for the clinical testing of a food additive. *Am J Clin Nutrit* 46: 204–215, 1987.
46. Leon AS, Hunninghake DB, Bell C, et al: Safety of long-term large doses of aspartame. *Arch Int Med* 149:2318–2324, 1989.
47. Shaywitz BA, Anderson GM, Novotny EJ, Ebersole JS, Sullivan CM, Gillespie SM: Aspartame has no effect on seizures or epileptiform discharges in epileptic children. *Ann Neurol* 35:98–103, 1994.
48. Wolf-Novak LC, Stegink LD, Brummel MC, et al: Aspartame ingestion with and without carbohydrate in

phenylketonuric and normal subjects: Effect on plasma concentrations of amino acids, glucose, and insulin. *Metabolism* 39:391–396, 1990.

49. Mackey SA, Berlin CM Jr: Effect of dietary aspartame on plasma concentrations of phenylalanine and tyrosine in normal and homozygous phenylketonuric patients. *Clin Pediatr* 31:394–399, 1992.

50. Trefz F, deSonneville L, Matthis P, Benninger C, Lanz-Englert B, Bickel H: Neuropsychological and biochemical investigations in heterozygotes for phenylketonuria during ingestion of high dose aspartame (a sweetener containing phenylalanine). *Hum Genet* 93:369–374, 1994.

51. Wolraich ML, Lindgren SD, Stumbo PJ, Stegink LD, Appelbaum MI, Kiritsy MC: Effects of diets high in sucrose or aspartame on the behavior and cognitive performance of children. *N Engl J Med* 330:301–307, 1994.

52. Shaywitz BA, Sullivan CM, Anderson GM, Gillespie SM, Sullivan B, Shaywitz SE: Aspartame, behavior, and cognitive function in children with attention deficit disorder [see comments]. *Pediatrics* 93:70–75, 1994. Comment in: *Pediatrics* 93:127–128, 1994. Comment in: *Pediatrics* 94:576, 1994.

53. Conners CK: The acute effects of caffeine on evoked response, vigilance, and activity level in hyperkinetic children. *J Abnorm Child Psychol* 7:145–151, 1979.

54. Nehlig A, Debry G: Consequences on the newborn of chronic maternal consumption of coffee during gestation and lactation: A review. *J Am Coll Nutr* 13:6–21, 1994.

55. Nehlig A, Debry G: Potential teratogenic and neurodevelopmental consequences of coffee and caffeine exposure: A review on human and animal data. *Neurotoxicol Teratol* 16:531–543, 1994.

56. American Psychiatric Association: *Diagnostic and Statistical Manual of Mental Disorders*, ed 4. Washington, DC: American Psychiatric Association Press, 1994.

57. Greden JF, Fontaine P, Lubetsky M, et al: Anxiety and depression associated with caffeinism among psychiatric inpatients. *Am J Psychiatry* 134:963–966, 1978.

58. Gilliland K, Andress D: Ad lib caffeine consumption, symptoms of caffeinism and academic performance. *Am J Psychiatry* 138:512–514, 1981.

59. Boulenger JP, Uhde TW, Wolff EA, et al: Increased sensitivity to caffeine in patients with panic disorder. *Arch Gen Psychiatry* 41:1067–1071, 1984.

60. Eaton WW, McLeod J: Consumption of coffee or tea and symptoms of anxiety. *Am J Public Health* 74:66–68, 1984.

61. Snyder SH: Adenosine as a mediator of the behavioral effects of xanthines, in Dews PB (ed): *Caffeine*. New York, Springer-Verlag, 1984.

62. Schnackenberg RC: Caffeine as a substitute for schedule II stimulants in hyperkinetic children. *Am J Psychiatry* 130:796–798, 1973.

63. Huestis RD, Arnold LE, Smeltzer DJ: Caffeine versus methylphenidate and d-amphetamine in minimal brain dysfunction: A double-blind comparison. *Am J Psychiatry* 132:868–870, 1975.

64. Leviton A: Behavioral correlates of caffeine consumption by children. Paper presented at the 60th Annual Meeting of the American Academy of Pediatrics, New Orleans, 1991. *Clin Pediatr* 31:742–750, 1992.

65. Rapoport JL, Berg CJ, Ismond DR, et al: Behavioral effects of caffeine in children:Relationship between dietary choice and effects of caffeine challenge. *Arch Gen Psychiatry* 41:1073–1079, 1984.

66. Wurtman RJ, Wurtman JJ (eds): *Nutrition and the Brain*. New York, Raven Press, 1979, vol 3.

67. Eisenberg J, Asnis GM, van Praag HM, et al: Effect of tyrosine on attention deficit disorder with hyperactivity. *J Clin Psychiatry* 49:193–195, 1988.

68. Colquhoun ID: Attention deficit/hyperactive disorder: A dietary/nutritional approach. *Ther Care Educ* 3:159–172, 1994.

69. Goyer RA: Nutrition and metal toxicity. *Am J Clin Nutr* 61(Suppl.):646S–650S, 1995.

70. Wasserman GA, Graziano JH, Factor-Litvak P, Popovac D, Morina N, Musabegovic A, Vrenezi N, Capuni-Paracka S, Lekic V, Preteni-Redjepi E, et al: Consequences of lead exposure and iron supplementation on childhood development at age 4 years. *Neurotoxicol Teratol* 16:233–240, 1994.

71. Benton D, Roberts G: Effect of vitamin and mineral supplementation on intelligence of a sample of schoolchildren. *Lancet* 1:140–143, 1988.

72. Crombie IK, Todman J, McNeill G, et al: Effect of vitamin and mineral supplementation on verbal and non-verbal reasoning of schoolchildren. *Lancet* 335:744–747, 1990.

73. Nelson M, Naismith DJ, Burley V, et al: Nutrient intakes, vitamin/mineral supplementation and intelligence in British schoolchildren. *Br J Nutr* 64:13–22, 1990.

74. Benton D, Buts JP: Vitamin/mineral supplementation and intelligence. *Lancet* 335:1158–1160, 1990.

75. Schoenthaler SJ, Amos SP, Eysenck HJ, et al: Controlled trial of vitamin-mineral supplementation: Effects on intelligence and performance. *Pers Individ Differ* 12:351–362, 1991.

76. Benton D, Cook R: Vitamin and mineral supplements improve the intelligence scores and concentration of six-year-old children. *Pers Individ Differ* 12:1151–1158, 1991.

77. Nelson M, Paul AA: Unpublished work, described in Committee on Medical Aspects of Food Policy, Dietary Sugars and Human Disease: Department of Health Report on Health and Social Subjects No. 37. London, HMSO.

78. Lipton MA, Mailman RB, Nemeroff CB: Vitamins, megavitamin therapy, and the nervous system, in Wurtman RJ, Wurtman JJ (eds): *Nutrition and the Brain*. New York, Raven Press, 1979, vol 3.

79. Aman MG, Singh NN: Vitamin, mineral and dietary treatments, in Aman MG, Singh NN (eds): *Psychopharmacology of the Developmental Disabilities*. New York, Springer-Verlag, 1988.

80. Haslam RH, Dalby JT, Rademaker AW: Effects of megavitamin therapy on children with attention deficit disorders. *Pediatrics* 74:103–111, 1984.

81. Arnold LE, Christopher J, Heustis RD, et al: Megavitamins for minimal brain dysfunction. *JAMA* 240:2642–2643, 1978.

82. Kershner J, Hawke W: Megavitamins and learning disorders: A controlled double-blind experiment. *J Nutr* 109:819–826, 1979.

83. Cott A: Megavitamins: The orthomolecular approach to behavioral disorders and learning disabilities. *Acad Ther* 7:245–258, 1972.

84. Rimland B: An orthomolecular study of psychotic children. *J Orthomol Psychiatry* 3:371–377, 1974.

85. Rimland B, Calloway E, Dreyfus P: The effect of high doses of vitamin B6 on autistic children: A double-blind crossover study. *Am J Psychiatry* 135:472–475, 1978.

86. Aman MG, VanBourgondien ME, Wolford PL, Sarphare G: Psychotropic and anticonvulsant drugs in subjects with autism: Prevalence and patterns of use. *J Am Acad Child Adolesc Psychiatry* 34:1672–1681, 1995.

87. Aman MG, Kern RA: The efficacy of folic acid in fragile X syndrome and other developmental disabilities. *J Child Adolesc Psychopharmacol* 1:285–295, 1990.

88. Kozlowski BW: Megavitamin treatment of mental retardation in children: A review of effects on behavior and cognition. *J Child Adolesc Psychopharmacol* 2:307–320, 1992.

89. Pollitt E, Leibel RL, Greenfield DB: Iron deficiency and cognitive test performance in preschool children. *Nutr Behav* 1:137–146, 1983.

90. Moser-Veillon PB: Zinc: Consumption patterns and dietary recommendations. *J Am Diet Assoc* 90:1089–1093, 1990.

91. Colquhoun I, Bunday S: A lack of essential fatty acids as a possible cause of hyperactivity in children. *Med Hypotheses* 7:673–679, 1981.

92. Arnold LG, Votolato NA, Kleykamp D, Baker GB, Bornstein RA: Does hair zinc predict amphetamine improvement of ADD/hyperactivity? *Int J Neurosci* 50:103–107, 1990.

93. Needleman HL: The neurobehavioral consequences of low lead exposure in childhood. *Neurobehav Toxicol Teratol* 4:729–732, 1982.

94. Needleman HL: Low-level lead exposure in the fetus and young child. *Neurotoxicology* 8:389–394, 1982.

95. Needleman HL: The persistent threat of lead: A singular opportunity. *Am J Pub Health* 79:643–645, 1989.

96. Needleman HL, Gunnoe C, Leviton A, Reed R, Peresie H, Maher C, Barrett P: Deficits in psychologic and classroom performance of children with elevated dentine lead levels. *N Engl J Med* 300:689–695, 1990.

97. Milar CR, Schroeder SR, Mushak P, et al: Failure to find hyperactivity in preschool children with moderately elevated lead burden. *J Ped Psychol* 1:85–95, 1981.

98. Thatcher RW, McAlaster R, Lester ML, et al: Comparisons among EEG, hair minerals and diet predictions of reading performance in children, in White SJ, Teller V (eds): *Annals of the New York Academy of Sciences*. New York, New York Academy of Sciences, 1984 vol. 425 pp 421–423.

99. Lewis M, Worobey J, Ramsay DS, McCormack MK: Prenatal exposure to heavy metals: Effect on childhood cognitive skills and health status. *Pediatrics* 89:1010–1015, 1992.

100. Marlowe M: The violation of childhood: Toxic metals and developmental disabilities. *J Orthomol Med* 10:79–86, 1995.

101. Feingold B: *Why Your Child Is Hyperactive*. New York, Random House, 1975.

102. Harley JP, Ray RS, Tomasi L, et al: Hyperkinesis and food additives: Testing the Feingold hypothesis. *Pediatrics* 61:818–828, 1978.

103. Goldstein S, Ingersoll B: Controversial treatments for children with ADHD and impulse disorders, in Koziol LF, Stout CE, Ruben DH (eds): *Handbook of Childhood Impulse Disorders and ADHD: Theory and Practice*. Springfield, Ill, Charles C. Thomas, 1993, p. 236.

104. Kaplan BJ, McNicol J, Conte RA, et al: Dietary replacement in preschool-aged hyperactive boys. *Pediatrics* 83:7–17, 1989.

105. Egger J, Carter CM, Graham PJ, et al: Controlled trial of oligoantigenic treatment in the hyperkinetic syndrome. *Lancet* 1:540–545, 1985.

106. Boris M, Mandel FS: Foods and additives are common causes of the attention deficit hyperactive disorder in children. *Ann Allergy* 72:462–468, 1994.

107. Schwab EK, Conners CK: Nutrient-behavior research with children: Methods, considerations, and evaluation. *J Am Diet Assoc* 86(3):319–326, 1986.
108. Rowe KS, Rowe KJ: Synthetic food coloring and behavior: A dose response effect in a double-blind, placebo-controlled, repeated-measures study. *J Pediatr* 125:691–698, 1994.
109. Shrader WA: EPD History, Theory, and Results [on-line]. 1996. Available: http://www.tiac.net/users/kkv/epd-general.shtml
110. Egger J, Stolla A, McEwen LM: Controlled trial of hyposensitisation in children with food-induced hyperkinetic syndrome [see comments]. *Lancet* 339:1150–1153, 1992.
111. Krieger I: *Pediatric Disorders of Feeding, Nutrition, and Metabolism.* New York, John Wiley & Sons, 1982.

15

Anxiolytics, Sedatives, and Miscellaneous Drugs

JOHN SCOTT WERRY, M.D., and MICHAEL G. AMAN, Ph.D.

I. INTRODUCTION

This chapter contains discussions of anxiolytics and sedatives and several miscellaneous drugs that do not fit naturally into the remaining drug chapters. Included here are reviews of central nervous system (CNS) depressants (such as the benzodiazepines), antihistamines and anticholinergics, and atypical anxiolytics. Under the rubric of "miscellaneous drugs," we have included clonidine and guanfacine, melatonin, hypericin, tryptophan and 5-hydroxytryptophan, fenfluramine, the β-blockers, and the opiate antagonists.

II. ANXIOLYTICS AND SEDATIVES

A. Anxiolytics and Sedatives Defined

Here, the term anxiolytic will be restricted to those drugs whose primary purpose is to relieve anxiety arising in normal life or in nonpsychotic psychiatric disorders (such as those classified in DSM or ICD as the anxiety, adjustment, and somatoform disorders or allied disorders; see Chapter 7). This somewhat arbitrary definition distinguishes anxiolytics from other drugs used in the treatment of anxiety but developed primarily for psychotic or severe mood disorders, such as antipsychotics (neuroleptics) or antidepressants (see Chapters 9 and 10). Sedation is an old term that includes any reduction of the level of arousal by chemical means. Since this can now be achieved in a variety of neurochemical ways with correspondingly different clinical pictures, sedation lacks precise meaning. The term

JOHN SCOTT WERRY, M.D. • University of Auckland, Auckland, New Zealand.   **MICHAEL G. AMAN, Ph.D.** • The Nisonger Center for Mental Retardation and Developmental Disabilities, Ohio State University, Columbus, Ohio 43210-1296.

Practitioner's Guide to Psychoactive Drugs for Children and Adolescents (Second Edition), Werry and Aman, eds. Plenum Publishing Corporation, New York, 1999.

sedative has acquired a somewhat more specific meaning in pharmacology, referring to drugs used primarily to induce sleep, although it would be better if this term were now replaced by modern terms like hypnotic (i.e., sleep-inducing drug).

There are three main groups of anxiolytic–sedative drugs: (1) CNS depressants, (2) antihistaminic/anticholinergic sedatives, and (3) atypical anxiolytics, a relatively new group.

The social, recreational, and illicit use of these drugs is described in Chapter 11; their use as antimanic drugs is covered in Chapter 9, and as antiepileptics (anticonvulsants) in Chapter 12. Here, only their pharmacology relevant to anxiolysis and their clinical use in anxiety, sleep, and related disorders will be presented. Much of what follows here is a distillate of four highly recommended monographs.[1-4]

B. CNS Depressants

1. Pharmacology

a. Classification and Action

The term CNS depressant encompasses a wide class of mostly highly lipid soluble gases, liquids, and solids—medical, commercial, industrial, and illicit—united by their capacity to slow neuronal excitability by interfering with ionic flows (most notably chloride) across membranes,[5,6] resulting in increased resistance to depolarization and hence to induction and passage of the nerve impulse. CNS depressants achieve this in one of two ways. The first is by a direct effect on the membrane, probably physicochemical, related to high lipid solubility,[6] which produces an effect on all nervous (and other) tissue. As a result, drugs that act by this mechanism are called general CNS depressants.[5] Alcohol is the prototypical drug in this class. The second way is by affecting specific receptors. Drugs which affect receptors that, as in the case of GABA receptors, are not uniformly distributed throughout the brain and other tissues produce a limited effect and are thus called selective CNS depressants[5] (often known popularly as minor tranquilizers). Benzodiazepine drugs are typical of this group, and although the mechanism is different, the net effect is similar to that of general depressants, namely, a reduction in ionic flux[7,8] raising the threshold to excitation. The difference between general and selective depressants in therapeutic dosage is more apparent than real. Their basic pharmacological similarity is evidenced by their cross-tolerance or their ability to serve as substitutes for one another in dependence and withdrawal (see Chapter 11). However, in overdose, the selective depressants are clinically distinctive because saturation of the target receptors limits their action, whereas the general depressants go on increasing their effect in a dose-dependent way, leading to coma and/or death. Thus, the therapeutic ratio of selective CNS depressants is very high, while that of the general depressants is almost always low (nitrous oxide is an exception), which makes them potentially dangerous drugs.

Although the somewhat different modes and sites of action among the various CNS depressants will likely cause important inter- and intraclass differences, more is to be gained by grouping all these substances together as having basically similar clinical effects and differing only in their toxicology and pharmacokinetics. There is a vast amount of knowledge that is currently divided into parcels among different medical specialties—anesthesiology, epileptology, alcohol and substance abuse, and psychopharmacology—according to the application of the substance. This unfortunately prevents a consolidation of knowledge. For example, had the similarity of the benzodiazepines to alcohol and the barbiturates been kept in mind, the widespread problem of benzodiazepine dependence might have been avoided. Similarly, a knowledge of the general properties of all CNS depressants might have led to an earlier recognition of behavioral and cognitive toxicity of the antiepileptics phenobarbital and phenytoin (see Chapter 12). Anesthesiology has much knowledge that could have assisted in an earlier understanding of inhalant abuse (see Chapter 11).

b. Use

The use to which this wide group of substances is put is determined to a large extent by the speed of onset and duration of their action. Gaseous or highly volatile substances are used in anesthesia or for a quick "buzz" by adolescents, since they can be inhaled and then enter the pulmonary circulation and the brain in a few seconds. This effect will disappear quickly as the substance is taken up by lipid (fat) tissues throughout the rest of the body (Chapter 2). Inhaled substances will not be discussed further here since, in children and adolescents, their only psychoactive use is as drugs of abuse (Chapter 11).

The therapeutic choice of substance will be dictated by safety and the time frame of action. Short-acting drugs are preferred for anesthesia and in the management of insomnia, and longer-acting ones for the relief of dysfunctional anxiety that generally lasts for much of the day. Because benzodiazepines offer a high level of safety and a wide variety of durations of effect [from 2 to 4 hr with triazolam (Halcion®) or days with chlordiazepoxide (Librium®)], they have very properly displaced all other traditional anxiolytic–sedative drugs [such as barbiturates, meprobamate (Equanil®), chloral hydrate, or paraldehyde] except for antihistamines in very young children (see Section II.C). They are not, however, without adverse effects (see Sections II.B.4 and II.B.6), and so the search for better anxiolytics goes on. Most of the newer developments such as zopiclone (Imovane®), though not benzodiazepines, are similar selective depressants and offer no real advance, but there are a few new atypical anxiolytics, such as buspirone (BuSpar®), that are truly different (see below).

c. Types, Potencies, and Pharmacokinetics

In Table 1 the benzodiazepines in common use are summarized as now classified[1] two-dimensionally by (1) potency (high and low) and (2) elimination half-life [short (<14 hr) and long; for most long-half-life benzodiazepines (including diazepam), the half-life is at least 20 hr]. The importance of this classification is that it predicts certain significant adverse actions—notably, risk of rebound symptoms and dependency—and hence dictates clinical usage. There is little difference in efficacy among the various benzodiazepines, but there is a great deal of difference in potency (i.e., milligram dose; see Chapter 2). For example, a normal adult dose of triazolam (Halcion®) is about 0.125 mg, whereas that of diazepam (Valium®) is 50–100 times higher.

Oral absorption is somewhat unpredictable (Chapter 2), but most benzodiazepines are quickly and sufficiently absorbed with peak blood concentrations, especially in children, occurring in about 15–30 min.[5] Some, such as oxazepam and clonazepam, are only slowly absorbed so that their peak concentrations in blood may take several hours to build up. Intramuscularly administered drug (except possibly lorazepam)[3] is irregularly absorbed and should be used only when essential oral medication is refused. Intravenous use, though rapid and effective, is potentially dangerous, because very high brain concentrations are rapidly attained, and is unlikely to be justifiable in children or adolescents in any but most exceptional situations such as status epilepticus.

TABLE 1. Benzodiazepines[a]

Class	Daily dose[b] (mg/kg)	Active metabolities[c]
I. Long half-life (>13 hr)/high potency		
Clonazepam (Klonopin®, Rivotril®)	0.007–0.05	No
II. Long half-life (>13 hr)/low potency		
Chlordiazepoxide (Librium®)	0.2–0.5	Yes
Diazepam (Valium®)	0.07–0.5	Yes
Clorazepate (Tranxene®)	0.2–0.8	Yes
Flurazepam (Dalmane®)	0.2–0.4	Yes
Nitrazepam (Mogadon®)	0.06–0.14	No
III. Short half-life (<13 hr)/high potency		
Lorazepam (Ativan®)	0.014–0.08	No
Alprazolam (Xanax®)	0.014–0.08[d]	No
Triazolam (Halcion®)	0.0017–0.007	No
IV. Short half-life (<13 hr)/low potency		
Oxazepam (Serax®, Serapax®)	0.14–1.7	No
Temazepam (Restoril®, Euhypnos®)	0.2–0.4	No

[a]Refs. 1, 4, 5, and 8.
[b]Doses are for adults[1] converted to mg/kg by dividing by 70. Doses and indications have not been established in children or adolescents.
[c]Clinical action may be longer than elimination half-life where active metabolites are produced.
[d]Upper limit of range for alprazolam is for panic disorder only.

After absorption, the pharmacokinetics become rather complex.[1,5] Distribution into highly perfused lipid tissues like the brain is rapid, but after a single dose effects may disappear quite quickly as other, less vascular tissues such as fat stores take up the drug more slowly. Also, some benzodiazepines, such as diazepam, show a secondary peak after about 6–12 hr, suggestive of enterohepatic recirculation. Inactivation occurs in the liver, and a pharmacodynamic equilibrium will be ultimately achieved as expected after about 4–5 half-lives (Chapter 2), but this may not reflect the time frame of actual clinical actions because of the production of active metabolites with some benzodiazepines (e.g., diazepam to nordiazepam to oxazepam), which may prolong detectable effect up to 100 hr. Much of the original data on duration of action were misleading since they were based on a single dose before lipid stores are saturated and/or active metabolites produced. The drugs that produce no or only trivial active metabolites are lorazepam, oxazepam, temazepam, alprazolam, triazolam, and nitrazepam.[1,4]

Action of benzodiazepines is thought to be rapidly reversible and accurately reflects the actual concentration of the drug or its active metabolites at receptor sites.

i. **Route of Administration.** In psychotropic use, benzodiazepines should be given only orally. Intravenous use is for medical emergencies, and, except with lorazepam,[3] intramuscular absorption is poor and slower than oral.[5] If a drug is given at intervals about equal to the half-life (approximately 24 hr for long-acting), then peak and nadir blood levels will vary by 50%. Because there is a narrow relationship between anxiolytic and sedative blood levels (about 1:2), it is therefore desirable to give benzodiazepines in smaller divided doses two (long-acting) to four (short-acting) times daily to prevent these surges in blood level.[5]

ii. **Choice of Benzodiazepine.** On the whole, low-potency, long-acting drugs like diazepam (Valium®) should be preferred since their adverse effects have been far better researched[1] and most of the indications for the use of these drugs in adults are for sustained anxiety. They are the only benzodiazepines currently accepted by the U.S. Food and Drug Administration (FDA) for use in children under 12 years.[9] Also, the high-potency and/or short-acting drugs are suspected of presenting more problems of dependence, rebound, and withdrawal.[1] In the case of sleep disturbances, however, a short-acting drug may be preferable, particularly if it is to be given for only a very few days. Clonazepam, a high-potency, long-half-life benzodiazepine, seems to have become rather popular in psychiatry lately. There is no good pharmacological reason for this, and there is much to recommend staying with better-studied drugs such as diazepam, over which clonazepam has no apparent clear advantages.

iii. Dosage and Duration. These have not been established for children and adolescents, so in Table 1 those recommended as "usual" for adults[1] have been converted to milligrams per kilogram on the basis of an assumed 70-kg adult weight and rounded downward. As such, and since a child's metabolism is faster than an adult's (Chapter 2), these doses are conservative, except for alprazolam, for which the upper range may be indicated only in panic disorder (probably rare in children).[10] Doses cited are only those found likely to be necessary in average adults. Therefore, begin with a much lower dose— say, 25% of the minimum daily dose in Table 1—and (except in emergencies or anticipated short-term use) increment slowly over intervals of several days (say, 5–7) to allow time for accumulation in fat stores and the production of active metabolites. Since problems of dependence and discontinuance are highly correlated with length of administration, benzo-diazepines should not be used in excess of 4 months,[1] and shorter periods are desirable. As ever in medicine, the objective is to give the smallest therapeutic dose for the shortest time, but this is particularly important with anxiolytics since both duration and dose are correlated with adverse effects.

2. Clinical Indications

There are no established indications for the use of these drugs in psychiatric disorders in children and adolescents. However, there are indications in the adult literature and from some uncontrolled clinical impressions that there may be some small role for their use in special instances as follows.

a. Anxiety Disorders

It is worth noting that the main pharmacological agents used for the treatment of anxiety disorders and most of the more creative and recent research are not with benzo-diazepines but with other drugs such as antidepressants[11] (see Chapter 9). There have been several reviews of clinical studies of anxiolytics in children,[7,9,11–14] some quite recent. These latter have been mostly reiterative, adding little new information largely because there is nothing much in the recent literature apart from an occasional letter to the editor or uncontrolled impressions. All have concluded that, while there is a strong literature attesting to the value of benzodiazepines in the treatment of adults with anxiety disorders,[1,5,15] there are very few reliable data on children or adolescents. Although there are some studies[9,12,16,17] that suggest a beneficial effect, most of these are uncontrolled and include diagnostic heterogeneity.[7,12] Despite being valuable in research for deciding whether to proceed to conduct properly controlled studies, those without placebo are of highly dubious value from a clinical point of view since anxiety is among the most placebo-responsive symptoms. While there are some recent reports of the possible value of benzo-diazepines in anxiety disorders (e.g., alprazolam and clonazepam in panic and separation anxiety disorder[7]), sometimes reflected in reviews,[11,13,16] the few properly controlled studies cast doubt on this. For example, one study[16] showed that while alprazolam produced improvement in children with overanxious or avoidant disorder, it was little better than placebo. A more recent double-blind, crossover study of clonazepam in various anxiety disorders in children yielded equivocal results (and many side effects, primarily behavioral irritability and sedation, though the authors suggest that the latter may have been an artifact of the speed of titration).[18]

In the absence of good data for children and adolescents, it could be argued that extrapolation of the indications for adults—panic, generalized anxiety, and possibly social phobic disorder[15]—should be made. However, in addition to the negative findings from the controlled studies in children above, there are some complexities to this extrapolation. (1) Anxiety disorders seen most often in children and adolescents are in a developmentally distinct group—separation anxiety, overanxious, and avoidant disorders—which have not (yet) been shown to be identical or continuous with those of adults.[12,19] (2) In those adult disorders that occur most commonly in children and adolescents, such as simple phobic disorders and obsessive–compulsive disorder, benzodiazepines are not indicated[15] since other types of drugs or behavioral therapy are preferred.[20,21] (3) Panic disorder, in which benzodiazepines may be indicated as a second line of treatment after antidepressants,[5,15] is rare in children and probably infrequent in adolescents,[10] but this does not seem to stop some clinicians from seeing it everywhere. (4) Although studies in adults have shown anxiolytics to be superior to placebo in generalized anxiety and possibly social phobic disorder, their effect is largely symptomatic. It has been known from animal experiments and from clinical studies in behavior therapy[20,21] for many years that the only cure for nonpsychotic anxiety is extinction through exposure to the anxiogenic situation with prevention of escape/avoidant behavior. Although benzodiazepines may provide relief and theoretically may assist behavioral or extinction procedures, they mute but do not cure anxiety. (5) Despite the fact that benzodiazepines have been shown to be helpful in controlled trials in adults, one also has to ask what the risk is for children and adolescents. The question is whether it is prudent to introduce children and adolescents to the chemical way of dealing with anxiety or to potentially dependency-producing drugs (and ones that can affect basic learning processes),[1] at such a vulnerable age.

b. Sleep Disorders

Nonorganic sleep disorders in children[22,23] are most common in infants and toddlers and can be divided into (1) difficulty falling asleep, (2) waking usually after nightmares, (3) night terrors and somnambulism, which occur during deep or slow-wave sleep and are characterized by resistance to comforting and by amnesia next morning, and (4) disorders of the sleep—wake cycle seen in adolescents after a series of late nights.

Benzodiazepines have the ability to both induce and sustain sleep, but not without some cost. They suppress the normal architecture of sleep, and this produces a subjective sensation of not having slept as well as in natural sleep. Children have a reputation for actually being made more irritable and hyperactive with sedatives (see Chapter 12).[24] Since sleep disturbances are often chronic or recurrent, repeated use is likely. With all except the ultrashort-acting benzodiazepines, this will produce some degree of daytime sedation (if the half-life is 12 hr, then after 24 hr one-quarter of the drug will still be present). Though theoretically more suitable, ultrashort-acting drugs like triazolam and alprazolam are prone to produce "rebound" symptoms even after only a few weeks of use,[1] and there is a particular danger of dependency and withdrawal with repeated use. They may also lower the threshold of tolerance in caretakers for future bouts of sleep disturbance.

Although there is little doubt that benzodiazepines and other sedatives are used widely in children and adolescents for sleep disorders,[22,24] neither their value nor their safety has been tested. They cannot be described as established for this use as a recent review might seem to suggest.[9] Not settling and night waking are relatively easily dealt with by behavioral or other simple psychological methods,[22,23] and those who cannot be so treated almost certainly require proper psychiatric investigation and treatment.[24] In severe or difficult cases, there may be a place for benzodiazepines given for 3–5 days but only to facilitate a nonpharmacological treatment program[25] or where there is good evidence to suggest that the episode of insomnia is acute and likely to be short-lived. However this use is, as yet, unsubstantiated.

Night terrors and somnambulism (classified as partial arousals)[25] have the best rationale for pharmacotherapy in that benzodiazepines suppress stage 4 sleep, during which they occur, but this is vitiated by the facts that these two disorders are (1) much more distressing to parent than to child and (2) unpredictable and infrequent in occurrence (say, not more than once a week), which hardly justifies keeping a child under constant medication with its consequent risks. A recent review of sleep disorders[25] suggests that though benzodiazepines (e.g., clonazepam beginning at 0.5 mg) can decrease the number of partial arousals, this use should be reserved for the most severe cases and for "breaking the cycle" in combination with other, nonpharmacological treatments. It should also be noted that there are other medications such as antidepressants which can be used for this purpose.[25]

c. Excited/Aggressive States

Long-acting benzodiazepines like diazepam or clonazepam have been used in adults with some success in excited states[3] associated with mania (Chapter 9) and schizophrenia.[26] In both instances, a reduction in the amount of antipsychotic medication needed to control behavior has been reported. However, this is not without some objection. First, the combination of antipsychotics with depressant drugs acts synergistically to enhance CNS depression, and when high doses are needed—which is likely to be the case in excited states—these two types of drugs, which separately have very high therapeutic ratios, together may cause toxicity. Second, alcohol and drug abuse are very often comorbid with these psychotic states, and it could be imprudent to use drugs of abuse and dependency like benzodiazepines, especially in children and teenagers, who may thus be introduced precociously to these drugs. Third, there is always the possibility with benzodiazepines of disinhibition or actually making some patients more rather than less excited—this has been demonstrated to occur in children.[27] Fourth, if parenteral administration is required, only lorazepam[3] is other than poorly absorbed. Finally, especially in children and adolescents, the correct treatment may not be more pharmacotherapy[3] but better nursing care or other psychosocial procedures. However, in very disturbed patients (especially psychotic adolescents) who do not respond quickly and well to antipsychotics and who have no history of drug abuse, and/or in emergencies, this combination may be considered, even though there are no data except for adults.

Benzodiazepines have been tried in recurrent aggressive outbursts in mentally retarded adolescents, in hostile delinquents, and in hospitalized children with conduct disorder.[27] While improvement was reported in the first two groups, it would seem inappropriate to be giving drugs with potential for abuse to delinquents. In the study with children, unacceptable behavioral toxicity and paradoxical increases in aggression were noted. Thus, at present, there is little support for the use of these drugs in nonpsychotic excited/ aggressive states or in conduct disorder in children and adolescents.

d. Tic Disorders

The use of benzodiazepines in the treatment of tic disorders is perhaps the only really substantive new development of the use of these drugs in child and adolescent psychiatry, and, again, it is supported by only one uncontrolled study, the authors of which urge caution as to the preliminary nature of their findings.[28] It should also be noted that the subjects had both tics and attention-deficit hyperactivity disorder (ADHD) and that the use of clonazepam that was found to be helpful was as an adjunct to clonidine.

3. Prescribing Guidelines

a. Deciding to Prescribe

The lack of good data to support the use of benzodiazepines in children and adolescents and the risk of adverse effects (especially impairment of learning) means that, at the moment, anxiety disorders in children and adolescents cannot be regarded as established indications for benzodiazepines or other CNS depressant drugs. FDA guidelines set varying age limits for different benzodiazepines—none for clonazepam, 6 months for diazepam, 6 years for chlordiazepoxide, 12 years for lorazepam, and 18 years for alprazolam.[9] However, these limits are arbitrary and not based on well-conducted studies or any good rationale. Practitioners will have to make their own decisions about the validity of adult data for children and whether to try benzodiazepines in any patient. This decision must be based on whether (1) the relief sought is likely to be accomplished without adverse effects, (2) the drug can be discontinued within a short period (say, a maximum of 2 months) since benzodiazepines are unsuited to long-term use,[1] (3) the severity of the anxiety is disabling, (4) less invasive and/or curative psychosocial methods, such as supportive psychotherapy or behavior therapy, have failed or are impracticable, (5) parental supervision of medication is adequate, (6) there are no hidden pressures on the child (or more likely adolescent) to abuse drugs, and (7) there is no likelihood of alcohol consumption, which will augment any effects.

However, for the practitioner who has mentally worked through these and other general principles set out in Chapter 1 and has decided that anxiolytics are indeed justified, guidelines are offered below. Issues of informed consent and assent (Chapters 1 and 6) and careful evaluation of effect (Chapter 5) and adverse effects (Chapters 4 and 5) are not detailed as they are not specific to anxiolytics but are part of prescribing in general. The American Psychiatric Association Task Force Report[1] is strongly recommended for further reading, as it contains the distilled wisdom of 30 years' experience with benzodiazepines in adults. One review[9] gives detailed practical information for children and adolescents (who are not covered in the Task Force Report), although the underlying data base for this somewhat optimistic review has to be recognized as extremely thin.

4. Effects

a. CNS

All but insignificant clinical effects of benzodiazepines (and other true sedatives) stem from their effect on the brain, which is to depress excitability of nerve tissue.[7,8] As a result, all produce a dose-dependent progressive depression of brain function, although with selective depressants this plateaus short of fatal coma because of receptor saturation.

   i. Neurophysiologically. This depression is seen in blocking of the EEG to brainstem activating system stimulation, depressing spinal reflexes, raising the seizure threshold, and depressing afterdischarges in the limbic system, mild depressing of REM sleep, and suppression of stage 4 sleep with prolongation of total sleep time.[5] The production of any significant degree of muscle relaxation is debatable, despite its widespread clinical assumption.[5]

   ii. Behaviorally. The depression of brain function is seen as progressively affecting, in a dose-dependent way, the level of consciousness, beginning with the most quintessentially human characteristics of intellect and social judgment as well as motor coordination. This does not preclude the use of sedatives in medicine, any more than it precludes the use of alcohol in civilized society; it is merely a matter of proper cost–benefit accounting. For example, antiepileptic drugs, all of which are CNS depressants, can in therapeutic doses suppress disabling seizures without noticeable detriment to most children (see Chapter 12). If the behavior seen socially with the prototypical CNS depressant, alcohol, is kept in mind, then there will be little difficulty in remembering what these effects are and how they proceed in a dose-dependent way. In particular, the effects of benzodiazepines and other sedatives will be greatly influenced by the social setting and the prevalent mood state of the individual. In quiet states, sleep is likely to intervene at a low dose, and in worried states only at a higher dose. In group situations, laudable bonhomie is likely to prevail, but when conflict arises, this can change quickly to hostility or panic. Since children were typically given sedatives when frightened by unfamiliar situations like hospitals or while upset and resisting sleep, it is little wonder that the pediatric literature is replete with anecdotal accounts and occasional demonstrations of "paradoxical" actions of drugs like phenobarbital in which the child became more, rather than less, aroused (see Chapter 12). For example, a recent study of clonazepam in children with anxiety disorders found behavioral disinhibition and irritability to be a major problem.[18]

   Though much is made of the ability of benzodiazepines to achieve anxiolysis without sedation, both are essentially part of the same process of CNS depression, and the gap between the two is quite narrow—as measured by blood levels.[5] Further, this gap will narrow or widen depending on the state of arousal of the individual and the social stimulation. Only in higher doses or occasional individuals will true intoxication with its lurching gait, slurred speech, sedated mien, and drunken behavior be seen. While this may be common with self-administered alcohol, it should be an unusual occurrence with benzodiazepines and, if seen, a sign that dosage is excessive. Also, unlike alcohol, benzodiazepines do not cause dangerous vomiting as unconsciousness supervenes because they lack both the gastric irritation and neurotoxic metabolite (acetaldehyde). Fortunately, with the benzodiazepines, overdose does not go as far as life-threatening, and it is almost impossible to kill oneself with these drugs provided they are taken orally and without any other drugs.

   iii. Psychomotor Function. In contrast to anticonvulsants (Chapter 12) and stimulants (Chapter 8), there have been few systematic studies of the psychomotor effects of benzodiazepines and other sedative drugs in children and adolescents in therapeutic doses[8,9] (see also Chapter 11). However, there is no reason to suppose that young people will be any less vulnerable to the well-documented effects seen in adults. The American Psychiatric Association Task Force on Benzodiazepine Dependence[1] summarized the principal impairments as occurring in memory, psychomotor speed, motor coordination, and sustained attention, whereas well-learned functions and untimed tasks appear unaffected. These effects are complex and unpredictable, being affected by dose, route of administration, vulnerability (especially advanced age and, presumptively, brain damage), duration of administration, and state of arousal. Where the patient is highly anxious, there may be some improvement, but the findings are inconsistent, although the only two studies in children and adolescents did show mild improvement on benzodiazepines.[16,17]

There are two possible effects on memory: (1) impairment of consolidation or delayed recall, which may be found even when there is no evidence of sedation or other psychomotor impairment, and (2) anterograde amnesia (blackouts), which usually occurs after acute, higher intravenous dosage but also in association with alcohol and with high-potency, short-acting drugs like triazolam. Conversely, discontinuation of benzodiazepines is associated with subjective reports and limited laboratory evidence of improved function.

b. Other Body Systems

The benzodiazepines are almost without effect on any other body systems, especially in normal dosages.[8] There is some mild depression of function in the respiratory and cardiovascular systems, but it is of little clinical significance. The lack of, or clinically insignificant, effect on muscle tone has been noted above.[5]

5. Drug Combinations

The most deliberated uses of benzodiazepines in combination with other drugs are with clonidine in Tourette's disorder comorbid with ADHD[28] and with antipsychotics in excited manic and psychotic states. One major group of investigators reports usefulness in combination with antidepressants in anxiety disorders such as obsessive–compulsive disorder but offers no direct evidence to support this claim other than their clinical experience.[29] Otherwise, there is little evidence of other useful combinations, though the lack of apparent interest in the benzodiazepines in pediatric psychopharmacology makes it difficult to make any definitive statements at this time.

6. Side Effects

Most side effects are predictable but unwanted effects of the drug (1) at the upper end of CNS depression or sedation in higher doses or (2) in individuals unduly sensitive to normal clinical dosage. They have been discussed in detail in Section II.B.4: behavioral disinhibition, hyperactivity, irritability, aggressiveness, sedation, intoxication similar to that produced by alcohol, slowing of psychomotor function, and impairment of memory, other cognitive functions, and motor coordination. It should be noted that in contrast to adults, behavioral disinhibition with irritability may be conspicuous in children.

In addition to these exaggerations of normal effects, abuse, dependence, withdrawal (i.e., anxiety, insomnia, tremor, restlessness, irritability, muscle tension, sweating, nausea, and seizures),[1] and rebound symptoms (i.e., exacerbation of original symptoms appearing rapidly after dicontinuance)[1] are now recognized as major problems with these drugs. These adverse effects have been discussed in Chapter 11 and in much useful detail in the American Psychiatric Association Task Force Report.[1] Even so, the overwhelming majority of adults (there are no data on children or adolescents) who are prescribed benzodiazepines use them safely—at least, the low-potency benzodiazepines. The high-potency drugs are newer and as yet inadequately studied in this respect.[1] Suffice it to say here (see Chapter 11) that problems of this sort are most likely to occur with (1) the high-potency and/or short-acting drugs (see Table 1), (2) higher dosages such as those used in panic disorder, (3) continuous use for 4 months or more, (4) abrupt rather than graduated discontinuance, and (5) abuse of other drugs and especially alcohol.[1]

7. Interactions

Care is needed in using benzodiazepines with any other "sedating" agent or drug, including antihistamines and anticholinergics commonly used in children, but especially alcohol. There are also important interactions with anticonvulsants used in children; benzodiazepines cause raising of valproate and lowering of carbamazepine blood levels, whereas phenobarbital causes rises in the level of benzodiazepines. Benzodiazepines may increase heterocyclic antidepressant blood levels and, by sedation, mask signs of developing toxicity. Fluoxetine and other specific serotonin reuptake inhibitors (SSRIs) are powerful inhibitors of some hepatic enzymes, and this may cause rises in benzodiazepine levels. There may be an augmentation of disinhibiting effects by monoamine oxidase inhibitors (MAOIs). However, apart from the interaction with other sedating drugs and substances, most of the interactions are infrequent or of unestablished clinical significance. For further discussion of interactions, see Ref. 30.

8. Management of Overdoses

On their own, unlike traditional sedatives and hypnotics, all benzodiazepines are not normally life-threatening in overdose since, because of the indirect action through GABA receptors, true coma is uncommon.[8] However, in combination with other CNS depressant drugs such as alcohol and other psychiatric drugs such as antidepressants, they can be fatal. It is often difficult to be sure that only one type of drug has been taken, and so anyone who has taken an overdose requires, as a minimum, assessment by a doctor and may require a hospital assessment, depending on his or her condition. When the person is unconscious, this is nearly always a sign that other drugs have been taken too and a medical emergency obtains to apply such life-support and remedial care as is required and appropriate. Toxicological blood examinations can be helpful but take some time so that emergency care must be dictated by the clinical state of the person. Recovery times will be related to the half-life of the particular benzodiazepine taken.

C. Antihistamines and Anticholinergics

Historically and in pediatrics, anticholinergics and especially antihistamines have figured large in dealing with sleep disorders and fussiness in infants and very young children[31] However, there have been almost no new allusions to their use and no proper studies in the last five years, though there is no reason to doubt that their widespread use continues.

The precise cause of the sedating effect of these drugs is unknown[32,33] although most are muscarinic anticholinergics, which are sedating, so that this seems the most likely explanation.[33] This type of sedation has been poorly studied, but it almost certainly differs qualitatively from that produced by CNS depressants[33] in lacking the progressive CNS depression. In view of the important role of acetylcholine in cognition and memory, these drugs may be disruptive or even deliriant in higher doses. It is well known from ophthalmology, where these drugs are used widely, and from belladonna poisoning that atropine and other anticholinergics can precipitate delirium, especially in children and the elderly.

The most popular drugs are hydroxyzine (Atarax®, Vistaril®), diphenhydramine (Benadryl®), promethazine (Phenergan®), and (outside the United States) trimeprazine (Vallergan®). The last two are phenothiazines, structurally very similar to chlorpromazine except for differences in the side chain, which attenuate any antipsychotic or dopamine-blocking action. Only diphenhydramine is short-acting (4–6 hr). Despite the frequency with which these drugs are used by pediatricians and family doctors,[31,34] they have been the subject of very few systematic studies, although these do show a modest degree of improvement and parent acceptability.[9,34] However, these drugs do not usually eliminate night waking entirely and, unlike behavioral methods,[21,22] have the disadvantage that when discontinued, the problem usually recurs.[34] The short-acting diphenhydramine may show no prolongation of duration of sleep, but the other antihistamines in common use have the disadvantage that they continue to act throughout most of the waking day. Since these drugs depend on the anticholinergic effect, they are likely to show rapid loss of sedative effect, as seen with other anticholinergic drugs such as the low-potency antipsychotics or some of the antidepressants, where, of course, this tolerance is seen as an advantage.

Sleep disorders in young children are extremely exhausting and aversive for parents, and, although behavioral methods are greatly to be preferred, there may be occasions where antihistamines may be useful on a short-term or intermittent basis, especially when the disturbance is acute and/or occurs in the context of minor illness or upset, or when parents are at the breaking point. Doses reported are 1 mg/kg for diphenhydramine (Benadryl®) and 30–60 mg for trimeprazine in infants and toddlers.[34] There are no good data on other agents.

Curiously—since atropinic effects like dry mouth are unpleasant—these are also drugs of abuse (e.g., benztropine, datura), possibly for the deliriant effect (see Chapter 11). Thus, there is a good reason for avoiding their use in adolescents. They also interact synergistically with all other "sedating" drugs and augment atropinic effects of anticholinergic drugs, including a number of other psychoactive drugs like antidepressants and antipsychotics.

These drugs are relatively nontoxic though not without unpleasant adverse effects. In overdosage, they produce atropinic side effects such as dry skin and mouth, dilated pupils, and, extremely, a dramatic atropinic delirium, which can be fatal though only exceptionally. Treatment is usually supportive and will depend on the dose taken and the clinical state of the patient. Anyone in a delirium or coma requires urgent medical care, particularly since this suggests that other drugs may have been taken as well and that makes the situation potentially much more serious.

D. Atypical Anxiolytics

Buspirone is the most important of the atypical anxiolytics. Its receptor profile is quite different from that of benzodiazepines in that it is without any effect on GABA receptors but acts primarily at dopamine, and 5-HT$_{1A}$ receptors.[5,7] Like carbamazepine (Tegretol®), it also increases firing in the brainstem adrenergic (arousal) system,[9] which may explain its lack of sedation. It is also said to be free of cognitive depression and of abuse and dependency potential.[3,7,9] The source of its anxiolytic action is obscure. It has a short half-life (2–11 hr) with no active metabolites.[7,9]

Although initial trials in adults suggested that the anxiolytic properties of buspirone were equal to those of the benzodiazepines, there has been a waning of enthusiasm for what looked initially to be a substantial improvement on the benzodiazepines.[3] Some of this may be that unlike the benzodiazepines, the optimal effect takes up to 3–4 weeks to emerge.[3,7,9] There are only a very few case reports and open studies in children and adolescents, so doses and indications are not well established. In adults, buspirone has been useful in generalized, anticipatory, and situational anxiety, and therefore in children it could be predicted to be possibly helpful in generalized anxiety, avoidant, and phobic disorders.[7,9] There have been a number of studies in children and/or adolescents mostly with various anxiety disorders though also with mood, externalizing, autistic, or self-injury problems.[7,35–40] Most are positive case reports and/or uncontrolled studies. Side effects reported are mild and transitory and include nausea, headaches, drowsiness, and overexcitement, though in one study[38] two children developed a drug-dependent psychosis. As in adults, the drug is probably without effects on cognitive function.[35] Care is needed if buspirone is used with MAOIs since hypertension has been reported.[9]

Doses derived from adults (divided by 70 to convert them to milligrams per kilogram) would be 0.2–0.6 mg/kg per day, subdivided for twice- to thrice-daily administration. However, in the largest and best study,[35] the doses were somewhat higher, beginning at 5 mg daily and increased weekly as needed to a maximum of 20 mg. The average dose was around 18 mg daily compared with recommended doses for adults of 20–30 mg.

Since buspirone lacks adequate study in children and adolescents, it cannot at this stage be recommended other than for cautious use in children and adolescents.[9,35] Its lack of side effects of the type that cause concern about the benzodiazepines suggests that cautious, properly controlled exploration is desirable, especially regrading its use in severe anxiety disorders and self-injurious and externalizing behavior where other measures have failed.

Unlike most other anxiolytic drugs, buspirone does not interact synergistically with alcohol and other depressant drugs,[41] but it should be used with care with other psychiatric drugs nevertheless. In overdosage, care should be supportive appropriate to the clinical state. However, as far as is known, it is not lethal alone.

E. Summary of Anxiolytics and Sedatives

Anxiolytics have been surprisingly little studied in children and adolescents and thus have no firmly established role or dosage in children and adolescents. The lack of comparability between the more common adult and child anxiety disorders limits the extrapolation of findings from adults to children. Also, since children and adolescents are active learners, adolescents are often exposed to pressures to abuse drugs, and there are pharmacological similarities and cross-tolerance with alcohol, the benzodiazepines are not drugs to be prescribed lightly. Experience with adults suggests that when anxiety is particularly severe and disabling, benzodiazepines may have an effective and safe place as very short term (less than 1–2 months) palliative-only treatments while better methods of treatment are put in place or until the crisis passes. The use of any kind of anxiolytic or sedative in sleep disorders is not well proven, and in infants there will usually be safer and faster ways than pharmacotherapy to deal with the problem. However, there may be an occasional place for antihistamines on a short-term basis. In very disturbed psychotic behavior, adjunctive use of benzodiazepines with antipsychotics or antimanic drugs may be useful in crisis management and reduce the amount of the other drugs required to maintain behavioral control.

Because of its more benign pharmacological profile, the atypical anxiolytic buspirone is worth studying in proper clinical trials.

III. MISCELLANEOUS DRUGS

A. α_2 Agonists (Clonidine, Guanfacine)

1. Pharmacology

The role of the antihypertensive agent clonidine (Catapres®) in psychopharmacology was the subject of a comprehensive review in 1990 which is particularly useful in discussing its pharmacology.[42] It acts as an α_2-adrenergic antagonist which, in lower dosages, stimulates presynaptic autoreceptors, leading to inhibition of the release of noradrenaline, lowering blood serotonin, and increasing dopamine turnover. In the brain it produces immediate reduction in arousal by inhibiting the locus coeruleus, the hub of the noradrenergic activating system, and there are effects on dopaminergic and serotonergic systems as well. However, in high dosages it has direct adrenergic effects as well, which may negate the blocking actions for which it is used primarily in medicine. There is some discrepancy between its half-life (about 12 hr) and its duration of action observed in psychotropic applications (2–4 hr). A transdermal slow-release preparation has been developed to try to prolong this short action.

Guanfacine, a longer-acting analogue, introduced around 1976,[43] has attracted recent interest in pediatric psychopharmacology. Although it is rather similar to clonidine, guanfacine is said to have greater tissue penetration, be more selective in targeting brain α_2 receptors, and, if anything, improve rather than depress cognition.[43] It also is less liable to produce rebound adrenergic symptoms (headache, anxiety, tremors, abdominal pain, sweating, tachycardia) on sudden withdrawal, possibly because of its longer half-life (24 hr).[44]

2. Dosage

For clonidine, standardized daily doses are 3–4 µg/kg for ADHD and 3–5 µg/kg for Tourette's disorders; these doses are achieved slowly over several weeks.[45] In children, it is recommended to begin with 0.05 mg (half a 0.1-mg tablet) and increase by half a tablet (0.05 mg) every third or fourth day while closely monitoring for side effects.[42,46] Others[43] suggest that in a sensitive minority of children fewer side effects will result if a quarter of a tablet (0.025 mg) is used instead. The extra tablets are given at 4-hr intervals. The total daily dose should not exceed 0.15–0.3 mg though higher doses have been reported. These doses usually do not produce sedation or hypotension, provided they are built up slowly.[45] Psychoactive effects may last only 2–4 hr[42] though this may be more true of sedation than other effects. One practitioner has claimed that the rate of absorption of oral clonidine can be extended by having the pharmacy mix pulverized clonidine tablets with a methylcellulose extended-release polymer and inserting the mix in gelatin capsules.[47] A transdermal preparation is available, but local allergic reactions are said to occur in about 30% of cases.[46] Stabilization is first achieved on oral medication, and then a change is made to the size of patch that delivers the same amount as the oral dose each day (3.5 cm², 0.1 mg/day; 7.0 cm², 0.2 mg/day; 10.5 cm², 0.3 mg/day).[47] One source claims that transdermal administration minimizes all except the cutaneous side effects of clonidine.[48] Steady state is reached on the fourth day with the skin patch, and blood pressure is said to return to pretreatment values over 3–4 days after the removal of the patch.[48] Guanfacine has double the half-life and longer action.

Guanfacine has been given in regimens of 0.5 mg at bedtime increasing by 0.25–0.5 mg every 5–7 days to a mean effective dosage of 1.27 mg (0.0225 mg/kg) given in two divided doses.[43] Hunt et al.[49] used higher dosages—0.5 mg with similar increments every third day and three divided doses with a mean dosage of 3.2 mg daily, or 0.091 mg/kg. Horrigan and Barnhill[43] have pointed out that they achieved a similar effect with over half to one-quarter that dosage. Pending further evidence therefore, the more conservative regimen is preferable. This study incidentally also points to the value of expressing doses in milligrams per kilogram. While the total daily dosages differed only by a factor of 2, the mg/kg difference was fourfold owing to differences in ages in the two groups.

3. Clinical Indications

Because of its ability to reduce arousal and cause a type of sedation, clonidine has been tried as a psychoactive agent in adults in a variety of conditions of presumed high arousal—aggression, manic episodes, the anxiety disorders (panic, social phobic, and posttraumatic stress disorders), tic disorders, and insomnia—as well as for side effects of some psychotropic drugs, such as akathisia due to antipsychotic drugs (see Chapter 10). Despite some favorable case reports or open studies,[15,42] clonidine does not seem to have found much clinical acceptance in adults so far[3,15] except in alcohol and substance withdrawal[3] (Chapter 11) and in tic disorders such as Tourette syndrome.[42,45]

There has been a phenomenal growth in the use of the α_2-agonists for managing ADHD, sleep problems, and a variety of other conditions in children over the last few years. Swanson et al.[50] reported that there was a fivefold increase in the number of prescriptions for clonidine between 1992 and 1995, with approximately 150,000 clonidine prescriptions in 1994 for ADHD alone. However, despite the upsurge in the use of this drug, there is a remarkable lack of data attesting to its efficiency for any psychiatric application except, perhaps, Tourette syndrome.

In summary, despite a dearth of controlled studies,[43,51] in children and adolescents, there has been a significant increase in psychotropic use of this group of drugs since 1990. Though most of this has occurred in ADHD and Tourette's syndrome,[42] the use of clonidine to treat a wide range of conditions and symptoms has attracted, and continues to attract, attention and this interest seems likely to grow.

4. Probable/Possible Indications

a. ADHD

A highly influential study[52] showed clonidine to be rather similar to methylphenidate except that it was more effective against hyperactivity than attentional deficits, suggesting that it might be better reserved for use with grossly overactive children where stimulants had not achieved a good result. Despite the flawed nature of this study, and the fact that one of the authors pointed out elsewhere the need for replication,[42] the use of clonidine in ADHD seems to have soared, spurred on by a handful of favorable open or case studies and two somewhat less favorable controlled studies.[51]

In the best controlled study to date, desipramine and clonidine were compared with placebo in 34 children with ADHD and comorbid Tourette syndrome.[53] Parent ratings of hyperactivity and tics failed to indicate superiority of clonidine over placebo. Teacher ratings of hyperactivity did show limited benefit with clonidine, but desipramine emerged as the stronger treatment in the eyes of both parents and teachers.

Complementing these studies are two uncontrolled ones of guanfacine,[43,49] both of which suggest that it too may have value in the treatment of ADHD. In their overview of the studies, Swanson et al[51] concluded that clonidine is probably effective in treating some of the symptoms of ADHD though the size of the effect is probably only around 20% and considerably less than suggested by the studies. There is also a possibility that guanfacine, in addition to being longer-acting, may have fewer side effects though this needs much more substantiation. The effectiveness of the α_2-adrenergic agonists may be greater when ADHD is comorbid with tic/Tourette's disorder.[28]

b. Tourette's Disorder

There are at least seven open and four controlled studies of the use of clonidine in patients with Tourette's disorder (all ages), but they yield conflicting results, the reported improvement ranging from in excess of 70% to nil.[42,47,53] Much of the reported improvement in Tourette's disorder may well be behavioral rather than an improvement in the tics themselves. Nevertheless, clonidine is worth trying in this very distressing disorder, either on its own or in combination with antipsychotics when the latter fail, are only partially successful, or produce unacceptable side effects.[45] When used in combination, effective doses of both drugs are said to be lower than when either is used alone.[45] It is posited that there is a subgroup of patients with Tourette's disorder which is more responsive, but attempts to define such a subgroup have so far failed.[47]

c. Autism

One group documented significant gains with oral clonidine in parent ratings of hyperactivity and teacher ratings of irritability, hyperactivity, and repetitive speech in 8 autistic children.[54] Others reported significant improvement in physician ratings of stereotypic behavior and in global impressions of change in 7 boys and men treated with the transdermal patch.[55] An uncontrolled trial also described moderate decreases in hyperactivity with oral clonidine in 7 children with autism.[56] Again, given the severity of this disorder, the α_2-agonists may be worth considering in difficult cases.

d. Sleep Problems (Including Those Due to Stimulants)

Most of the reports on this use are clinical and anecdotal case reports. There are two summarizing papers which include clinical experience with 62 children and adolescents (with ADHD and most with difficulty falling asleep) and valuable management information as well as theoretical speculation on the use of clonidine in both primary sleep disturbances associated with ADHD and sleep problems secondary to stimulant medication.[57,58] There was a high level of improvement in both primary- and secondary-type sleep problems, and this persisted for as long as three years, though regular increases in dose were required. As the authors pointed out, improvement was based solely on parental reports and there is a need for proper clinical trials before what looks like a promising use can be confirmed.

e. Aggression

There is a small number of case reports on the use of clonidine in serious aggression in a variety of diagnostic disorders such as conduct disorder and ADHD.[51,59–61] All report substantial improvement. However, the size of the improvement, not uncommon in uncontrolled studies in general, suggests that an unknown but substantial component is probably due to placebo/expectancy effects and selection bias.[51]

f. Stuttering

Observations made initially in patients with Tourette's disorder suggested that clonidine might aid stuttering, but a single controlled study failed to support this—certainly for stuttering in general and in ADHD.[62]

g. Anxiety Disorders

Clonidine has been used in adults for anxiety disorders such as panic and obsessive–compulsive disorders. It is said to have improved sleep disturbance and overarousal, but there are no good studies.[13] A recent review of the pharmacotherapy of anxiety disorders in children does not mention clonidine.[12]

5. Effects

Physical effects are largely adrenolytic, and since they are usually unwanted, they are described as side effects below. However, one man's meat is another's poison, and these very side effects in psychiatric use are utilized in the management of hypertension and alcohol and drug withdrawal states. The main therapeutic use of these drugs is as antihypertensive agents. Hypotension is achieved through stimulation of the baroceptors, not through adrenolysis; thus, unlike that occurring with other psychoactive drugs such as antipsychotics and antidepressants (Chapters 9 and 10), the hypotension is not orthostatic in type (i.e., only on standing up). However, as is not too unusual in pharmacotherapy, side effects in one disorder may be useful therapeutically in another. Thus, it is the adrenolytic actions, especially on the CNS, that are used psychotropically. Paradoxical adrenergic effects may occur in higher doses and in sensitive individuals (e.g., vasoconstriction, increased activity).[43,63] There may be effects on the pituitary axis[64] though these await confirmation.

Apart from tics, where the effects may be more on motor than phonic ones,[47] there seems general agreement that behavior and emotions most affected by these drugs are those which represent hyperarousal (hyperactivity, aggression, insomnia). Frank sedation can occur especially at the beginning of therapy and can be captured advantageously for the treatment of insomnia. There is also a variable effect on mood, which may range from depression to irritability. Occasionally, paradoxical hyperactivity may occur.[43]

Very few data are available as to cognitive effects. Although it seems reasonable to speculate that the commonly described sedation might result in impairment, this has not been reported in the only two studies to look at clonidine and cognitive functioning. In one report, clonidine was said to have no effects on a "neuromaturational battery,"[49] and in a larger, well-controlled investigation no effects were found on a series of cognitive tests.[53] Unfortunately, the cognitive findings were not tabulated in either of these reports, so it is not possible to examine the data for likely trends.

Hunt et al.[42] state quite emphatically that clonidine has no effects on distractibility though rating scale changes suggest otherwise. Interestingly, guanfacine had been shown to improve driving skills marginally in adults[43] and equally improved rating scale measures of inattention in both open studies in children with ADHD.[43,49] However, this should not be taken as proof that either or both drugs do improve cognition. Proper controlled laboratory studies such as have been used extensively with the stimulants are now required.

6. Side Effects, Toxic Effects, and Contraindications

Side effects, toxic effects, and contraindications have been discussed in detail in reviews.[42,63] In adults treated for hypertension, the most common side effects of clonidine are dry mouth and sedation.[65] Also noted are adrenergic rebound type symptoms (headache, palpitations, tension, sweating, stomachache, tremor) on sudden cessation. Sedation, when not used as the principal action (e.g., in Tourette's disorder), can be a problem.[46] Other side effects reported occasionally are irritability, insomnia, headache, dizziness, and, of course, hypotension. Depression has also been reported.[42] As noted, guanfacine may prove to have fewer side effects in view of its narrower profile of action[43] though most of the side effects reported seem much the same.

Some occasional cardiac effects in both adults and children have also been reported, which is hardly surprising given that these drugs have profound effects on that system. These include cardiac arrhythmias, bradycardia, and other electrocardiogram (ECG) abnormalities[66] and, according to another report, first-degree heart block and nonconducted P waves.[67] The clinical significance of these changes in those without preexisting cardiac disease is unclear.[68] Nevertheless, as Popper notes,[68] it makes good sense to examine pulse rate and blood pressure routinely, which is a simple enough procedure for office practice. Popper also recommends "screening" children with known preexisting cardiac abnormalities before clonidine therapy and during dose increase of any cardioactive medication. The question naturally arises as to the safety of clonidine–methylphenidate combinations, as the two drugs are used quite frequently in clinical practice. Popper[68] comments that there are *theoretical* reasons to be concerned about combining clonidine and methylphenidate but that there is no scientific evidence to support (or discredit) the safety and efficacy of the combination. In order to avoid hypertension/tachycardia rebound (or overshooting), Popper recommends that children and their parents be advised of the need to adhere strictly to the prescribed dose times.

There is one report of two cases of precocious puberty associated with clonidine use[64] though this may have been the cause of the aggression for which clonidine was given.

7. Interactions

The most important interaction for pediatric psychopharmacological use is with tricyclic antidepressants and trazodone. These drugs may reduce the efficacy of the α^2-adrenergic agonists, and vice versa.[30] However, this problem may be more theoretical than real since their combined use, as in ADHD, seems common[57] and without problems.[69] β-Adrenergic blockers, on withdrawal of the α_2-adrenergic blockers first, may cause sympathetic overreaction. There is also said to be some possible potentiation of alcohol and other sedating drugs, and lithium may reduce the effect of clonidine somewhat.[30]

8. Combinations

Clonidine seems often to be used in combination especially with neuroleptics[29] in Tourette's disorder and with methylphenidate and antidepressants in ADHD.[29] The objective is to enhance efficacy or to reduce dosage and hence side effects or, in the case of methylphenidate, to treat the putative, though disputed, side effect of insomnia. There is one report of its use in combination with fluoxetine in obsessive–compulsive disorder.[70] Also, there is another of use with clonazepam in Tourette's disorder resistant to clonidine alone, where it was found to affect tics but not ADHD symptoms.[28] There was some augmentation of sedative effects, but these were said to dissipate.

Although there was a momentary flurry of concern about possible dangers in association with methylphenidate, this seems to have been overexaggerated,[68] though as the number of concurrent drugs used increases, so does the possibility for serious interactions.[50] However, there is little proper controlled information about combined use,[63] so that due caution needs to be exercised. As Fenichel[71] points out, if there is more systematic study of combinations before clinicians begin to use them widely, it would be easier to discount suggestions of problems when they arise.

9. Overdose

Clonidine is one of the drugs most commonly implicated in toxicological admissions to intensive care units for young children in the United States.[63,72] The main symptoms which have a rapid onset (within 1 hr) include serious cardiovascular and respiratory problems.[63,73] Lethargy, bradycardia, miosis (pupillary constriction), hypotension, hypothermia, and respiratory depression are reported to occur. There is also a suggestion that the initial effect may be adrenergic and mask the more serious decrease in sympathetic activity. Treatment recommended includes decontamination, treatment of bradycardia and hypotension with atropine, and intravenous fluid therapy or IV dopamine.[73] However, for most practitioners the best course to follow is emergency, life-support transport and admission to a hospital with intensive care if needed.

10. Summary

α_2-Agonists are among the drugs that have shown the greatest increase in popularity in pediatric psychopharmacology in the last few years. Regrettably, they also illustrate one of the more persistent problems in pediatric psychopharmacology in that clinical enthusiasm tends greatly to outstrip proper study of indications, efficacy, and safety. Any conclusions have to be highly tentative. On the positive side, side effects in normal dosage with slow buildup and in healthy children appear to be relatively benign (though significant cardiovascular effects cannot be discounted, especially in those with preexisting cardiovascular disease). Thus, the use of α_2-agonists in difficult cases not responding well to other frontline drugs may be justifiable.

Clonidine and guanfacine may sometimes be helpful as an adjunctive or as primary treatment in Tourette's disorder and also in ADHD where stimulants are ineffective or contraindicated though there are better drugs to try first (such as antidepressants). They may be more helpful in combination with methylphenidate when there is coexistent tic or Tourette's disorder though there is then need for monitoring for cardiovascular side effects. There is also an increasing but unproven use of these drugs for sleep disturbances, including those induced by stimulants. Clinical rumor suggests that they may have some role to play in aggression though usually when this is seen in combination with ADHD. They also have a role to play in drug and alcohol withdrawal states. Use in anxiety disorders awaits demonstration. Guanfacine may offer improvements over clonidine in terms of length of action and fewer side effects such as sedation. Transdermal patches can offer advantages in prolonging action, but there is quite a high frequency of local allergic cutaneous responses. Overdosage should be regarded as a medical emergency.

The undoubted and growing popularity of these drugs demands considerably more effort at proper study to seek whether clinical observations are correct or, as so often in the past, the chimera of expectancy and enthusiasm.

B. Melatonin

Melatonin has captured the imagination of the New Age public recently as a purported remedy for aging and, indeed, most things that ail human beings. However, its possible use in children and adolescents with behavioral problems is considerably narrower, though still unproven. There are a number of useful reviews, from which most of what follows has been drawn.[74,75] Most of the interest in psychopathology has been in seasonal aspects of affective disorder and sleep regulation.

1. Physiology

The physiological roles of melatonin are described in Refs. 74 and 76. Melatonin is a hormone (chemical messenger) secreted by the pineal gland. Secretion is low until age 3 months, when it achieves adult levels. It then remains constant until levels begin to decay slowly in later life to reach near zero in the very old. Secretion is under adrenergic control (stimulatory) and is linked to light (low secretion) and dark phases (high secretion), which in animals governs light-dependent seasonal events such as the onset of reproductive behavior and circadian rhythms. In animals, melatonin governs to some degree the onset of puberty and, when given exogenously, may delay the onset of puberty. It also has an apparently unrelated role as a powerful scavenger of free hydroxyl radicals, which are highly damaging to tissue.

In humans, the role of melatonin is poorly elucidated, with extrapolations from animal experiments running considerably ahead of empirical demonstration. Anatomically, the connections between the pineal and the parts of the pituitary responsible for secretion of sex hormones have been lost in humans (along with the seasonality of the breeding cycle) though the daily phases in secretion of melatonin remain. Any relationship to the onset of puberty is dubious, and in adult females the menstrual cycle appears quite unrelated to melatonin levels. However, the lack of relationships may well be less true of abnormal states.

Most of the legitimate interest in humans centers on the relationship of melatonin to circadian rhythms and its disruptions, such as jet lag and delayed-onset sleep (sometimes seen in adolescence) and other abnormalities of the sleep–wake cycle, and to some psychiatric disorders such as seasonal affective disorder. A finding in animals that melatonin excretion can be influenced not only by light but by electromagnetic waves has raised questions about possible disruptions in humans increasingly exposed to this environmental influence. The rather histrionic popular ascribing of antiaging powers to melatonin comes from imaginative overelaborations of the observations of the decline in melatonin secretion in old age and of its putative scavenging effects on damaging hydroxyl radicals.

2. Pharmacology

Melatonin is a derivative of the dietary essential amino acid tryptophan (see below) but most proximately of 5-hydroxytryptamine (serotonin). It is almost completely inactivated by hydroxylation in the liver. Synthetic melatonin can be safely administered by all routes and in a variety of forms. Peak plasma concentrations occur around 60–150 min after administration. The elimination half-life is very short (30–53 min). (For a detailed discussion of the pharmacology of melatonin, see Ref. 74.)

Melatonin is not yet approved by the FDA though the widespread use of the substance by the public and doubts about the purity and safety of the commercially available preparation are forcing some drug-licensing bodies (e.g., in New Zealand) to register it as a drug. Some of the concerns about safety have arisen because melatonin is related to tryptophan, and when that drug was marketed unregulated, it contained contaminants that caused eosinophilia–myalgia syndrome.[77]

3. Effects and Indications

The main effect of melatonin is inconstant drowsiness, an effect that it shares with its more remote precursor, tryptophan (see below). It may have the power to reset sleep rhythms. Rather conflicted effects on anterior pituitary hormones (growth hormone, prolactin), and on luteinizing hormone in mature females, have been noted. Prepubertal children show less constant changes in prolactin.[74] No effects on testosterone have been observed in adult males.

Melatonin currently has no proven clinical indications though there have been studies in adults to suggest that it may have value in jet lag and disorders of the sleep–wake cycle.[78] There are case reports of its successful use to adjust the sleep–wake cycle in blind children,[74,78,79] in children with various psychiatric diagnoses,[76] and in neurologically multiply disabled children.[80] As noted, the drug is supposed to work by resetting the biological clock and, in theory, should need to be given only for a few days. However, nonpharmacological methods such as retraining and light therapy[78] may be effective and are currently less controversial. Dosages in children and adolescents have varied hugely from 2 mg to 250 mg, but most have been in the range of 3–10 mg.[75,77,80]

There are changes in melatonin in affective disorders, and it was hoped that these changes might serve not only as a marker for depression but also as the basis for a treatment where melatonin was low. Unfortunately, melatonin has proven ineffective.[75] There are also changes in melatonin secretion in anorexia and bulimia[81] but, so far, these have no pharmacotherapeutic applications.

4. Unwanted/Toxic Effects

Melatonin has been given by a wide variety of routes and in a wide range of doses, some very high, including in children and adolescents, without any adverse effects except mild drowsiness.[74,80] However, further work is needed to fully establish its safety.

5. Summary

At this stage, any psychoactive role for melatonin is unclear though careful, proper investigation of its role in disturbances of the sleep–wake cycle in infants, children, and adolescents seems warranted, especially in cases which do not respond to simpler measures and/or appear to be the result of brain disturbances.

C. Hypericin (St. John's Wort)

St. John's wort is an herbal extract from *Hypericum perforatum* flowers, found commonly in Europe and Asia on heath and other dry lands. It contains a number of substances. Hypericin is one compound, but there are many others, including caffeinelike substances. It may have monoamine oxidase-inhibiting or other monoamine-enhancing properties (see Chapter 9). Widely sold in health stores in many countries and of exploding popularity, it has been used by the medical profession in Germany (where the laws for licensing drugs are more relaxed than those in the United States and other Western countries) for the treatment of depression.[82] So far it has not been used in children, but there is little doubt that, because of its "stimulant" properties, it soon will be, so it is included here. There are over 50,000 references to St. John's wort on the World Wide Web, nearly all of which are impressionistic, assertive, or alternative medicine rather than truly medical.

A metaanalysis[83] of 23 randomized clinical trials (nearly all from Germany) has shown a modest antidepressant activity similar to that of the tricyclic antidepressants and superior to placebo. However, the studies leave much to be desired in terms of careful diagnosis of the subjects and proper dosages of tricyclics. Further, it is doubtful that many of the patients in these trials had severe depression or even a true depression.[82] Side effects seemed rather similar to those of tricyclic antidepressants. In New Zealand, St. John's wort is classified as a noxious weed, because it can cause severe photosensitization of the skin in fair-skinned domestic animals. However, according to one manufacturer,* this side effect has not been observed in humans though the manufacturer states that "in rare instances and especially in fair skinned people, (the possibility of) photosensitization cannot be completely excluded." The manufacturer also states that this is only likely to occur when the dose taken is 30–50 times that recommended.

The conclusions are that while hypericin shows promise as an alternative treatment for mild depression for those who prefer natural medicines, it requires much more testing using proper standards.[82,83] It is marketed as Kira® by Lichter Pharma in Berlin, who recommend no more than four weeks of treatment. The manufacturer provides a product information booklet, which is unusual among product literature for herbal remedies for its approximation to the medical standard and is recommended to those who wish to use it.

Current enthusiasm for hypericin is part of a widespread belief that anything that is herbal or "natural" is superior to orthodox medical products. This belief, embraced even by those who are well educated and supposedly intelligent, is ignorant of both the history of medicine and the canons of common sense. Orthodox medicine used natural products for thousands of years. When one of the authors (J.S.W.) began his career, extracts of thyroid and of digitalis were still in common use, and even these have been replaced by pure synthesized products. Use of the latter has eliminated the problems of wide variation in potency and deterioration of active substances. However, the success of a tiny handful of natural products like those two (or the oft-quoted quinine for malaria) has obscured the fact that the vast majority was useless or dangerous. The latest examples of dangerous effects have been seen in the toxic effects of some of the vitamins and the Jakob–Creutzfeldt dementia resulting from the use of "naturally obtained" growth hormone.

What medicine has done in the last 100 years is to take the tiny handful of natural remedies that seemed to work and test, refine, and then synthesize those that survived rigorous testing. Thus, instead of resorting to the natural preparations, which are something

---

*Thompson Nutrition, personal communication to J.S. Werry, December 22, 1997.

of a pharmacological lottery in terms of strength, purity, and active substances, medicine uses only what is demonstrably pure, effective, and safe. Medicine accepts that there is a necessary trade-off between efficacy and safety, which must be weighed against the severity of the illness, and that occasional unforeseen effects may arise, so that new drugs should be carefully monitored for several years after introduction. Also, the medical profession is constrained to report to the appropriate government agency any significant or unexpected side effects at any time, even with well-established drugs. No such safeguards exist for herbal remedies. Thus, and for the additional reason that the theoretical rationale for many herbal medicines is in fact false, the safest and most effective way to prevent and treat disease is still through orthodox medical diagnosis and treatment.

The popularity of herbal remedies and unorthodox medical practices has to be seen against the backdrop of anti-intellectual populism—a persistent theme in Western democracies—which tends to view government, business, and established professions with partly well-earned but grossly exaggerated suspicion. It is also a sad reflection on the failure of the education system to instill a proper understanding of how medical knowledge is weighed and established through the scientific method. Such knowledge actually empowers people in the management of their health and makes them resistant to quackery. What makes the situation currently rather more dangerous than formerly is that, with modern communication methods such as satellite television and the World Wide Web, hocus-pocus medicine can be promulgated instantaneously to millions around the world.

In summary, hypericin is unusual among herbal remedies in that it has had more investigation and is more responsibly marketed than most. It may prove to have a place in the management of mild depression and dysthymia. Side effects seem similar to those of low-dosage tricyclics. There have been no reports of fatalities. However, proper testing and isolation of the active substance and purification of the product are required. Its use in children is not currently recommended.

D. L-Tryptophan and 5-Hydroxytryptophan

L-Tryptophan (L-Trp) is an essential amino acid, and 5-hydroxytryptophan (5-OH-Trp) is its metabolite on the path to synthesis of serotonin (5-hydroxytryptamine). There is evidence directly from blood, CSF, or urine studies or inferred from the therapeutic effect of serotonergic antidepressant drugs like fluoxetine or clomipramine (Chapter 9) that some psychiatric and allied disorders are associated (in some cases) with lowered levels of serotonin; these include bipolar mood disorder, major depression, autism, Down's syndrome, Tourette syndrome, obsessive–compulsive disorder, and self-mutilation.[84,85] L-Trp has been tried in adults primarily in depression,[85] in bipolar disorders,[86] and in insomnia,[3] where the results were promising. However, the drug has been withdrawn by the U.S. FDA because of over 1300 cases of eosinophilia–myalgia syndrome, although this may have been due to a contaminant rather than the drug itself.[3] It is hepatotoxic in animals.

5-OH-Trp has been tried in Down's syndrome and in autistic children without success and in Lesch–Nyhan syndrome (a congenital metabolic disorder marked by mental retardation, movement disorders, and self-mutilation) and Tourette syndrome with equivocal results.[84] There is some evidence that 5-OH-Trp may be an antidepressant in its own right.[85] Ordinarily, both 5-OH-Trp and L-Trp should not be used with serotonergic drugs because they may induce a serious serotonin syndrome (Chapter 9) resembling the neuroleptic malignant syndrome (Chapter 10).

In summary, while both these drugs are of interest, they currently have no proven role in the treatment of children and adolescents and there is concern about potential toxicity.

E. Fenfluramine

This book goes to press just as a major controversy is brewing over fenfluramine's safety. *There are concerns that fenfluramine and its near relative, dexfenfluramine, may cause valvular disease and/or primary pulmonary hypertension. Because of these concerns, both drugs were withdrawn from the market in December of 1997. This is discussed later under "Side Effects and Toxicity."* Nevertheless, due to high interest in and considerable research on fenfluramine, we have retained this section. It is also possible that the fears of an association with heart disease may prove to be unfounded or that any association may be sufficiently weak that the drug may be returned to market one day.

1. Pharmacology

Fenfluramine (Pondimin®, Ponderax®) is an amphetamine analogue that was originally used as an adjunct in the treatment of obesity. However, unlike the amphetamines, fenfluramine is predominantly serotoninolytic rather than catecholaminergic, causes CNS depression, and is thought to have little abuse potential.[86]

Following oral administration, fenfluramine is well absorbed, with an absorption half-life of about 1.2 hr.[86] Plasma half-life is approximately 20 hr in adults,[86] and steady-state levels are therefore reached after 3–4 days. Most excretion is via the kidneys and depends on urinary flow and pH.[86] The principal metabolite is norfenfluramine, which is said to have very similar effects to the parent drug in animal studies.[86]

Fenfluramine increases glucose uptake in muscle and reduces blood glucose levels.[86] Decreases have been reported in plasma cholesterol levels, but this may be due to reduced food consumption from anorexia. With long-term treatment, fenfluramine may reduce linear growth velocity, although short-term studies of growth hormone have found conflicting results.[86] Clinical studies show reductions in blood pressure, and the action of certain antihypertensive drugs may be increased.[86]

CNS effects include a sedative-type effect on the waking electroencephalogram (EEG).[86] Chronic administration of fenfluramine in adults has produced reductions in REM sleep, increases in number of arousals, changes in slow-wave sleep, and reports of poorer quality of sleep.[86]

2. Clinical Indications

a. Autism

Fenfluramine has been extensively researched in children with autism, with over 35 publications. The rationale has been that about 30–40% of subjects with autism show high levels of serotonin in blood.[87–89] A similar, although perhaps stronger, pattern is seen in nonautistic subjects with idiopathic mental retardation, who, as a group, exhibit increases in whole-blood serotonin that are often positively correlated with severity of mental retardation.[87] Nevertheless, as far as pharmacotherapy is concerned, the greatest interest to date has been in autistic subjects.[90] Since fenfluramine is a serotonin-depleting agent in blood, this eventually led investigators to try the drug in autistic subjects on the presumption that the excessive serotonin may be etiologically significant in autism and/or that it may be contributing to the severe behavioral problems seen so commonly in these children.[91] The original report on three cases treated with fenfluramine suggested major gains in IQ performance and improvements in behavioral symptoms,[91] and this led to an upswing of research with the drug, which has been reviewed critically elsewhere.[87,88]

The predominant findings from studies of fenfluramine in autistic children are as follows. (1) Almost all studies have reported substantial reductions in whole-blood serotonin, usually on the order of 50%. (2) Although IQ and adaptive behavioral changes were found in some of the earliest reports, there was little support for this from well-controlled studies. (3) Stereotypic and ritualistic behaviors and social interaction may improve. (4) Overactivity, inattention, and distractibility were often significantly improved.[86] Speech, communication, or other language indicators showed little or no gain.[90]

Thus, there are indications of improvement with fenfluramine, mainly in the area of stereotypic/ritualistic, inattentive, and hyperactive behaviors; however, changes have shown up in only some of the 35 reports, so responding appears to be somewhat idiosyncratic. One criticism made about many of these studies is that the measures of treatment effectiveness were often coarse (e.g., IQ and adaptive behavior scales) so that more subtle effects on target behaviors (e.g., activity level) were often neglected.[87]

b. ADHD

One study assessed three doses of fenfluramine in hyperactive (ADHD) children of normal IQ.[92] In contrast to findings in autistic children, no clinical or cognitive changes were detected.

c. Mental Retardation

Three recent group studies have tried fenfluramine in mentally retarded patients. In one, significant improvements in children, adolescents, and adults with Prader–Willi syndrome were noted in weight loss, food-related behavior, and aggression.[93] In the second, fenfluramine caused significant changes compared with placebo in children with mental retardation and ADHD.[94] Improvements occurred on parent and teacher ratings of irritability, conduct problems, and hyperactivity and in memory performance on a color-matching task. In the third, fenfluramine resulted in improved ratings of hyperactivity and irritability by parents and teachers of children with ADHD.[95] Fenfluramine also caused improved attention on a vigilance task, reduced seat activity, and consistently longer response times on computer-controlled learning tasks.[96] If anything, the findings with mentally retarded subjects without autism appear to be stronger than those with autistic subjects, and its clinical effects in children with both ADHD and mental retardation seem to be reasonably well established.

3. Clinical Usage

a. Dosage

Most studies have used standardized doses of 1.5 mg/kg per day divided into morning and evening doses. The first study with hyperactive mentally retarded children used a gradual scheme in which dose was started at 0.5 mg/kg per day for 1 week, increased to 1.0 mg/kg per day for 1 week, and finally raised to 1.5 mg/kg per day.[94] Because of drowsiness, a few of the 28 children could not tolerate the final dose, and one child the intermediate dose, so that gradually increasing dosage appears to be more appropriate than using a single weight-determined dose. Following a comparison study of 1.0, 1.5, and 2.0 mg/kg per day of fenfluramine, the investigators recommended a gradual phase-in of fenfluramine up to 1.5 mg/kg per day, given in two divided doses, for the majority of children.[95]

b. Side Effects and Toxicity

The most commonly reported side effects with fenfluramine include anorexia/weight loss, lethargy/sedation, and irritability.[87] Sleep difficulties and agitation have also been reported in a few subjects and gastrointestinal symptoms and dizziness have been reported occasionally. However, most of these side effects will abate somewhat with lower dosage.

The main concern about fenfluramine is that it may be associated with valvular disease and/or primary pulmonary hypertension. One study[97] reported on 24 women who took the combination of fenfluramine and phentermine (popularly called "fen-phen") for obesity. All 24 had valvular disease (including unusual valvular morphology and leakage) and 8 of the women had newly documented pulmonary hypertension. Two other articles[98,99] also reported valvulopathy associated not only with fen-phen but also with fenfluramine and dexfenfluramine monotherapy.

One FDA notice[100] on the World Wide Web reported on 101 cases of valvulopathy associated with these diet drugs: 85 patients previously took fen-phen, 3 took fenfluramine alone, 9 took dexfenfluramine alone, and 4 took fen-phen and dexphenfluramine at different times. The same notice[100] reported on 271 "asymptomatic" patients who had taken fen-phen and were subsequently given echocardiograms. Eighty-six cases (32%) met the investigative criteria for valvular leakage; both aortic and mitral regurgitation were found but aortic was more common. At the time of this writing, Wyeth-Ayerst, the manufacturer, is conducting a study of 400 patients who previously took fen-phen, 400 who took dexfenfluramine, and 400 who took neither.[100] Hopefully, this and related research will soon resolve whether there is a causal link between fenfluramine and heart disease or only an apparent link due to other factors, such as higher morbidity in obese patients.[101]

Finally, fenfluramine has long been a controversial drug because of studies suggesting irreversible neurochemical changes when laboratory animals are given large doses of the drug. For example, early studies reported an irregular shape and intense dark staining throughout cells in a serotonergic cell group in the brains of laboratory rats.[102] More recently, it has been reported that doses from 12.5 to 100 mg/kg per day produced long-lasting depletions of serotonin in the brains of rats, guinea pigs, and rhesus monkeys.[103] From observations such as these, some conclude that fenfluramine might cause permanent depletions of brain serotonin in humans.

However, there are counter arguments.[87] (1) The weight-corrected doses in most animal studies are many times larger than those used in children and thus may not be relevant to the clinical context. (2) There are large interspecies differences in behavioral and physiological responses to fenfluramine, so that animal data may not be applicable to human beings. (3) Some researchers have been unable to replicate the findings even in laboratory animals. (4) We have been unable to locate any data showing functional losses, even in laboratory animals treated with very large doses. (5) The drug has now been on the market for 25 years, and there are no data indicating long-lasting neurological effects in obese patients or in autistic youngsters who have received it for appreciable periods.

4. Overdose

According to the *Physicians' Desk Reference* (PDR),[104] the following may accompany fenfluramine overdose: agitation or drowsiness, confusion, flushing, tremor, fever, sweating, stomachache, hyperventilation, dilated/nonresponsive pupils, tachycardia, and exaggerated or depressed reflexes. At higher doses still, convulsions, coma, and ventricular extrasystoles may occur, culminating in ventricular fibrillation and cardiac arrest. The following steps have been reported in the PDR for managing fenfluramine overdose: (a) gastric lavage (but not drug-induced emesis) or, in the event of lockjaw, administration of muscle relaxants to enable gastric evacuation; (b) administration of activated charcoal after emesis/lavage to reduce fenfluramine absorption; (c) monitoring of vital signs and mechanical support if necessary; and (d) administration of diazepam or phenobarbital for convulsions, propranolol for tachycardia, and chlorpromazine for hyperpyrexia.

5. Summary

Obviously, the issue of neurotoxicity is important but unresolved. Clinically, the best policy may be to consider the use of fenfluramine only in children with well-defined mental retardation and in autism, and then only for specific target behaviors (such as hyperactivity) and only when other agents have failed. Fenfluramine should be continued only when there is evidence of substantial behavioral improvements. Disclosure to the parents of the controversial nature of this drug and its disputed neurotoxic effects is required, so that the parent can give informed consent (see Chapter 6). All of this is a moot point, of course, as long as the drug is off the market.

F. β-Adrenergic Blockers (β-Blockers)

1. Pharmacology

β-Adrenergic receptors are activated by adrenergic sympathetic nervous transmission and by endocrine (circulating) catecholamines such as noradrenaline. They are instrumental in producing what is known as the general alarm (or "fight or flight") reaction to stress.[104,105] β-Adrenergic blockers are synthetic adrenergic receptor-blocking agents.[106] About a dozen are listed by Neppe,[107] and 10 are approved by the U.S. FDA. Propranolol (Inderal®) is the prototype and is also available as long-acting (LA) capsules. Other β-blockers include atenolol, metoprolol, and nadolol.

β-Blockers can work on both β_1 and β_2 receptors. The former are found mainly in the heart and brain, whereas the latter are implicated in the functioning of vascular, bronchial, and gastrointestinal organs.[105–107] β-Blockers having β_1 blocking action tend to decrease heart rate, cardiac output, blood pressure, and maximal exercise tolerance.[108] They also have an antiarrhythmic effect on the heart. Metabolically, β-blockers can modify carbohydrate and fat metabolism, leading to hypoglycemia, especially in diabetics treated with insulin.[108] The β_2-blockers block the action of sympathomimetic amines, leading to increases in airway resistance, which is potentially dangerous in asthma, a common disorder in children.

The molecular size and degree of ionization at physiological pH differ little across the β-blockers, but there are differences in affinity for lipids.[107] Among the most lipid-soluble are propranolol, oxprenolol, and penbutolol, whereas atenolol, nadolol, and sotalol are not lipid-soluble.[107] Because the brain has a high lipid content, lipid solubility determines much of the potential for central actions,[107] although nadolol has been shown to have behavioral effects. With propranolol, peak absorption is reached in about 1–1½ hr. Most of the β-blockers have short half-lives, in the range of 2–9 hr, the exception being nadolol, which has a half-life of approximately 22 hr.[107] According to Neppe,[107] all β-blockers, regardless of half-life, must be given two to three times daily for psychiatric applications. Propranolol is metabolized in the liver or excreted unchanged by the kidneys.[107] It is heavily bound to protein (90–95%) in plasma.[107]

2. Clinical Indications

The most common uses for the β-blockers are for treating cardiovascular conditions in adults, but they have been used in at least 34 disorders (mostly in adults), many of which are psychiatric.[107] In adults the most accepted psychiatric use of β-blockers is for anxiety disorders with marked somatic components, such as palpitations and tremor. Generalized anxiety disorder, panic disorders, and agoraphobia have been the conditions most frequently treated and researched with β-blockers.[107] There is literature that suggests that propranolol is useful in managing recurrent migraines.[109,110] Other conditions in which they have been tried include schizophrenia, rage in chronic organic brain syndrome, alcoholism, stuttering, akathisia, and certain tremors.[107] Only use in children and adolescents will be discussed here. A recent review[111] listed akathisia (a side effect of antipsychotics; Chapter 10) as a probable indication for β-blockers, and aggressive dyscontrol in brain-damaged patients, anxiety disorders, and migraine as conjectural applications.

a. Aggression

A recent review looked at the use of β-blockers in youngsters and developmentally disabled patients having aggressive disorders.[105] Subjects had a variety of symptoms and/or disorders, including conduct disorder, intermittent explosive disorder, impulsive assaultive behavior, self-injurious behavior, and organic personality disorder. None of the 11 studies was properly controlled, and objective or standardized measures were generally lacking. Of the combined total of 99 subjects, 78% were regarded as showing a positive response to either propranolol or nadolol. Of 62 participants who had mental retardation, 81% were reported as responding.

Improvements were seen in reduced rage outbursts, verbal and physical assaults and agitation and increased frustration tolerance. In developmentally disabled subjects, self-injury and ritualistic behavior were also said to be decreased.[105] One study reported that presumed brain damage associated with mental retardation was predictive of a positive outcome,[112] although this association was not seen in other studies.[105] The same study also found more bradycardia in nonresponders than in responders.[112] Two studies used the noncentrally acting nadolol instead of propranolol, but the degree of improvement appeared to be equal.[105] Four studies that included only children and adolescents had a mean dose of 150 mg/day of propranolol, which is far lower than the dose levels that have been recommended and used for treating aggression in adults.[105]

As noted, these studies were uncontrolled, and many participants were already taking neuroleptics, concentrations of which are known to be increased with propranolol. Case reports suggesting beneficial effects on self-injury and aggression continue to appear,[113–115] although there are still no properly controlled group studies of the β-blockers. Hence, the use of β-blockers for treating aggression in youngsters remains experimental, although there is enough positive evidence in the literature to justify some much-needed well-controlled research.

b. Anxiety

The literature on the use of β-blockers for treating adults with anxiety disorders is sparse, especially given that these drugs have been available for well over two decades.[115]

One review concluded that propranolol may be effective (as a second-line treatment) for generalized anxiety disorders, particularly those accompanied with somatic symptoms.[115] The β-blockers have not been well researched in panic disorders, and the findings thus far are not encouraging for that application.[116] We were able to find only one study of these drugs in children, this being a poorly controlled study of propranolol in children with posttraumatic stress disorder (PTSD).[117] Propranolol, titrated to 2.5 mg/kg per day, improved affective, cognitive, and physiological symptoms associated with PTSD. Obviously, the literature base is much too narrow to draw any conclusions with respect to the use of β-blockers for treating anxiety in youngsters, and hence any use should be regarded as experimental.

3. Clinical Usage

a. Dosage

One author recommends starting with 10 mg twice daily and increasing dosage by 10–20 mg every 3–4 days.[111] A review found that mean doses for controlling aggression were much lower than those cited in the adult literature (120–214 mg/day versus 520 mg and more per day in adults).[105] Many recommend raising dosage until there is an obvious decrease in blood pressure or heart rate.[105,111] Blood pressure should be maintained above 90/60 and heart rate above 60 beats/min.[111]

b. Side Effects

Side effects are, in decreasing order of approximate frequency of occurrence, Raynaud's phenomenon, bradycardia, bronchoconstriction, sexual impotence, depression/dysphoria, congestive heart failure, hallucinations, hypotension, vomiting/nausea, diarrhea, insomnia/nightmares, dizziness, and hypoglycemia.[107,111]

c. Contraindications

Contraindications include cardiorespiratory conditions (such as asthma, congestive heart failure, or angina), insulin-dependent diabetes, vascular disease, renal disease, and hyperthyroidism.[105]

d. Interactions

The β-blockers interact with a large number of other agents.[111] They may increase concentrations or the effects of the following: phenothiazines, clonidine, phenytoin, calcium-blocking agents, anesthetics, lidocaine, epinephrine, monoamine oxidase inhibitors, and thyroxine. β-Blockers may decrease the effects of insulin and oral diabetes agents. Molindone and cimetidine may increase the effects of β-blockers. Finally, smoking, nonsteroidal anti-inflammatory analgesics, oral contraceptives, and carbamazepine may decrease the effects of β-blockers.[111]

e. Overdose

Common symptoms of β-blocker overdose include hypotension, bradycardia, prolonged AV conduction times, widened QRS complexes, seizures, and psychiatric depression.[108] Common therapeutic steps include (a) evacuation of gastric contents, (b) managing bradycardia with atropine (also with a cardiac pacemaker if necessary), (c) treating hypotension with an adrenergic agonist (e.g., epinephrine), and (d) administration of digitalis for cardiac failure.

4. Summary

β-Blockers are best indicated in psychiatry for drug-induced tremor or akathisia but may be tried in episodic dyscontrol of aggression and anxiety with marked somatic symptoms. They should not be used where there is asthma or cardiorespiratory disease.

G. Opiate Blockers

1. Pharmacology

Two agents with relatively pure opiate blocking properties are naloxone (Narcan®) and naltrexone (Trexan®), which act by competitive binding at opioid receptors.[104] Both reduce the subjective effects of opiate narcotics and help to reverse respiratory and cardiovascular depression in overdose with opiates.[118] The use of these agents in narcotic abuse and dependency, where they are employed to reverse respiratory depression or test for dependency, is discussed in Chapter 11.

Naloxone is available only in solution for parenteral use. When given intravenously, it is active within 1–2 min, its plasma half-life is about 1 hr, and its duration of action is 1–4 hr.[118] Naltrexone is maximally absorbed within about 1 hr and has a half-life of about 4 hr, but it produces a major metabolite that has a half-life of about 13 hr.[104] Most of the naltrexone (95%) is converted in the liver to metabolites, and these are excreted by the kidneys.

The pharmacological effects depend on whether the patient has taken another opioid-like agent. In normal adults free of exogenous opiates, doses of up to 12 mg of naloxone produce no subjective effects, but very large doses (up to 24 mg) cause slight drowsiness.[118] Tolerance to the opiate antagonist properties and physical and psychological dependence are said not to occur.[118]

2. Clinical Indications

a. Self-Injury

There has been considerable speculation that opiate blockers may have a role in treating patients, usually those with mental retardation and/or autism, who have high rates of self-injury. Two competing hypotheses that implicate the opiate system have been put forward.[119,120] In the first, it is posited that such individuals have an abnormally high threshold for pain and, as a result, a higher probability of serious injury when self-injury is used as a form of self-stimulation or attention getting.[120] The competing hypothesis suggests that self-injury may be reinforcing, presumptively because it leads to the highly rewarding release of endogenous opioids.[120] The use of opiate blockers follows logically from both these models. In the former, opiate blockers should reverse the pathologically altered pain threshold, thereby making any self-inflicted injury more painful and aversive. In the latter model, opiate blockers should minimize any euphoric effects caused by release of endogenous opioids and thus remove any positive reinforcement contingent upon self-injury.

The effects of naloxone and naltrexone in self-injurious subjects with developmental disabilities have been reviewed elsewhere,[120–123] although conclusions differ somewhat. The more conservative views[121,122] will be summarized here. The majority of early reports included only one or two subjects each, although one had 18.[124] About half of the case reports were positive in outcome, but the controlled comparisons were less successful. Large therapeutic effects were seen infrequently, and many of the studies had important deficiencies. In addition to lack of placebo control in one-third of the reports, the observations of treatment effects were brief in duration in a further one-third of the reports.[122] Self-injurious behavior is known to be highly variable in some individuals, and the brief observation time employed may have caught the patient during a quiescent period.

Recently, at least four group studies of reasonable sample size appeared, but their results were conflicting. In two of the studies,[125,126] the findings were positive. In one of these, 13 of 21 subjects (62%) showed at least a 25% reduction in self-injury.[126] However, the other two studies failed to observe significant effects with doses of 1.0 mg/kg per day)[127] and 100 mg/day (mean = 1.61 mg/kg per day).[128]

In summary, there has been tremendous interest in the opiate blockers for the troublesome problem of self-injury in patients with developmental disabilities. Unfortunately, all of the pre-1993 publications involved very small groups of patients, and the more recent larger-scale studies appear to be in some disagreement. Only naltrexone is suitable for outpatient treatment, as naloxone can only be given by injection. Clearly, this area still requires further studies, hopefully with sizable groups of patients. Naltrexone appears to have promise for managing self-injury, although this use is still clinically experimental, and it is still unknown whether naltrexone is more effective than other therapeutic agents.

b. Autism

Endogenous opioids can produce autistic-like behavior in animals (e.g., isolation, impaired clinging to the mother, insensitivity to pain).[122] This has led to suggestions that opiate blockers might have a role in treating autistic children.[84,129,130] One early study, using graduated acute doses of naltrexone in 10 autistic children,[131] indicated improvements in autistic behavior and hyperactivity and possible changes in self-injury. However, the study was open and did not control for time or placebo effects. Another acute-dose study[132] observed significant improvements on acetometer readings and attention during play but no changes in core features of autism with a dose of 40 mg (mean = 1.96 mg/kg). A large-scale trial of naltrexone, given in doses of 1.0 mg/kg per day, documented modest effects on activity and on ratings of hyperactivity but no improvements in other clinical areas such as socialization.[127] In another well-controlled trial, all improvements were confined to reduced ratings of hyperactivity.[133]

The clear impression to emerge is that naltrexone may be helpful for managing hyperactivity in some children with autism, but it does not seem to have a reliable effect on other aspects of the disorder. The drug may have some role in reducing severe hyperactivity in appropriately selected children, although it is unknown how naltrexone would compare with other drugs, such as the psychostimulants, in this respect.

3. Clinical Usage

a. Dosage

A range of 0.5–2.0 mg/kg per day has been used for the treatment of self-injury. Early studies suggested that therapeutic response improved with dosage up to 1.5 mg/kg per day, but with a reversal thereafter. However, others suggested that reductions in self-injury were greatest with the highest dose used (2.0 mg/kg per day).[124,126] In the autism studies employing acute dosing, doses in the range of 0.5–2.0 mg/kg were used.[131] Both studies employing longer dosing intervals used a standardized dose of 1.0 mg/kg per day, usually given in the morning.

b. Side Effects

The most common side effects in adults include difficulty sleeping, anxiety, nervousness, stomachaches, nausea, low energy, muscle/joint pain, and headaches.[104] Several of the studies on self-injury suggest that opiate blockers may cause sedation, drowsiness, and anxiolysis.[122] As stress may exacerbate self-injury, this nonspecific property may account for some of the therapeutic effects attributed to these drugs. One group monitored 13 autistic children during acute doses of naltrexone (0.4, 1.0, 1.5, and 2.0 mg/kg) and failed to find any significant changes in heart rate, blood pressure, mean arterial blood pressure, axillary body temperature, ECG parameters, or liver enzymes.[134] However, they recommended routine monitoring of liver function in any child receiving chronic naltrexone treatment.

c. Contraindications

Contraindications are largely related to opioid dependency or treatment and include the following: (1) patients in acute opioid withdrawal, (2) presence of hepatitis or liver failure, (3) patients receiving opioid analgesics, and (4) opioid dependence.[104]

d. Overdose

According to the *Physicians Desk Reference*,[104] there is no documented clinical experience with naltrexone overdosage in human beings. In the laboratory, lethal doses produce clonic/tonic convulsions and/or respiratory failure in rodents. The PDR recommends symptomatic treatment with close supervision.

4. Summary

Opiate antagonists may have a role in treatment of self-injury in mentally retarded patients. They may also reduce symptoms of hyperactivity in autism, although further studies are needed to establish this as an indication.

IV. SUMMARY

This chapter reviews a diverse collection of agents, many of which have CNS depressant properties in common. The agents discussed are largely experimental at present, and all are underresearched. With certain exceptions (e.g., clonidine for tic disorders and naltrexone for self-injury), specific applications are generally lacking for their use in children and adolescents. However, by extension of data from adult populations, certain probabilistic uses can be hazarded for sedative–hypnotic drugs in younger persons. Likewise, preliminary data exist that suggest possible limited roles for the miscellaneous agents discussed. Many of these agents have therapeutic promise, but our knowledge is at a relatively rudimentary stage. All of the agents covered require careful, prospective, well-controlled studies to evaluate their efficacy.

ACKNOWLEDGMENTS. Work on this chapter was supported in part by a research contract from the U.S. National Institute of Mental Health (Grant MH NO1 MH80011 and 90 DD).

REFERENCES

1. American Psychiatric Association: *Benzodiazepine Dependence, Toxicity, and Abuse: A Task Force Report.* Washington, DC, American Psychiatric Press, 1990.
2. Gilman AG, Rall TW, Nies AS, et al (eds): *Goodman and Gilman's The Pharmacological Basis of Therapeutics*, ed 8. New York, Pergamon Press, 1990.
3. Gelenberg AJ, Bassuk EL, Schoonover SC (eds): *The Practitioner's Guide to Psychoactive Drugs*, ed 3. New York, Plenum Press, 1991.
4. Greenblatt DJ, Shader, RI: *Benzodiazepines in Clinical Practice.* New York, Raven Press, 1974.
5. Baldessarini RJ: Drugs and the treatment of psychiatric disorders, in Gilman AG, Rall TW, Nies AS, et al (eds): *Goodman and Gilman's The Pharmacological Basis of Therapeutics*, ed 8. New York, Pergamon Press, 1990, pp 383–435.
6. Kennedy SK, Longnecker DE: History and principles of anesthesiology, in Gilman AG, Rall TW, Nies AS, et al (eds): *Goodman and Gilman's The Pharmacological Basis of Therapeutics*, ed 8. New York, Pergamon Press, 1990, pp 269–284.
7. Kutcher SP, Reiter S, Gardner DM, et al: The pharmacotherapy of anxiety disorders in children and adolescents. *Psychiatr Clin North Am* 15:41–68, 1992.
8. Rall TW: Hypnotics and sedatives; ethanol, in Gilman AG, Rall TW, Nies AS, et al (eds): *Goodman and Gilman's The Pharmacological Basis of Therapeutics*, ed 8. New York, Pergamon Press, 1990, pp 345–382.
9. Coffey BJ: Anxiolytics for children and adolescents: Traditional and new drugs. *J Child Adolesc Psychopharmacol* 1:57–86, 1990.
10. Klein DF, Mannuzza S, Chapman T, et al: Child panic revisited. *J Am Acad Child Adolesc Psychiatry* 31:112–116, 1992.
11. Bernstein GA, Borchardt CM: Anxiety disorders of childhood and adolescence: A critical review. *J Am Acad Child Adolesc Psychiatry* 30:519–532, 1991.
12. Allen AJ, Leonard H, Swedo SE: Current knowledge of medications for the treatment of childhood anxiety disorders. *J Am Acad Child Adolesc Psychiatry* 34:976–986, 1995.
13. Bernstein GA, Perwien AR: Anxiety disorders, in Riddle MA (ed): Pediatric psychopharmacology. *Child Adolesc Clin North Am* 4:305–322, 1995.
14. Popper DW: Psychopharmacological treatment of anxiety disorders in adolescents and children. *J Clin Psychiatry* 54(suppl):52–63, 1993.
15. Roy-Byrne PP, Wingerson D: Pharmacotherapy of anxiety disorders, in Tasman A, Riba MB (eds): *American Psychiatric Press Review of Psychiatry.* Washington, DC, American Psychiatric Press, 1992, vol 11, pp 260–284.
16. Simeon JG, Ferguson HB, Knott V, et al: Clinical, cognitive, and neurophysiological effects of alprazolam in children and adolescents with overanxious and avoidant disorders. *J Am Acad Child Adolesc Psychiatry* 31:29–33, 1992.
17. Aman MG, Werry JS: Methylphenidate and diazepam in severe reading retardation. *J Am Acad Child Psychiatry* 21:31–37, 1982.
18. Graae F, Milner J, Rizzotto L. et al: Clonazepam in childhood anxiety disorders. *J Am Acad Child Adolesc Psychiatry* 33:372–376, 1994.
19. Werry JS: Overanxious disorder: A review of its taxonomic properties. *J Am Acad Child Adolesc Psychiatry* 30:533–544, 1991.
20. Brown TA, Hertz RM, Barlow DH: New developments in cognitive-behavioral treatment of anxiety disorders, in Tasman A, Riba MB (eds): *American Psychiatric Press Review of Psychiatry.* Washington, DC, American Psychiatric Press, 1992, vol 11, pp 285–306.
21. Werry JS, Wollersheim JP: Behavior therapy with children and adolescents: A twenty year overview. *J Am Acad Child Adolesc Psychiatry* 28:1–18, 1989.
22. Richman N, Douglas J, Hunt H, et al: Behavioural methods in the treatment of sleep disorders: A pilot study. *J Child Psychol Psychiatry* 26:581–590, 1985.
23. Horne J: Sleep and its disorders in children. *J Child Psychol Psychiatry* 33:473–487, 1992.

24. Dahl RE: The pharmacologic treatment of sleep disorders. *Psychiatr Clin North Am* 15:161–178, 1992.
25. Dahl RE: Child and adolescent sleep disorders, in Riddle MA (ed): Pediatric psychopharmacology. *Child Adolesc Clin North Am* 4:323–341, 1995.
26. McClellan JM, Werry JS: Schizophrenia. *Psychiatr Clin North Am* 15:131–148, 1992.
27. Campbell M, Gonzalez NM, Silva RR: The pharmacologic treatment of conduct disorders and rage outbursts. *Psychiatr Clin North Am* 15:69–85, 1992.
28. Steingard RJ, Goldberg M, Lee D, et al: Adjunctive clonazepam treatment of tic symptoms in children with comorbid tic disorders and ADHD. *J Am Acad Child Adolesc Psychiatry* 33:394–399, 1994.
29. Wilens T, Spencer T, Biederman J, et al: Combined pharmacotherapy: An emerging trend in pediatric psychopharmacology. *J Am Acad Child Adolesc Psychiatry* 34:110–112, 1995.
30. Ciraulo DA, Shader RI, Greenblatt DJ, et al: *Drug Interactions in Psychiatry.* Baltimore: Williams & Wilkins, 1989.
31. Werry JS, Carlielle J: The nuclear family, suburban neurosis, and iatrogenesis in Auckland mothers of young children. *J Am Acad Child Psychiatry* 22:172–179, 1982.
32. Garrison JC: Histamine, bradykinin, 5-hydroxytryptamine and their antagonists, in Gilman AG, Rall TW, Nies AS, et al (eds): *Goodman and Gilman's The Pharmacological Basis of Therapeutics*, ed 8. New York, Pergamon Press, 1990, pp 575–599.
33. Werry JS: Anticholinergic sedatives, in Burrows GD, Werry JS (eds): *Advances in Human Psychopharmacology*. Greenwich, Conn, JAI Press, 1980, pp 19–42.
34. Richman N: A double-blind drug trial of treatment in young children with waking problems. *J Child Psychol Psychiatry* 26:591–598, 1985.
35. Simeon J, Knott VJ, DuBois C, et al: Buspirone therapy of mixed anxiety disorders in childhood and adolescence: A pilot study. *J Child Adolesc Psychopharmacol* 4:159–170, 1994.
36. Gross MD: Buspirone in ADHD with ODD [letter]. *J Am Acad Adolesc Psychiatry* 34:1260, 1995.
37. Mandoki M: Buspirone treatment of truamatic brain injury in a child who is highly sensitive to adverse effects of psychotropic medications. *J Child Adolesc Psychopharmacol* 4:129–139, 1994.
38. Soni P, Weintraub AL: Buspirone associated mental changes. *J Am Acad Adolesc Psychiatry* 31:1098–1099, 1992.
39. Realmuto GL, August GJ, Garfinkel BD: Clinical effect of buspirone in autistic children. *J Clin Psychopharmacol* 9:122–125, 1989.
40. Zwier KJ, Rao U: Buspirone use in an adolescent with social phobia and mixed personality disorder (Cluster A type). *J Am Acad Adolesc Psychiatry* 33:1007–1011, 1994.
41. Gelenberg AJ, Bassuk EL, Schoonover SC: *Practitioner's Guide to Psychoactive Drugs* ed 3. New York, Plenum, 1991, pp 199–200.
42. Hunt RD, Capper L, O'Connell P: Clonidine in child and adolescent psychiatry. *J Child Adolesc Psychopharmacol* 1:87–102, 1990.
43. Horrigan JP, Barnhill LJ: Guanfacine for treatment of attention deficit hyperactivity disorder. *J Child Adolesc Psychopharmacol* 5:215–223, 1995.
44. Gerber JG, Nies AS: Antihypertensive agents and the drug treatment of hypertension, in Gilman AG, Rall TW, Nies AS, Taylor P (eds): *Goodman and Gilman's The Pharmacological Basis of Therapeutics*, ed 8. New York, Pergamon Press, 1990.
45. Cohen DJ, Riddle MA, Leckman JF: Pharmacotherapy of Tourette's syndrome and associated disorders. *Psychiatr Clin North Am* 15:109–130, 1992.
46. Chapple PB, Leckman JF, Riddle MA et al: The pharmacological treatment of tic disorders, in Riddle MA (ed): Pediatric psychopharmacology. *Child Adolesc Clin North Am* 4:197–216, 1995.
47. Horacek HJ: Clonidine extended-release capsules as an alternative to oral tablets and transdermal patches. *J Child Adolesc Psychopharmacol* 4:211–212, 1994.
48. Lowenthal DT, Matzek KM, MacGregor TR: Clinical pharmacokinetics of clonidine. *Clin Pharmacokinet* 14:287–310, 1988.
49. Hunt RD, Arnsten A, Asbell MD: An open trial of guanfacine in the treatment of attention deficit hyperactivity disorder in boys. *J Am Acad Child Adolesc Psychiatry* 34:50–54, 1995.
50. Swanson JM, Flockhart D, Udrea D, et al: Clonidine in the treatment of ADHD: Questions about safety and efficacy. *J Child Adolesc Psychopharmacol* 5:301–304, 1995.
51. Swanson JM, Udrea D, Cantwell D, et al: Clonidine in the treatment of children with ADHD I: Efficacy. Personal communication, 1995.
52. Hunt RD, Minderaa RB, Cohen DJ: Clonidine benefits children with attention deficit disorder and hyperactivity: Report of a double-blind placebo-crossover therapeutic trial. *J Am Acad Child Psychiatry* 24:617–629, 1985.

53. Singer HS, Brown J, Quaskey S, et al: The treatment of attention deficit hyperactivity disorder in Tourette's Syndrome: A double blind placebo-controlled study with clonidine and desipramine. *Pediatrics* 95:74–81, 1995.
54. Jaselskis CA, Cook EH, Fletcher KE, et al: Clonidine treatment of hyperactive and impulsive children with autistic disorder. *J Clin Psychopharmacol* 12:322–327, 1992.
55. Fankhauser MP, Karumanchi VC, German ML, et al: A double-blind, placebo-controlled study of the efficacy of transdermal clonidine in autism. *J Clin Psychiatry* 53:77–82, 1992.
56. Ghaziuddin M, Tsai L, Ghaziuddin N: Clonidine for autism [letter to the editor]. *J Child Adolesc Psychopharmacol* 2, 1992.
57. Prince JB, Wilens TE, Biederman J, et al: Clonidine for sleep disturbances associated with attention deficit hyperactivity disorder: A systematic chart review of 62 cases. *J Am Acad Child Adolesc Psychiatry* 35:599–605, 1996.
58. Wilens T, Biederman J, Spencer T: Clonidine for sleep disturbances associated with attention deficit hyperactivity disorder. *J Am Acad Child Adolesc Psychiatry* 33:424–426, 1994.
59. Kemph JP, Devane CL, Levin GM, et al: Treatment of aggressive children with clonidine: Results of an open pilot study. *J Am Acad Child Adolesc Psychiatry* 32:577–581, 1993.
60. Schvehla TJ, Mandoki MW, Sumner GS: Clonidine therapy for comorbid attention deficit hyperactivity disorder and conduct. *South Med J* 87:692–695, 1994.
61. Stowe JK, Kreusi MJP, Lelio DF: Psychopharmacology of aggressive states and features of conduct disorder, in Riddle MA (ed): Pediatric psychopharmacology. *Child Adolesc Clin North Am* 4:359–380, 1995.
62. Althaus M, Vink HJ, Minderaa, RR et al: Lack of effect of clonidine on stuttering in children. *Am J Psychiatry* 152:1087–1089, 1995.
63. Swanson JM, Udrea D, Cantwell D, et al: Clonidine in the treatment of children with ADHD II: Side effects. Personal communication, 1995.
64. Levin GM, Burton-Teston K, Murphy T: Development of precocious puberty in two children treated with clonidine for aggressive behavior. *J Child Adolesc Psychopharmacol* 3:127–131, 1993.
65. Hoffman BB, Lefkowitz RJ: Catehcolamines and sympthomimetic drugs, in Gilman AG, Rall TW, Nies AS, et al (eds): *Goodman and Gilman's The Pharmacological Basis of Therapeutics*, ed 8. New York, Pergamon Press, 1990.
66. Chandran KSK: ECG and clonidine. *J Am Acad Child Adolesc Psychiatry* 33:1351–1352, 1994 .
67. Dawson PM, Zanden JAV, Werkman SW, et al: Cardiac dysrhythmia with use of clonidine in explosive disorder. DICP, *The Annals of Pharmacotherapy* 23:465, 1989.
68. Popper CW: Combining methylphenidate and clonidine: Pharmacologic questions and news reports about sudden death. *J Child Adolesc Psychopharmacol* 5:157–167, 1995.
69. Wilens T, Biederman J: Safety of clonidine and nortriptyline [letter]. *J Am Acad Child Adolesc Psychiatry* 33:142–143, 1994.
70. Geller DA, Biederman J, Reed ED, et al: Similarities in response to fluoxetine in the treatment of children and adolescents with obsessive–compulsive disorder. *J Am Acad Child Adolesc Psychiatry* 34:36–44, 1995.
71. Fenichel RR: Combining methylphenidate and clonidine: The role of post-marketing surveillance. *J Child Adolesc Psychopharmacol* 5:155–156, 1995.
72. Henretig FM: Special considerations in the poisoned pediatric population. *Emerg Med Clin North Am* 12:549–567, 1994.
73. Wiley JF, Wiley CC, Torrey SB, et al: Clonidine poisoning in young children. *J Pediatr* 116:654–658, 1990.
74. Cavallo A: The pineal gland in human beings: Relevance to pediatrics. *J Pediatr* 123:844–851, 1993.
75. Webb SM, Puig-Domingo M: Role of melatonin in health and disease. *Clin Endocrinol* 42:221–234, 1995.
76. Reiter RJ: The pineal gland and melatonin in relation to aging: A summary of theories and of the data. *Exp Gerontol* 30:199–212, 1995.
77. Masters KJ: Melatonin for sleep problems [letter]. *J Am Acad Child Adolesc Psychiatry* 35:704, 1996.
78. Regestein QR, Pavlova M: Treatment of delayed sleep phase syndrome. *Gen Hosp Psychiatry* 17:335–345, 1995.
79. Palm L, Bleenow G, Wetterberg: Correction of a non-24-hour sleep/wake cycle by melatonin in a blind retarded boy. *Ann Neurol* 29:336–339, 1991.
80. Jan JE, Espezel H, Appleton RE: The treatment of sleep disorders with melatonin. *Dev Med Child Neurol* 36:97–107, 1994.
81. Kennedy SH: Melatonin disturbances in anorexia nervosa and bulimia. *Int J Eat Dis* 16:257–265, 1994.
82. DeSmet PA, Nolen WA: St. John's wort as an antidepressant [editorial]. *Br Med J* 313:241–245, 1996.
83. Linde K, Ramirez G, Mulrow CD, Pauls A, Weidenhammer W, Melchart D: St John's wort for depression—an overview and meta-analysis of randomised clinical trials. *Br Med J* 313:253–258, 1996.

84. Sokol MS, Campbell M: Novel psychotropic agents in the treatment of developmental disorders, in Aman MG, Singh NN (eds): *Psychopharmacology of the Developmental Disorders*. Berlin, Springer-Verlag, 1988, pp 146–167.
85. Goodwin FK, Jamison KR: *Manic–Depressive Illness*. London, Oxford University Press, 1990, pp 622–653.
86. Pinder RM, Brogden RN, Sawyer PR, et al: Fenfluramine: A review of its pharmacological properties and therapeutic efficacy in obesity. *Drugs* 10:241–328, 1975.
87. Aman MG, Kern RA: Review of fenfluramine in the treatment of the developmental disabilities. *J Am Acad Child Adolesc Psychiatry* 28:549–565, 1989.
88. Campbell M: Annotation: Fenfluramine treatment of autism. *J Child Psychol Psychiatry* 29:1–10, 1988.
89. DuVerglas G, Banks SR, Guyer KE: Clinical effects of fenfluramine on children with autism: A review of the research. *J Autism Dev Disord* 18:297–308, 1988.
90. Gillberg C, Aman MG, Reiss A: Fenfluramine, in Reiss S, Aman MG (eds.): *Psychotropic Medications and Developmental Disabilities: The International Consensus Handbook*. Columbus, Ohio, The Nisonger Center UAP, 1998.
91. Geller E, Ritvo ER, Freeman BJ, et al: Preliminary observation on the effect of fenfluramine on blood serotonin and symptoms in three autistic boys. *N Engl J Med* 307:165–169, 1982.
92. Donnelly M, Rapoport JL, Potter WZ, et al: Fenfluramine and dextroamphetamine treatment of childhood hyperactivity: Clinical and biochemical findings. *Arch Gen Psychiatry* 46:205–212, 1989.
93. Selikowitz M, Sunman J, Pendergast A, et al: Fenfluramine in Prader—Willi syndrome: A double blind, placebo controlled trial. *Arch Dis Child* 65:112–114, 1990.
94. Aman MG, Kern RA, McGhee, et al: Fenfluramine and methylphenidate in children with mental retardation and ADHD: Clinical and side effects. *J Am Acad Child Adolesc Psychiatry* 32:851–859, 1993.
95. Aman MG, Kern RA, Osborne P, et al: Fenfluramine and methylphenidate in children with mental retardation and borderline IQ: Clinical effects. *Am J Ment Retard* 101:521–534, 1997.
96. Aman MG, Kern RA, Osborne P, et al: Fenfluramine and methylphenidate in children with mental retardation and borderline IQ: Cognitive effects. Unpublished manuscript, Ohio State University, 1998.
97. Connolly HM, Crary JL, McGoon MD, et al: Valvular heart disease associated with fenfluramine–phentermine. *N Engl J Med* 337:581–588, 1997.
98. Graham DJ, Green L: Further cases of valvular heart disease associated with fenfluramine-phentermine. *N Engl J Med* 337:635, 1997.
99. Cannistra LB, Davis SM, Bauman AG: Valvular disease associated with dexfenfluramine. *N Engl J Med* 337:636., 1997.
100. FDA analysis of cardiac valvular dysfunction with use of appetite suppressants. http://www.fda.gov/cder/news/slide/index.htm.
101. Johannes L, Langreth R: Diet drugs' side effects are still a mystery. *The Wall Street Journal*, September 18, 1997, pp. B1, B5.
102. Harvey JA, McMaster SE: Fenfluramine: Evidence for a neurotoxic action on midbrain and a long-term depletion of serotonin. *Psychopharmacol Commun* 1:217–228, 1975.
103. Schuster CR, Lewis M, Seiden LS: Fenfluramine: Neurotoxicity. *Psychopharmacol Bull* 22:148–151, 1986.
104. *Physicians' Desk Reference*, ed 46. Oradell, NJ, Medical Economics Co, 1992.
105. Arnold LE, Aman MG: Beta blockers in mental retardation and developmental disorders. *J Child Adolesc Psychopharmacol* 1:361–373, 1991.
106. Fraser WI, Ruedrich S, Kerr, M et al: Beta-adrenergic blockers, in Reiss S, Aman MG (eds): *Psychoactive Medications and Developmental Disabilities: The International Consensus Handbook*. Columbus, Ohio, The Nisonger Center UAP, 1998.
107. Neppe VM: *Innovative Psychopharmacotherapy*. New York, Raven Press, 1989.
108. Hoffman BB, Lefkowitz, RJ: Adrenergic receptor antagonists, in Gilman AG, Rall TW, Nies AS, et al (eds): *Goodman and Gilman's The Pharmacological Basis of Therapeutics*, ed 8. New York, Pergamon Press, 1990, pp 221–243.
109. Holroyd KA, France JL, Cordingley GE, et al: Enhancing the effectiveness of relaxation–thermal biofeedback training with propranolol hydrochloride. *J Consult Clin Psychol* 2:327–330, 1995.
110. Holroyd KA, Penzien DB, Cordingley G: Propranolol in the management of recurrent migraine: A meta-analytic review. *Headache* 31:333–340, 1991.
111. Coffey BJ: Anxiolytics for children and adolescents. Traditional and new drugs. *J Child Adolesc Psychopharmacol* 1:57–83, 1990.
112. Kuperman S, Stewart MA: Use of propranolol to decrease aggressive outbursts in younger patients. *Psychosomatics* 28:315–319, 1987.

113. Connor DF: Nadolol for self-injury, overactivity, inattention, and aggression in a child with pervasive developmental disorder. *J Child Adolesc Psychopharmacol* 4:101–111, 1994.

114. Lang C, Remington D: Case study: Treatment with propranolol of severe self-injurious behavior in a blind, deaf, retarded adolescent. *J Am Acad Child Adolesc Psychiatry* 33:265–269.

115. Schmidt JG, Dombovy ML, Watkins K: Treatment of viral encephalitis organic personality disorder and autistic features with propranolol: A case report. *J Neurol Rehab* 9:45–45, 1995.

116. Hayes PE, Schultz SC: Beta-blockers in anxiety disorders. *J Affect Dis* 13:119–130, 1987.

117. Famularo R, Kinscheroff R, Fenton T: Propranolol treatment for childhood post-traumatic stress disorder, acute type. *Am J Dis Child* 142:1244–1247, 1988.

118. Jaffe JH, Martin WR: Opioid analgesics and antagonists, in Gilman AG, Rall TW, Nies AS, et al (eds): *Goodman and Gilman's The Pharmacological Basis of Therapeutics*, ed 8. New York, Pergamon Press, 1990, pp 485–521.

119. Sandman CA, Datta PC, Barron J, et al: Naloxone attenuates self-abusive behavior in developmentally disabled clients. *Appl Res Ment Retard* 4:5–11, 1983.

120. Sandman CA: The opiate hypothesis in autism and self-injury. *J Child Adolesc Psychopharmacol* 1:237–248, 1990/1991.

121. Aman MG: Efficacy of psychotropic drugs for reducing self-injurious behavior in the developmental disabilities. *Ann Clin Psychiatry* 5:171–188, 1993.

122. Aman MG: Pharmacotherapy in the developmental disabilities: New developments. *Aust N Z J Dev Disabil* 17:183–199, 1991.

123. Sandman CA, Thompson T, Barrett R, et al: Opiate blockers, in Reiss S, Aman MG (eds): *Psychotropic Medications and Developmental Disabilities: The International Consensus Handbook*. Columbus, Ohio, The Nisonger Center UAP, 1998.

124. Hetrick W, Taylor D, Touchette P, et al: Treatment of self-injurious behavior with naltrexone: Effects in SIB, learning, and neurological function. Paper presented at the Gatlinburg Conference on Research and Theory in Mental Retardation and Developmental Disabilities, Key Biscayne, Fla, 1991.

125. Thompson T, Hackenberg T, Cerutti D, et al: Opioid antagonist effects on self-injury in adults with mental retardation: Response form and location as determinants of medication effects. *Am J Ment Retard* 99:85–102, 1994.

126. Sandman CA, Hetrick WP, Taylor DV, et al: Naltrexone reduces self-injury and improves learning. *Exp Clin Psychopharmacol* 1:1–17, 1993.

127. Campbell M, Anderson LT, Small AM, et al: Naltrexone in autistic children: Behavioral symptoms and attentional learning. *J Am Acad Child Adolesc Psychiatry* 32:1283–1291, 1993.

128. Willemsen-Swinkles SH, Buitelaar JK, Nijhof GJ, et al: Failure of naltrexone hydrochloride to reduce self-injurious and autistic behavior in mentally retarded adults. *Arch Gen Psychiatry* 52:766–773, 1995.

129. Deutsch SI: Rationales for the administration of opiate antagonists in treating infantile autism. *Am J Ment Defic* 90:631–635, 1986.

130. Sahley TL, Panksepp J: Brain opioids and autism: An updated analysis of possible linkages. *J Autism Dev Disabil* 17:201–216, 1987.

131. Campbell M, Overall JE, Small AM, et al: Naltrexone in autistic children: An acute open dose range tolerance trial. *J Am Acad Child Adolesc Psychiatry* 28:200–206, 1989.

132. Willemsen-Swinkels SH, Buitelaar JK, Weijnen FG, et al: Placebo-controlled acute dosage naltrexone study in young autistic children. *Psychiatry Res* 58:203–215, 1995.

133. Kolmen BD, Feldman HM, Handen BL, et al: Naltrexone in young autistic children: A double-blind placebo-controlled crossover study. *J Am Acad Child Adolesc Psychiatry* 34:223–231, 1995.

134. Herman BH, Asleson GS, Powell A, et al: Cardiovascular and other physical effects of acute administration of naltrexone in autistic children. *J Child Adolesc Psychopharmacol* 3:157–168, 1993.

Psychoactive Medications Grouped by Drug Class and Foods Studied for Psychoactive Effects

Drug and class	Trade name(s)
CNS stimulants	
amphetamine	Benzedrine®
deanol	Deaner®
dextroamphetamine (D-amphetamine)	Dexedrine®
dextroamphetamine/amphetamine[a]	Adderall®
levoamphetamine (L-amphetamine)	Cydril®
methamphetamine	Desoxyn®
methylphenidate	Ritalin®
pemoline	Cylert®
Neuroleptics (antipsychotics, "major tranquilizers")	
Phenothiazines	
chlorpromazine	Largactil®, Thorazine®
fluphenazine (decanoate)	Prolixin®, Modecate®
mesoridazine	Serentil®
peracetazine	Quide®
pericyazine	Neulactil®
perphenazine	Trilafon®
pipothiazine palmitate	Piportil®
prochlorperazine	Compazine®, Stemetil®
promazine	Sparine®
thioridazine	Mellaril®
trifluoperazine	Stelazine®
Thioxanthenes	
chlorprothixene	Taractan®, Tarasan®
flupenthixol (decanoate)	Depixol®
thiothixene	Navane®
Benzisothiazolyl piperazines	
ziprasidone	Zeldox®

Practitioner's Guide to Psychoactive Drugs for Children and Adolescents (Second Edition), Werry and Aman, eds. Plenum Publishing Corporation, New York, 1999.

Drug and class	Trade name(s)
Neuroleptics (antipsychotics, "major tranquilizers") (*cont.*)	
Benzisoxazoles	
risperidone	Risperdal®
Butyrophenones	
droperidol	Droleptan®
haloperidol	Haldol®, Serenace®
pipamperon	Dipiperon®
Dibenzothiazepines	
quetiapine	Seroquel®
Dibenzoxazepines	
loxapine	Loxitane®
Dihydroindolones	
molindone	Moban®
Diphenylbutylpiperidines	
pimozide	Orap®
Dibenzodiazepines	
clozapine	Clozaril®, Leponex®
Thienobenzodiazepines	
olanzapine	Zypexa®
sertindole	Serlect®
Antiparkinson drugs[b]	
amantadine	Symmetrel®
benztropine	Cogentin®
biperiden	Akineton®
diphenhydramine	Benadryl®
ethopropazine	Parsidol®
procyclidine	Kemadrin®
trihexyphenidyl	Artane®
Antidepressant drugs	
Tricyclics	
amitriptyline	Elavil®, Amitril®, Endep®
clomipramine	Anafranil
desipramine	Norpramin®, Pertofrane®
doxepin	Sinequan®, Adapin®
imipramine	Tofranil®, Janimine®, Dumex®
nortriptyline	Pamelor®, Aventyl®, Allegron®
protriptyline	Vivactil®, Concordin®
trimipramine	Surmontil®
Atypical antidepressants	
amoxapine	Asendin®
bupropion	Wellbutrin®
maprotiline	Ludiomil®
Selective serotonin reuptake inhibitors (SSRIs)	
fluoxetine	Prozac®
fluvoxamine	Luvox®
paroxetine	Paxil®
sertraline	Zoloft®
Serotonin agonists and antagonists	
nefazadone	Serzone®
trazodone	Desyrel®
Serotonin-norepinephrine dual reuptake inhibitor	
venlafaxine	Effexor®
Monoamine oxidase inhibitors (MAOIs)	
isocarboxazid	Marplan®
moclobemide	Aurorix®

Drug and class	Trade name(s)
Antidepressant drugs (*cont.*)	
Monoamine oxidase inhibitors (MAOIs) (*cont.*)	
phenelzine	Nardil®
selegiline	Deprenyl®
tranylcypromine	Parnate®
Novel antidepressants	
mirtazapine	Remeron®
Other	
hypericum extract (active ingredient in St. John's wort)	Kira®
Mood stabilizers (antimanics)	
carbamazepine[c]	Tegretol®
clonazepam[c]	Klonopin®, Rivotril®
lithium carbonate	Eskalith®, Lithane®, Lithobid®, Lithonate®, Lithotab®
lithium citrate	Cibalith-S®
valproic acid[c]	Depakote®, Depakene®, Epilim®
Antiepileptics (anticonvulsants)	
Barbiturates	
mephobarbital	Mebaral®
phenobarbital	Gardenal®, Luminal®
primidone	Mysoline®
Hydantoins	
ethotoin	Peganone®
mephenytoin	Mesantoin®
phenytoin	Dilantin®
Succinimides	
ethosuximide	Zarontin®
methsuximide	Celontin®
phensuximide	Milontin®
Benzodiazepines	
clonazepam[c]	Klonopin®, Rivotril®
clorazepate[c]	Tranxene®
diazepam[c]	Valium®
lorazepam[c]	Ativan®
GABA agonists	
tiagabine	Gabitril®, Tiabex®
valproic acid/divalproex	Depakene®, Depakote®, Epilim®
vigabatrin (γ-vinyl GABA)	Sabril®
Membrane-acting or multiple mechanisms	
carbamazepine	Tegretol®
felbamate	Felbatol®
gabapentin	Neurotin®
lamotrigine	Lamictal®
topiramate	Topamax®
New/under development	
clobazam	
flunarizine	Sibelium®
GW 534	
loreclezole	
oxcarbazepine	
progabide	Gabren®
remacemide	
rufinamide	
stiripentol	
zonisamide	

Drug and class	Trade name(s)
Sedative-hypnotics	
Antihistamines	
diphenhydramine	Benadryl®
hydroxyzine	Atarax®, Vistaril®
promethazine	Phenergan®
trimeprazine	Temaril®, Vallergan®
Benzodiazepines ("minor tranquilizers")	
alprazolam	Xanax®
chlordiazepoxide	Librium®
clonazepam[c]	Klonopin®, Rivotril®
clorazepate[c]	Tranxene®
diazepam[c]	Valium®
flurazepam	Dalmane®
lorazepam[c]	Ativan®
nitrazepam	Mogadon®
oxazepam	Serax®, Serapax®
prazepam	Verstran®
temazepam	Restoril®, Euhypnos®
triazolam	Halcion®
Benzodiazepine analogues	
zopiclone	Imovane®
Atypical anxiolytics	
buspirone	BuSpar®
Other	
alcohol	
chloral hydrate	Noctec®
melatonin	Melatonex®, Somniset®
meprobamate	Equanil®, Miltown®
secobarbital	Seconal®
α_2-adrenergic agonists	
clonidine	Catapres®, Combipres®
guanfacine	Tenex®
Opiate blockers	
naloxone	Narcan®
naltrexone	Trexan®
β blockers	
acebutolol	Sectral®
atenolol	Tenoretic®, Tenormin®
bisoprolol	Zebeta®
esmolol	Brevibloc®
labetolol	Normodyne®
metoprolol	Lopressor®, Toprol®
nadolol	Corgard®
oxprenolol	Oxanol®, Trasicor®
penbutolol	Levatol®
propranolol	Inderal®, Inderide®
sotalol	Betapace®, Sotacor®, Sotalex®
timolol	Blocadren®, Timoptic®
Nootropics	
aniracetam	Draganon®, Reset®, Sarpul®
etiracetam	
nefiracetam	
oxiracetam	Neuromet®, Neuractiv®
piracetam	Avigilen®, Nootropil®, Nootropyl®, others[d]
pramiracetam	Neupramir®, Remen®
rolziracetam	

Drug and class	Trade name(s)
Miscellaneous	
Fenfluramine (serotoninolytic agent) (withdrawn from the market)	Pondimin®, Ponderax®
5-Hydroxytryptophan (serotonin precursor)	
L-tryptophan (serotonin precursor) (off the market in the United States)	
Foods and and substances present in food	
Foods/derivatives	
aspartame	Equal®, NutraSweet®
caffeine	
chocolate	
choline	
sugar	
tryptophan	
tyrosine	
Food additives	
benzoic acid	
monosodium glutamate	
tartrazine	
Vitamins/minerals	
iron	
vitamin B_6	
zinc	

[a]Dextroamphetamine saccharate, dextroamphetamine sulfate, amphetamine aspartate, amphetamine sulfate.
[b]Drug belongs to more than one clinical group.
[c]Frequently used to treat extrapyramidal side effects of neuroleptic drugs; seldom used as psychotropic drugs.
[d]Cerebroforte®, Cerebrospan®, Cetam®, Dinagen®, Encefalux®, Encetrop®, Euvifor®, Gabacet®, Genogris®, Memo-Puren®, Nootron®, Nootrop®, Normabrain®, Norzetam®, Pirroxil®, Psycoton®, Stimucortex®.

Major Psychoactive Medications Ordered by Trade Name

Trade name	Generic name	Class
Adapin®	doxepin	Antidepressant
Adderall®	dextroamphetamine/amphetamine	CNS stimulant
Akineton®	biperiden	Antiparkinson
Allegron®	nortriptyline	Antidepressant
Amitril®	amitriptyline	Antidepressant
Anafranil®	clomipramine	Antidepressant
Artane®	trihexyphenidyl	Antiparkinson
Asendin®	amoxapine	Antidepressant
Atarax®	hydroxyzine	Sedative–hypnotic
Ativan®	lorazepam	Sedative–hypnotic, antiepileptic
Aurorix®	moclobemide	Antidepressant
Aventyl®	nortriptyline	Antidepressant
Avigilen®	piracetam	Nootropic
Benadryl®	diphenhydramine	Sedative–hypnotic, antiparkinson
Benzedrine®	amphetamine	CNS stimulant
Betapace®	sotalol	β-Blocker
Blocadren®	timolol	β-Blocker
Brevibloc®	esmolol	β-Blocker
BuSpar®	buspirone	Sedative–hypnotic (anxiolytic)
Catapres®	clonidine	Antihypertensive, α_2-adrenergic agonist
Celontin®	methsuximide	Antiepileptic
Cerebroforte®	piracetam	Nootropic
Cerebrospan®	piracetam	Nootropic
Cetam®	piracetam	Nootropic
Cibalith-S®	lithium citrate	Mood stabilizer/antimanic
Clozaril®	clozapine	Neuroleptic
Cogentin®	benztropine	Antiparkinson
Combipres®	clonidine	Antihypertensive, α_2-adrenergic agonist
Compazine®	prochlorperazine	Neuroleptic
Concordin®	protriptyline	Antidepressant
Corgard®	nadolol	β-Blocker
Cydril®	levoamphetamine	CNS stimulant
Cylert®	pemoline	CNS stimulant
Dalmane®	flurazepam	Sedative–hypnotic
Deaner®	deanol	CNS stimulant

Practitioner's Guide to Psychoactive Drugs for Children and Adolescents (Second Edition), Werry and Aman, eds. Plenum Publishing Corporation, New York, 1999.

Trade name	Generic name	Class
Depakene®	valproic acid	Antiepileptic, mood stabilizer/antimanic
Depakote®	valproic acid	Antiepileptic, mood stabilizer/antimanic
Depixol®	flupenthixol (decanoate)	Neuroleptic
Deprenyl®	selegiline	Antidepressant
Desoxyn®	methamphetamine	CNS stimulant
Desyrel®	trazodone	Antidepressant
Dexedrine®	dextroamphetamine (D-amphetamine)	CNS stimulant
Dilantin®	phenytoin	Antiepileptic
Dinagen®	piracetam	Nootropic
Dipiperon®	pipamperon	Neuroleptic
Draganon®	aniracetam	Nootropic
Droleptan®	droperidol	Neuroleptic
Dumex®	imipramine	Antidepressant
Elavil®	amitriptyline	Antidepressant
Encefalux®	piracetam	Nootropic
Encetrop®	piracetam	Nootropic
Endep®	amitriptyline	Antidepressant
Epilim®	valproic acid	Antiepileptic, mood stabilizer/antimanic
Equanil®	meprobamate	Sedative–hypnotic
Eskalith®	lithium carbonate	Mood stabilizer/antimanic
Euhypnos®	temazepam	Sedative–hypnotic
Euvifor®	piracetam	Nootropic
Felbatol®	felbamate	Antiepileptic
Gabacet®	piracetam	Nootropic
Gabitril®	tiagabine	Antiepileptic
Gabren®	progabide	Antiepileptic
Gardenal®	phenobarbital	Antiepileptic
Genogris®	piracetam	Nootropic
Halcion®	triazolam	sedative–hypnotic
Haldol®	haloperidol	Neuroleptic
Imovane®	zopiclone	Sedative–hypnotic
Inderal®	propranolol	β-Blocker
Inderide®	propranolol	β-Blocker
Janimine®	imipramine	Antidepressant
Kemadrin®	procyclidine	Antiparkinson
Klonopin®	clonazepam	Antiepileptic, sedative–hypnotic, mood stabilizer/antimanic
Lamictal®	lamotrigine	Antiepileptic
Largactil®	chlorpromazine	Neuroleptic
Leponex®	clozapine	Neuroleptic
Levatol®	penbutolol	β-Blocker
Librium®	chlordiazepoxide	Sedative–hypnotic
Lithane®	lithium carbonate	Mood stabilizer/antimanic
Lithobid®	lithium carbonate	Mood stabilizer/antimanic
Lithonate®	lithium carbonate	Mood stabilizer/antimanic
Lithotab®	lithium carbonate	Mood stabilizer/antimanic
Lopressor®	metoprolol	β-Blocker
Loxitane®	loxapine	Neuroleptic
Ludiomil®	maprotiline	Antidepressant
Luminal®	phenobarbital	Antiepileptic
Luvox®	fluvoxamine	Antidepressant
Marplan®	isocarboxazid	Antidepressant
Mebaral®	mephobarbital	Antiepileptic
Melatonex®	melatonin	Sedative–hypnotic
Mellaril®	thioridazine	Neuroleptic
Memo-Puren®	piracetam	Nootropic

Trade name	Generic name	Class
Mesantoin®	mephenytoin	Antiepileptic
Milontin®	phensuximide	Antiepileptic
Miltown®	meprobamate	Sedative–hypnotic
Moban®	molindone	Neuroleptic
Modecate®	fluphenazine (decanoate)	Neuroleptic
Mogadon®	nitrazepam	Sedative–hypnotic
Mysoline®	primidone	Antiepileptic
Narcan®	naloxone	Opiate blocker
Nardil	phenelzine	Antidepressant
Navane®	thiothixene	Neuroleptic
Neulactil®	pericyazine	Neuroleptic
Neupramir®	pramiracetam	Nootropic
Neuractiv®	oxiracetam	Nootropic
Neuromet®	oxiracetam	Nootropic
Neurotin®	gabapentin	Antiepileptic
Noctec®	chloral hydrate	Sedative–hypnotic
Nootron®	piracetam	Nootropic
Nootrop®	piracetam	Nootropic
Nootropil®	piracetam	Nootropic
Nootropyl®	piracetam	Nootropic
Normabrain®	piracetam	Nootropic
Normodyne®	labetolol	β-Blocker
Norpramin®	desipramine	Antidepressant
Norzetam®	piracetam	Nootropic
Orap®	pimozide	Neuroleptic
Oxanol®	oxprenolol	β-Blocker
Pamelor®	nortriptyline	Antidepressant
Parnate®	tranylcypromine	Antidepressant
Parsidol®	ethopropazine	Antiparkinson
Paxil®	paroxetine	Antidepressant
Peganone®	ethotoin	Antiepileptic
Pertofrane®	desipramine	Antidepressant
Phenergan®	promethazine	Sedative–hypnotic
Piportil®	pipothiazine palmitate	Neuroleptic
Pirroxil®	piracetam	Nootropic
Ponderax®	fenfluramine	Serotoninolytic agent
Pondimin®	fenfluramine	Serotoninolytic agent
Prolixin®	fluphenazine (decanoate)	Neuroleptic
Prozac®	fluoxetine	Antidepressant
Psycoton®	piracetam	Nootropic
Quide®	peracetazine	Neuroleptic
Remen®	pramiracetam	Nootropic
Remeron®	mirtazapine	Antidepressant
Reset®	aniracetam	Nootropic
Restoril®	temazepam	Sedative–hypnotic
Risperdal®	risperidone	Neuroleptic
Ritalin®	methylphenidate	CNS stimulant
Rivotril®	clonazepam	Antiepileptic, sedative–hypnotic, mood stabilizer/ antimanic
Sabril®	vigabatrin (γ5-vinyl GABA)	Antiepileptic
Sarpul®	aniracetam	Nootropic
Seconal®	secobarbital	Sedative–hypnotic
Sectral®	acebutolol	β-Blocker
Serapax®	oxazepam	Sedative–hypnotic
Serax®	oxazepam	Sedative–hypnotic
Serenace®	haloperidol	Neuroleptic

Trade name	Generic name	Class
Serentil®	mesoridazine	Neuroleptic
Serlect®	sertindole	Neuroleptic
Seroquel®	quetiapine	Neuroleptic
Serzone®	nefazadone	Antidepressant
Sibelium®	flunarizine	Antiepileptic
Sinequan®	doxepin	Antidepressant
Somniset®	melatonin	Sedative–hypnotic
Sotacor®	sotalol	β-Blocker
Sotalex®	sotalol	β-Blocker
Sparine®	promazine	Neuroleptic
Stelazine®	trifluoperazine	neuroleptic
Stemetil®	prochlorperazine	Neuroleptic
Stimucortex®	piracetam	Nootropic
Surmontil®	trimipramine	Antidepressant
Symmetrel®	amantadine	Antiparkinson
Taractan®	chlorprothixene	Neuroleptic
Tarasan®	chlorprothixene	Neuroleptic
Tegretol®	carbamazepine	Antiepileptic, mood stabilizer/antimanic
Temaril®	trimeprazine	Sedative–hypnotic
Tenex®	guanfacine	α_2-Adrenergic agent
Tenoretic®	atenolol	β-Blocker
Tenormin®	atenolol	β-Blocker
Thorazine®	chlorpromazine	Neuroleptic
Tiabex®	tiagabine	Antiepileptic
Timoptic®	timolol	β-Blocker
Tofranil®	imipramine	Antidepressant
Topamax®	topiramate	Antiepileptic
Toprol®	metoprolol	β-Blocker
Tranxene®	clorazepate	Sedative–hypnotic, antiepileptic
Trasicor®	clorazepate	β-Blocker
Trexan®	naltrexone	Opiate blocker
Trilafon®	perphenazine	Neuroleptic
Valium®	diazepam	Sedative–hypnotic, antiepileptic
Vallergan®	trimeprazine	Sedative–hypnotic
Verstran®	prazepam	Sedative–hypnotic
Vistaril®	hydroxyzine	Sedative–hypnotic
Vivactil®	protriptyline	Antidepressant
Wellbutrin®	bupropion	Antidepressant
Xanax®	alprazolam	Antidepressant, sedative–hypnotic
Zarontin®	ethosuximide	Antiepileptic
Zebeta®	bisoprolol	β-Blocker
Zeldox®	ziprasidone	Neuroleptic
Zoloft®	sertraline	Antidepressant
Zypexa	olanzapine	Neuroleptic

Not all drugs listed are approved for use in children or in all countries.

Index

Neurotin®: *see* Gabapentin
Nicotine: *see* Tobacco
Nifedipine, 9, 266, 277
Night terrors, 200
  benzodiazepines in, 439
Niridazole, psychotropic side effects, 403
Nisonger Child Behavior Rating Form, 111, 112,
    137, 139
Nitrazepam, 436, 474; *see also* Anxiolytics, Seda-
    tive-hypnotics
Nitrous oxide, 340; *see also* Inhalants
Noctec®: see Chloral hydrate
Nomifensine, 9; 253; *see also* Antidepressants
Noncompliance: *see* Compliance
Nonsteroidal antiinflammatory drugs (NSAIDs),
    psychotropic side effects, 398, 401
Nootron®: *see* Piracetam
Nootrop®: *see* Piracetam
Nootropil®: *see* Piracetam
Nootropyl®: *see* Piracetam
Nootropics, 414–416, 474
Noradrenalin, *see also individual drugs*; Cellular ac-
    tion
  in ADHD, 186–187
  in anxiety disorders, 199
  in eating disorders, 194–195
  in enuresis, 201
  in mood disorders, 189–190
  and tricyclic antidepressants, 242
Norepinephrine, 214
Norephedrine, psychotropic side effects, 401
Normabrain®: *see* Piracetam
Normodyne®: *see* Labetolol
Norpramin®: *see* Desipramine
Nortriptyline, 251–255, 258, 472; *see also* Antide-
    pressant drugs
  nursing, 4
Novel Antidepressants, 472
Norzetam®: *see* Piracetam
NutraSweet®: see Aspartame

Obsessive–compulsive disorder (OCD)
  antidepressants in, 260, 270
  benzodiazepines in, 438
  biochemical correlates, 199
  diagnostic features, 198
  instruments for assessing, 131–132
  pharmacotherapy of, 198
Occupational therapy, 4
Off-label use of medication, 179
Olanzapine, 9, 299, 301, 308, 471; *see also*
    Neuroleptics
Opiates
  abuse of, 347–349
  psychotropic side effects, 401–406
Opiate blockers, 462–464
  contraindications, 464
  dose, 462–463

Opiate blockers (*cont.*)
  indications, 462–463
  management of overdose, 464
  pharmacology, 462
  side effects, 464
  in treatment of opiate abuse, 348–349
Oppositional defiant disorder; *see* Aggression; Con-
    duct disorder
  assessment, 117
  diagnostic features, 187–188
  pharmacotherapy, 188
Oral contraceptives: *see* Contraceptives;
    Corticosteroids
Orap®: *see* Pimozide
Organic anxiety syndrome, 406
  causes of psychosis, 71
  psychiatric disorders: *see* Medical drugs
Organ imaging, tests in assessment, 94–95
Over-the-counter drugs: *see* Herbal remedies
Overanxious disorder, *see also* Generalized Anxiety
    Disorder
  benzodiazepines in, 438
  pharmacotherapy of, 196
Overdosage of medication, treatment of: *see* Individ-
    ual drugs
Over-prescribing, 51
Overt Aggression Scale, 118
Oxalamine, psychotropic side effects, 398
Oxanol®: *see* Oxprenolol
Oxazepam, 435, 436, 474; *see also* Anxiolytics Sed-
    ative-hypnotics
Oxcarbazepine, 473; *see also* Antiepileptics
Oxiracetam, 474; *see also* Nootropics
Oxyprenolol, 459, 474; *see also* β-blockers

Paired associate learning, 147; *see also* Performance
    tests
Pamelor®: *see* Nortriptyline
Panic disorder, 197
  benzodiazepines in, 438
  instruments for assessing, 132
Paraldehyde, 9, 435; *see also* Anxiolytics, CNS de-
    pressants
Pargyline, 265; *see* MAOI antidepressants
Parkinsonian side effects, 313
Parnate®: *see* Tranylcypromine
Paroxetine, 251–253, 255, 256, 268, 269, 272–273,
    472; *see also* SSRI antidepressant drugs
Parsidol®: *see* Ethopropazine
Paxil®: *see* Paroxetine
PCP, 344
Pediatric(s)
  behavioral, 4–5
  definition, 4
  neurology, 4
Peer Conflict Scale, 110, 118, 119, 120
Peer Nomination Inventory of Depression (PIND),
    125, 126